Cancer Prevention and Management through Exercise and Weight Control

NUTRITION AND DISEASE PREVENTION

Published Titles

Genomics and Proteomics in Nutrition
Carolyn D. Berdanier, Ph.D., Professor Emerita, University of Georgia, Athens, Watkinsville, Georgia
Naima Moustaid-Moussa, Ph.D., University of Tennessee, Knoxville, Tennessee

Perinatal Nutrition: Optimizing Infant Health and Development
Jatinder Bhatia, M.B.B.S., Medical College of Georgia, Augusta, Georgia

Soy in Health and Disease Prevention
Michihiro Sugano, Ph.D., Professor Emeritus at Kyushu University, Japan

Nutrition and Cancer Prevention
Atif B. Awad, Ph.D., Department of Exercise and Nutrition Science, State University of New York, Buffalo, New York
Peter G. Bradford, Ph.D., Department of Pharmacology and Toxicology, School of Medicine and Biomedical Science, State University of New York, Buffalo, New York

Cancer Prevention and Management through Exercise and Weight Control
Anne McTiernan, Fred Hutchinson Cancer Research Center, Seattle, Washington

Cancer Prevention and Management through Exercise and Weight Control

Edited by ANNE McTIERNAN

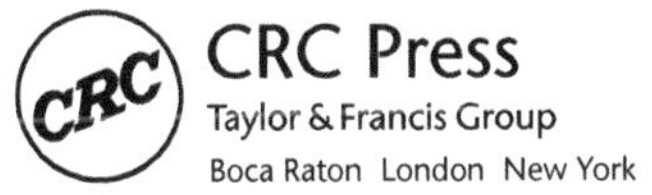

CRC Press is an imprint of the
Taylor & Francis Group, an informa business
A TAYLOR & FRANCIS BOOK

CRC Press
Taylor & Francis Group
6000 Broken Sound Parkway NW, Suite 300
Boca Raton, FL 33487-2742

First issued in paperback 2019

ISBN-13: 978-1-57444-907-5 (hbk)
ISBN-13: 978-0-367-39155-3 (pbk)

Library of Congress Card Number 2005048618

Library of Congress Cataloging-in-Publication Data

Cancer prevention and management through exercise and weight control / edited by Anne McTiernan.
p. cm. – (Nutrition and disease prevention 5)
Includes bibliographical references and index.
ISBN 1-57444-907-9 (alk. paper)
1. Cancer – Nutritional aspects. 2. Obesity – Complications. 3. Cancer – Prevention. 4. Cancer – Exercise therapy. 5. Weight loss. I. McTiernan, Anne. II. Series.

RC268.45.C362 2005
616.99'405—dc22 2005048618

Visit the Taylor & Francis Web site at
http://www.taylorandfrancis.com

and the CRC Press Web site at
http://www.crcpress.com

Foreword

Homo sapiens survived the rigors of the African savannah and migrated to the rest of the globe because of the capacity and the need to move. We evolved as a nomadic species that lived by cunning and mobility, not by specialized skills and tools of the predator (no slicing teeth, no slashing claws) or by the herd behavior and acceleration of the herbivore. Movement, to gather and hunt through the day and to spread far and wide over longer time scales, has helped define who and what we are.

Even when we abandoned our gatherer–hunter lifestyle for the settled agricultural life, we moved — to plant, to weed, to reap, to protect the crops, to defend the village. The industrial laborer and the miner, like the agricultural laborer, earned their bread by the sweat of their brows. Only in the last hundred years has a significant proportion of humanity — and it is a greater proportion every day — ceased to move to earn a wage.

There is a price to pay: with lack of physical activity comes obesity, particularly when accompanied by a remarkable abundance of food and the insatiable desire of the food manufacturers to push ever increasing consumption. With obesity come the diseases that we used to think of as the diseases of affluence. However, these increasingly afflict the urban poor in the developed and developing world; they are better thought of as the diseases of inertia.

Mostly we think of cardiovascular disease and diabetes in this context, but it is increasingly clear that cancer is also a disease of inertia. In this book, a broadly multidisciplinary group presents the evidence and provides the recommendations.

The antidote to diseases of inertia is movement — let's move!

John Potter, M.D., Ph.D.
Dr. Potter is senior vice president and director of the Division of Public Health Sciences, Fred Hutchinson Cancer Research Center, Seattle, Washington, and professor of epidemiology, University of Washington. He is internationally known for his work on the role of diet and nutrition in cancer and served as chair of the World Cancer Research Fund committee that produced the 1997 report, *Food, Nutrition and the Prevention of Cancer: A Global Perspective.* He is author or coauthor of more that 350 scientific papers and book chapters. He is co-editor-in-chief of *Cancer Epidemiology, Biomarkers and Prevention* and is currently U.S. representative and chair of the Science Council, International Agency for Research on Cancer, Lyon, France. He serves on the U.S. National Cancer Institute's Board of Scientific Advisors and is a member of the U.S. National Cancer Policy Board, Institute of Medicine, National Academy of Sciences.

Preface

Many clinicians, researchers, and lay public associate an expanding waistline and a couch-potato lifestyle with increased tendency to develop cardiovascular disease and some of its risk factors (diabetes, hypertension, hypercholesterolemia). These lifestyle factors, however, also play into the etiology and prognosis of several types of cancers, which is important in the clinical and public health areas. It is important to public health because cancer is a common disease (one in two men and one in three women will develop cancer in their lifetime) and overweight or obesity and sedentary behavior are extremely common and becoming more so (two thirds of American adults are overweight or obese, and three quarters do not meet the minimal recommendations for 30 minutes of aerobic activity per day). It is important to medicine because a marked increase in a consistent risk factor will mean an increase in number of cancer cases unless some other widespread prevention factor negates this effect.

In addition, the implications for poorer prognosis in affected individuals means that treating oncologists and other health care providers will need to develop new and better therapies to deal with the declining prognosis in this large segment of the population. Clinicians should be aware that, because two thirds of the American population is overweight or obese and being overweight increases risk for cancer, the vast majority of cancers in the future will occur in overweight and obese individuals.

The association between obesity and a sedentary lifestyle with risk for cancer has been appreciated for several decades. Only in the past 10 years or so, however, has the strength and consistency of this association been apparent. This is largely due to two things: (1) the increase in prevalence in overweight, obesity, and sedentary lifestyles; and (2) an increase in the number of epidemiological studies focusing on these associations.

The American Cancer Society estimates that a third of all cancer deaths could be prevented through avoidance of obesity and sedentary lifestyles. The World Health Organization's International Agency for Research on Cancer estimates that 25 to 30% of several cancers could be prevented if individuals avoided lifetime weight gain and obesity and participated in regular physical activity. These same organizations and several clinical groups are now recognizing the important role that physical activity can play in improving quality of life in cancer patients and survivors. This area is new, so there is great need for a definitive textbook that provides the scientific background and evidence supporting these relationships, as well as clinical guidelines for bringing physical activity and weight control into cancer prevention and treatment practices throughout the world.

We are very fortunate to have a world-class roster of authors for this text. The chapter authors have been chosen because they are the top researchers in the field of obesity, physical activity, and cancer.

Section I focuses on the research methods used in assessing the associations between physical activity, energy balance, and cancer risk and prognosis. Observational epidemiological studies can provide important information about relationships among these variables. More definitive evidence of the effect of changing behaviors, with resulting change in level of adiposity and amount of energy expended, is provided through randomized clinical trials. Dr. Prentice, principal investigator of the Women's Health Initiative Clinical Coordinating Center and a world expert on nutrition and cancer describes the benefits and drawbacks of each of these study design methods.

The measurement of energy balance and physical activity are far from straightforward. Energy balance involves the interplay among energy intake, energy expenditure, and metabolic rate. Genetic, age, and gender factors also play an important role. Defining what exactly energy balance is and what aspects of excessive adiposity are most pertinent to cancer and determining how much physical activity a person is actually doing are all great challenges requiring the concerted input of measurement experts. Drs. Ainsworth and Coleman present the intricacies of exercise and physical activity measurement, and Dr. Irwin describes the pluses and minuses of the many ways of assessing body composition.

The role of physical activity in the incidence of individual cancers is the focus of Section II. In a comprehensive literature review, Drs. Patel and Bernstein write about the intriguing data pointing to a role of exercise and physical activity in reducing risk for breast cancer. They compare and contrast the types of epidemiological studies and the role of exercise and physical activity in premenopausal and postmenopausal breast cancer. The many studies on exercise, physical activity, and colon cancer are reviewed by Dr. Slattery, who summarizes how exercise plays a role in colon cancer etiology. She also reviews the evidence regarding the association between physical activity and rectal cancer occurrence. Dr. Friedenreich elegantly summarizes the state of knowledge on the associations between exercise and prostate cancer risk, pointing out why the associations are not yet firm and suggesting future research pathways.

Section III focuses on mechanisms that may explain the inverse association between physical activity and incidence of several cancers. Dr. McTiernan reviews the effect of exercise on sex hormones, which has relevance for several hormone-related cancers such as breast, endometrium, and prostate. Dr. Frank reviews the role of exercise in reducing insulin resistance and hyperinsulinemia; insulin has been shown to promote tumor cells *in vitro*, and persons with high insulin levels have increased risk for some cancers and reduced prognosis once diagnosed with breast cancer. Ms. Wetmore and Dr. Ulrich review the literature on the complicated associations between physical activity and several markers of immune function, especially ones that may be relevant to cancer occurrence or prognosis. Dr. Martínez describes the effect of exercise on prostaglandins, which may in part explain the consistent findings of reduced colon cancer risk among active, compared with sedentary, persons. Drs. Thompson, Jiang, and Zhu describe the animal model research that has defined the role of excess adiposity and of energy restriction on tumorogenesis. The current state of human intervention studies on physical activity and cancer biomarkers is presented by Dr. McTiernan. Dr. Rankinen reviews the intriguing new field of genetics, physical activity, and cancer, which may help to define persons who may be helped with activity in terms of cancer risk.

Section IV focuses on the breadth and depth of knowledge on the effect of overweight and obesity on cancer incidence. Dr. Ballard-Barbash presents the state of knowledge regarding the effects of weight, adiposity, lifetime weight change, and risk of breast cancer in premenopausal and postmenopausal women. Drs. Kaaks and Lukanova present similar information for the effect of increasing adiposity on the development of endometrial cancer. Drs. Michaud and Giovannucci present the emerging data linking increased adiposity with increased risk for pancreatic cancer. The new and increasing body of knowledge regarding the effect of obesity on esophageal cancer is presented by Drs. Hoyo and Gammon. Dr. Slattery reviews the role of overweight and obesity in the etiology of colon cancer.

Section V reviews the mechanisms that might explain the association between adiposity and incidence of several cancers. Drs. Kaaks and McTiernan describe the role of adipose tissue in the production and metabolism of sex hormones, which is important for several hormone-related cancers such as breast, endometrium, and prostate cancers. Dr. Blackburn presents the state of knowledge regarding obesity and insulin resistance, taking from the extensive depth of information available from diabetic research results. Drs. Priest and Church present data on the effect of adiposity on cytokines and inflammatory markers that may have particular relevance for cancer. The important role of animal studies in shedding light on the effect of exercise on biology related to cancer formation is described in depth by Dr. Colbert. Drs. Tworoger and McGrath present the emerging body of literature on the genetics of obesity as it pertains to cancer incidence.

Section VI concentrates on the importance of physical activity on aspects of quality of life and prognosis for many cancer patients. Dr. Winters-Stone describes the studies that have examined the effect of exercise and physical activity on fatigue in breast cancer patients and survivors. Dr. Courneya, Ms. Campbell, Ms. Karvinen, and Ms. Ladha describe studies that have explored the effect of exercise on quality of life in colon and other cancer patients. Drs. Abrahamson and Gammon describe the emerging information on the role of physical activity in cancer prognosis and suggest biological mechanisms that might explain the association.

Section VII presents information on the role of overweight and obesity on prognosis of several cancers. Dr. Goodwin reviews the many studies that have examined the effect of adiposity on breast cancer recurrence and survival and presents suggested mechanisms for such relationships. Dr. Rock presents results of recent studies pointing to a role of adiposity on survival and recurrence in patients with colon, prostate, and other cancers.

The final section, Section VIII, gives the reader clues to how the information presented in the rest of the book might be implemented at the individual, clinical, and public health levels. Dr. Fogelholm writes on the use of exercise and physical activity in weight control at the individual level. Dr. Heber and Ms. Bowerman provide information on dietary and other methods of energy balance for overweight and obese persons. Dr. Bull describes population-level initiatives to increase physical activity in population settings. Dr. Pronk provides insight into disseminating exercise and diet interventions into the primary care setting. Drs. Schwartz and Winters-Stone provide advice on initiating and maintaining increased exercise and physical activity in cancer patients and survivors. Finally, Drs. Chlebowski, Geller, Harvie and Howell provide guidance on incorporating exercise and diet recommendations into clinical oncology practice.

We hope that this volume provides a comprehensive review of the roles of energy balance, physical activity, and cancer incidence and prognosis. The epidemic of overweight and obesity and the increasing prevalence of sedentary lifestyles will have an impact on the magnitude and quality of the cancer problem around the globe. Viewed differently, knowing that energy balance is so important to the risk and prognosis from cancer may be an important incentive for the general public, persons at high risk, and cancer patients and survivors to increase physical activity, reduce excess weight, and maintain energy balance lifelong.

Anne McTiernan, M.D., Ph.D.
Fred Hutchinson Cancer Research Center
Seattle, Washington

Acknowledgments

I am very grateful, first and foremost, to the authors who made this volume possible. They are all cutting-edge, prominent researchers in obesity, exercise science, and cancer research. I appreciate their carving time into their busy schedules to produce such excellent bodies of work for this book.

For her many and excellent hours of hard work, attention to detail, and organization, I thank my administrative assistant, Jennifer Becker. She kept the other authors and me on schedule, and always with a cheerful "can do" attitude.

I am very grateful to the editors and staff at Taylor & Francis, who had the foresight to see a volume on physical activity, weight, and cancer as being of great interest in the scientific and clinical communities. Joette Lynch, Production project editor, provided outstanding editorial work. Erika Dery, Editorial Project Development project coordinator, was extremely helpful throughout the process of putting this volume together. I also appreciate the careful oversight of Barbara Norwitz, our contact editor.

I thank the many women and men, with and without a history of cancer, who have contributed their time and efforts to our studies. They are the true pioneers in this developing field.

I am very grateful, also, to the leadership and guidance of the U.S. National Cancer Institute, the American Cancer Society, and the International Agency for Research on Cancer in sponsoring research on physical activity, obesity, and cancer. They provide the means to give guidance on healthy lifestyles for preventing cancer and its sequelae.

Finally, the Fred Hutchinson Cancer Research Center has provided the resources for investigating the associations between lifestyle and cancer risk and prognosis to many researchers. I appreciate this support and that of all of the institutions of this volume's authors.

Editor

Anne McTiernan, M.D., Ph.D., is a faculty member in the Division of Public Health Sciences at the Fred Hutchinson Cancer Research Center in Seattle, Washington, and a research professor in the University of Washington Schools of Medicine and Public Health and Community Medicine. At the Fred Hutchinson Cancer Research Center, she is director of the Prevention Center, which includes an ambulatory clinic, exercise testing and training facility, and human nutrition laboratory. She received her medical training at New York Medical College and her primary care internal medicine training at the University of Washington. She received her Ph.D. in epidemiology from the University of Washington.

Dr. McTiernan's research focuses on identifying ways to prevent new or recurrent breast cancer and colorectal cancer with a particular focus on physical activity and obesity. She is principal investigator of several clinical trial and cohort studies investigating the associations among exercise, diet, body weight, hormones, and risk for cancer incidence and prognosis. Dr. McTiernan is also a coinvestigator in the Women's Health Initiative coordinating center.

Dr. McTiernan has published widely in major medical journals, including the *New England Journal of Medicine, the Journal of the American Medical Association, the Journal of the National Cancer Institute,* and *Cancer Research*. She is lead author of the book, *Breast Fitness: An Optimal Exercise and Health Plan for Reducing Your Risk of Breast Cancer*, St. Martin's Press, 2000. Dr. McTiernan is also an editor of the *Journal of Women's Health and Medscape Women's Health*. She has served on several national and international health advisory boards and working groups including the International Agency for Research on Cancer's Cancer Prevention Handbooks of Cancer Prevention Vol. 6: Weight Control and Physical Activity; the 2002 American Cancer Society Guidelines for Nutrition and Physical Activity and Prevention of Cancer; and the 2003 Expert Committee on Nutrition and Physical Activity during and after Treatment. Dr. McTiernan is an elected fellow in the American College of Sports Medicine, the North American Association for the Study of Obesity, and the American College of Epidemiology.

Dr. McTiernan is widely sought as a speaker for professional and lay audiences. She has delivered keynote, plenary, and educational talks at several national and international meetings, including the North American Association for the Study of Obesity, the American College of Sports Medicine, the International Symposium on Women's Health and Menopause, the Ireland/Northern Ireland/National Cancer Institute Cancer Consortium, Seminar on Obesity and Cancer, and the American Society for Clinical Oncology. She regularly presents scientific findings to clinical and lay audiences at cancer centers and medical centers across the U.S. She is frequently interviewed and quoted in various media including CNN, NBC (Today Show), ABC, MSNBC, NPR, *The New York Times*, *Parade Magazine*, and various other print media and magazines.

Contributors

Page E. Abrahamson
Cancer Epidemiology Program, Breast Cancer Program
Department of Epidemiology
Chapel Hill, North Carolina

Barbara E. Ainsworth
Department of Exercise and Nutritional Sciences
San Diego State University
San Diego, California

Rachel Ballard-Barbash
Division of Cancer Control and Population Sciences
National Cancer Institute
Bethesda, Maryland

Leslie Bernstein
Department of Preventive Medicine and
USC/Norris Comprehensive Cancer Center
University of Southern California
Los Angeles, California

George Blackburn
The Center for the Study of Nutrition Medicine
Harvard Medical School
Beth Israel Deaconess Medical Center
Boston, Massachusetts

Susan Bowerman
UCLA Center for Human Nutrition
Los Angeles, California

Fiona Bull
Loughborough University
School of Sports and Exercise Science
Loughborough Leicestershire, United Kingdom

Kristin L. Campbell
University of Alberta
Edmonton, Alberta, Canada

Rowan T. Chlebowski
University of California
Harbor–UCLA Research
Oakland, California

Timothy S. Church
Cooper Institute
Dallas, Texas

Lisa H. Colbert
Department of Kinesiology
Comprehensive Cancer Center
University of Wisconsin
Madison, Wisconsin

Karen J. Coleman
Department of Health Promotion
Graduate School of Public Health
San Diego State University
San Diego, California

Kerry S. Courneya
University of Alberta
Edmonton, Alberta, Canada

Mikael Fogelholm
UKK Institute for Health Promotion Research
Tampere, Finland

Laura Lewis Frank
University of Washington School of Medicine
Department of Psychiatry and Behavioral Sciences
Geriatric Research, Education and Clinical Center (GRECC)
VA Puget Sound Health Care System
Seattle/Tacoma, Washington

Christine M. Friedenreich
Division of Population Health and Information
Tom Baker Cancer Centre
Calgary, Alberta, Canada

Marilie D. Gammon
Cancer Epidemiology Program, Breast Cancer Program
Department of Epidemiology
Chapel Hill, North Carolina

Michelle L. Geller
University of California
Harbor–UCLA Research
Oakland, California

Edward Giovannucci
Department of Epidemiology
Harvard School of Public Health and Department of Medicine
Channing Laboratory
Harvard Medical School and Brigham and Women's Hospital
Boston Massachusetts

Pamela J. Goodwin
Mount Sinai Hospital
Toronto, Ontario, Canada

Michelle Harvie
CRUK Department of Medical Oncology
Christie Hospital
Manchester, England

David Heber
UCLA Center for Human Nutrition
Los Angeles, California

Anthony Howell
CRUK Department of Medical Oncology
Christie Hospital
Manchester, England

Cathrine Hoyo
Department of Community and Family Medicine
Duke Comprehensive Cancer Center
Durham, North Carolina

Melinda Irwin
Department of Epidemiology and Public Health
Yale School of Medicine
New Haven, Connecticut

Weiqin Jiang
Cancer Prevention Laboratory
Colorado State University
Fort Collins, Colorado

Rudolf Kaaks
Hormones and Cancer Team
International Agency for Research on Cancer
Lyon, France

Kristina H. Karvinen
University of Alberta
Edmonton, Alberta, Canada

Aliya B. Ladha
University of Alberta
Edmonton, Alberta, Canada

Annekatrin Lukanova
Department of Obstetrics and Gynecology
New York University School of Medicine
New York, New York

María Elena Martínez
Arizona Cancer Center
Mel and Enid Zuckerman Arizona College of Public Health
University of Arizona
Tucson, Arizona

Monica McGrath
Channing Lab
Harvard University
Boston, Massachusetts

Anne McTiernan
Fred Hutchinson Cancer Research Center, Cancer Prevention
Department of Medicine, School of Medicine, University of Washington
Seattle, Washington

Dominique S. Michaud
Harvard School of Public Health
Department of Epidemiology
Boston, Massahcusetts

Alpa V. Patel
Department of Epidemiology and Surveillance Research
American Cancer Society
Atlanta, Georgia

Ross L. Prentice
Division of Public Health Sciences
Fred Hutchinson Cancer Research Center
Seattle, Washington

Elisa L. Priest
Cooper Institute
Dallas, Texas

Nicolaas P. Pronk
HealthPartners Research Foundation
Minneapolis, Minnesota

Tuomo Rankinen
Pennington Biomedical Research Center
Human Genomics Laboratory
Baton Rouge, Louisiana

Cheryl L. Rock
Family and Preventive Medicine
UCSD Cancer Center
La Jolla, California

Anna L. Schwartz
University of Washington
Biobehavioral Nursing and Health Systems
Seattle, Washington

Martha L. Slattery
Family and Preventive Medicine
The University of Utah, School of Medicine
Salt Lake City, Utah

Henry J. Thompson
Cancer Prevention Laboratory
Colorado State University
Fort Collins, Colorado

Shelley Tworoger
Channing Lab
Harvard University
Boston, Massachusetts

Cornelia M. Ulrich
Cancer Prevention
Fred Hutchinson Cancer Research Center
Department of Epidemiology
University of Washington, School of Public Health and Community Medicine
Seattle, Washington

Belinda Waltman
The Center for the Study of Nutrition Medicine
Harvard Medical School
Beth Israel Deaconess Medical Center
Boston, Massachusetts

Catherine M. Wetmore
Department of Epidemiology
University of Washington, School of Public Health and Community Medicine
Seattle, Washington

Kerri Winters-Stone
Oregon Health and Sciences University
School of Nursing
Portland, Oregon

Zongjian Zhu
Cancer Prevention Laboratory
Colorado State University
Fort Collins, Colorado

Contents

Section I

Research Methods

1 Observational Studies and Intervention Trials in Exercise, Diet, and Cancer Prevention Research

Ross L. Prentice

CONTENTS

INTRODUCTION

This chapter is concerned with the strengths and weaknesses of, and the role played by, major observational and interventional study designs in cancer prevention through exercise and weight control research agenda. Because the research study design issues tend to be similar for the prevention of cancer and for other major chronic diseases, the discussion is broadened to the role of these study designs in chronic disease prevention. Also, issues related to physical activity assessment have much in common with those for dietary assessment, and energy balance is central to weight control, so the discussion also highlights issues arising in the study of diet and nutrition and chronic disease prevention.

A major goal of a research program aimed at weight control and chronic disease prevention is the development of evidence-based preventative recommendations for the general population and for its major subgroups, along with the development of practical approaches to satisfying such recommendations. Pharmaceutical approaches also have a role among chronic disease prevention tools for persons for whom behavioral strategies may be insufficient. In either case, preventative recommendations need to have an overriding focus on overall health benefits vs. risks, with important implications for research designs and emphases.

From the obesity epidemic in the United States and other Western countries, and from the strong associations between overweight and obesity and the incidence and mortality from cancer [1] and other chronic diseases, it seems evident that Western societies are suffering a tremendous disease burden owing to unfavorable physical activity and dietary consumption patterns. However, available recommendations concerning the amount and type of physical activity [2–5] and nutrient consumption and dietary patterns [5–8] have been only modestly influenced by chronic disease prevention considerations, because of limitations in available research data. Related to this, research that aims to develop and test behavioral interventions and strategies for improving physical activity and dietary patterns for individuals or communities tends to be hampered by a lack of consensus on desirable intervention goals.

Indeed, the development of practical physical activity and dietary recommendations that may help to reverse overweight, obesity, and chronic disease trends is a most challenging research aim, though many opportunities are currently available. The obvious epidemiological approach to gaining the requisite knowledge involves comparing persons with various physical activity and dietary patterns in respect to subsequent weight changes and chronic disease event rates. In fact, cohort studies, along with other observational designs, do constitute a mainstay approach in exercise and nutritional epidemiology. However, epidemiological research on these patterns is attended by some important issues that can cast aspersions on the reliability and interpretation of reported associations.

OBSERVATIONAL STUDIES OF PHYSICAL ACTIVITY AND DIETARY PATTERNS

Confounding

The first issue concerning the reliability and interpretation of observational studies in these areas is classical epidemiological confounding. For example, persons sustaining a high level of physical activity over much of their lifespan may differ in many biobehavioral respects from more sedentary persons. These may, for example, include socioeconomic factors, skill level in sports, aspects of physical functioning and emotional status, and dietary habits. Insofar as these factors also relate to weight maintenance and chronic disease risk, they need to be recognized, accurately measured, and properly included in data analysis to avoid confounding. In fact, such comprehensive confounding control is rarely practical, so there is always some uncertainty, for example, as to whether a reported association of a physical activity pattern with a chronic disease risk is attributable in part to corresponding uncontrolled differences in diet or other potential confounding factors.

Very similar confounding issues attend dietary patterns, with physical activity as an important potential confounder. Additionally, studies aimed at elucidating the relationship of the consumption of specific nutrients or foods to chronic disease risk need to acknowledge potential confounding by other nutrients and food that may be highly correlated with those under investigation.

"Exposure" Assessment Measurement Error

An equally important issue in physical activity and dietary epidemiology concerns "exposure" assessment. Physical activity is typically self-reported by means of records, logs, or recalls. The instruments used may have demonstrated some degree of repeatability in populations of interest, but the accuracy, and measurement properties more generally, are usually unknown. Alternatively, physical activity is sometimes indirectly assessed using physiological methods. For example, measures of cardiopulmonary fitness, such as maximum oxygen output volume, have been used to produce estimates of normal physical activity [9], although such measures may be insensitive to low-intensity or longer term activity levels.

Most observational studies, however, rely on self-reported physical activity assessments obtained using personal interviews or mailed questionnaires that ask the respondent to recall historic information; this is used to construct physical activity estimates over time. Clearly, such physical activity estimates may include substantial measurement error. Statistical approaches to accommodating such measurement error [10] almost universally assume a classical measurement model in which the assessment, Z, relates to the targeted actual physical activity, X (e.g., average METs/day over the past decade), via

$$Z = X + e \tag{1.1}$$

where the measurement error term e is assumed to be statistically independent of X and independent of other study subject characteristics and confounding factors.

Unfortunately, these methods will generally not yield accurate estimates of association between physical activity and disease risk if a more complex measurement model is required. For example, if overweight or obese persons tend to perceive and report physical activity differently than do normal or underweight persons, biased associations can be expected. Similarly, if physical activity reporting depends on age, ethnicity, socioeconomic factors, social desirability factors, or dietary patterns, bias can be expected to the extent that these factors are related to the outcomes under study.

Note that this issue of systematic bias in physical activity assessment is quite distinct from the confounding issue cited previously. For example, suppose that, in a cohort study of physical activity in relation to breast cancer risk, overweight women tend to report greater physical activity than leaner women, although their actual physical activity tends to be somewhat less. Such systematic bias in assessment will distort and may even reverse the direction of the estimated physical activity and disease risk association. The inclusion of an indicator variable for overweight in a regression analysis of breast cancer risk, which may be considered to prevent confounding, cannot be expected to resolve the distortion caused by systematic bias in physical activity assessment.

The use of objective measures of physical activity, at least in a subset of the study cohort, provides potential to avoid major biases due to measurement error. An objective measure is one in which the measurement error is independent of study subject characteristics or other confounding factors. For example, the maximum oxygen output volume previously mentioned may plausibly satisfy this criterion. Additionally, the objective measure should adhere to the classical measurement model (Equation 1.1) so that the assessment measures the targeted quantity, X, aside from random error. This may be a difficult criterion to satisfy because potential objective measures of physical activity may often be insensitive, incomplete, or variable over time in their response to specific physical activity patterns.

The doubly labeled water measure of energy expenditure [11] provides a valuable tool for objectively measuring physical activity. The rates of recovery of two nonradioactive isotopes in urine, following bolus consumption in the form of doubly labeled water, allows carbon dioxide production, and thus energy expenditure, to be estimated accurately over a short-term (typically 2 weeks) period. Subtraction of basal metabolic energy expenditure, as determined by indirect calorimetry, yields an assessment of physical activity-related energy expenditure that plausibly adheres to Equation 1.1 as an estimate of actual (short-term) energy expenditure. The costs of this approach (specifically of the doubly labeled water) are such that it is not a practical approach for all members of a study cohort, which typically includes tens of thousands of study subjects if rare diseases are under study. Rather, such a procedure can only be applied to a modest subset of cohort members. The relationship between the objective measure and self-report measures can then be used to calibrate the self-report measures on the remainder of the cohort, and the calibrated values play a fundamental role in analyses to associate physical activity-related energy expenditure to disease risk.

To date, the doubly labeled water method has evidently not been used in large epidemiological cohort studies of physical activity, at least not on the scale required for the calibration procedure just mentioned. The doubly labeled water measure has received greater use, however, in nutritional epidemiology, in which the estimate of energy expenditure can reasonably be equated to short-term energy consumption among weight-stable persons. For example, the National Cancer Institute's Observing Protein and Energy Nutrition (OPEN) Study [12,13] used the doubly labeled water method, along with urinary nitrogen [14], as an objective recovery measure [15] of protein consumption among 484 men and women aged 40 to 69; this project studied the structure of measurement error in commonly used dietary self-report instruments, including a food frequency questionnaire and a 24-hour dietary recall.

A Nutrient Biomarker Study among 544 women is currently nearing completion within the dietary modification component of the Women's Health Initiative Clinical Trial among nearly 48,835 postmenopausal women [16]. In that context, energy consumption, X, will be related to disease risk using the measurement model, Equation 1.1, for the doubly labeled water measure, Z, along with the measurement model [17]:

$$W = a + bX + cV + dX \otimes V + r + u \tag{1.2}$$

for the food frequency energy consumption estimate W, where V represents factors such as obesity, age, or ethnicity that may affect how a person reports dietary consumption, the term $X \otimes V$ allows the influence of these factors on reporting to depend on actual consumption X, r represents a person-specific bias (random effect) term, u represents random error, and all variates on the right side of Equation 1.1 and Equation 1.2 are assumed to be statistically independent.

Observational Study Reliability

In addition to the avoidance of confounding, and the need for a suitable measurement error model, observational studies of physical activity and diet in relation to chronic disease risk require the selection of representative study subjects from the target population and outcome ascertainment that is unrelated to study exposures. It is reasonable to ask how related potential sources of bias should affect one's evaluation and interpretation of the reliability of observational study reports describing associations, or lack thereof, between some aspect of exercise and diet and the risk of a chronic disease. In fact, the many ways to present measures of these exposures and to slice exposure ranges tend to reduce study reliability unless the authors have adhered to a prespecified analysis plan.

The overall question of study reliability is, however, often difficult to answer. The discussion section of observational study reports often runs down a list of potential biases, and the authors give their opinions as to why each bias is not expected to be of importance. Indeed, decades of intensive risk factor studies using cohort or case-control designs for a number of chronic diseases, along with the development of corresponding analytic procedures, have put the epidemiologist in a position to make a serious effort to control confounding. The extent to which the inclusion of standard disease risk factors, as determined by questionnaire, in logistic regression or Cox regression analyses guards against confounding by poorly measured potential confounding factors is unclear. Such factors include those related to physical activity or diet, or biobehavioral factors. However, typical observational study confounding factors should go some distance in reducing the source of bias.

Exposure measurement error, on the other hand, is much less explored in terms of plausible magnitude of impact on observational study results in the exercise and diet arena. There has been some study of energy consumption reporting as a function of body weight. In one sizeable study, energy consumption on food diaries tended to be substantially less than corresponding doubly labeled water estimates among obese persons, with little difference among normal weight persons [18]. Studies of breast cancer occurrence in the U.K. find rather different relationships to dietary fat intake, depending on the type of dietary assessment instrument applied [19]. The OPEN study [13] reported positive assessment error correlations for energy and protein between a food frequency instrument and 24-hour dietary recalls. This finding reduces the plausibility that a self-report assessment can serve as a "reference instrument" that adheres to Equation 1.1 for the purpose of calibrating a food frequency assessment in a cohort study analysis. These studies are not definitive, but they do raise the measurement error issue as one that needs to be resolved if nutrition and physical activity observational studies are to have a clear and direct interpretation.

INTERVENTION TRIALS OF PHYSICAL ACTIVITY AND NUTRITION

Intervention Trial Features and Challenges

Given the challenges associated with observational studies in physical activity and nutritional epidemiology, why not go directly to the randomized controlled trial of physical activity or dietary interventions and cancer incidence among healthy persons? Indeed, disease rate comparisons will not be confounded by prerandomization factors, whether or not they can be measured well or even recognized. Furthermore, such comparisons do not depend on physical activity or dietary assessment for their validity although such assessments for the randomized groups as a whole are needed for trial interpretation. In addition, an intervention trial setting can provide an excellent context for outcome ascertainment that is common across intervention groups.

These types of considerations have caused the randomized, controlled trial to be the central study design in most therapeutic research settings. However, disease prevention research has some critical practical limitations. Specifically, because the outcomes targeted for prevention have low incidence rates over a trial follow-up period of a few years' duration, preventative trials typically need to be very large scale, perhaps in the tens of thousands. Difficult logistics and great expense typically attend such large trials, so a handful at most can be supported at a given point in time. Furthermore, the physical activity or dietary changes to be tested may be difficult to maintain over the several years that may be required to affect chronic disease risk by a detectable amount. Also, a range of other behavioral changes may accompany the changes targeted by the interventions under study, thus reducing the etiologic, but perhaps not the public health, implications of trial results.

For the reasons just outlined, proposals to conduct full-scale intervention trials for chronic disease prevention are often met with skepticism and resistance. Critics may examine trial cost estimates and consider the number of individual research grants that could be supported by the requisite amount of funding. Others may question whether the underlying hypothesis or the intervention to achieve study goals has been developed with sufficient care and thoroughness. These are important issues that proponents of a prevention trial must adequately address before a randomized controlled trial can proceed.

Intermediate Outcome Trials

One response to the cost and logistics issue associated with a full-scale intervention trial having disease outcomes is the use of short-term responses, which may be altered as a part of a carcinogenesis or other disease pathway, as an intervention trial outcome variable. For example, a recent exercise intervention trial [20] was conducted in 173 sedentary, overweight postmenopausal women randomly assigned to a moderate-intensity exercise program or to a control (self-selected physical activity) group; outcomes included serum hormone concentrations and body fat distribution [21,22]. This type of physical activity trial, as well as small-scale human nutrition intervention trials, has an important place in the chronic disease prevention research agenda.

With a varied set of meaningful intermediate outcomes, such trials can provide much insight into the disease prevention potential of an intervention and a context for developing intervention procedures that can achieve physical activity and dietary goals and maintain them over the typical trial follow-up period of a few months. Intermediate outcome trials, however, are generally not a sufficient replacement for a full-scale trial; in a number of contexts, favorable intermediate outcome changes have been shown not to convey meaningful disease prevention benefits, and interventions may have unsuspected consequences for outcomes other than those targeted for prevention. Thus, appropriate forums are needed to identify the most promising and timely physical activity and nutrition interventions for full-scale testing.

Sources of Hypotheses and Interventions

Sources of intervention hypotheses in the exercise and nutrition area include observational studies and therapeutic trials. Both sources are valuable. As explained earlier, observational studies may lack specificity due to highly correlated patterns of the consumption of various nutrients and may lack reliability more generally. Furthermore, observational studies may not be well configured to examine the health effects of changes in physical activity or dietary patterns and usually are not concerned with methods and procedures to achieve exercise or dietary goals. On the other hand, therapeutic trials cannot be expected to yield interventions that act predominantly at the early stages of disease development and may infrequently focus on behavioral interventions.

For example, preclinical trials of physical activity and diet in rodent systems can provide valuable insights into interventions that may have favorable effects on cancer processes (e.g., carcinogen metabolism, hormone regulation, cell division and differentiation, apoptosis, and cell-cycle regulation) and on processes relevant to other chronic diseases. An interesting special case is provided by studies of dietary restriction in rodents in relation to disease risk and longevity [23,24]. These types of trials, which typically involve a moderate number of animals and a few months' duration, can inform the small-scale human intervention trials mentioned previously.

In both settings, the ongoing development of high-dimensional genotyping, gene and protein expression, and metabolomic approaches provides the opportunity for specific and comprehensive hypothesis development activities. Hypothesis development initiatives need to target a medical model that tailors interventions to a person's genotype as well as specific exposures and characteristics and, equally importantly, a public health model that aims to develop physical activity and nutrition recommendations and interventions applicable to major segments of the general population.

RESEARCH NEEDS AND AGENDA

Methodology Development

In a number of chronic disease prevention settings, one has extensive observational data along with one or more randomized controlled trials, and the results (at least superficially) disagree between the two sources. These provide a particular opportunity to assess study design and analysis properties and to identify approaches to strengthening each type of study. For example, in the nutrition area, observational studies of beta-carotene consumption in relation to the incidence of lung and other cancers suggested important preventative potential [25,26]; however, subsequent controlled trials found no effect [27] or an apparently adverse effect [28,29] of beta-carotene supplementation. It remains unclear whether the observational studies were too nonspecific to allow favorable lung cancer trends to be attributed to this specific nutrient or were otherwise misleading, or whether consumption at low levels in food is beneficial but higher level supplementation is harmful. Similarly, observational studies indicating lower colorectal cancer incidence among persons consuming low-fat, high-fiber diets were not supported by subsequent trials of colorectal adenoma recurrence prevention using wheat bran fiber [30] or a low-fat eating pattern [31]. These trials again raise questions about the specificity and reliability of the observational studies, as well as about the utility and necessary follow-up duration in adenoma recurrence trials.

A striking example of an apparent observational vs. trial discrepancy arises in studies of combined postmenopausal hormone therapy and coronary heart disease, in which observational studies [32] suggest a 40 to 50% reduction in incidence; however, a recent randomized controlled trial [33] found an incidence rate elevation over a 5.6-year intervention period. Although studies are still under way [34] to explain such discrepancy, an important aspect seems to be a hazard ratio function that is elevated early, but subsequently declines and may reverse direction. Available trial data were highly influenced by the early elevation, although such available observational data depend predominantly on follow-up that begins some years after hormone therapy initiation.

The identification of study design and analysis procedures that can avoid these types of discrepancies is an important research goal in the physical activity, diet, and chronic disease prevention research area. The manner and extent to which discrepancies can be resolved and avoided also will help identify the complementary role to be played by observational studies and full-scale intervention trials.

Hypothesis Development and Initial Testing

The potential of exercise and dieting changes to improve health and prevent chronic disease risk is such that it merits attention and best efforts of the public health-oriented research community. Additional basic and clinical science efforts are needed to identify interventions for testing in human populations. Also, too few research groups are configured to carry out the small-scale exercise or nutrition intervention trials, with a comprehensive set of outcomes, out of which a specific intervention for full-scale testing may arise. Although observational study of exercise and dietary factors with disease risk is substantial, studies that use biomarkers in a fundamental way in association tests are particularly needed.

Generation and Evaluation of Full-Scale Trial Proposals

A standing forum comprising a broad cross-section of pertinent scientists is needed to stimulate and evaluate timely, scientifically defensible proposals for full-scale prevention trials. For example, such a forum could arise from an NIH-sponsored cooperative group of investigators with interest and expertise in basic, clinical, and population aspects of nutrition and physical activity, and in health-related outcomes [35]. This group could conduct early phase studies, evaluate concepts from the broader scientific community for new studies, and facilitate the translation of such concepts into full proposals for peer review.

ACKNOWLEDGMENTS

This work was partially supported by grant CA53996. This chapter draws on the substance and report [35] from a recent workshop, Nutrition and Physical Activity and Chronic Disease Prevention: Research Strategies and Recommendations, and the author is indebted to workshop participants for helpful discussions.

REFERENCES

1. Calle EE, Rodriquez C, Walker–Thurmond K, Thun MJ. Overweight, obesity, and mortality from cancer in a prospectively studied cohort of U.S. adults. *N Engl J Med*, 348, 1625, 2003.
2. U.S. Department of Health and Human Services. *Physical Activity and Health: a Report of the Surgeon General.* Atlanta GA: U.S. Department of Health and Human Services, Centers for Disease Control and Prevention, National Center for Chronic Disease Prevention and Health Promotion, 1996.

3. International Agency for Research on Cancer. *IARC Handbook of Cancer Prevention*, V6, *Weight Control and Physical Activity.* Lyon, IARC Press, 2002.
4. Brown JK, Byers T, Doyle C, Courneya KS, Demark–Wahnefried W, Kushi LH, McTieman A, Rock CL, Aziz N, Bloch AS, Eldridge B, Hamilton K, Katzin C, Koonce A, Main J, Mobley C, Morra ME, Pierce MS, Sawyer KA. Nutrition and physical activity during and after cancer treatment: an American Cancer Society guide for informed choices. *CA Cancer J Clin*, 53, 268, 2003.
5. Institute of Medicine (IOM). *Dietary Reference Intakes for Energy, Carbohydrate, Fiber, Fat, Fatty Acids, Cholesterol, Protein and Amino Acids.* A report of the Food and Nutrition Board, Institute of Medicine of the National Academies, Washington D.C.: National Academics Press, 2002.
6. National Research Council (NRC). *Recommended Dietary Allowances*, 10th ed. Report of the Subcommittee on the Tenth Edition of the RDAs. Food and Nutrition Board and the Commission on Life Sciences. Washington D.C.: National Academy Press, 1989.
7. Anonymous. Guidelines on diet, nutrition and cancer prevention: reducing the risk of cancer with healthy food choices and physical activity. *CA Cancer J Clin*, 46, 325, 1996.
8. National Research Council. *Diet and Health. Implications for Reducing Chronic Disease Risk.* Washington D.C.: National Academy Press, 1989.
9. Balady GJ, Berra KA, Golding LA, Gordon NF, Mahler DA, Myers JN, Sheldahl LM, Grais IM, Herbert DL, Herbert WG, Swain DP, Tokarczyk SL, Young AJ. *ACSM's Guidelines for Exercise Testing and Prescription.* 6th ed. Philadelphia (PA): Lippincott Williams & Wilkins; 2000.
10. Carroll RJ, Ruppert D, Stefanski LA. *Measurement Error in Nonlinear Models.* New York: Chapman & Hall, 1995.
11. Schoeller DA. Validation of habitual energy intake. *Public Health Nutr*, 5, 883, 2002.
12. Subar AF, Kipnis V, Troiano RP, Midthune D, Scholler DA, Bingham S, Sharbaugh CO, Trabulsi J, Runswick S, Ballard-Barbash R, Sunshine J, Schatzkin A. Using intake biomarkers to evaluate the extent of dietary misreporting in a large sample of adults: the OPEN Study. *Am J Epidemiol*, 158, 1, 2003.
13. Kipnis V, Subar AF, Midthune D, Freedman LS, Ballard–Barbash R, Troiano RP, Bingham S, Schoeller DA, Schatzkin A, Carroll RJ. Structure of dietary measurement error: results of the OPEN biomarker study. *Am J Epidemiol*; 158, 14, 2003.
14. Bingham SA. Biomarkers in nutritional epidemiology. *Public Health Nutr*, 5, 821, 2002.
15. Kaaks R, Ferrari P, Ciampi A, Plummer M, Riboli E. Uses and limitations of statistical accounting for random error correlations, in the validation of dietary questionnaire assessments. *Public Health Nutr*, 5, 969, 2002.
16. Women's Health Initiative Study Group. Design of the Women's Health Initiative Clinical Trial and Observational Study. *Control Clin Trials*, 19, 61, 1998.
17. Prentice RL, Sugar E, Wang CY, Neuhouser M, Patterson R. Research strategies and the use of nutrient biomarkers in studies of diet and chronic disease. *Public Health Nutr*, 5, 977, 2002.
18. Heitmann BL, Lissner L. Dietary underreporting by obese individuals: is it specific or nonspecific? *Br Med J*, 311, 986, 1995.
19. Bingham SA, Luben R, Welch A, Wareham N, Khaw KT, Day N. Are imprecise methods obscuring a relationship between fat and breast cancer? *Lancet*, 362, 212, 2003.
20. McTiernan A, Ulrich CM, Yancey D, Slate S, Nakamura H, Oestreicher N, Bowen D, Yasui Y, Potter J, Schwartz R. The Physical Activity for Total Health (PATH) Study: rationale and design. *Med Sci Sports Exercise*, 31, 1307, 1999.
21. Irwin ML, Yasui Y, Ulrich CM, Bowen D, Rudolph RE, Schwartz RS, Yukawa M, Aiello E, Potter JD, McTiernan A. Effect of exercise on total and intra-abdominal body fat in postmenopausal women. *JAMA*, 289, 323, 2003.
22. McTiernan A, Tworoger SS, Ulrich CM, Yasui Y, Irwin ML, Rajan KB, Sorensen B, Rudolph RE, Bowen D, Stanczyk FZ, Potter JD, Schwartz RS. Effect of exercise on serum estrogens in postmenopausal women: a 12-month randomized controlled trial. *Cancer Res*, 64, 2923, 2004.
23. Shi H, Vigneau–Callahan K, Shestopalov I, Milbury PE, Matson WR, Kristal BS. Characterization of diet-dependent metabolic serotypes: primary validation of male and female serotypes in independent cohorts of rats. *J Nutr*, 132, 1039, 2002.
24. Berrigan D, Perkins SN, Haines DC, Hursting SD. Adult-onset calorie restriction and fasting delay spontaneous tumorigenesis in p53-deficient mice. *Carcinogenesis*, 23, 817, 2002.

25. Ziegler RG, Mayne ST, Swanson CA. Nutrition and lung cancer. *Cancer Causes Control*, 7, 157, 1996.
26. Greenberg ER, Baron JA, Karakas MR, Stukel TA, Nierenberg DW, Stevens MM, Mandel JS, Haile RW. Mortality associated with low plasma concentration of beta carotene and the effect of oral supplementation. *JAMA*, 275, 699, 1996.
27. Hennekens CH, Buring JE, Manson JE, Stampfer M, Rosner B, Cook NR, Belanger C, LaMotte F, Gaziano JM, Ridker PM, Willett W, Peto R. Lack of effect of long-term supplementation with beta carotene on the incidence of malignant neoplasms and cariovascular disease. *N Engl J Med*, 334, 1145, 1996.
28. Alpha-Tocopherol, Beta Carotene Cancer Prevention Study Group. The effect of vitamin E and beta carotene on the incidence of lung cancer and other cancers among male smokers. *N Engl J Med*, 330, 1029, 1994.
29. Omenn GS, Goodman GE, Thornquist MD, Balmes J, Cullen MR, Glass A, Keogh JP, Meyskens FL, Valanis B, Williams JH, Barnhart S, Hammar S. Effects of a combination of beta carotene and vitamin A on lung cancer and cardiovascular disease. *N Engl J Med*, 334, 1150, 1996.
30. Alberts DA, Martinez ME, Roe DJ, Guillen-Rodriguez JM, Marshall JR, van Leeuwen JB, Reid ME, Ritenbaugh C, Vargas PA, Bhattacharyya AB, Earnest DL, Sampliner RE. Lack of effect of a high-fiber cereal supplement on the recurrence of colorectal adenomas. *N Engl J Med*, 342, 1156, 2000.
31. Schatzkin A, Lanza E, Corle D, Lance P, Iber F, Caan B, Shike M, Weissfeld J, Burt R, Cooper MR, Kikendall JW, Cahill J. Lack of effect of a low-fat, high-fiber diet on the recurrence of colorectal adenomas. *N Engl J Med*, 342, 1149, 2000.
32. Stampfer M, Colditz G. Estrogen replacement therapy and coronary heart disease: a quantitative assessment of the epidemiologic evidence. *Prev Med*, 20, 47, 1991.
33. Writing Group for the Women's Health Initiative Investigators. Risks and benefits of estrogen plus progestin in healthy postmenopausal women. Principal results from the Women's Health Initiative randomized controlled trial. *JAMA*, 288, 321, 2002.
34. Prentice RL, Langer R, Stefanick M, Howard Bv, Pettinger M, Anderson G, Barad D, Curb JD, Kotchen J, Kuller L, Limacher M, Wachtawski-Wende J, for the Women's Health Initiative Investigators. Combined postmenopausal hormone therapy and cardiovascular disease: toward resolving the discrepancy between observational studies and the Women's Health Initiative clinical trial. To appear, *Am J Epidemiol*, 2005.
35. Prentice RL, Willett WC, Greenwald P, Alberts D, Bernstein L, Boyd NF, Byers T, Clinton SK, Fraser G, Freedman L, Hunter D, Kipnis V, Kolonel LN, Kristal BS, Kristal A, Lampe JW, McTiernan A, Milner J, Patterson RE, Potter JD, Riboli E, Schatzkin A, Yates A, Yetley E. Nutrition and physical activity and chronic disease prevention: research strategies and recommendations. *J Natl Cancer Inst*, 96, 1276, 2004.

2 Physical Activity Measurement

Barbara E. Ainsworth and Karen J. Coleman

CONTENTS

OVERVIEW

Despite the available research and the known benefits of physical activity, 45% of U.S. adults do not accumulate a sufficient amount of physical activity to derive health benefits and 16% do not engage in any physical activity during their leisure time [1]. Because many health experts attribute the obesity epidemic [2] and elevated risks for some chronic diseases to physical inactivity [3], a priority has been placed on the use of valid and reliable measures to assess all levels of physical activity [3,4]. This is especially true for understudied populations such as ethnic minorities and women [5].

Numerous reviews of physical activity assessment have been conducted in the past decade, including several for self-report [6–8], objective activity monitoring [9,10], and cancer studies [11,12]. In 1999, the Cooper Aerobics Institute held a conference specifically for the measurement of physical activity, the proceedings of which were published in a special supplement of *Research Quarterly for Exercise and Sport* [13]. In addition, a reference text for the assessment of physical activity was also recently published [9].

This chapter is limited to the methods used to assess physical activity using direct and indirect measures. For the purposes of this review, direct measures are considered "real time" in that they assess physical activity concurrently with the activity. Direct measures include physical activity records, observation, and activity monitors. Indirect methods assess physical activity retrospectively and include self-report questionnaires, structured recall interviews, focus groups, and ethnographic life-history methods. Using direct and indirect methods to assess physical activity is growing in popularity [9,14] and is recommended by most physical activity researchers as a more comprehensive way of indexing a person's physical activity.

CONCEPTUAL FRAMEWORK

LaMonte and Ainsworth [15] present a conceptual framework for the measurement of movement as a global construct. The construct has two dimensions: physical activity (a behavior) and energy expenditure (the energy cost of the behavior). Both dimensions can be measured using the direct and indirect methods depicted in Figure 2.1. This review is limited to the measurement of physical activity and not energy expenditure. However, the measurement of energy expenditure is often used to infer physical activity, especially when measures like doubly labeled water and activity monitors are used. This partly reflects the controversy in public health about whether a minimal level of energy expenditure or bodily movement leads to the protective benefits of physical activity [3,4].

Activity monitors often provide estimates of energy expenditure and bodily movement; when they are validated, they are compared to actual energy expenditure, not body movement (an exception is with pedometers that have actual number of steps counted by observers) [9]. Self-report is much more complex because no objective assessment of bodily movement is made. Instead, the type, duration, frequency, and intensity are assessed; this may be used to estimate energy expenditure and then related to health outcomes [15].

DIRECT PHYSICAL ACTIVITY ASSESSMENT METHODS

Activity Monitors/Motion Sensors

The four basic types of activity monitors: (1) measure acceleration (accelerometers); (2) measure the movement of the body up and down when a person lifts the feet off the ground (pedometers); (3) monitor heart rate; and (4) measure changes in body temperature. An accelerometer detects acceleration and deceleration in one or more planes of motion (vertical, longitudinal, and medial). A uniaxial accelerometer measures acceleration in the vertical plane, and biaxial and triaxial accelerometers are sensitive to movements in two and three dimensions, respectively. When these devices detect movement, an electric current proportional to the degree of acceleration is generated

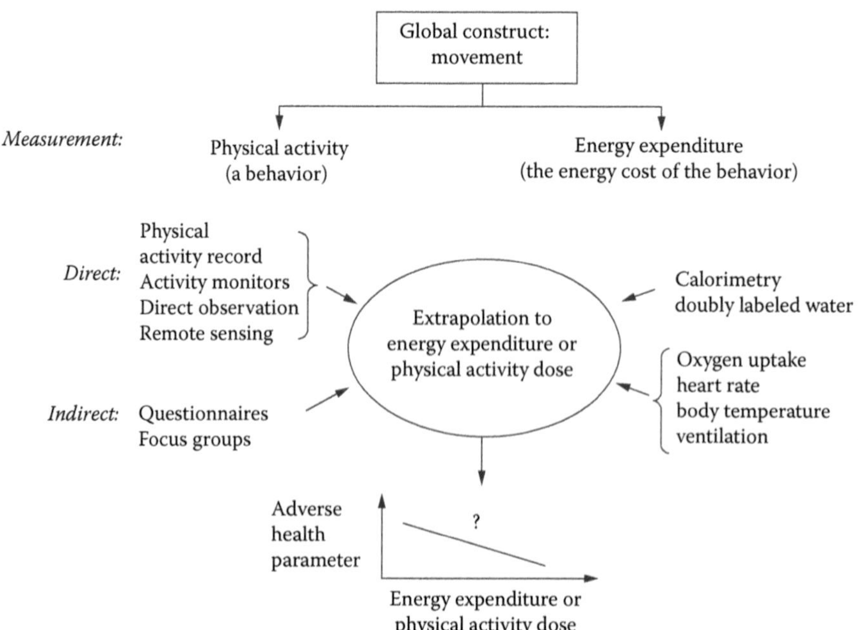

FIGURE 2.1 Conceptual framework for the measurement of a global construct for *Movement*.

within the motion sensor. Because acceleration increases in several dimensions with faster movements, theoretically, accelerometers should accurately determine energy expenditure across a wide range of exercise intensities [16].

There are a myriad of activity monitors available for research [9]. Triaxial accelerometers include the TriTrac R3D (Professional Products Inc., Madison, WI), the RT3 Tri-axial Research Tracker (Stayhealthy Inc., Monrovia, CA), and the Tracmor (available from Klaus Westerterp, Maastricht University, Maastricht, The Netherlands). The RT3 Tri-axial Research Tracker is the third generation of the TriTrac models. The two most common uniaxial accelerometers are the Caltrac (Muscle Dynamics, Torrence, CA) and the Computer Science Applications (CSA) monitor (Shalimar, FL), now known as the MTI Actigraph (Fort Walton Beach, FL). The new generation models are not the same as the old models and thus validity and reliability should be assessed separately for these new devices [17]. The BioTrainer-Pro (IM Systems, Baltimore, MD) is the only stand-alone biaxial accelerometer currently available for research.

At least 13 different pedometers are available for research [18]; however, to date, the Yamax models (New Lifestyles, Inc., Lee's Summit, MO) are the most accurate. Although many heart rate monitors are commercially available, almost all studies have been done using Polar models (Polar Electro Inc., New York) because of their ability to store large amounts of information [19]. Finally, the SenseWear Armband (BodyMedia Inc., Pittsburgh, PA) is a new device that contains a biaxial accelerometer, a heart rate receiver, and a thermocoupler with the unique capability of measuring heat production.

Which monitor is "best" depends a great deal on the target population, the monetary resources of the project, the time and labor available to the project, and the research questions. No activity monitor provides the type of activity engaged in, and thus some kind of self-report must always accompany the monitor if this is an important research question. The accelerometers can store up to 30 days of minute-to-minute activity; however, they cost approximately $500 per monitor and hours of labor and computer programming are necessary to consolidate data into meaningful intensity, frequency, and duration information. The BioTrainer Pro has demonstrated the poorest validity for the measurement of energy expenditure (and thus physical activity) of all the available accelerometers [17,20]; the CSA (now referred to as the MTI Actigraph) with the Freedson correction for energy expenditure [21] and the TriTrac R3D [17,22] have the best validity.

Pedometers provide the most user friendly and economical approach ($10 to $20 each) to activity monitoring. In addition, they are often excellent sources of immediate feedback for participants [10]. However, they cannot "store" daily activity data, so participants must record their steps each day, and they have limited validity in assessing any activities that are not related to walking [23]. Finally, although expensive ($500 each), the SenseWear Armband may have some promise as a research tool. It seems to be a valid indicator of energy expenditure at a variety of walking speeds [17,24] and its position on the upper arm avoids the extraneous movement common to accelerometers worn around the waist [25].

Direct Observation

One of the most accurate, comprehensive direct measures of physical activity is systematic observation [9,26]. Information can be collected about the type, intensity, duration, and frequency of any observable physical activity [9,26]. This field has been almost exclusively devoted to the observation of school-aged children's physical activity [27–29]. The two main systems used in research are the System for Observing Fitness Instruction Time (SOFIT), its newest variant, the System for Observing Play and Physical Activity in Youth (SOPLAY) [30,31], and the Children's Activity Rating Scale (CARS) [32]. These tools have been extensively validated in a variety of settings including the classroom [33], physical education [34], and after school [35].

Almost no data on behavioral observation in adults are available. Most of this work has been done to examine people's walking and bicycling behavior [36,37]. Given the utility of behavioral observation in providing detailed information about all aspects of physical activity — especially descriptions of type — this area should be more extensively developed in adult and elderly populations.

Physical Activity Records

Physical activity records provide a detailed account of activities done within a given period of time [8]. Records are useful in identifying the type, duration, and frequency of activities and may take the form of a written diary or record book, dictation into a tape recorder, or by recalling the prior days' activities in the presence of a trained interviewer. Physical activity records have been used to describe activity patterns in populations [38–41] and to validate physical activity questionnaires [42]. Irwin and colleagues [43] provide detailed instructions in the use of a physical activity record.

The precision of physical activity records has been studied using doubly labeled water. Irwin et al. [43] compared recorded physical activity in the form of estimated energy expenditure with doubly labeled water kilocalories obtained during a 7-day period, showing difference in kilocalorie estimates on the order of 7.9 ± 3.2% kcal. Unfortunately, physical activity records have many drawbacks, mostly concerning the large participant burden and limited application to people with low-literacy skills. Recording physical activity can interfere with daily activities, resulting in poor compliance to study protocols. In addition, physical activity records share with qualitative data the expense of time in coding descriptive information into quantitative data. However, with the refinement of hand-held tape recorders, palm pilots with voice- and handwriting-recognition software to facilitate recording and coding of physical activity records, the drawbacks related to participant burden and data management may be minimized [44]. Advancements in voice-recognition software will eliminate the need for writing altogether, increasing the use of physical activity records in low-literacy populations [45].

Physical Activity Logs

Physical activity logs are checklists used to record the type and duration of activities performed during intermittent periods of the day or at the end of a single day. A good example is the Bouchard Physical Activity Log [39], which has users check the type and intensity of activity that they complete every 15 minutes during a specific period of the day. Another example is the Ainsworth Physical Activity Log that has users review a list of activities at the end of each day and estimate the total duration in hours and/or minutes during which they performed each activity [8]. Physical activity logs can be tailored for specific research or practice settings to reflect the purposes of a study or to highlight specific activities performed. For example, a walking log may focus only on walking activities performed in specific settings, such as occupation, transportation, household, and leisure settings [46]. These logs may also be tailored to monitor physical activity during clinical trials to track the types and amounts of activity performed in supervised and free-living settings.

Physical activity logs have advantages over detailed records in that they substantially reduce the burden of recording for the participants. However, the trade-off comes with the limitation that physical activity logs provide less detailed information about specific activities performed and are subject to recall bias; thus, they may not be as accurate as direct detailed records.

INDIRECT PHYSICAL ACTIVITY ASSESSMENT METHODS

Physical Activity Questionnaires

Physical activity questionnaires are most commonly used to assess physical activity behaviors in epidemiological studies of health-related outcomes and in some clinical and intervention research settings. Ainsworth et al. [6], LaMonte et al. [8], Welk [9], and Kriska et al. [47] provide a good overview of most physical activity questionnaires used in health-related research. Questionnaires can be classified as global, self-administered recall, interview-administered recall, and quantitative history instruments.

Global Questionnaires

Global questionnaires are short instruments that provide a general classification of one's physical activity status as active or inactive. The questionnaires are usually very short and often reflect participation in structured exercise. They provide few details about specific patterns and types of physical activity performed. Several validated questionnaires are available in the public domain with 1-month test–retest reliabilities from r = 0.80 to 0.90 [47]. Validity is on the order of r = 0.30 when compared with cardiorespiratory fitness, activity monitors, and physical activity records [42]. Because global questionnaires are short and easy to construct, many researchers develop global questions designed to meet specific study needs. These questionnaires may or may not be validated and, if not validated, their accuracy in classifying people by physical activity levels is unknown.

Self-Administered Recall Questionnaires

Self-administered recall questionnaires assess the frequency and duration of specific activities for 1 to 2 weeks in the past. The questionnaires may be completed in person, by postal mail, or by e-mail. Examples of two commonly used self-administered questionnaires are the Paffenbarger College Alumni Questionnaire [48] and the International Physical Activity Questionnaire [49]. The former is a postal mail questionnaire that assesses the frequency and duration of walking, stair climbing, and sports and recreational activities performed in the past week. Adjustments are made for the number of weeks per year during which the sports and recreational activities are performed. A summary score (physical activity index) in kilocalories per week is computed from the intensity, frequency in days per week, and duration in hours or minutes per event for each activity recalled. The International Physical Activity Questionnaire assesses the hours per day and days per week spent in various moderate and vigorous intensity activities, walking activities, and sedentary activities. The International Physical Activity Questionnaire has been evaluated in international settings and is available for download in various languages at www.ipaq.ki.se.

Scoring protocols for recall questionnaires vary widely, ranging from simple ordinal scales that reflect participation levels (inactive, insufficiently active, sufficiently active, highly active) to comprehensive scores that reflect the intensity, frequency, and duration of reported activities (MET-minutes, MET-hours, kilocalories). Many studies have assessed the reliability and validity of recall questionnaires; most have 1-month test–retest reliability in cross-sectional settings on the order of r = 0.60 to 0.75 and r = 0.30 for validity against actual measures of energy expenditure, activity monitors, and physical activity records [47].

Limitations in the use of recall questionnaires relate to errors in recall that may result in biased measures of physical activity. For example, Rzewnicki and colleagues [50] noted overreporting of vigorous activities on the International Physical Activity Questionnaire when it was compared with other physical activity assessment methods. This suggests that care be taken in selecting self-administered questionnaires as the primary method of measuring physical activity, especially if the purpose is to assess changes in physical activity in research studies.

Interview-Administered Physical Activity Recall Questionnaires

Interview-administered recall questionnaires provide information about the type, frequency, intensity, and duration of physical activity performed during a brief period in the past, ranging from 24 hours to 7 days. Technically, any self-administered physical activity recall questionnaire can be administered by an interviewer. This is often the case when the study involves low-literacy populations. Interview protocols differ from self-administered physical activity recall questionnaires in that they generally use a series of questions and probes asked by a trained interviewer over the telephone or in person. As a participant answers the interviewer's questions, the information is recorded on a form tailored for the specific setting. The advantage of this interview method is that clarification can be obtained about a person's physical activity and a great deal of detail can be obtained about all elements of the behavior.

Two of the most common interview-administered physical activity recall protocols are the Seven-Day Physical Activity Recall and the Previous Day Physical Activity Recall. The Seven Day Physical Activity Recall is one of the most widely used and validated measures of self-reported physical activity [9], and has undergone several revisions [51,52]. It has been used with adults [53], minorities [54,55], and adolescents [56]. Participants are asked to recall their sleep, and moderate, hard, and very hard physical activities for morning, afternoon, and evening hours in the past 7 days. Activities are then summarized in 10- to 15-minute blocks in weekend, weekday, work, and nonwork categories.

The Previous Day Physical Activity Recall was developed for use with school-aged children [57,58]. Older children can self-administer this recall method, but, for younger children (less than 10 years old), the Previous Day Physical Activity Recall is administered by an interviewer. Physical and sedentary activities are recorded in 30-minute blocks by type and intensity, using a list of activities and illustrations to help children with their self-report.

As with self-administered recall questionnaires, recall interviews of physical activity are affected substantially from recall bias. This is especially problematic with moderate intensity activities that do not seem to make the same impression in participant memories as more intense physical activities [59]. Evidence suggests that activities recalled from the first day in the Seven-Day Physical Activity Recall are not any more accurate than those recalled from the last day in the interview [54]. This is primarily because of the extensive probing and memory cues used in the interview protocol. In addition, no studies using the Seven-Day Physical Activity Recall in the elderly have been published. Although decrements in memory occur with advanced age, the Seven-Day Physical Activity Recall protocol lends itself well to a variety of memory-enhancement exercises [59] that could substantially improve physical activity recall in this group of adults.

Quantitative History Questionnaires

Quantitative history questionnaires assess physical activity for a long period in the past, usually from 1 year to a lifetime, and assess the frequency and duration of multiple types of physical activity. The questionnaires may be age or activity specific [60–63] and may be used to assess physical activity behaviors associated with specific outcomes such as cancer [64] or cardiovascular disease [65].

A well-known quantitative history questionnaire is the Minnesota Leisure-Time Physical Activity Questionnaire used in the Multiple Risk Factor Intervention Trial [66] and in various other settings [47]. The Minnesota Leisure Time Physical Activity Questionnaire is an interviewer-administered questionnaire that has respondents check one of 74 activities performed within the past year. For each activity checked, respondents indicate the number of months per year, times per month, and average hours and minutes during which they were active.

To date, only one quantitative history questionnaire has proven effective in demonstrating physical activity changes in response to behavior change interventions [63]: the Community Healthy Activities Model Program for Seniors (CHAMPS) questionnaire. This questionnaire was developed to assess changes in the weekly frequency and duration of various physical activities performed by older men and women. The questionnaire has adequate validity and reliability and is stable in measuring physical activity over a 6-month period [63].

Quantitative history recall questionnaires are limited by the difficulty in validating the questionnaires because it is often impossible to obtain objective measures of physical activity from long periods in the past, especially for instruments that assess lifetime physical activity. Reliability is generally acceptable [47,64]. Lifetime questionnaires have the greatest utility in the study of the impact of physical activity on diseases that have a long latency period between the exposure and outcomes, such as cancer and osteoporosis.

Qualitative Physical Activity Assessment

Despite advancements in the quantitative assessment of physical activity, researchers still do not understand why some adults engage in physical activity and others do not. Physical activity researchers have also had great difficulty to date creating culturally appropriate and age- and gender-specific instruments. Part of the reason for this is that they are not engaging in systematic instrument development with populations who are consistently identified as physically inactive [5]. Instead, researchers often use whatever seems to have the highest published validity, reliability, and ease of use and then "adapt" it for use with the studied populations. This may be ineffective when they are trying to identify physical activity patterns of distinct population groups [67].

Qualitative data collection methods are particularly suited to the study of physical activity behaviors in understudied populations. Focus groups and ethnographic interviews are two of many qualitative data collection methods. Focus groups have their foundations in business market research and are conducted in groups of eight to ten participants purposely selected from the target population to come together and discuss a particular topic area [68]. A group moderator guides participants through a brief script of approximately three to five questions about a particular topic, with probes used to better understand the responses. Traditionally, the focus groups are audio-recorded (sometimes also videotaped) and then the audiotapes are transcribed verbatim for later analysis. Several studies have used this approach to explore physical activity in a variety of ethnic groups [5,69] and then used the information to develop quantitative surveys to measure physical activity [70].

The best self-report tool that currently exists for exploring the determinants of physical activity in a culturally relevant way is the life-history ethnographic interview [71]. Although developed for cultural anthropology investigations, this procedure has increasingly been applied to the study of health-related behaviors [72,73]. Much of the work in this area has focused on elucidating explanatory models of health and disease in minority cultures [74]. Investigators have applied ethnographic interviewing to the study of ethnic minority women's explanatory models of weight management [72,75] and physical activity [75,76].

WHEN TO USE PHYSICAL ACTIVITY ASSESSMENT METHODS

Many methods to assess physical activity in research and practice settings have been presented. The methods vary in complexity and the amount of information given. The use of a specific instrument should reflect the needs for the research or practice setting. For population studies and national surveillance systems, global or short-recall questionnaires are the preferred method because they are short, easy for respondents to understand, and relatively simple to score. On the other hand, experimental studies are better suited for the use of activity monitors, physical activity records and logs, and/or observation systems to assess physical activity because they provide a higher level of precision needed to quantify the effects of the intervention in modifying physical activity behaviors. Using a combination of questionnaires and direct methods to assess physical activity will substantially increase the amount of information obtained about a target population's physical activity. Finally, when working with a new population, it is best to begin with qualitative data collection methods to assess physical activity and then proceed to tailored instrument creation, instead of adapting an existing questionnaire for a new population without an understanding of the cultural context for physical activity in that population.

CONCLUSIONS

Numerous methods to assess physical activity provide information about the type, frequency, intensity, and duration of an activity performed. Ideally, direct methods of physical activity assessment should be used instead of indirect methods because they avoid bias associated with poor recall. However, it is not always possible to use direct methods based on the setting and study design. When questionnaires are used to assess physical activity, care should be taken to use instruments with the highest validity and reliability for the population group to be studied. Furthermore, questionnaires that are effective in detecting changes in physical activity behaviors should be used in pre–post experimental study designs. When possible, combinations of direct and indirect methods should be used to maximize the information obtained about participants' physical activity.

REFERENCES

1. Macera, C.A. et al. Prevalence of physical activity, including lifestyle activities among adults — United States, 2000–2001, *Morb. Mort. Wkly. Rep.*, 52, 764, 2003.
2. Mokdad, A.H. et al. The continuing epidemics of obesity and diabetes in the United States. *JAMA*, 286, 1195, 2001.
3. United States Department of Health and Human Services. *Physical Activity and Health: a Report of the Surgeon General.* Atlanta, GA: U.S. Department of Health and Human Services, Centers for Disease Control and Prevention, National Center for Chronic Disease Prevention and Health Promotion, 1996.
4. Pate, R.R. et al. Physical activity and public health: a recommendation from the Centers for Disease Control and Prevention and the American College of Sports Medicine. *JAMA*, *273*, 402, 1995.
5. Masse, L. et al. Measuring physical activity in minority women: issues and ideas. *J. Women's Health*, 7, 57, 1998.
6. Ainsworth, B.E., Montoye, H.L., and Leon, A.S. Methods of assessing physical activity during leisure and at work, in *Physical Activity, Fitness, and Health: International Proceedings and Consensus Statement*, Bouchard, C., Shephard, R.J., and Stephens, T., Eds., Human Kinetics, Champaign, IL, 1994, chap. 4.
7. LaMonte, M.J. and Ainsworth, B.E. Field assessment of physical activity and energy expenditure, in *Nutritional Assessment of Athletes*, Driskell, J.A. and Wolinsky, I., Eds., CRC Press, Washington, D.C., 2002, chap. 10.
8. LaMonte, M.J., Ainsworth, B.E., and Tudor–Locke, C. Assessment of physical activity and energy expenditure, in *Obesity — Etiology, Assessment, Treatment and Prevention,* Anderson, R.E., Ed., Human Kinetics, Champaign, IL, 2003, chap. 9.
9. Welk, G.J., Ed. *Physical Activity Assessments for Health-Related Research*, Human Kinetics, Champaign, IL, 2002.
10. Tudor–Locke, C. et al. Utility of pedometers for assessing physical activity. *Sports Med.*, 32, 795, 2002.
11. Irwin, M.L. and Ainsworth, B.E. Physical activity interventions following cancer diagnosis: methodological challenges to delivery and assessment. *Cancer Invest.*, 22, 30, 2004.
12. Ainsworth, B.E. et al. Measurement of physical activity in breast cancer research. *Cancer*, 83, 611, 1998.
13. Ainsworth, B.E. and Mahar, M., Eds. Proceedings from the 9th measurement and evaluation symposium of the Measurement and Evaluant Council of the American Association for Active Lifestyles and Fitness. *Res. Q. Exercise Sport*, 71, S1, 2000.
14. Strath, S.J. et al. Simultaneous heart rate-motion sensor technique to estimate energy expenditure. *Med. Sci. Sports Exercise*, 33, 2118, 2001.
15. LaMonte, M.J. and Ainsworth, B.E. Quantifying energy expenditure and physical activity in the context of dose–response. *Med. Sci. Sports Exercise,* 33, S370, 2001.

16. Welk, G.J. Use of accelerometry-based activity monitors to assess physical activity. In *Physical Activity Assessments for Health-Related Research*, Welk, G.J., Ed., Human Kinetics, Champaign, IL, 2002, chap. 8.
17. King, G. et al. Accuracy of the RT3, Tritrac-R3D, Biotrainer-Pro, and Sensewear Armband in measuring the energy cost of treadmill walking and running. *Med. Sci. Sports Exercise,* 36, 1244, 2004.
18. Schneider, P.L., Crouter, S.E., and Bassett, D.R. Pedometer measures of free-living physical activity: comparison of 13 models. *Med. Sci. Sports Exercise* 36, 331, 2004.
19. Crouter, S.E., Albright, C., and Bassett, D.R., Jr. Accuracy of polar S410 heart rate monitor to estimate energy cost of exercise. *Med. Sci. Sports Exercise*, 36, 1433, 2004.
20. Welk, G.J., Almeida J., and Morss, G. Laboratory calibration and validation of the Biotrainer and Actitrac activity monitors. *Med. Sci. Sports Exercise 35*, 1057, 2003.
21. Freedson, P.S., Melanson, E., and Sirard, J. Calibration of the Computer Science and Applications, Inc. accelerometer. *Med. Sci. Sports Exercise*, 20, 777, 1998.
22. Sherman, W.M. et al. Evaluation of a commercial accelerometer (Tritrac-R3 D) to measure energy expenditure during ambulation. *Int. J. Sports Med.* 19, 43–47, 1998.
23. Tudor–Locke, C.E. and Myers, A.M. Methodological considerations for researchers and practitioners using pedometers to measure physical (ambulatory) activity. *Res. Q. Exercise Sport*, 72, 1, 2001.
24. Fruin, M.L., and Rankin, J. W. Validity of a multisensor armband in estimating rest and exercise energy expenditure. *Med. Sci. Sports Exercise,* 36, 1063, 2004.
25. Westerterp, K.R. Physical activity assessment with accelerometers. *Int. J. Obes.*, 23, S45, 1999.
26. McKenzie, T.L. Observational measures of children's physical activity. *J. Sch. Health.* 61, 224, 1991.
27. Faucette, N., McKenzie, T.L., and Sallis, J.F. Self-contained versus team teaching: an analysis of a physical education intervention by classroom teachers. *J. Teach. Phys. Educ.,* 11, 268, 1992.
28. Mukeshi, M. et al. Validation of the Caltrac movement sensor using direct observation in young children. *Ped. Exercise Sci.*, 2, 249, 1990.
29. Welk, G.J., Corbin, C.B., and Dale, D. Measurement issues in the assessment of physical activity in children. *Res. Q. Exercise Sport,* 71, S59, 2000.
30. McKenzie, T.L., Sallis, J.F., and Nader, P.R. SOFIT: system for observing fitness instruction time. *J. Teach. Phys. Educ.,* 11, 195, 1991.
31. McKenzie, T.L. et al. Leisure-time physical activity in school environments: an observational study using SOPLAY. *Prev. Med.*, 30, 70, 2000.
32. Puhl, J., Greaves, K., Hoyt, M., and Baranowski, T. Children's Activity Rating Scale (CARS): description and calibration. *Res. Q. Exercise Sport,* 61, 26, 1990.
33. DuRant, R.H. et al. Evaluation of the Children's Activity Rating Scale (CARS) in young children. *Med. Sci. Sports Exercise,* 25, 1415, 1991.
34. Pope, R.P. et al. Validity of a revised system for observing fitness instruction time (SOFIT). *Ped. Exercise Sci.,* 14, 135, 2002.
35. Sleap, M. and Warburton, P. Physical activity levels of 5- to 11-year-old children in England: cumulative evidence from three direct observation studies. *Int. J. Sports Med.,* 17, 248, 1996.
38. Ainsworth, B.E. et al. Moderate physical activity patterns among minority women: the Cross-Cultural Activity Participation Study. *J. Women's Health*, 8, 805, 1999.
39. Bouchard, C. et al. A method to assess energy expenditure in children and adults, *Am. J. Clin. Nutr., 37,* 461, 1983.
40. Levin, S. et al. Intraindividual variation and estimates of usual physical activity. *Ann. Epidemiol.*, 9, 481, 1999.
41. Whitt, M.C. et al. Walking patterns in a sample of African American, Native American and Caucasian women: the Cross-Cultural Activity Participation Study. *Health Educ. Behav.*, 31, 45S, 2004.
42. Jacobs, D.R., Jr. et al. A simultaneous evaluation of ten commonly used physical activity questionnaires. *Med. Sci. Sports Exercise,* 25, 81, 1993.
43. Irwin, M.L., Ainsworth, B.E., and Conway JM. Determinants associated with over- and underestimation of physical activity in adult men. *Obes. Res.*, 9, 517, 2001.
44. Healey, J. Future possibilities in electronic monitoring of physical activity. *Res. Q. Exercise Sport*, 71, 137, 2000.
45. White, D.J., King, A.P., and Duncan, S.D. Voice recognition technology as a tool for behavioral research. *Behav. Res. Methods Instrum. Comput.,* 34, 1, 2002.

46. Coleman, K.J. et al. Providing sedentary adults with choices for meeting their exercise goals. *Prev. Med.,* 28, 510, 1999.
47. Kriska, A.M. et al. A collection of physical activity questionnaires for health-related research. *Med. Sci. Sports Exercise*, 29, S1, 1997.
48. Paffenbarger, R.S., Jr., Wing, A.L., and Hyde, R.T. Physical activity as an index of heart attack risk in college alumni. *Am. J. Epidemiol.*, 108, 161, 1978.
49. Craig, C.L., et al. International physical activity questionnaire: 12-country reliability and validity. *Med. Sci. Sports Exercise* 35, 1381, 2003.
50. Rzewnicki, R., Vanden Auweele, Y., and De Bourdeaudhuij, I. Addressing overreporting on the International Physical Activity Questionnaire (IPAQ) telephone survey with a population sample. *Pub. Health Nutr.*, 6, 299, 2003.
51. Blair, S.N. et al. Assessment of habitual physical activity by a seven-day recall in a community survey and controlled experiments. *Am. J. Epidemiol.,* 122, 794, 1985.
52. Gross, L.D. et al. Reliability of interviewers using the Seven-Day Physical Activity Recall. *Res. Q. Exercise Sport*, 61, 321, 1990.
53. Miller, D.J., Freedson, P.S., and Kline, G.M. Comparison of activity levels using the Caltrac accelerometer and five questionnaires. *Med. Sci. Sports Exercise*, 26, 376, 1994.
54. Hayden, H.A. et al. Evaluation of the telephone version of the seven-day physical activity recall. *Med. Sci. Sports Exercise*, 35, 801, 2003.
55. Rauh, M.J.D. et al. The reliability and validity of self-reported physical activity in an adult Latino sample. *Int. J. Epidemiol.,* 21, 966, 1992.
56. Sallis, J.F. et al. Seven-day recall and other physical activity self-reports in children and adolescents. *Med. Sci. Sport Exercise,* 25, 99, 1993.
57. Trost, S.G. et al. Validity of the Previous Day Physical Activity Recall (PDPAR) in fifth-grade children. *Ped. Exercise Sci.*, 11, 341, 1999.
58. Weston, A.T., Petosa, R., and Pate, R.R. Validation of an instrument for measurement of physical activity in youth. *Med. Sci. Sport Exercise*, 29, 138, 1997.
59. Durante, R. and Ainsworth, B.E. The recall of physical activity: using a cognitive model of the question-answering process. *Med. Sci. Sports Exercise,* 28, 1282, 1996.
60. Aaron, D.J. et al. Reproducibility and validity of an epidemiologic questionnaire to assess past year physical activity in adolescents. *Am. J. Epidemiol.,* 142, 191, 1995.
61. Ainsworth, B.E. et al. Evaluation of occupational activity surveys. *J. Clin. Epidemiol,* 9, 219, 1999.
62. Kriska, A.M. et al. The assessment of historical physical activity and its relation to adult bone parameters. *Am. J. Epidemiol.,* 127, 1053, 1988.
63. Stewart, A.L. et al. CHAMPS physical activity questionnaire for older adults: outcomes for interventions. *Med. Sci. Sports Exercise*, 33, 1126, 2001.
64. Friedenreich, C.M., Courneya, KS, and Bryant, H.E. The lifetime total physical activity questionnaire: development and reliability. *Med. Sci. Sports Exercise*, 30, 266, 1998.
65. Leon, A.S. et al. Leisure-time physical activity levels and risk of coronary heart disease and death. The Multiple Risk Factor Intervention Trial. *J. Am. Med. Assoc.* 6, 2388, 1987.
66. Taylor, H.L. et al. A questionnaire for the assessment of leisure time physical activities. *J. Chronic Dis.,* 31, 741, 1978.
67. Ainsworth, B.E. Issues in the assessment of physical activity in women. *Res. Q. Exercise Sport*, 71, S3, 2000. Errata sheet, *Res. Q. Exercise Sport,* 3, 1, 2000.
68. Krueger, R.A. and Casey, M.A. *Focus Groups: a Practical Guide for Applied Research.* 3rd ed. Sage Publications, Inc., New York, 2000.
69. Eyler, A.A. et al. Environmental, policy, and cultural factors related to physical activity in a diverse sample of women: The Women's Cardiovascular Health Network Project — summary and discussion. *Women's Health*, 36, 123, 2002.
70. Eyler, A.A. et al. Quantitative study of correlates of physical activity in women from diverse racial/ethnic groups: The Women's Cardiovascular Health Network Project — summary and conclusions. *Am. J. Prev. Med.*, 25, S93, 2003.
71. Goldman, R. et al. The life history interview method: applications to intervention development. *Health Ed. Behav.,* 30, 564, 2003.

72. Allan, J.D. Explanatory models of overweight among African American, Euro-American, and Mexican American women. *West. J. Nurs. Res.,* 20, 45, 1998.
73. McSweeney, J.C., Allan J.D., and Mayo, K. Exploring the use of explanatory models in nursing research and practice. *Image J. Nurs. Scholarship,* 29, 243, 1997.
74. Kleinman, A. *Patients and Healers in the Context of Culture: an Exploration of the Borderland between Anthropology, Medicine, and Psychiatry.* University of California Press, Berkeley, CA, 1980.
75. Coleman, K.J., Gonzalez, E.C., and Garcia, C.P. Modifying the physical activity recall interview to characterize the daily activities of Hispanic and Anglo women. *Meas. Phys. Educ. Exercise Sci.,* 4, 186, 2000.
76. Henderson, K.A. and Ainsworth, B.E. Perceptions of physical activity among older African American and Native American women. *Am. J. Public Health,* 93, 313, 2003.

3 Measurement of Body Fat and Energy Balance

Melinda Irwin

CONTENTS

INTRODUCTION

Obesity is an established risk factor for cancer and other chronic health problems such as cardiovascular disease and type-2 diabetes [1–3]. The prevalence of obesity is increasing among youths and adults in developed [4] and developing [5] countries. Presently, there is no precise clinical definition of obesity based on actual measures of body fat because of the difficulty of collecting such data. Consensus exists for an indirect measure of body fat, called body mass index (BMI). BMI is easily obtained and reliable for overweight and obese persons, and several studies [6,7] have shown that BMI is highly correlated with percent body fat.

In 1997, the World Health Organization developed a classification system for overweight and obesity based on grades of BMI values related to increasing risk of comorbidity. A BMI of between 25 and 29 was defined as overweight and a BMI of ≥ 30 was defined as obesity [8]. Recent estimates indicate that 34% of the adult American population is overweight and that 31% are obese [9].

The increasing prevalence of overweight and obesity among adults and children in the United States and around the world [10] has highlighted the need for accurate and reliable methods to assess body fat levels. An accurate assessment of body fat is necessary to identify properly a patient's health risk associated with an excessively low or high relative body fat. This assessment can then be used to estimate a patient's ideal body weight and develop an exercise and diet program. Periodic body fat measurements can be used to assess the effectiveness of exercise and diet interventions or monitor changes in body fat associated with growth or disease states. Thus, accurate and precise assessment methods that are sensitive enough to track small changes in body fat are essential for assessing the effects of intervention programs designed to decrease body fat.

Within the last decade, the accuracy and availability of body fat methodology has improved. Because body fat has been linked to numerous health conditions, there is a clinical need to measure percent body fat and fat distribution as well. Whatever the reason for assessing body fat, health educators, exercise physiologists, nutritionists, and other clinicians should have a general understanding of the most commonly used techniques for assessing body fat. A variety of methods are available to assess body fat, some direct and some less direct. Direct methods — also referred to in this chapter as laboratory-based methods — are used primarily in clinical research centers where accurate and precise measurements are essential. Methods such as densitometry, dual energy x-ray absorptiometry (DEXA), computed tomography (CT), magnetic resonance imaging (MRI), and ultrasound are examples of direct methods.

Indirect methods, also referred to in this chapter as field-based methods, provide estimates of body fat. These methods are based on assumptions regarding the density of fat mass and fat-free mass and the concentrations of water and electrolytes in the body. The accuracy and precision of indirect methods depend on their validation against results from direct methods. The adaptability and ease of use with large groups makes indirect methods applicable in epidemiological studies and in public health and obesity screening programs. Body weight, BMI, circumferences, skinfolds, and bioelectrical impedance (BIA) are examples of indirect methods.

The definition of laboratory or field methods can be somewhat arbitrary, but it is usually bound by the available resources, type and quality of information sought, and location of the study. Some other factors that should be considered when defining an ideal body fat method are: cost, training of operator, maintenance and operating costs, precision, and accuracy. If only weight and height are of interest, for example, these data can be obtained using only a scale and tape measure, and the sophisticated technologies described in the following sections are not needed. However, if the objective is to determine the body's fat mass or its internal (e.g., visceral, intramuscular) component, the more robust methods must be used.

The purpose of this chapter is to provide a brief overview of selected body fat methods that are most likely to be used in the lab or field for assessing body fat in large-scale epidemiological, clinical, or anthropometrical studies, examine their validity and reliability, and discuss the strengths and limitations of each method. The chapter is subdivided into laboratory methods and field methods. Several advanced methods, such as neutron activation, gamma resonance absorption, or whole-body potassium counting will not be presented here because they are not routinely used in human body fat studies [11]. Information beyond that presented in this chapter can be found in textbooks [12] and other peer-reviewed manuscripts [13,14].

LABORATORY METHODS

The most common laboratory methods for body fat assessment involve densitometry and imaging methods. These methods cannot be considered field methods for body fat analysis because of the high initial capital investment, the need for a highly trained technical staff, and the high annual maintenance and service costs. However, many scientists consider these methods the gold standards for precision and accuracy for body fat measurements.

Densitometry

The classical method of assessing body fat in vivo is densitometry. This method assumes that the body consists of two compartments, the fat mass (FM) and the fat free mass (FFM), so that weight = fat mass + fat free mass, each with its own specific and assumed constant density: 0.9007 g/cm^3 and 1.1000 g/cm^3, respectively. Determining the density of the body allows a calculation of the ratio of fat mass to fat free mass (the lower the density is, the more body fat a subject has); when body weight is known, the absolute and relative amounts of fat mass and fat free mass can be calculated. Density is weight divided by volume, and the methods that are now used to determine body volume are hydrodensitometry (also called underwater weighing, UWW) and air displacement plethysmography. Underwater weighing and air displacement plethysmography are strictly bound to a laboratory setting because the instruments are not portable.

Hydrodensitometry (Underwater Weighing)

Hydrodensitometry or underwater weighing was developed mainly as a means to measure body density to assess body fat. Because of its early development and widespread use, the measurement of body density, via underwater weighing, is often referred to as a gold standard for body fat measurements. Underwater weighing is based on Archimedes' principle: a body immersed in a fluid is buoyed by a force equal to the weight of the displaced fluid; thus, if a person's weight is measured in air and then when completely immersed in water, density can be calculated: density (g/cm^3) = weight (g)/volume (cm^3) = weight of body in air (g)/weight of body in air (g) – weight of body in water (g). Thus, underwater weighing, as the name implies, requires the subject to be completely submerged in water [15]. Additionally, the subject needs to remain relatively motionless underwater in order for a trained technician to get an accurate reading of the subject's underwater weight.

This procedure must be repeated multiple times for a valid and reliable reading. Generally, it is repeated until three trials within 100 g of each other are obtained. The average of these three trials is used as the underwater weighing for the calculation of body density [16]. Further adjustments are needed for water density, which depends on water temperature, and the volume of air in the respiratory system when the underwater weight is measured. This latter volume is normally the ventilated residual volume. The body density formula [17] is: body density = [(weight in air – weight in water)/water density] – residual volume. Body density is then converted to percent body fat using regression equations developed by Siri [18] or Brozek et al. [19]. For example, using Brozek's equation, if body weight (kg) is equal to unity with the two compartments represented as proportions such that fat mass – fat free mass = 1, then: 1/bone density = fat mass/fat mass density + fat free mass/fat free mass density. Using densities of 0.9007 [20] and 1.100 g/cm^3 [21] for fat mass and fat free mass, respectively, it can be shown that: % fat mass = [4.57/bone density] – 4.142 × 100. Body fat as a percentage of body weight calculated from the Siri equation is: % fat = [4.95/bone density– 4.50] × 100. The Siri and Brozek equations produce values within 1% body fat of each other.

For the residual volume correction, the recommended method is oxygen dilution with a closed-circuit spirometer system [22]. However, residual volume is not routinely performed but instead approximated using prediction equations. Unfortunately, predicted residual volume can result in residual volume variations that affect the estimation of percent body fat by as much as 8% [23]. Therefore, residual volume should not be predicted from age, height, body weight, or vital capacity. By comparison, errors associated with incorrect underwater weights and body weight fluctuations due to factors affecting hydration status are not as large, with a 2- to 3-kg weight fluctuation producing a change in relative body fat of only 1% [24]. Regarding the total cumulative error for percent body fat, it has been estimated to be on the order of 3 to 4% of body weight for the individual [25].

A major potential source of measurement error for this method is the formula used to convert body density to body fat. For years, the classic two-component models of Siri and Brozek have been the basis of underwater weighing estimates of % body fat. Both conversion formulas were based on direct analysis of a limited number of white male and female cadavers that did not necessarily represent the entire population. The Siri and Brozek conversion formulas assume that the density of fat mass and fat free mass density are constant for all individuals. Research documents that fat free mass density is not constant for all individuals, but rather varies with age, gender, body fatness, physical activity, and race/ethnicity [26]. Fat free mass changes from birth onward and the density of the fat free mass is thus likely not "constant" across the lifespan. Because of these limitations, underwater weighing cannot be considered a gold standard method. However, regarding precision, Ward et al. [27] reported good test–retest reliability ($r = 0.99$).

Underwater weighing has many flaws and may not be a practical technique for many subjects. Because subjects are required to exhale completely while submerged, this difficult maneuver requires a great deal of cooperation by the subject and the overall measurement period is quite time consuming (e.g., ~10 trials for a total of ~30 min). Another limitation of underwater weighing is that it is difficult for an overweight or obese person to submerge. Underwater weighing also may not be easy to undertake with elderly or physically disabled persons or individuals with diseases. Furthermore, to ensure an accurate measure of body volume from underwater weighing, residual volume requires a skilled technician and is difficult, and sometimes impossible, for some subjects to perform. Lastly, the underwater weighing instrumentation is priced moderately and requires high maintenance and a well-trained operator. These limitations have shown that this method is not suited for laboratory-based body fat methods.

Air Displacement Plethysmography

The overall density of the human body may be measured using water displacement, i.e., underwater weighing, or air displacement. For years, UWW has been considered by some experts as a gold standard method. However, because of the limitations noted earlier, a new technique for measuring body density and, in turn, body fat has been developed has the potential to become a field method. The instrument used is the Bod Pod® (Life Measurement Instruments, Inc., Concord, CA). The Bod Pod is a large, egg-shaped fiberglass chamber. This method is based on air displacement plethysmography (ADP) and uses the relationship between pressure and volume to derive body volume. The physical design and the operating principles of air displacement plethysmography have been described in detail elsewhere [28].

The instrument [28] consists of two chambers; the subject sits in one chamber and the other serves as a reference. With the subject in one chamber, the door is closed and sealed, the pressure increased slightly, and a diaphragm, separating the two chambers, is oscillated to alter the volumes slightly. The classic relationship of pressure vs. volume at a fixed temperature is used to solve for the volume of the subject chamber. The volumes of the two chambers are varied slightly and the difference in air pressure is recorded. The subject's body volume is calculated using corrections for isothermal properties of the air in the lungs and near the skin's surface.

From the subject's perspective, the procedures are quite simple. Wearing minimal clothing (e.g., a bathing suit) so as not to alter body surface area calculations, swim cap (to minimize isothermal air trapped within the hair), and nose clip, the subject enters and sits in the fiberglass chamber for two trials of approximately 45 sec each. The Bod Pod is sealed, and the subject breathes normally for 20 sec while body volume is measured. The subject is then connected to a breathing tube that is connected to the reference chamber in the rear of the Bod Pod to measure thoracic gas volume. The subject resumes tidal breathing through the tube. After three breathing cycles, a valve in the circuit momentarily occludes the airway. At this point, the subject gently "puffs" by alternately contracting and relaxing the diaphragm. This effort produces small pressure fluctuations in the airway and chamber that are used to determine thoracic gas volume. This value is used to correct body volume for thoracic gas volume. The body volume is equal to the volume of air in an empty chamber minus the volume of air remaining in the chamber after the subject enters it. The percent body fat is then calculated using the Siri equation [18].

Studies using air displacement plethysmography have shown very good agreement with the underwater weighing method in healthy adults and children [29,30]. This may prove to be a more valid and reliable method than underwater weighing, especially for older adults, physically challenged individuals, and those afraid of being submerged underwater. Air displacement plethysmography has been reported to be a highly reliable method for determining percent body fat in adult humans [31]. Although not significantly different, the same-day test–retest reliability of the air displacement plethysmography was slightly better than it was for underwater weighing, with the average coefficients of variation being 1.7 and 2.3% for air displacement plethysmography and underwater weighing, respectively. The mean difference in percent body fat between the two methods was only 0.3% ($r = 0.96$, SEE = 1.81%). However, at the individual level differences were quite large, with 95% confidence intervals ranging from –9% to +7% body fat [32].

Air displacement plethysmography is a quicker, more convenient, and an easier test to administer than underwater weighing (i.e., less technical expertise required); therefore, it has the potential to reduce technician error. The air displacement plehtysmography method involves little effort on the part of the subject, thereby reducing within-subject error. Another advantage is that the subject does not need to be submerged under water, although he or she still needs to wear a swimsuit and cap. Another advantage is that the measurement time is only a few minutes.

Disadvantages or limitations of air displacement plethysmography are that the devices of this method are limited to persons who are "moderately" obese at best — i.e., someone with a BMI > 30 may be difficult to assess. Another major drawback of air displacement plethysmography is the high cost of the instrument [33]. The same assumptions for converting body density to percent body fat that limit underwater weihing also exist for air displacement plethysmography. Thus, even if all the technical limitations can be corrected, the question of the physiological accuracy of using a common fat free mass density among individuals still remains. The assumption of a fixed density will produce a larger error of fat free mass than the cumulative technical errors associated with the density measurement. Thus, without additional knowledge of the density of the fat free mass, underwater weighing and air displacement plethysmography techniques may best serve to identify outliers in a population.

Imaging Techniques

Three major techniques are used for imaging of the body: dual energy x-ray absorptiometry (DEXA), computed tomography (CT), and magnetic resonance imaging (MRI). Many scientists consider these methods the standards for precision and accuracy for body fat measurements [34,35]. Furthermore, DEXA, CT, and MRI provide the only presently fully accepted approach for measuring body fat distribution [36]. However, a significant advantage of CT and MRI is the ability to assess not only abdominal body fat, but also the important visceral adipose tissue compartment and intramuscular fat — information that is presently not available with any other body fat methods. Recently, ultrasound has been used as a technique for assessing body fat, specifically visceral adipose tissue.

DEXA

DEXA is a relatively new technique developed in the 1980s mainly to diagnose osteoporosis. When DEXA is applied, a subject, lying supine on a padded table, is scanned (two-dimensionally) from head to toe with x-rays of two energy levels [37]. Based on the different attenuation coefficients of minerals and soft tissue on the one hand, and of soft tissue between lean mass and fat mass on the other, the composition of the body can be calculated in terms of bone mineral, lean tissue, and fat tissue. Fat mass, as well as bone mineral content and lean tissue mass, is derived according to computer algorithms provided by the manufacturer [38]. Most important, the attenuation of soft tissue can now be measured rather than assumed, as is the case with underwater weighing and air displacement plethysmography. The average skin dose of radiation is 1 to 3 mrad per DEXA scan [39], which is comparable to the skin exposure from a week of environmental background radiation (about 3.5 mrad/week) [40].

At present, three manufacturers provide DEXA devices measuring body fat: Hologic Inc. (Waltham, MA), Lunar Radiation Corp (Madison, WI), and Norland Medical Systems (Fort Atkinson, WI). The DEXA instruments from different manufacturers are unique in implementation but based on the same theoretical principles. DEXA devices are composed principally of a generator emitting x-rays of two energies, a scanning table, a detector, and a computer system. The fundamental physical principle behind DEXA is presented in a review by Genton et al. [41]. Percent body fat has been shown to vary among manufacturers [42], the data collection mode (pencil beam vs. array beam), and the software version used to analyze the data [43].

Only the DEXA manufacturers have developed standard software that can measure body fat. Furthermore, the physical limitations of weight, length, thickness, and width also vary with each manufacturer and type of DEXA machine. For example, weight limitations are 100 and 136 kg for current Lunar and Hologic machines, respectively, and appropriate for a person of average height (178 cm) and a maximum BMI of between 31 and 43. However, these manufacturers have a body width restriction of about 60 to 66 cm, and Lunar has a body thickness limit of 26 cm. These limits are a function of the available table scan area of the machines. Thus, bodies of many obese individuals are too wide or thick to receive a whole-body DEXA scan with current machines, although some innovative adaptations, such as scanning an obese person twice, have been proposed [44].

Although DEXA was originally used to measure bone density and total body fat, recent improvements in software allow it to determine abdominal fat mass. Glickman et al. [45] examined the validity and reliability of DEXA to measure abdominal fat accurately in 65 men and women aged 18 to 72 using a Lunar DPX-IQ scanner. Multislice CT scans were performed between L1 and L4 vertebral bodies. Abdominal total tissue mass (7.07 ± 1.96 kg vs. 7.48 ± 1.87 kg, $p = 0.02$) and abdominal fat mass (2.22 ± 1.63 kg vs. 2.99 ± 1.99 kg, $p < .0001$) were significantly lower as measured by DEXA compared to CT. However, Bland–Altman analysis demonstrated good concordance between DEXA and CT for abdominal total tissue mass (i.e., limits of agreement = –1.56 to 2.54 kg) and fat mass (i.e., limits of agreement = –0.40 to 1.94 kg). DXA also showed excellent reliability ($R = 0.94$ and 0.97 for total abdominal and abdominal fat mass).

Although DEXA was found to be reliable and reproducible in the estimation of abdominal adipose tissue, it does not allow the visual distinction between visceral and subcutaneous fat tissue. However, combining DEXA and waist circumference data accounted for 84% of the variance in CT-derived visceral adipose tissue (VAT), providing researchers with a method to estimate VAT using DEXA. The equation to predict VAT is: VAT (g) = DEXA L1–L4 fat mass (0.31) + WC (7.03).

DEXA is highly reliable, with repeated measurements over 1 day in the same subject demonstrating CVs of about 0.8% for fat [46]. Mazess et al. [47] reported excellent short-term precision for DEXA. Ten measurements each on 12 subjects were conducted over a period of 1 week. The authors reported a precision error for fat mass equal to 1.4%. The short- and long-term precision of DEXA was assessed by Johnson and Dawson–Hughes [48]. They scanned subjects six times initially and then again 9 months later. The CV for fat mass was 2.7% at the start of the study and 1.7% after 9 months.

Many studies have now examined DEXA accuracy in animals and humans. DEXA fat estimates in species ranging widely in body size are highly correlated with corresponding criterion estimates, such as chemical analysis of cadavers. Good agreement is also present between percent body fat estimates obtained by underwater weighing and DEXA [49]. In studies that compared underwater weighing to DEXA, investigators have found DEXA to be a better predictor of mean percent body fat than underwater weighing [50]. DEXA may have the greatest sensitivity to changes in body fat with exercise. In a study by Houtkooper et al. [51] in which postmenopausal women (n = 76) were exercise-trained, SDs for changes in body fat were the smallest for DEXA estimates. Consequently, the estimates of percent body fat from DEXA had the smallest variability and therefore, when compared with results from underwater weighing, were the most sensitive measures for detecting small changes in body fat in this sample of women.

The DEXA model is an important advance in body fat methodology. DEXA is an attractive alternative to underwater weighing and air displacement plethysmography as a reference method because it is a safe, noninvasive method that involves only a small radiation dose and is accurate and precise [52]. DEXA is rapid (most scans are completed in 10 min), requires minimal subject cooperation, and, most importantly, accounts for individual variability in fat free mass. It is also less affected by and therefore less prone to the errors associated with the underlying assumptions inherent in UWW and ADP. DEXA evaluations are relatively inexpensive to carry out. The greatest advantage of DEXA over other laboratory methods may be the ability to assess regional as well as total body fat and analyze separate compartments of the body.

Because DEXA does not rely on the assumption of a two-component model (i.e., fat mass and fat free mass) to provide estimates of body fat and does not depend on subject performance, it is sometimes regarded as a standard against which other methods can be validated. However, like most other methods for measuring body fat, DEXA is also subject to errors [53]. Limitations of DEXA are the high initial capital investment, the need for a highly trained technical staff, and the high annual maintenance and service costs. Also, tissue depth has an impact on the total attenuation of the body, so the method has different accuracy in obese persons compared with lean persons [54]. In summary, owing to its nature, the method is not suitable for most field studies. Nevertheless, DEXA is a safe, quick, accurate, and reliable method for measuring body fat in the majority of the population.

Computed Tomography (CT)

CT has been considered the most accurate and reproducible technique of body fat measurement [55], particularly abdominal adipose tissue. Since 1990, CT has been proposed as the gold standard method to quantify abdominal obesity [55]. Despres and Lamarche [56] observed that a visceral fat area of 130 cm^2 was associated with a high risk of cardiovascular events in 213 men and 190 women. More recently, a visceral adipose tissue $\geq$ 106 cm^2 was associated with an elevated risk [57] in 233 persons.

The use of CT and MRI (see later section) allows for three-dimensional information of body fat. In contrast to DEXA, the information is obtained on a tissue level, rather than a chemical level, so adipose tissue rather than chemical body fat is determined. For comparison, adipose tissue can be converted to body fat assuming that 80% of adipose tissue is fat. CT and MRI can be used to get information on total body fat; however, because of the radiation and/or price of measurements, they are usually used to obtain information on body fat distribution (employing single scans at the L4–L5 level).

From the subject's perspective, CT is quite simple. The subject lies on a padded table for scanning. One scan is usually performed using a lateral-view radiograph of the skeleton (abdominal area) to establish the position of the L4–L5 space within 1.0 mm. A second scan is then performed at the L4–L5 space (at 125 kV and with a slice thickness of 8 mm). Ideally, following the scanning, one technician then measures the subcutaneous and intra-abdominal fat areas using a commercial software application (e.g., Slice-O-Matic from Tomovision, Montreal, Quebec, Canada) that identifies and measures each of the areas of interest by tracing lines around them and computing the circumscribed areas.

Although available for nearly 30 years, CT was only minimally applied in body fat research because of expense and radiation exposure [58]. The importance of CT is that the method produces cross-sectional images of tissue-system level components at predefined anatomic locations, via a rotating x-ray tube and detector, which moves in a perpendicular plane to the subject. The CT x-rays are attenuated as they penetrate tissues and Fourier analysis or filtered back-projection is used in reconstructing the image. Image analysis software then allows estimation of the adipose tissue, skeletal muscle, and other tissue-system level component pixels. Pixels, or "picture elements," translate to respective tissue areas. The CT number assigned to each pixel is a measure of photon attenuation relative to air and water [59]. Air, adipose tissue, nonadipose lean tissues, and skeleton pixels all have characteristic CT number ranges. Acquiring images at predefined intervals and then integrating tissue component areas permits reconstruction of whole-body components such as skeletal muscle mass [60].

CT can now quantify the mass of all major organs and tissues. The CT images can also be used to separate the total adipose tissue mass into its subcutaneous and visceral components, or the lean tissues into skeletal muscle and visceral or organ mass.

Reconstruction of total body mass and separate organ masses based on scans along the length of the body at 10-cm intervals has been shown to have excellent accuracy (<1% error) and precision (<1%) [61]. It has also been shown that CT provides a more accurate determination of visceral adipose tissue than MRI does (see next section) [62]. Extensive validation studies for CT include human and animal cadavers. Rossner et al. [63] compared adipose tissue estimates by CT with corresponding planimetry measurements of corresponding band-sawed slices from two male cadavers. Strong correlations were present between the two types of area estimates ($r = 0.77$ to 0.94).

Strengths and limitations of CT are discussed next with those of MRI.

Magnetic Resonance Imaging (MRI)

MRI is based on interaction between nuclei of hydrogen atoms and magnetic fields produced and controlled by the MRI's instrumentation. Protons have a magnetic moment that causes them to function as small magnets. Under usual conditions in the earth's weak magnetic field, these magnetic moments are randomly oriented, and they tend to cancel each other. When a subject is placed inside the scanner's high-field strength magnet proton, magnetic moments tend to align longitudinally to the external magnet's field. A pulsed radio-frequency field is then applied to body tissues, causing some of the aligned hydrogen protons to absorb energy [64]. Several excellent reviews of the practical aspects of the MRI measurement have been presented previously [65,66].

To obtain MRI data, the subject is positioned in the magnet's bore in a prone or supine position. Typically, a 320-mm region of the body is imaged in a single acquisition. The time required to obtain multiple (i.e., seven) images is the same as that required to obtain a single image. Therefore, in most MRI studies, multiple images of a given region are obtained in a single acquisition. Depending on the pulse frequency used, the time needed for an abdominal image can take 8 to 10 min or more, although recent technological advances may have reduced this time to ~30 sec per slice [67]. For a whole-body measurement, a series of multiple scans along the length of the body is needed, which may require the subject to be in the magnet's bore for 30 min or longer.

Cross-sectional abdominal images obtained with MRI allow for separation of the SAT from the visceral adipose tissue compartment. The coefficient of variation for repeated measures of subcutaneous adipose tissue ranges from 1 to 10% [68]. The coefficient of variation for visceral adipose tissue estimates is higher — 6 to 11% — as a result of measurement errors associated with respiratory motion. Human cadaver studies were used by Abate et al. [69] to examine the validity of MRI SAT and visceral adipose tissue estimates. The overall agreement between dissection weight and MRI-estimated adipose tissue weights was 6% or 0.08 kg.

Some consideration should be given to whether to use CT or MRI to characterize the adipose tissue content and distribution in humans. There is generally good agreement between CT- and

MRI-derived measures of regional body fat [70], and both methods are highly reproducible and reliable [71,72]. The lower coefficient of variation of CT compared to MRI is usually ascribed to a shorter image acquisition time, and CT is thus less vulnerable to image artifacts produced by gastrointestinal tract movement [73].

A limitation to CT and MRI is that access to the scanners is limited and cost in most centers is prohibitive. Additionally, the time required for analysis of the images can be substantial. Although the scan times for CT are shorter than for MRI, with MRI there is no ionizing radiation, making the acquisition of multiple images more practical. However, if the pixel resolution required for routine CT scans can be relaxed, the dose can be significantly reduced. Studies have shown that a ten-scan image of the trunk region can be obtained with an effective dose of <0.3 mSv, which is about 1/25 that of a routine clinical CT scan [74]. It would be quite difficult to collect MRI and CT data from many of the obese because they are too large for the opening in the magnet or the scanner. In summary, CT and MRI provide the only presently fully accepted approach for estimating the important visceral adipose tissue compartment [36].

Ultrasound

CT and MRI have been considered the most accurate and reproducible techniques of body fat measurement, particularly abdominal adipose tissue. However, both are costly and time-consuming measures and involve exposure to radiation. Because of these limitations, alternative methods, such as ultrasound, are being used to assess fat distribution and to estimate intra-abdominal fat deposition.

In 1990, Armellini et al. [75] proposed the use of ultrasound for the quantification of visceral adiposity as an alternative technique to CT. Ultrasound allows the individual visualization of subcutaneous and intra-abdominal fat. In addition, ultrasound is a noninvasive and quick method with good reproducibility rates (<1%) and lower costs than CT scans [76]. However, specific equipment and a well-trained examiner are required. Ultrasonography is performed using a high-resolution ultrasonographic system and a 7.5- or 3.5-MHz probe. Subjects are examined in the supine position with all frozen images obtained immediately after respiration to avoid the influence of the respiratory status.

Recently, Ribeiro–Filho et al. [76] compared ultrasound for the assessment of visceral adipose tissue as an alternative to CT and also to establish cut-off values to define visceral adiposity based on ultrasound. The study enrolled 100 women, 20 to 65 years of age. Ultrasound procedures were performed using a 3.5-MHz probe located 1 cm from the umbilicus. Two ultrasound measurements of intra-abdominal and subcutaneous fat were taken. The coefficient of variation for ultrasound was 0.8%. A correlation of $r = 0.71$ ($p < .0001$) was found between CT-determined visceral fat and ultrasound. Total fat (visceral plus subcutaneous) determined by ultrasound correlated with total fat area determined by CT ($r = 0.65$, $p < .001$).

Similar correlations were observed in studies by Kim et al. [77] and Stolk et al. [78]. Visceral obesity by ultrasound showed a diagnostic concordance of 74% with CT. An ultrasound value of 6.90 cm for visceral distance was found as a diagnostic cut-off for visceral obesity. A noninvasive and less expensive method such as ultrasound may facilitate identification of high-risk patients and allow earlier interventions.

FIELD METHODS

A number of methods are available for field purposes. Field methods rely on statistical relationships between easily measurable parameters and a method of reference (e.g., lab-based methods). The validity of these methods is less compared with the laboratory methods, mainly because more assumptions are made on top of those already held for the method of reference. The advantage is that the method is portable and inexpensive, although information on an individual level is not very valid or reliable.

Body Mass Index

Body mass index (BMI), defined as weight/height^2, is the most commonly used field method. For population studies, BMI is generally accepted as a measure of body fatness [79]. Body weight is usually measured to the nearest 0.1 kg using a beam balance and body height is usually measured to the nearest 0.5 cm using a stadiometer.

The World Health Organization cut-off points of BMI for overweight and obesity are based on observational studies of the relationship between BMI and morbidity (in particular, cardiovascular disease and diabetes) and mortality [80]. Because no studies relate directly measured body fat to morbidity and mortality, no clear cut-off points for obesity, based on body fat measurements, are known. Based on the relationship between BMI and percent body fat, one can calculate that, in adults, a BMI value of 30 corresponds to about 25% body fat in males and 35% body fat in females [81]. Because body fat generally increases and fat free mass decreases with increasing age, older subjects will have a higher percent body fat than young subjects of the same BMI [82].

Variations in percent body fat for the same BMI may also be caused by variations in physical activity, fitness, body build, diet, and race or ethnicity [83]. For the same BMI, physically inactive or unfit men and women on average have slightly greater fat mass than physically active or fit men and women [84]. Exercise intervention studies have also demonstrated that, when performed for a sufficient duration, aerobic exercise in the absence of a change in BMI is associated with reductions in total fat mass [85], subcutaneous adipose tissue [86], and visceral adipose tissue [87]. In studies by Irwin et al. [88] and Janssen et al. [89], aerobic exercise training with little or no change in body weight or BMI was associated with significant reductions in total fat mass and visceral adipose tissue fat.

Although the World Health Organization and U.S. Center for Disease Prevention and Control recommend BMI as a measure of percent body fat [90], recent findings have challenged the assumption that BMI has the same meaning in all racial or ethnic groups [91]. A recent meta-analysis of the relationship between BMI and percent body fat among Chinese, Ethiopians, Indonesians, Polynesians, Thais, American blacks, and American whites revealed that people of different ethnic groups had significantly different BMIs at the same levels of body fat, age, and gender [92]. Possible reasons for ethnic differences in the relationship between BMI and percent body fat include differences in fat free mass, the distribution of subcutaneous adipose tissue, and limb length relative to trunk size [93]. These findings suggest that estimates of body fat from BMI may produce systematic errors across different ethnic groups.

The distinct advantages of using BMI to assess body fat are that it is portable, noninvasive, and inexpensive; requires little training and little maintenance and operating costs; and is very precise (if measured). Other advantages of BMI are that it has available extensive national reference data, has established direct relationships with levels of body fat and with morbidity and mortality, and is highly predictive of future risk for overweight and obesity. Weight and BMI are useful in monitoring the treatment of overweight and obesity because they are sensitive to positive progress in response to treatment. Weight is easily monitored and tracked at home. One clear advantage for using BMI in adults is that height remains somewhat constant during most of adulthood, so longitudinal examinations based on BMI reflect mainly changes in weight.

Limitations of BMI are that an increased BMI does not show which body compartment (fat or lean mass) is inadequate and cannot differentiate subcutaneous adipose tissue from visceral adipose tissue. Another limitation is the accuracy of BMI in assessing body fatness for the individual [94]. Measured body weight, height, and BMI are limited in accuracy; however, there is even greater concern related to self-reported estimates of these measures. Studies have shown that women and men, especially obese persons, tend to underreport their body weight and that men tend to overreport height [95,96]. Underreporting weight and overreporting height lead to an underestimate of BMI and body fat. In summary, although BMI has its limitations, it remains a simple measure to obtain and is used widely in large-scale studies, including international studies for long follow-up periods to assess disease risk.

Circumferences

Due to the ease and feasibility of body circumference measurements, they are often used in large-scale epidemiological studies and when more elaborate methods of assessing body fat are unavailable. Circumference measurements involve placing a tape measure around a specific body segment. Using a flexible, plastic-coated tape measure with a spring-loaded handle enables the clinician to reproduce the tension on the end of the tape measure, thereby increasing reliability and precision. An often used tape measure, the Gulick II (Lafayette Instrument Co, Lafayette, IN) has a tension meter attached so that the tape's tension can be standardized during measurement. Several studies found that waist circumference is more closely associated with visceral adipose tissue than is either waist-hip-ratio or BMI [97,98]. In a guide about obesity treatment published by the U.S. National Institutes of Health, waist circumference and BMI were suggested as the most available and reliable means of identifying obesity, establishing the risks related to it, and monitoring its treatment [99].

The U.S. National Institutes of Health guide suggests that the waist circumference measurement be taken just above the iliac crest. However, in the literature, 14 different descriptions of the site for waist circumference measurements exist [100,101]. Overall, these sites can be organized into four groups defined by specific anatomic landmarks:

- Immediately below the lowest ribs
- At the narrowest waist
- At the midpoint between the lowest rib and iliac crest
- Immediately above the iliac crest

The narrowest waist is the most frequently recommended site. However for some subjects, there is no single narrowest point because of a large amount of abdominal fat or extreme thinness.

Wang et al. [102] made comparisons between waist circumference measurements at the four sites with the hope of developing a universally accepted method of measuring waist circumference. The reproducibility of the waist circumference measurements was very high for both sexes in all four sites. The Intra-class correlations (ICCs)were all $r > 0.996$. The four sites had CVs < 1%. An important finding of the study is that waist circumference values measured at any of the four commonly used sites are almost equally associated with total body fat and central fat in each sex.

Men and women with waist circumference values ≤ 102 and ≤ 88 cm, respectively, are considered to have a normal waist circumference, whereas men and women with waist circumference values > 102 and > 88 cm, respectively, are considered to have a high waist circumference [103]. However, Lemieux et al. [104] concluded that a waist circumference cut-off point of 100 cm should be used for subjects aged ≤ 40 years and 90 cm in subjects aged > 40 years for men and women. They based their calculation on the absolute amount of visceral fat measured using a CT scan and the cut-off point of 130 cm^2 as the reference value. The above-mentioned waist cut-off points best corresponded to the specified amount of visceral fat. However, of note is the fact that there are differences between waist circumference indices of visceral fat and the actual amount of visceral fat as measured by CT or MRI are different among different ethnic groups. Albu et al. [105] showed that, for the same amount of fat mass, obese black women had significantly less visceral fat and a lower visceral fat-to-subcutaneous fat ratio for any given waist–hip circumference ratio than white women.

Being meticulous with site location and measurement is critical for accurate and reliable measures. The reproducibility of waist circumference measurements at any site depends on the observer's skill. A potential source of measurement error for all waist circumference sites is incorrectly positioning the tape measure on the subject's body. It is critical that the observer position the tape around the subject's body in a plane that is perpendicular to the long axis of the body. Reproducibility can be increased by giving special attention to positioning the subject, using anatomic landmarks to locate measuring sites, taking readings with the tape measure directly in contact with the subject's skin without compression, and keeping the tape at 90 degrees to the long axis of the body [106].

Given that most members of the population cannot readily calculate their BMI [107] and that this difficulty is compounded by the inaccuracy of self-reported height and weight measurements [95,96], waist circumference is a preferred measure of adiposity. Approximately 20% of adults are classified in the incorrect BMI category on the basis of self-reported height and weight [96]. By comparison, only 2% of men and women are classified in the incorrect waist circumference category (e.g., low, moderate, or high) on the basis of self-measured waist circumference [108].

In summary, strengths of using circumference measures are that they can always be measured regardless of body size or fatness. Waist circumference is strongly correlated with visceral adipose tissue and can easily be interpreted. This makes it a suitable candidate for an optimal indicator of abdominal obesity.

Skinfolds

The third most commonly used field method to assess body fatness is based on skinfold measurements of the subcutaneous fat layer using inexpensive calipers. Skinfold thickness is accepted as a body fatness predictor for two reasons: about 40 to 60% of total body fat is in the subcutaneous adipose tissue region of the body, and skinfold thickness can be directly measured using a well-calibrated caliper. There are more than 19 sites for measuring skinfold thickness. The triceps site has been used more frequently than other sites because it is easy to access, is reproducible, and can measure wide differences among people. The skinfold technique involves pinching the skin with the thumb and forefinger, pulling it away from the body slightly, and placing the calipers on the fold. Thus, skinfold measures the thickness of two layers of skin and the underlying subcutaneous adipose tissue .

To standardize skinfold measurements, guidelines for anatomical location of skinfold sites and measurement technique have been published [109]. Four different calipers have been used: Adipometer, Harpenden, Holtain, and Lange. Lange is the most widely used. The calipers have been calibrated measuring ranges up to 60 mm. Interobserver error is a major issue in measuring skinfolds [110]. Standardized methodology, including positioning of the instrument, a well-trained data collector, and practicing until results are consistent, can increase reproducibility. Special attention to locating the site, grasping the skin, and assuring that the caliper is at a 90 degree angle relative to the grasped skinfold are essential for high reproducibility.

Due to its relative low cost and simplicity, the measurement of skinfold is a popular method of estimating body density; more than 100 skinfold prediction equations have been published. One of the most popular and widely used skinfold equations is that developed by Jackson and Pollock [111]. This generalized equation was developed on a heterogeneous sample of 308 men ranging in age from 18 to 61 years and cross-validated on a similar sample of 95 men. The regression model was developed from the sum of seven skinfold sites (chest, midaxillary, triceps, subscapula, abdomen, suprailium, and thigh, r = 0.90, SEE = 0.0078 g/cc). A high correlation was found between the sum of seven skinfold sites and the sum of three skinfold sites, so another equation using just three skinfold sites (chest, abdomen, and thigh) was developed (r = 0.91, SEE = 0.0077 g/cc). A similar model and generalized equations using the same sum of seven skinfold sites (r = 0.85, SEE = 0.0083 g/cc) and a different set of three skinfold sites (triceps, thigh, and suprailium, r = 0.84, SEE = 0.0086 g/cc) were developed from a heterogeneous sample of 249 women ages 18 to 55 years and cross-validated on a sample of 82 women [112].

Because the skinfold method indirectly measures the thickness of subcutaneous adipose tissue, certain basic relationships are assumed [113]. One is that skinfold is a good measure of subcutaneous adipose tissue. Hayes et al. [114] showed a good relationship between mean fat thickness estimated from 12 skinfold sites and MRI. For men, the correlations between skinfold and MRI ($r = 0.88$) was significant. A second assumption is that the distribution of the fat subcutaneously and internally is similar for all individuals. The validity of this assumption is questionable. Older subjects have less subcutaneous adipose tissue than their younger counterparts. Also, lean individuals have a higher proportion of internal fat, and the proportion of fat located internally decreases as overall body fatness increases [115]. Additionally, race could be a factor, with African Americans storing a greater percentage of total body fat internally compared to whites.

A third assumption for the skinfold method is that a good relationship exists between subcutaneous adipose tissue and total body fat. It is estimated that SAT makes up one third of total fat [116]. However, Lohman noted that subcutaneous adipose tissue can range from 20 to 70% of total body fat depending on such biological factors as age, sex, and degree of fatness. A fourth assumption is that a relationship is present between skinfold sites and body density. This relationship is linear for homogenous samples. A linear regression line will fit the data well only within a narrow range of body fatness values [117].

The precision of the skinfold data has been shown to be highly variable and operator dependent. The accuracy of this method has been questioned when assessing body fat of the individual. The accuracy and precision of skinfold measurements are affected by the technician's skill, type of skinfold caliper, and subject factors [118]. It is difficult, even for highly skilled technicians, to measure the skinfold thickness of obese individuals accurately. Often, the subject's skinfold thickness exceeds the maximum aperture of the caliper, and the jaws of the caliper may slip off the fold during the measurement. Therefore, skinfolds should not be used to measure body fat of obese subjects.

In summary, the skinfold method requires a considerable amount of technical skill, being meticulous with site location and measurement, and restriction to populations from whom the prediction equation was derived. Although it is an excellent field method to use on lean subjects, it is difficult to obtain reliable and accurate readings on older subjects with less connective tissue or obese individuals with large folds. The availability of skinfold calipers capable of larger measurements would not be a significant improvement because of the physical difficulty of picking up a very large skinfold on an obese adult.

Bioelectrical Impedance

The bioelectrical impedance method is widely applied in the field as a means of estimating fat free mass [119], total body water, and total body fat. Bioelectrical impedance is based on the premise that when a low-level electrical current is passed through the body at a fixed frequency (50 kHz) [120], the voltage drop between two electrodes is proportional to the body's fluid volume in that region of the body. This, in turn, is used to estimate fat-free and fat masses. Bioelectrical impedance is based on the principle that lean tissue, which contains large amounts of water and electrolytes, is a good electrical conductor, and that fat, which is anhydrous, is a poor conductor. Therefore, the greater the total body water and fat free mass are, the less resistance to the flow of the electric current occurs.

For healthy adults, the water content of fat free mass is relatively constant: 0.732 per kg [121]. Thus, any measurement technique based on the assay for total body water indirectly provides an estimate for fat free mass. The body's percentage of fat can be defined as % fat = 100 × (weight – fat free mass of total body fat)/wt. The voltage produced between two electrodes is measured with a BIA analyzer. Most bioelectrical impedance systems include body fat software based upon descriptive models. Two commonly used bioelectrical impedance analyzers are the RJL System (Detroit, MI) and Vahalla Scientific (San Diego, CA).

The biolelectrical impedance measurement is a relatively simple procedure. The subject lies supine on a nonconducting surface with arms and legs abducted at an angle of 30 to 45 degrees from the trunk. Source electrodes are placed at the wrist and at the ankle so that a weak alternating current undetectable by the subject can be passed through the body. The voltage drop is measured and the resistance calculated while the current is kept constant. The actual measurement procedure for the subject is relatively easy and can be performed within a few minutes. Resistance is recorded to the nearest ohm and used in prediction equations to estimate total body fat or fat free mass.

A major source of error for the bioelectrical impedance method is intraindividual variability in whole-body resistance due to factors that affect the subject's state of hydration. Taking resistance measures 2 to 4 h after a meal decreases resistance and is likely to overpredict fat free mass by almost 1.5 kg [122]. On the other hand, dehydration increases resistance, resulting in a 5.0-kg underestimate of fat free mass [123]. The accuracy and precision of the bioelectrical impedance measurements are also affected by instrumentation, technician skill, subject factors, and environmental factors [124]. Thus, the accuracy of bioelectrical impedance results and their interpretation should be used with caution [125]. Another concern with bioelectrical impedance is that it is an indirect method and must be calibrated with a reference assay. The number of bioelectrical impedance calibration equations that have been developed is approaching the level observed for the skinfold method.

In a review, Kushner [126] reported the mean CV of multiple resistance measurements taken on the same subject in the same day ranges from 0.3 to 2.8%. When measured over days or weeks, intraindividual variability ranged from 0.8 to 3.6%. Kushner and Schoeller [127] reported intraindividual variations in bioelectrical impedance measurements to average 1.3 and 2.2% for within-day and week-to-week measurements, respectively.

bioelectrical impedance is an attractive method of body fat assessment because it is quick, relatively inexpensive, does not require a high degree of technician skill, yields results immediately, and does not intrude on the subject's privacy. However, because the bioelectrical impedance method is based on impedance to electrical current flow, the subject's state of hydration can influence the results; thus, strict guidelines for standardizing hydration levels prior to bioelectrical impedance testing need to be followed [109].

Although the practical measurement of bioelectrical impedance is easy, a number of factors influence the measurements and, even after careful standardization of the measurement procedure, there remain factors for which one cannot easily control remain. One source of error is the distribution of body water between the intra- and extracellular spaces. Furthermore, body impedance depends on body and skin temperature, body posture during measurement, skin humidity (skin resistivity), and whether the subject is in the fasting state or took strenuous exercise before the measurements. For all these reasons, prediction equations for body fat based on impedance are highly population specific and are clearly different between males and females and age groups (as a result of body water distribution). Using inadequate prediction equations can lead to high bias and, in lean subjects, often results in negative values for percent body fat. Changes in body fat have been studied by bioelectrical impedance and other techniques in many publications. The results are not consistent.

ENERGY BALANCE

Energy balance is the difference between energy intake and energy expenditure. If energy intake is greater than energy expenditure (i.e., positive energy balance) over a prolonged period of time, increases in body fat may occur. To measure energy balance, scientists and clinicians measure energy intake and expenditure via direct (e.g., doubly labeled water) and indirect (e.g., questionnaires and diaries) methods [128]. Assessment of energy intake and expenditure is beyond the scope of this chapter; however, Chapter 2 discusses assessment of energy expenditure and physical activity in detail. Information beyond that presented in this chapter and Chapter 2 can be found in other peer-reviewed manuscripts [129,130].

TABLE 3.1
Summary of Laboratory- and Field-Based Body Fat Methods

Body fat method	Strengths	Limitations
Underwater Weighing	Good reliability	Need skilled technician
		Fat free mass not constant
		Subject needs to go under water
		Great deal of subject cooperation
		Difficult with obese subjects and elderly
		High instrumentation maintenance
		Time consuming
Air Displacement Plethysmography	Quick	Subject needs to wear swimsuit
	Convenient	Cannot measure obese subjects
	Easy to administer	High cost of instrumentation
	Good reliability	Fat free mass not constant
DEXA	High reliability	Radiation exposure
	High validity	Body fat varies among brands
	Quick	
	Safe	
	Small radiation dose	
	Minimal subject cooperation	
	Able to assess regional body fat	
CT	High reliability	Expensive
	High validity	High radiation dose
	Able to measure SAT	Limited access to scanners
	Short scan times	
MRI	High reliability	Expensive
	High validity	Limited access to machines
	No radiation exposure	Time consuming (compared to CT)
Ultrasound	Good reliability	Limited access to machines
	Good validity	More expensive than field methods
	No radiation exposure	
	Noninvasive	
BMI	Good reliability	Not valid on individual level
	Portable	Does not differentiate fat mass and fat free mass
	Inexpensive	
	Little training required	
Skinfolds	Portable	Poor reliability
	Inexpensive	Poor validity
		Cannot measure obese subjects
		Fat free mass not constant
Waist Circumference	Good reliability	Meticulous with site location
	Portable	Does not differentiate subcutaneous adipose tissue and visceral adipose tissue
	Inexpensive	
	Strongly correlated with VAT	
	Quick	
Bioelectrical Impedance	Portable	Poor reliability
	Quick	Poor validity
		Assumes constant total body water

SUMMARY

It does not appear that the present epidemic of overweight and obesity will disappear in the near future. The ability to diagnose and treat obesity is limited, in part, by the ability to assess body fat. This chapter reviewed many of the existing body fat measures and their strengths and limitations (see Table 3.1). The precision and accuracy errors reported for the various measurement techniques are presented in Table 3.2. Direct, or laboratory-based, body fat methods, when performed at their best, have an error of at least 2 to 3% body fat when compared with results from other methods [131]. With indirect, or field-based, methods, an error rate of 5% body fat is presently the best that can be expected, and an error of between 5 and 10% is more realistic.

It is hoped that the information presented in this review will aid the clinician and researcher in selecting the most appropriate body fat measure for their needs and objectives. Generally, laboratory methods are more precise than the field methods; however, they are also more expensive and more time intensive, and require a higher degree of technical training and skill. Numerous factors need to be considered prior to selecting a method for body fat assessment:

- Cost
- Ease of operation
- Technician training
- Subject cooperation and comfort
- Number of subjects and time available for assessment
- Purpose of the assessment
- Size of the individual
- Whether the assessment will be conducted on multiple occasions to assess changes in body fat

No single method is best; rather, the clinician or researcher must weigh the practical considerations of assessment needs with the limitations of the methods. Regardless of the instrument chosen, the method is only as good as the measurement technique and prediction or conversion formula applied. It is imperative that the clinician follow the standard guidelines and protocols associated with each method to limit measurement error.

TABLE 3.2
Precision and Accuracy of Different Body Fat Measurement Techniques

Body fat method	Precision (%)[a]	Accuracy (%)[b]	Ref.
Underwater Weighing	2–3	>5	132
Air Displacement Plethysmography	2–6	>5	132, 133
DEXA	1–3	2–4	46, 48, 132, 134
CT	1–2	1–2	61, 135
MRi	1–2	1–2	135
Ultrasound	1–2	4–5	76
BMI	1–2	>5	136
Waist Circumference	1–2	>5	102, 137
Skinfolds	>5	>5	138
Bioelectric Impedence	>5	>8	132

[a]Reproducibility for repeat measurements.
[b]Accuracy for absolute body fat estimate.

REFERENCES

1. Melanson KJ, McInnis KJ, Rippe JM, Blackburn G, Wilson PF. Obesity and cardiovascular disease risk: research update. *Cardiol Rev.* 2001; 9:202–207.
2. Visscher TL, Seidell JC. The public health impact of obesity. *Ann Rev Public Health.* 2001; 22:355–375.
3. Grundy SM. Metabolic complications of obesity. *Endocrine J.* 2000; 13:155–165.
4. Kuczmarski RJ, Flegal KM, Campbell SM, Johnson CL. Increasing prevalence of overweight among US adults: The National Health and Nutrition Examination Surveys, 1960 to 1991. *JAMA.* 1994; 274:205–211.
5. Popkin BM. An overview on the nutrition transition and its health implications: the Bellagio meeting. *Public Health Nutr.* 2002; 5:93–103.
6. Gallagher D, Visser M, Sepulveda D, Peirson RN, Harris T, Heymsfield SB. How useful is BMI for comparison of body fatness across age, sex and ethnic groups? *Am J Epidemiol.* 1996; 143:228–239.
7. Deurenberg P, Yap M, Van Staveren WA. BMI and percent body fat: a meta-analysis among different ethnic groups. *Int J Obesity.* 1998; 22:1164–1171.
8. World Health Organization. Obesity: preventing and managing the global epidemic. World Health Organization Program of Nutrition. 1998. Geneva.
9. Flegal KM, Carroll MD, Ogden CL, Johnson CL. Prevalence and trends in obesity among U.S. adults, 1999–2000. *JAMA.* 2002; 288:1723–1727.
10. Troiano RP, Flegal KM, Kuczmarski RJ, Campbell SM, Johnson CL. *Arch Pediatr Adolesc Med.* 1995; 149:1085–1091.
11. Ellis KJ. Human body composition: *in vivo* methods. *Physiol Rev.* 2000; 80:649–680.
12. Ellis KJ, Yasumura S, Morgan WDE (Editors). In Vivo *Body Composition Studies.* London: Institute of Physical Sciences in Medicine, 1987.
13. Heymsfield SB, Wang Z, Baumgartner RN, Ross R. Human body composition: advances in models and methods. *Ann Rev Nutr.* 1997; 17:527–558.
14. Ellis KJ. Human body composition: *in vivo* methods. *Physiol Rev.* 2000; 80(2):649–680.
15. Behnke AR, Feen BG, Welham WC. The specific gravity of healthy men. Body weight and volume as an index of obesity. *JAMA.* 1942; 118:495–498.
16. Bonge D, Donnelly JE. Trials to criteria for hydrostatic weighing at residual volume. *RQES* . 1989; 60:176–179.
17. Buskirk ER. Underwater weighing and body density: a review of procedures. In: Brozek J, Henschel A, Eds. Techniques for measuring body composition. Washington, D.C.: National Academy of Sciences — National Research Council, 1961; 90–106.
18. Siri W. *Techniques for Measuring Body Composition.* Vol. 61. Brozek J, Henshcel A (Eds.). National Academy Press: Washington, D.C., 1961.
19. Brozek J, Grande F, Anderson J, Keys A. Densitometric analysis of body composition: revision of some quantitative assumptions. *Ann NY Acad Sci.* 1963; 110:113–140.
20. Fidanza F, Keys A, Anderson JT. Density of body fat in man and other mammals. *JAP.* 1953; 6:252–256.
21. Brozek J, Grande F, Anderson J, Keys A. Densitometric analysis of body composition: revision of some quantitative assumptions. *Ann NY Acad Sci.* 1963; 110: 113–140.
22. Wilmore JH, Vodak PA, Parr RB, Girandola RN, Billing JE. Further simplification of a method for determination of residual volume. *MSSE* . 1980; 12:216–218.
23. Katch FI, Katch VL. Measurement and prediction errors in body composition assessment and the search for the perfect equation. *RQES* . 1980; 51:249–260.
24. Pollock ML, Wilmore JH. Exercise in *Health and Disease: Evaluation and Prescription for Prevention and Rehabilitation* (2nd ed.). Philadelphia: Saunders, 1990.
25. Heymsfield SB, Wang J, Kehayias S, Heshka S, Lichtman S, Pierson RN. Chemical determination of human body density in vivo: relevance to hydrodensitometry. *Am J Clin Nutr.* 1989; 50: 1282–1289.
26. Williams DE, Going SB, Massett MP, Lohman TG, Bare LA, Hewitt MJ. Aqueous and mineral fractions of the fat-free body and their relation to body fat estimates in men and women aged 49–82 years. In K.J. Ellis, JD Eastman (Eds.). *Human Body Composition*: in Vivo *Methods, Models, and Assessment.* New York: Plenum, 1993; 109–113.

27. Ward A, Pollock ML, Jackson AS, Ayres JJ, Pape G. A comparison of body fat determined by underwater weighing and volume displacement. *Am J Phys.* 1978; 234:E94–E96.
28. Dempster P, Aitkens S. A new air displacement method for the determination of human body composition. *MSSE* . 1995; 27:1692–1697.
29. McCrory MA, Mole PA, Gomez TD, Dewey KG, Bernauer EM. Body composition by air displacement plethysmography by using predicted and measured thoracic gas volumes. *JAP* . 1998; 84:1475–1479.
30. Lockner DW, Heyward VH, Baumgartner RN, Jenkins KA. Comparison of air displacement plethysmography, hydrodensitometry, and dual x-ray absorptiometry for assessing body composition in children 10 to 18 years of age. *Ann NY Acad Sci.* 2000; 904:72–78.
31. McCrory MA, Gomez TD, Bernauer EM, Mole PA. Evaluation of a new air displacement plethysmograph for measuring human body composition. *MSSE* . 1995; 27:1686–1691.
32. Demerath EW, Guo SS, Chumlea WC, Towne B, Roche AF, Siervogel RM. Comparison of percent body fat estimates using air displacement plethysmography and hydrodensitometry in adults and children. *Int J Obesity.* 2002; 26:389–397.
33. Wagner DR, Heyward VH, Gibson AN. Validation of air displacement plethysmography for assessing body composition. *MSSE.* 2000; 1339–1343.
34. Chettle DR, Fremlin JH. Techniques of *in vivo* neutron activation analysis. *Phys Med Biol.* 1984; 29:1011–1043.
35. Ellis KJ. Human body composition: *in vivo* methods. *Physiol Rev.* 2000; 80:649–680.
36. Abate N, Burns D, Peshock RM, Garg A, Grundy SM. Estimation of adipose tissue mass by magnetic resonance imaging: validation against dissection in human cadavers. *J Lipid Res.* 1994; 35:1490–1496.
37. Pietrobelli A, Formica C, Wang ZM, Heymsfield SB. Dual energy x-ray absorptiometry body composition model: review-of concepts. *Am J Phys.* 1996; 271:E941–E951.
38. Houtkooper LB, Going SB, Sproul J, Blew RM, Lohman TG. Comparison of methods for assessing body composition changes over 1 year in postmenopausal women. *Am J Clin Nutr.* 2000; 72:401–406.
39. Lang P, Steiger P, Faulkner K, Gluer C, Genant HK. Osteoporosis: current techniques and recent developments in quantitative bone densitometry. *Radiologic Clinics North Am.* 1991; 29:49–76.
40. Lukaski HC. Soft tissue composition and bone mineral status: evaluation by dual energy x-ray absorptiometry. *J Nutr.* 1993; 123:438–443.
41. Genton L, Hans D, Kyle U, Pichard C. Dual energy x-ray absorptiometry and body composition: Differences between devices and comparison with reference methods. *Nutrition.* 2002; 18:66–70.
42. Kistorp CN, Svednsen OL. Body composition analysis by dual energy x-ray in female diabetics differ between manufacturers. *Eur J Clin Nutr.* 1997; 51:449–454.
43. Lohman TG. Dual energy x-ray absorptiometry. In *Human Body Composition.* AF Roche, SB Heymsfield, TG Lohman (Eds.). Champaign, IL: Human Kinetics, 1996; 63–78.
44. Tataranni PA, Ravussin E. Use of dual-energy x-ray absorptiometry in obese individuals. *Am J Clin Nutr.* 1995; 62:730–734.
45. Glickman SG, Marn CS, Supiano MA, Dengel DR. Validity and reliability of dual energy x-ray absorptiometry for the assessment of abdominal obesity. *JAP.* 2004; 10:1152–1162.
46. Ellis KJ. Selected body composition methods can be used in field studies. *Am Soc Nutr Sci.* 2001; 1589S–1595S.
47. Mazess RB, Barden HS, Bisek JP, Hanson J. Dual energy x-ray absorptiometry for total body and regional bone mineral and soft tissue composition. *Am J Clin Nutr.* 1990; 51:1106–1112.
48. Johnson J, Dawson–Hughes B. Precision and stability of dual energy x-ray absorptiometry measurements. *Calcified Tissue Int.* 1991; 49:174–178.
49. Van Loan MD, Mayclin PL. Body composition assessment: dual energy x-ray absorptiometry compared to reference methods. *Eur J Clin Nutr.* 1992; 46:125–130.
50. Friedl KE, DeLuca JP, Marchitelli LJ, Vogel JA. Reliability of body fat estimations from a four-compartment model by using density, body water, and bone mineral measurements. *Am J Clin Nutr.* 1992; 55:764–770.
51. Houtkooper LB, Going SB, Sproul J, Blew RM, Lohman TG. Comparison of methods for assessing body composition changes over 1 y in postmenopausal women. *Am J Clin Nutr.* 2000; 72:401–406.
52. Mazess RB, Barden HS, Bisek JP, Hanson J, Dual energy x-ray absorptiometry for total body and regional bone mineral and soft tissue composition. *Am J Clin Nutr.* 1990; 51:1106–1112.

53. Van Loan MD. Is dual energy x-ray absortiopmetry ready for prime time in the clinical evaluation of body composition? *Am J Clin Nutr.* 1998; 68:1155–1156.
54. Nakata Y, Tunaka K, Mizuki T. Body composition measurement by DXA differs between two analysis modes. *J Clin Densitom.* 2004; 7(4):443–447.
55. Rossner S, Bo WJ, Hiltbrandt E. Adipose tissue determinations in cadavers — a comparison between cross-sectional planimetry and computed tomography. *Int J Obesity.* 1990; 14:893–902.
56. Despres JP, Lamarche B. Effects of diet and physical activity on adiposity and body fat distribution: implications for the prevention of cardiovascular disease. *Nutr Res Rev.* 1993; 6:137–159.
57. Nicklas BJ, Penninx BW, Ryan AS, Berman DM, Lynch NA, Dennis KE. Visceral adipose tissue cutoffs associated with metabolic risk factors for coronary heart disease in women. *Diabetes Care.* 2003; 26(5):1413–1420.
58. Sjostrom L. A computer-tomography based multicomponent body composition technique and anthropometric predictions of lean body mass, total, and subcutaneous adipose tissue. *Int J Obesity.* 1991; 15:19–30.
59. Despres JP, Ross R, Lemieux S. Imaging techniques applied to the measurement of human body composition. In: *Human Body Composition*, AF Roche, SB Heymsfield, TG Lohman, Eds. Champaign, IL: Human Kinetics, 1996; 149–166.
60. Ross R, Leger L, Morris D, de Guise J, Guardo R. Quantification of adipose tissue by MRI: relationship with anthropometric variables. *JAP.* 1992; 72:787–795.
61. Rossner S, Bo WJ, Hiltbrandt E, Hinson W, Karstaedt N, Santago P, Sobol WT, Crouse JR. Adipose tissue determinations in cadavers — a comparison between cross-sectional planimetry and computed tomography. *Int J Obesity.* 1990; 14:893–902.
62. Despres JP, Ross R, Lemieux S. Imaging techniques applied to the measurement of human body composition. In: *Human Body Composition*, AF Roche, SB Heymsfield, TG Lohman, Eds. Champaign, IL: Human Kinetics, 1996; 149–166.
63. Rossner S, Bo WJ, Hiltbrandt E. Adipose tissue determinations in cadavers — a comparison between cross-sectional planimetry and computed tomography. *Int J Obesity.* 1990; 14:893–902.
64. Heymsfield SB, Wang Z. Human body composition: advances in models and methods. *Ann Rev Nutr.* 1997; 17:527–558.
65. Kvist H, Chowdhury B, Grangard U, Tylen U, Sjostrom L. Total and visceral adipose tissue volumes derived from measurements with computed tomography in adult men and women: predictive equations. *Am J Clin Nutr.* 1988; 48:1351–1361.
66. Van Der Kooy K, Seidell J. Techniques for the measurement of visceral fat: a practical guide. *Int J Obesity.* 1993; 17:187–196.
67. Despres JP, Ross R, Lemieux S. Imaging techniques applied to the measurement of human body composition. In: *Human Body Composition*, AF Roche, SB Heymsfield, TG Lohman, Eds. Champaign, IL: Human Kinetics, 1996; 149–166.
68. Heymsfield SB, Ross R, Wang ZM, Frager D. Imaging techniques of body composition: advantages of measurement and new uses. In *Emerging Technologies for Nutrition Research.* Washington, D.C.: National Academy Press, 1997; 1–25.
69. Abate N, Burns D, Peshock RM, Garg A, Grundy SM. Estimation of adipose tissue mass by magnetic resonance imaging: validation against dissection in human cadavers. *J Lipid Res.* 1994; 35:1490–1496.
70. Seidell JC, Bakker CJ, van der Kooy K. Imaging techniques for measuring adipose tissue distribution: a comparison between computed tomography and 1.5-T magnetic resonance. *Am J Clin Nutr.* 1990; 51:953–957.
71. Ross R, Shaw KD, Martel Y. Adipose tissue distribution measured by magnetic resonance imaging in obese women. *Am J Clin Nutr.* 1993; 57:470–475.
72. Thaete FL, Colberg SR, Burke T, Kelley DE. Reproducibility of computed tomography measurement of visceral adipose tissue area. *Int J Obesity.* 1995; 19:464–467.
73. Gerard EL, Snow RC, Kennedy DN. Overall body fat and regional fat distribution in young women: quantification with MR imaging. *Am J Roentgenol.* 1991; 157:99–104.
74. Starck G, Lonn L, Cederblad A, Alpsten M, Sjostrom L, Ekholm S. Dose reduction for body composition measurements with CT. *Appl Radiat Isotopes.* 1998; 49:561–564.
75. Armellini F, Zamboni M, Rigo L et al. The contribution of sonography to the measurement of intra-abdominal fat. *J Clin Ultrasound.* 1990; 18:563–567.

76. Ribeiro–Filho FF, Faria AN, Azjen S, Zanella M, Ferreira SR. Methods of estimation of visceral fat: advantages of ultrasonography. *Obesity Res.* 2003; 11(12):1488–1494.
77. Kim SK, Hae JK, Kyu YH et al. Visceral fat thickness measured by ultrasonography can estimate not only visceral obesity but also risks of cardiovascular and metabolic diseases. *Am J Clin Nutr.* 2004; 79:593–599.
78. Stolk RP, Meijer R, Mali W et al. Ultrasound measurements of intraabdominal fat estimate the metabolic syndrome better than do measurements of waist circumference. *Am J Clin Nutr.* 2003; 77:857–860.
79. Deurenberg P, Yap M, van Staveren WA. Body mass index and percent body fat: a meta analysis among different ethnic groups. *Int J Obesity.* 1998; 22:1164–1171.
80. WHO. Obesity: Preventing and managing the global epidemic. Report on a WHO Consultation on obesity, Geneva, June 3–5, 1997, WHO/NUT/NCD/98.1, WHO, Geneva, Switzerland, 1998.
81. WHO. Physical status: the use and interpretation of anthropometry. Technical Report Series 854. WHO, Geneva, Switzerland, 1995.
82. Gallagher D, Visser M, Sepulveda D, Pierson RN, Harris T, Heymsfield SB. How useful is BMI for comparison of body fatness across age, sex, and ethnic groups? *Am J Epidemiol.* 1996; 143:228–239.
83. Deurenberg P, Deurenberg–Yap M, Wang J. The impact of body build on the relationship between body mass index and percent body fat. *Int J Obesity.* 1999; 23:537–542.
84. Kyle UG, Gremion G, Genton L. Physical activity and fat-free and fat mass as measured by bioelectrical impedance in 3853 adults. *MSSE.* 2001; 33:576–584.
85. Anderson B, Xu XF, Rebuffe–Scrive M, Terning K, Krotkiewski M, Bjorntorp P. The effects of exercise training on body composition and metabolism in men and women. *Int J Obesity.* 1991; 15:75–81.
86. Mourier A, Gautier JF, De Kerviler E et al. Mobilization of visceral adipose tissue related to the improvement in insulin sensitivity in response to physical training in NIDDM. Effects of branched-chain amino acid supplements. *Diabetes Care.* 1997; 20:385–391.
87. Schwartz RS, Shuman WP, Larson V. The effect of intensive endurance exercise training on body fat distribution in young and older men. *Metabolism.* 1991; 40:545–551.
88. Irwin ML, Yasui Y, Ulrich C, Bowen D, Rudolph R, Schwartz R, Yukawa M, Aiello E, Potter J, McTiernan A. Effect of exercise on total and intra-abdominal body fat in postmenopausal women: a randomized controlled trial. *JAMA.* 2003; 289(3):323–330.
89. Janssen I, Katzmarzyk PT, Ross R, Leon AS, Skinner JS, Rao DC, Wilmore JH, Rankinen T, Bouchard C. Fitness alters the associations of BMI and waist circumference with total and abdominal fat. *Obesity Res.* 2004; 12(3):525–537.
90. Seidell JC. Obesity, insulin resistance and diabetes: a world-wide epidemic. *Br J Nutr.* 2000; 83 (Suppl 1):S5–8.
91. Regional Office for the Western Pacific of the WHO, The International Association for the Study of Obesity and the International Obesity Task Force. The Asia–Pacific perspective: redefining obesity and its treatment. Sydney, Australia: Health Communications Australia Pty Limited; 2000.
92. Deurenberg P, Yap M, van Staveren WA. Body mass index and percent body fat: a meta analysis among different ethnic groups. *Int J Obesity.* 1998; 22:1164–1171.
93. Wagner DR, Heyward VH. Measures of body composition in blacks and whites: a comparative review. *Am J Clin Nutr.* 2000; 71:1392–1402.
94. Gallagher D, Visser M, Sepulveda D, Pierson R, Harris N, Heymsfield SB. How useful is body mass index for comparison of body fatness across age, sex, and ethnic groups? *Am J Epidemiol.* 1996; 143:228–239.
95. Nawaz H, Chan W, Abdulrahman M, Larson D, Katz DL. Self-reported height and weight: implications for obesity research. *Am J Prev Med.* 2001; 20:294–298
96. Spencer EA, Appleby PN, Davey GK, Key TJ. Validity of self-reported height and weight in 4808 EPIC–Oxford participants. *Public Health Nutr.* 2002; 5:561–565.
97. Han TS, Lean MEJ. Self-reported waist circumference compared with the waist watcher tape measure to identify individuals at increased health risk through intra-abdominal fat accumulation. *Br J Nutr.* 1998; 80:81–88.
98. Turcato E, Bosello O, Francisco V. Waist circumference and abdominal sagittal diameter as surrogates of body fat distribution in the elderly: their relation with cardiovascular disease risk factors. *Int J Obesity.* 2000; 24:1005–1010.

99. Ross R, Rissanen J, Hudson R. Sensitivity associated with the identification of visceral adipose tissue levels using waist circumference in men and women: effects of weight loss. *Int J Obesity.* 1996; 20:533–538.
100. Booth ML, Hunter C, Gore CJ, Bauman A, Owen N. The relationship between body mass index and waist circumference: implications for estimates of population prevalence of overweight. *Int J Obesity.* 2000; 24:1058–1061.
101. Lohman TG. *Anthropometric Standardization Reference Manual.* Champaign, IL: Human Kinetics, 1988; 28–80.
102. Wang J, Thornton JC, Burastero S. Comparison for body mass index and body fat percent among Puerto Ricans, blacks, whites, and Asians living in the New York City area. *Obesity Res.* 1996; 4:377–383.
103. Janssen I, Katzmarzyk PT, Ross R. Waist circumference and not body mass index explains obesity-related health risk. *Am J Clin Nutr.* 2004; 79:379–384.
104. Lemieux S, Prud'homme D, Bouchard C, Tremblay A, Despres JP. A single threshold value of waist girth identifies normal-weight and overweight subjects with excess visceral adipose tissue. *Am J Clin Nutr.* 1996; 64:685–693.
105. Albu JB, Murphy L, Frager DH, Johnson JA, Pi-Sunyer FX. Visceral fat and race-dependent health risks in obese nondiabetic premenopausal women. *Diabetes.* 1997; 46:456–462.
106. Lohman TG. *Anthropometric Standardization Reference Manual.* Champaign, IL: Human Kinetics, 1988; 28–80.
107. Lean ME, Han TS, Morrison CE. Waist circumference as a measure for indicating need for weight management. *Br Med J.* 1995; 311:158–161.
108. Han TS, Lean MEJ. Self-reported waist circumference compared with the waist watcher tape measure to identify individuals at increased health risk through intra-abdominal fat accumulation. *Br J Nutr.* 1998; 80:81–88.
109. Heyward VH. Evaluation of body composition. *Sports Med.* 1996; 22:146–156.
110. Lohman TG. *Anthropometric Standardization Reference Manual.* Champaign, IL: Human Kinetics, 1988; 28–80.
111. Jackson AS, Pollock ML. Generalized equations for predicting body density of men. *Br J Nutr.* 1978, 40:497–504.
112. Jackson AS, Pollock ML, Ward A. Generalized equations for predicting body density of women. *MSSE.* 1980; 12:175–182.
113. Heyward VH, Stolarczyk LM. *Applied Body Composition Assessment.* Champaign, IL: Human Kinetics, 1996.
114. Hayes PA, Sowood PJ, Belyavin A, Cohen JB, SMit FW. Subcutaneous fat thickness measured by magnetic resonance imaging, ultrasound, and calipers. *MSSE* . 1988; 20:303–309.
115. Lohman TG. Skinfolds and body density and their relation to body fatness: a review. *Hum Biol.* 1981; 53:181–225.
116. Lohman TG. Skinfolds and body density and their relationship to body fatness: a review. *Hum Biol.* 1981; 53:181–225.
117. Jackson AS. Research design and analysis of data procedures for predicting body density. *MSSE* . 1984; 16:616–620.
118. Heyward VH, Cook KL, Hicks VL, Jenkins KA, Quatrochi JA, Wilson W. Predictive accuracy of three field methods for estimating body fatness of nonobese and obese women. *Int J Sports Nutr.* 1992; 2:75–86.
119. Baumgartner RN, Chumlea WC, Roche AF. Bioelectrical impedance for body composition. *Exercise Sci Sports Sci Rev.* 1990; 18:193–224.
120. National Institutes of Health. Bioelectrical impedance analysis in body composition measurement. NIH technology assessment conference statement. Bethesda, MD, 1994; 1–35.
121. Wang J, Thornton JC, Burastero S, Heymsfield SB, Pierson RN. Bio-impedance analysis for estimation of total body water, and fat-free mass in white, black, and Asian adults. *Am J Hum Biol.* 1995; 7:33–40.
122. Deurenberg P, Weststrate JA, Paymans I, van der Kooy K. Factors affecting bioelectrical impedance measurements in humans. *Eur J Clin Nutr.* 1988; 42:1017–1022.

123. Lukaski HC. Use of the tetrapolar bioelectrical impedance method to assess human body composition. In *Human Body Composition and Fat Distribution*. Waginegen. The Netherlands: Euronut, 1986; 143–158.
124. Heyward VH, Cook KL, Hicks VL, Jenkins KA, Quatrochi JA, Wilson W. Predictive accuracy of three field methods for estimating body fatness of nonobese and obese women. *Int J Sports Nutr.* 1992; 2:75–86.
125. Heyward VH. Practical body composition assessment for children, adults, and older adults. *Int J Sports Nutr.* 1998; 8:285–307.
126. Kushner RF, Schoeller DA. Estimation of total body water by bioelectrical impedance analysis. *Am J Clin Nutr.* 1986; 44:417–424.
127. Kushner RF, Schoeller DA. Estimation of total body water by bioelectrical impedance analysis. *Am J Clin Nutr.* 1986; 44:417–424.
128. Hill J, Melanson E. Overview of the determinants of overweight and obesity: current evidence and research issues. *MSSE* . 1999; 31(11 Suppl):S515–21.
129. Neuhouser M, Patterson R, Kristal A, Rock C. Validity of short food frequency questionnaires used in cancer chemoprevention trials: results from the Prostate Cancer Prevention Trial. *CEBP* 1999; 8(8):721–725.
130. Lamonte M, Ainsworth B. Quantifying energy expenditure and physical activity in the context of dose response. *MSSE* . 2001; 33(6 Suppl):S370–378.
131. Lukaski H. Methods for the assessment of human body composition: traditional and new. *Am J Clin Nutr.* 1987; 46:537–556.
132. Ellis KJ. Selected body composition methods can be used in field studies. *Am Soc Nutr Sci.* 2001 ; 1589S–1595S.
133. Demerath EW, Guo SS, Chumlea WC, Towne B, Roche AF, Siervogel RM. Comparison of percent body fat estimates using air displacement plethysmography and hydrodensitometry in adults and children. *Int J Obesity.* 2002; 26: 389–397.
134. Wagner DR, Heyward VH. Techniques of body composition assessment: a review of laboratory and field methods. *RQES.* 1999; 70(2):135–146.
135. Shen W, Wang Z, Punyanita M, Lei J, Sinav A, Kral J, Imielinska C, Ross R, Heymsfield SB. Adipose tissue quantification by imaging methods: a proposed classification. *Obesity Res.* 2003; 11(1):5–16.
136. Deurenberg P, Yap M. The assessment of obesity: methods for measuring body fat and global prevalence of obesity. *Baillieres Clin Endo Metab.* 1999; 13 (1):1–11.
137. Janssen I, Katzmarzyk PT, Ross R, Leon AS, Skinner JS, Rao DC, Wilmore JH, Rankinen T, Bouchard C. Fitness alters the associations of BMI and waist circumference with total and abdominal fat. *Obesity Res.* 2004; 12(3):525–537.
138. Wang J, Thornton JC, Kolesnik S, Pierson RN. Anthropometry in body composition. *Ann NY Acad Sci.* 2001; 12:200–208.

Section II

Physical Activity and Cancer Incidence

4 Physical Activity and Cancer Incidence: Breast Cancer

Alpa V. Patel and Leslie Bernstein

CONTENTS

Physical activity has been proposed as a modifiable risk factor for breast cancer primarily because of its effects on steroid sex hormones. Physical activity also may influence breast cancer risk through its influence on energy balance, weight control, insulin sensitivity, and immune function. To date, at least 50 observational studies have been conducted to examine the association between some measure of recreational or occupational physical activity and breast cancer risk. The majority of studies have observed an inverse association between physical activity and breast cancer risk. In this chapter, we first consider the mechanisms that may account for lower breast cancer risk among physically active women and then review studies of recreational and occupational physical activity in relation to breast cancer risk. Finally, we comment on the importance of timing, frequency, duration, and intensity of physical activity in determining breast cancer risk.

BIOLOGICAL MECHANISMS

Physical Activity and Estrogen

Evidence exists that estrogen is critical in the development of breast cancer through increased proliferation of epithelial breast cells. In *in vitro* [1,2] and *in vivo* [3] studies, estradiol, considered the most potent and active form of estrogen, has been shown to increase mitotic activity of breast epithelial cells. By increasing mitoses, estrogens act to promote breast cell proliferation and thus increase the possibility of mutations, including those that are carcinogenic. Thus, cumulative lifetime exposure to estrogen is a key factor in determining a woman's breast cancer risk [4,5].

During reproductive years, particularly during adolescence, high levels of moderate and vigorous physical activity have an impact on markers of ovarian hormone exposure, resulting in delayed menarche, increased likelihood of secondary amenorrhea and irregular or anovulatory menstrual cycles, and shortened luteal phases of the menstrual cycle; thus, physical activity is associated with reduced levels of estradiol, progesterone, and follicle-stimulating hormone (FSH) [6–11]. In part due to the effects of physical activity, these factors would result in a reduction in lifetime ovulatory cycles and cumulative estrogen and progesterone exposure, therefore potentially reducing risk of breast cancer. Although the majority of early studies were conducted in athletes, increasing evidence suggests ovarian function also is altered in recreational athletes through lower mean hormone levels and longer anovular menstrual cycle length [9,10,12–14].

After menopause, production of estrogen from the ovaries is negligible, resulting in a dramatic decrease of circulating estrogen levels compared to premenopausal women. Studies in normal weight women have shown that estrogen levels decline to approximately one-third of the lowest premenopausal levels [15]. The main endogenous source of postmenopausal estrogen production is from the peripheral conversion of androstenedione to estrone in adipose tissue. Women who are physically active during their postmenopausal years have decreased levels of serum estrone, estradiol, and androgens (androstenedione and testosterone) that are precursors to estrogens [16–19]. An association between physical activity and increased levels of sex hormone-binding globulin (SHBG) also has been observed [20]. However, the association between the various hormones and physical activity in postmenopausal women has not been as consistent as that found for premenopausal women, and several studies have found no clear association between hormone levels [21,22] or urinary hormone metabolites [23] and physical activity.

Because aromatization of androstenedione to estrone takes place in fatty tissue, a larger amount of estrogen is produced by heavier postmenopausal women compared to thinner women [24]. Consequently, obesity and weight gain are well-established risk factors for postmenopausal breast cancer [25–28]. High levels of physical activity have been associated with lower weight, lower BMI, and weight loss [16,20,21,29]. Thus, the effects of physical activity in postmenopausal women may be due to direct suppression of hormone levels or indirect because physical activity affects body weight.

Physical Activity and Insulin Sensitivity

Insulin and insulin-like growth factor (IGF)-I have been implicated in carcinogenesis because they play a role in stimulating cell proliferation and inhibiting apoptosis [30]. Increased levels of insulin specifically also may increase breast cancer risk because they have been associated with decreased levels of SHBG and, consequently, higher levels of free estradiol — that is, estradiol that is not inactivated through binding to SHBG [31]. Some epidemiological studies support a positive association between insulin levels and breast cancer risk [32,33]. High levels of insulin also are associated with decreased levels of insulin-like growth factor binding protein-I (IGFBP-I) that may result in a higher level of unbound IGF-I [34].

Insulin-like growth factor I also has been shown *in vitro* to act as a mitogen in breast cell lines and synergistically with estradiol to promote mitosis [35–37], and to play a role in promoting breast cell differentiation and transformation and in suppressing apoptosis [35]. Epidemiological studies have suggested that high IGF-I levels are associated with increased risk of premenopausal breast cancer [38–40].

Two major determinants of insulin resistance are abdominal obesity and physical inactivity. Regular physical activity has been associated with increased insulin sensitivity and decreased levels of serum insulin, independent of its impact on body weight [20,41,42]. Therefore, it may reduce the risk of breast cancer. Previous studies support a positive relationship between obesity and IGF-I levels [42], but current evidence does not allow clear conclusions to be drawn regarding a possible association between physical activity, independent of body weight, and IGF-I levels [42,43].

Physical Activity and Immune Function

Changes in immune function may also mediate the relationship between physical activity and breast cancer risk. Some researchers have observed that physical activity heightens immune response and may reduce risk of chronic disease by increasing production of natural killer (NK) cells that contribute to immune defense [44,45]. This hypothesis is not specific to breast cancer, but would explain a protective role of physical activity in most cancers.

The immune response hypothesis may be particularly relevant to breast cancer because recent evidence suggests that estrogen suppresses NK cell activity [46–48]; therefore, higher levels of estrogens and suppressed NK cell activity may interact to increase breast cancer risk in inactive women. Consequently, women who are physically active may be at a decreased risk of breast cancer because they have a higher production of NK cells as well as lower levels of estrogen. However, little work specifically has been done to define the role of immune function in breast carcinogenesis, particularly the potential mediation between immune function and hormones.

Physical Activity, Energy Balance, and Weight Control

Maintenance of normal body weight throughout a woman's adult years is one of the few known modifiable risk factors for breast cancer that occurs after the menopause. Increased physical activity has been consistently associated with lower body mass index (BMI kg/m^2) and weight maintenance. Weight maintenance is achieved through energy balance in which energy intake equals energy expenditure, resulting in no net change of stored energy in the body. High energy intake coupled with low expenditure leads to excess storage of adipose tissue and results in obesity [49]. As previously stated, excess adiposity (high BMI) and the accumulation of adipose tissue over time (weight gain) are associated with increased risk of breast cancer among postmenopausal women [25–28]. In addition to influencing estrogen production directly, the lack of energy balance resulting in excess adipose tissue is associated with many other potential breast cancer risk factors, such as:

- Insulin resistance [50,51]
- Increased levels of IGF-I [51]
- Increased levels of aromatase activity, resulting in increased total estradiol [52]
- Decreased levels of SHBG, resulting in increased levels of free estradiol [20,52]
- Immunosuppression [53]

Therefore, promotion of normal weight maintenance through energy balance, increased physical activity, and reduced caloric intake may be an effective approach to reducing the risk of breast cancer [54,55].

PREVIOUS LITERATURE

Recreational Physical Activity

To date, 16 prospective cohorts [56–71], 22 population-based case-control studies [72–93], and four hospital-based case-control studies [94–97] have examined the relationship between recreational physical activity and breast cancer risk. Seven studies yielded more than one publication [62,67,70,82,85,88,97–107]; consequently, only the most recent report from each study has been used to reference each study. Additionally, a study by Enger et al. [108] combined and analyzed subjects from two different previously cited studies [72,106] and therefore was not considered as a separate study population.

Overall, most studies suggest that physically active women have a lower risk of developing breast cancer than physically inactive women. A 20 to 80% reduction in risk with physical activity has been reported in 12 cohort studies [57–62,64,65,67–69,71]; 16 population-based case control studies [72–74,78–86,88,90,91,93] observed a reduction in risk ranging from 20 to 70% and three hospital-based case control studies [95–97] generally reported a 20 to 30% reduction in risk (Table 4.1).

The association between physical activity and breast cancer also is consistent across different populations and countries. Studies conducted in Australia [73], various countries across Europe [58,80,81,95,96], Asia [78,84,97], and the U.S. and Canada [57,59–62,65,67,69,71,72,74,79, 82,83,85,86,88,90,91,93] have reported an inverse relationship between physical activity and breast cancer risk. Within U.S. studies, associations between physical activity and breast cancer were observed in multiethnic populations as well as specific subpopulations of white [57,59,69,86], black [83], Hispanic [86], and Asian–American women [93].

In some studies, the association between physical activity and breast cancer risk also has been assessed separately for *in situ* and invasive breast cancer as well as estrogen/progesterone receptor (ER/PR) positive and negative tumors. Although many previous studies include *in situ* and invasive breast cancer cases, only one study specifically examined the association between *in situ* breast carcinoma and exercise activity [91]. In one additional study, researchers examined the association between physical activity and breast cancer stratified by stage of disease and found risk reduction to be greater for localized invasive disease compared to *in situ* or regional/distant breast cancer [69]. Two studies also reported risk ratios separately for ER/PR positive and negative tumors, but neither found a difference in risk by ER/PR subtype [65,108].

The impact of physical activity on age at breast cancer onset also has been examined in some previous studies [57,109]. Physical activity, particularly in adolescence, was associated with significantly delayed onset of breast cancer in a case-only analysis of BRCA1 and BRCA2 mutation carriers [109]. In the Adventist Health Study, Fraser et al. observed age of onset for breast cancer was approximately 6.6 years earlier for women who were inactive at baseline compared to active women [57].

Quality of Data on Physical Activity

Questions regarding physical activity range from general questions such as "Do you get much exercise in things you do for recreation?" (NHANES-I questionnaire) [67] to very detailed reconstructed histories used in some case-control studies; these are based on lifetime calendars collecting information on duration, frequency, and intensity of physical activity that allow researchers to build exposure measures for different time periods throughout a woman's lifetime [72,85,88,91]. Some studies also collected information on frequency of various activities, but lacked individual information on duration and/or intensity [61,69,102]. In two other studies, physical activity was indirectly inferred through study design comparing athletes vs. nonathletes [62], or physical education teachers to language teachers [110]. Some questionnaires only allowed for a limited number of activities to be reported for each time period [84,94], so activity histories in these studies may have underestimated the actual activity level of extremely active women.

Summary measures based on the available information from questionnaire data were then used to compare women with higher levels of physical activity to those with lower levels or who were inactive. In some instances, the level of detail was minimal; women were classified only as having little, moderate, or much activity [67,96]. Other studies have collected the type of activity and hours per week of activity. In these studies, researchers have been able to examine activity level based on an intensity score, the metabolic equivalents of energy expended per hour of each individual activity (MET) [60,65,69,74,75,77,82,84–86,106]. However, these MET values are assigned to every individual participating in an activity and do not consider individual variation in the intensity of the activity, a function of skill and effort. In general, the MET values used are derived from the Compendium of Physical Activities [111] and this method of deriving MET-hours may result in misclassification of true energy expenditure.

TABLE 4.1
Previous Studies of Physical Activity and Breast Cancer

Study design (study date)	No. of cases	Pre- or postmenopausal	Type of activity	Timing of activity	How activity measured	Main findings	Author, date, and location
Retrospective cohort (1974–1979)	791	Combined	Occupational	Usual lifetime	Five levels based on Dept. of Labor codes	Levels 3–5 vs. level 1 PMR = 0.85 ($p< 0.05$)	Vena 1987, U.S. [126]
Hospital-based case-control (1979–1984)	241	Combined	Occupational	Lifetime	Energy expenditure and hours sitting based on job title	Sedentary vs. high = 0.7 (0.2–3.4), p-trend = 0.23	Dosemeci 1993, Turkey [125]
Prospective cohort (Framingham) (1954–1988)	117	Combined	Recreational	Baseline	Sleep, sedentary, light, moderate, and strenuous exercise h/day relative oxygen consumption	Q4 vs. Q1 1.6 (0.9–2.9)	Dorgan 1994, U.S. [56]
Population-based case-control (1983–1989)	545	Premenopausal	Recreational	Lifetime	Each activity, frequency, duration, type, age start and stopped recorded and used to calculate average lifetime h/week and specific time periods (e.g., 10 years after menarche)	3.8+ h/week vs. none = 0.42 (0.27–0.64), p-trend = 0.0001; p-trend for 10 years after menarche = 0.027	Bernstein 1994, U.S. [72]
Population-based case-control (1982–1984)	444	Both	Recreational	Baseline	H/week of light, moderate, and vigorous activities for winter and summer seasons to calculate kcal/week	>4000 kcal/week vs. none pre = 0.60 (0.30–1.17), p-trend = 0.09, post = 0.73 (0.44–1.20), p-trend = 0.32	Friedenreich 1995, Australia [73]

—continued

TABLE 4.1 (CONTINUED)
Previous Studies of Physical Activity and Breast Cancer

Study design (study date)	No. of cases	Pre- or postmenopausal	Type of activity	Timing of activity	How activity measured	Main findings	Author, date, and location
Hospital-based case-control (1987–1990)	617	Both	Strenuous recreational	Ages 15–21; 22–44; 45+	Report up to six activities (two at each age group)	3+ h/week vs. no at ages 15–21, pre = 0.7 (0.4–1.4), post = 1.0 (0.6–1.8); no report for other ages	Taioli 1995, U.S. [94]
Population-based case-control (1988–1990)	537	Combined and postmenopausal only	Recreational	Adulthood up to 2 years prior to interview	Calculated MET h/week from age started and stopped, frequency, and duration of each activity	Q5 vs. none all women = 0.9 (0.6–1.4) p-trend = 0.25, post women = 0.6 (0.4–1.0), p-trend = 0.009	McTiernan 1996, U.S. [74]
Prospective cohort (Adventist) (1977–1982)	218	Combined	Recreational and occupational combined	Baseline	Outside of work, at least 15 min of vigorous exercise three or more times per week and vigorous activity at work	"low" vs. "high" 1.46 (1.11–1.92)	Fraser 1997, U.S. [57]
Prospective cohort (National Health Screen. Service) (1974–1994)	351	Both	Recreational and occupational	Baseline, 3 and 5 years after baseline	Categories of level of activity (based on intensity and frequency) during leisure hours; four-point scale of level of occupational activity	Regular vs. sedentary recreational pre = 0.53 (0.25–1.14), post = 0.67 (0.41–1.10); heavy vs. sedentary occupational pre = 0.48 (0.24–0.95), post = 0.78 (0.52–1.18)	Thune 1997, Norway [58]

Population-based case-control (1983–1990)	747	Combined	Recreational	Ages 12–21 and 2 years prior to interview	Calculated MET h/week from age started and stopped, frequency, intensity, and duration of each activity	Two years prior 18+ vs. 0 MET/week = 0.95 (0.73–1.23), p-trend = 0.85; no assoc with age 12–21	Chen 1997, U.S. [75]
Population-based case-control (1989–1993)	157	Both	Recreational	Teens and 20s	Total h/week of strenuous and moderate activities in both time periods used to calculate kcal/week	650+ vs. 0 kcal/week in 20s for pre = 1.01 (0.54–1.87), p-trend = 0.876; 1100+ vs. 0 kcal/week for post = 0.53 (0.19–1.52), p-trend = 0.973; teen activity not associated	Hu 1997, Japan [76]
Population-based case-control (1988–1991)	4863	Combined	Occupational	Usual lifetime	Occupational titles categorized into four groups	Heavy vs. sedentary = 0.82 (0.63–1.08), p-trend = 0.007	Coogan 1997, U.S. (Coogan 1996 earlier report) [119,120]
Prospective cohort (Iowa 65+ Rural Health Study) (1982–1993)	46	Postmenopausal	Recreational	Baseline	Weekly or monthly walking, moderate or vigorous activity	High vs. inactive 0.2 (0.05–0.9), p-trend = 0.01	Cerhan 1998, U.S. [59]
Prospective cohort (College Alumni Health Study) (1962–1993)	109	Both	Recreational	Baseline	MET h/week calculated using h/week in stair climbing, blocks walked, sports	1000+ vs. <500 pre (age < 55) = 1.83 (0.77–4.31), post = 0.49 (0.28–0.86)	Sesso 1998, U.S. [60]
Population-based case-control (1990–1992)	1647	Both	Recreational	Ages 12–13, age 20, and year prior to interview	MET h/week calculated using frequency of moderate and vigorous activities at each time period	Average of all time periods Q4 v Q1 pre = 1.04 (0.84–1.28), post = 1.14 (0.34–3.83); no differences in any one time period	Gammon 1998, U.S. [77]

—continued

TABLE 4.1 (CONTINUED)
Previous Studies of Physical Activity and Breast Cancer

Study design (study date)	No. of cases	Pre- or postmenopausal	Type of activity	Timing of activity	How activity measured	Main findings	Author, date, and location
Hospital-based case-control (1991–1994)	2569	Both	Recreational and occupational combined	Recreational at ages 15–19, 30–39, and 50–59; occupational at ages 30–39	Composite of all activities based on h/week of leisure activities and sports and level of activity (sitting to very tiring) at job	Low vs. high pre = 1.39 (0.91–2.13), post = 1.61 (1.16–2.23)	Mezzetti 1998, Italy (reanalysis of D'Avanzo, 1996) [95,123]
Prospective cohort (Nurses Health Study I) (1976–1996)	3137	Combined	Recreational	Baseline every 2 years during follow-up	Average h/wk on moderate to vigorous activity; usual walking amount and pace; calc baseline only and long-term (updated) activity	7+ vs. <1 h/week long term = 0.82 (0.70–0.97), p-trend = 0.004; no difference between pre- and post-menopausal	Rockhill 1999, U.S. [61]
Prospective cohort (Swedish Cancer Registry) (1960–1989)	8281	Combined	Occupational	Baseline occupation	Occupational title classified by intensity as sedentary, light, medium, high	Sedentary vs. high 1.1 (1.0–1.2), p-trend = 0.1	Moradi 1999, Sweden [121]

Population-based case-control (1990–1997)	139	Both	Recreational and occupational	Lifetime	MET h/week calculated using regular sport or activity for at least 1 year in adulthood reported (type, frequency, number of years); usual occupation activity based on Baecke's work index (quintiles)	15.3+ vs. 0 MET/week pre = 0.32 (0.10–1.03), p-trend = 0.075, post = 0.49 (0.14–1.63), p-trend = 0.231; occupational Q4 vs. Q1 pre = 0.60 (0.16–2.28), p-trend = 0.680, post = 0.65 (0.22–1.94), p-trend = 0.464	Ueji 1999, Japan [78]
Population-based case-control (1993–1996)	863	Combined	Recreational	Age 12	Recalled chores and sports considered strenuous at age 12 (reported five levels of each activity)	14+ vs. <3 times/week active = 0.6 (0.3–1.1), p-trend = 0.07	Marcus 1999, U.S. [79]
Population-based case-control (1983–1986)	233	Combined	Occupational	Lifetime	Job title converted to one of five levels of activity based on Dept. of Labor	10+ yrs moderate/heavy vs. sedentary = 1.7 (0.9–3.3), p-trend = 0.26	Coogan 1999, U.S. [122]
Hospital-based case-control (1993–1998)	246	Combined	Recreational and occupational combined	Ages 15–19; 30–39; 50–59	Recreational: h/week of leisure time activities and sports; three levels of occupational activity	high vs. low: ages 15–19, R = 0.42 (0.26–0.69), p-trend = 0.001; ages 30–39, R = 0.50 (0.30-0.81), p-trend = 0.01; ages 50–59, R = 0.42 (0.22–0.80), p-trend = 0.001	Levi 1999, Switzerland [96]
Prospective cohort (Alumni Health Study) (1981–1996)	175	Combined	College athletes vs. nonathletes	College	College athletes vs. nonathletes	Athletes vs. non = 0.61 (0.44–0.84)	Wyshak 2000, U.S. (Frisch 1985 and Frisch 1987 earlier reports) [62,100,101]

—continued

TABLE 4.1 (CONTINUED)
Previous Studies of Physical Activity and Breast Cancer

Study design (study date)	No. of cases	Pre- or postmenopausal	Type of activity	Timing of activity	How activity measured	Main findings	Author, date, and location
Prospective cohort (Iowa Women's Health Study) (1986–1995)	1380	Postmenopausal	Recreational	Baseline	Frequency of regular moderate activity and regular vigorous activity	High vs. low = 0.95 (0.83–1.10)	Moore 2000, U.S. [63]
Population-based case-control (1986–1989)	918	Combined	Recreational and occupational	Lifetime	Vigorous activity for at least 6 months duration at age 10 and type of activity, start and end date, and frequency forward into adulthood to calculate MET h/week; converted job title to > or ≤ 80% sedentary	>6.3 vs. 0 average lifetime MET = 0.69 (0.50–0.94); no difference for each time point; high vs. low active = 0.84 (0.69–1.04)	Verloop 2000, Netherlands [80]
Population-based case-control (1993–1995)	2838	Postmenopausal	Recreational and occupational	Childhood (age <18 yrs), ages 18–30 and at interview; main lifetime occupation	Time spent on physical exercise/sport in each time period (h/week); converted job title by labor market board in Sweden	Never vs. 2+ h/week recent = 1.3 (1.1–1.5), p-trend = 0.005; age 18–30, p-trend = 0.07; childhood p-trend > 0.5; overall, no association with occupational activity	Moradi 2000, Sweden [81]

Population-based case-control (1988–1991)	4614	Combined	Recreational	Ages 14–18; 18–22	Strenuous activity or sports during both time periods, but not PE class; type of activity, number of mo per yr, and frequency of each to calculate frequency of activity per year and weighted MET score	Daily vs. none = 0.55 (0.39–0.78), p-trend = 0.002; same assoc using MET score	Shoff 2000, U.S. (Mittendorf 1995 earlier report) [82,103]
Population-based case-control	1184	Both	Recreational	Lifetime activity of at least 2 h/week	Frequency and duration of all episodes of regular (at least 2 h/week) activity to calculate lifetime, 10 yrs after menarche, menarche to age 39, age 40 to ref, and 10 years prior to ref MET h/week	17.6+ vs. 0 MET/week: pre ER+/PR+ = 0.60 (0.34–1.07), p-trend = 0.09, similar for other ER/PR groups; post: ER+/PR+ = 0.69 (0.42–1.13), p-trend = 0.16, similar for other ER/PR groups	Enger 2000, U.S. (combined reanalysis of Bernstein 1994 and Carpenter 1999) [72,106,108]
Prospective cohort (Netherlands Cohort Study) (1986–1993)	1208	Postmenopausal	Recreational and occupational	Baseline and history of sports; lifetime occupation	Frequency at baseline of walking, cycling, shopping, and sports/gym; report up to three sports in past; report of up to five jobs and job title used to calculate activity for longest held and most recent job	>90 vs. <30 min/d 0.76 (0.58–0.99), p-trend = 0.003; p-trend for past sports = 0.37; longest job > 12 vs. <8 kJ/min 0.83 (0.51–1.34); no assoc with most recent job	Dirx 2001, Netherlands [64]

—*continued*

TABLE 4.1 (CONTINUED)
Previous Studies of Physical Activity and Breast Cancer

Study design (study date)	No. of cases	Pre- or postmenopausal	Type of activity	Timing of activity	How activity measured	Main findings	Author, date, and location
Prospective cohort (Women's Health Study) (1992–1998)	411	Combined and postmenopausal separately	Recreational	Baseline	kJ/week calculated from eight groups of activities reported	6300+ vs. <840 kJ/week all = 0.80 (0.58–1.12), p-trend = 0.11, post = 0.67 (0.44–1.02), p-trend = 0.03)	Lee 2001, U.S. [65]
Prospective cohort (Finnish Adult Health Behavior Survey) (1979–1995)	332	Combined	Recreational	Baseline	Frequency of exercise at least 30 min that makes you at least mildly out of breath; and commute to/from work	Daily vs. <1/week = 1.01 (072–1.42)	Luoto 2001, Finland [66]
Prospective cohort (NHANES-I NHEFS) (1971–1992)	138	Both	Recreational	Baseline	Based on question, "When recreation, do you get much, moderate, little, no exercise?"	High vs. low pre (<50) = 1.19 (0.43–3.30), p-trend = 0.732; post (50+) = 0.33 (0.14–0.82), p-trend = 0.026	Breslow 2001, U.S. (Steenland 1995 and Albanes 1989 earlier reports) [67,98,99]
Nested case-control study (Black Women's Health Study) (1995–1999)	704	Both	Recreational	High school; ages 21, 30, and 40	H/week of strenuous activity during each time period	7+ vs. <1 h/week at age 21 = 0.5 (0.3–0.8), age 30 = 0.6 (0.3–0.9); age 40 = 0.3 (0.1–0.9); no association with high school	Adams–Campbell 2001, U.S. [83]

Population-based case-control (1996–1998)	1459	Both	Recreational and occupational	Ages 13–19 and last 10 years; lifetime occupation	Reported up to five activities per time period, duration and length of participation in each to calculate MET-h/day; reported each job held at least 3 years, duration, and h standing or walking	Regular adolescent and adult activity vs. none, pre = 0.57 (0.40–0.82), p-trend < 0.01, post = 0.36 (0.24–0.55), p-trend < 0.01; 6+ vs. <1 h/day standing/walking = 0.61 (0.48–0.77), p-trend < 0.01	Matthews 2001, China [84]
Population-based case-control (1995–1997)	1233	Both	Recreational and occupational combined	Lifetime	Recalled each activity's duration, frequency, length, and intensity to calculate MET-h/week for each time period and lifetime	Lifetime total activity 134.9+ vs. <86.MET/week/yr pre = 1.07 (0.72–1.61), p-trend = 0.50, post = 0.70 (0.52–0.94), p-trend = 0.003	Friedenreich 2001, Canada (Friedenreich 2001; Friedenreich 2001 earlier reports) [85,104,105]
Population-based case-control (1992–1994)	712	Both	Recreational	Year prior to reference date	Frequency of activity for at least 6 mo in year prior to reference date used to calculate MET-h/week	80+ vs. <25 MET/week for pre: Hisp = 0.29 (0.12–0.72), p-trend < 0.0001, non-Hisp = 1.13 (0.49–2.61), p-trend = 0.741; for post: Hisp = 0.38 (0.18–0.77), p-trend = 0.002, non-Hisp = 0.45 (0.24–0.85), p-trend = 0.019	Gilliland 2001, U.S. [86]

—continued

TABLE 4.1 (CONTINUED)
Previous Studies of Physical Activity and Breast Cancer

Study design (study date)	No. of cases	Pre- or postmenopausal	Type of activity	Timing of activity	How activity measured	Main findings	Author, date, and location
Population-based case-control (1998)	364	Combined	Recreational	Lifetime (ages 12–18, 19–34, 35–49, 50+)	Number of years, mo/yr, h/week of each activity used to calculate MET-h/week	Lifetime Q4 vs. Q1 = 1.10 (0.73–1.67), p-trend = 0.47; no association with any specific time period	Lee 2001, U.S. [87]
Prospective cohort (Swedish Twin Registry) (1967–1997)	506	Both	Recreational and occupational	Baseline	Reported exercise level (hardly any, light, regular, hard); reported level at work (sedentary, active, strenuous)	Regular vs. sedentary recreational pre = 1.3 (0.7–2.5), p-trend = 0.5, post = 0.6 (0.4–1.0), p-trend = 0.07; strenuous vs. sedentary occupational pre = 1.0 (0.4–2.1), p-trend = 0.1, post = 0.8 (0.5–1.3), p-trend = 0.3	Moradi 2002, Sweden [68]
Prospective cohort (CPS-II Nutrition Cohort) (1992–1997)	1520	Postmenopausal	Recreational	Year prior to baseline, 10 years prior to baseline, and age 40	1992 and age 40 report frequency of seven activities used to calculate MET-h/week; 1982 level as none, slight, moderate, heavy	Baseline 42+ vs. <7 = 0.71 (0.49–1.02), p-trend = 0.08; no association with age 40 or 1982	Patel 2003, U.S. [69]

Prospective cohort (Nurses Health Study II) (1989–1999)	849	Premenopausal	Recreational	High school, ages 18–22, baseline, and during f/u in 1991 and 1997	Report of up to eight activities in each time period to calculate MET-h/week	Recent activity: 27+ vs. <3 METs 1.04 (0.82–1.33), p-trend = 0.86; no association with high school or ages 18–22	Colditz 2003, U.S. (reanalysis of Rockhill, 1998 with longer follow-up) [70,102]
Prospective cohort (Finnish Teachers Study) (1967–2000)	465	Combined	Occupational	Baseline	Comparison of PE teachers vs. language teachers	PE vs. language teachers = 0.83 (0.63–1.09)	Rintala 2003, Finland (Pukkala 1993 and Vihko 1992 earlier reports) [110,117,118]
Prospective cohort (Women's Health Initiative) (1993–1998)	1783	Postmenopausal	Recreational	Baseline; ages 18, 35, and 50	Frequency, duration, and speed of activities used to calculate MET-h/week	40+ vs. none baseline = 0.78 (0.62–1.00), p-trend = 0.03	McTiernan 2003, U.S. [71]
Population-based case-control (1987–1989; 1992; 1995–1996)	1883	Postmenopausal	Recreational	Lifetime of at least 2 h/week	Each activity, frequency, duration, type, age started and stopped recorded and used to calculate average lifetime MET-h/week	Lifetime 17.6+ vs. 0 METs = 0.66 (0.48–0.90), p-trend = 0.07	Carpenter 2003, U.S. (extended analysis of Carpenter 1999) [88,106]

—continued

TABLE 4.1 (CONTINUED)
Previous Studies of Physical Activity and Breast Cancer

Study design (study date)	No. of cases	Pre- or postmenopausal	Type of activity	Timing of activity	How activity measured	Main findings	Author, date, and location
Population-based case-control (1986–1991)	740	Both	Recreational and occupational	Recreational activity at 2, 10, and 20 years before interview and age 16; lifetime occupation	Type and frequency of all activities that worked up a sweat at given time periods used to calculate h/yr; NCI physical activity job matrix used to convert each job held at least 1 year	Lifetime adult activity 546+ vs. 0 h/yr for pre = 1.07 (0.57–2.02) p-trend = 0.82, post = 0.78 (0.47–1.29) p-trend = 0.19; no assoc with any specific time period; % work years in moderate+ jobs 100% vs. 0%, pre = 1.02 (0.63–1.67) p-trend = 0.41, post = 1.55 (1.02–2.36) p-trend = 0.32)	Dorn 2003, U.S. [89]
Population-based case-control (1995–1998)	1593	Both	Recreational and occupational	Lifetime	Duration, frequency, and type of regular exercise through lifetime (at least 1 h/week for at least 4 mo/yr); daily living activities at least 20 min/day and limited to strenuous chores; using job title, each job held at least 1 year converted to activity level	Recreational: 20.8+ vs. <9.1 h/week pre = 0.74 (0.52–1.05); 21.7+ vs. <9.6 h/week post = 0.81 (0.64–1.02); moderate or strenuous jobs: 10.3+ vs. 0 h/week pre = 0.76 (0.53–1.10), 9.1+ vs. 0 h/week post = 0.70 (0.55–0.88)	John 2003, U.S. [90]

Population-based case-control (1999–2000)	360	Premenopausal	Recreational and occupational	Ages 12–19 and 20–30; lifetime occupation	Duration, intensity, and frequency of walking, cycling, household tasks, and 41 sports activities used to calculate MET-h/week; any job held at least 1 year classified and converted to MET-h/week	Recreational ages 12–30: 145.6+ vs. <70.4 MET/week = 0.94 (0.65–1.35), p-trend = 0.29; no difference in diff time periods; occupational METs: 35.1+ vs. <13.9 MET/week = 0.83 (0.59–1.18), p-trend = 0.56)	Steindorf 2003, Germany [92]
Population-based case-control (1995–1997)	501	Both	Recreational and occupational	Lifetime of at least 2 h/week; lifetime occupation	Frequency and duration of all episodes of activity (at least 2 h/week) to calculate lifetime, 10 yrs after menarche, menarche to age 39, age 40 to reference, and 10 years prior to reference; duration of up to three jobs converted by census	Lifetime 12+ vs. <3 MET/week: pre = 0.44 (0.25–0.78) p-trend = 0.004, post = 0.55 (0.33–0.92) p-trend = 0.003; Years held active jobs: 16+ vs. 0 = 0.63 (0.34–1.18) p-trend = 0.18	Yang 2003, U.S. [93]

—*continued*

TABLE 4.1 (CONTINUED)
Previous Studies of Physical Activity and Breast Cancer

Study design (study date)	No. of cases	Pre- or postmenopausal	Type of activity	Timing of activity	How activity measured	Main findings	Author, date, and location
Population-based case-control (1995–1998)	567	Combined (in situ breast cancer only)	Recreational	Lifetime	Each activity, frequency, duration, type, age started and stopped recorded and used to calculate average lifetime MET-h/week	MET/wk 32.+ vs. <3.0 = 0.65 (0.39–1.08), p-trend = 0.27; difference by timing of activity; for 10 yrs after menarche p-trend = 0.14, for ages 20–34 p-trend = 0.36, for 10 yrs before reference date, 4+ vs. no h/wk activity = 0.52 (0.33–0.80), p-trend = 0.03	Patel 2003, U.S. [91]
Hospital-based case-control (1988–2000)	2376	Both	Recreational	Year prior to interview	Frequency of physical activity (none, occasional, three to four times/mo, two-plus times/wk)	2+ times/wk vs. none, pre = 0.80 (0.64–1.00), p-trend = 0.129, post = 0.85 (0.69-1.04), p-trend = 0.131	Hirose 2003, Japan (Hirose 1995 earlier report) [97,107]
Hospital-based case-control (1997–1998)	257	Both	Occupational	Lifetime	Composite of occupational activity based on duration, frequency, and intensity	Moderate/high vs. sedentary: all = 0.71 (0.46–1.10) p-trend = 0.0001, age <55 = 1.04 (0.59–1.84), age 55+ = 0.40 (0.20–0.81)	Kruk 2003, Poland [124]

Despite the variety of questionnaire approaches, the range of detail obtained, and the paucity of information on intensity of physical activities collected, most epidemiological studies have observed an inverse association between recreational physical activity and breast cancer risk. However, the amount of physical activity needed to lower breast cancer risk by a certain percentage remains unclear.

The hypothesized biological mechanisms mediating an association between physical activity and breast cancer are based on observed physiological effects of moderate to vigorous exercise. However, no information is available regarding the direct physiological response to less intense activities. The effect of low-intensity activity (such as household activities, gardening, dancing, leisurely walking, or other activities with a MET score below 4) is still unclear, but may be of importance — particularly for postmenopausal breast cancer — because a large portion of activity among postmenopausal and elderly women is not vigorous [112].

Although previous studies have examined the association between leisure physical activity, such as walking, biking, swimming, and aerobics, not all studies have included the effects of other low-intensity activities, such as gardening, housework, or shopping, in their calculation of leisure physical activity; this may lead to an underestimation of true energy expenditure. A study examining the effect of retirement on leisure physical activity levels showed levels of recreational activity, including walking and household or gardening activity increased after retirement regardless of individuals' physical activity while they were working adults [112]. Therefore, in studies of postmenopausal breast cancer, especially those including some retired persons, inclusion of activities such as gardening or other housework may be important when calculating leisure activity levels.

Not only does the existing literature differ in the methods used to collect physical activity information, but studies also differ dramatically in the time frame of exposure. The time period of activity during a woman's life that is most important for predicting her breast cancer risk is still unclear because estrogen levels throughout a woman's life are key determinants of breast cancer risk among pre- and postmenopausal women. Lifetime recreational physical activity recording activity for every year of life [72,85,88,91], adolescent physical activity [62,64,71,72,79,82,84], and recent or baseline physical activity [57–61,64,65,69,71,74,84,86,88,97] have been associated with lower breast cancer risk. Studies examining risk more broadly for specific decades of life (asking a woman about activity in her teens, 20s, 30s, 40s, etc.) also have observed an inverse association with specific or all examined time periods [82,95,96].

Furthermore, studies have shown that even physical activity initiated after menopause can be beneficial in reducing breast cancer risk [59,69,71]. Women who are active as adolescents and young adults are generally more likely to engage in exercise activities later in life than women who were never active [113]; thus, it has been an epidemiological challenge to examine risk in women who are only active at one point in time. Therefore, even though it appears that physical activity at various points during a woman's lifetime (although affecting hormones and other potential mechanisms differently) may reduce risk of breast cancer, the important time periods for predicting risk remain unclear.

Epidemiological studies are also limited in their ability to measure lifetime or past physical activity without potential bias or misclassification of that past exposure because studies depend on the participant's ability to recall past activity accurately. Studies assessing the reliability of long-term recall of physical activity have shown that agreement between baseline and recalled activity was generally about 75% [114,115]. Participant characteristics, such as age, race, education, body weight, and marital status, have been shown to have little association with quality of recall of past physical activity [116]. The likelihood of recall bias has been minimized in many studies that have used validated lifetime calendars to aid study participants in recalling physical activity throughout their lifetime [72,85,88,91]. In cohort studies, the inability to recall past activity levels accurately would most likely be nondifferential, biasing risk estimates toward the null value; however, few cohort studies have attempted to obtain any historical information regarding physical activity [69–71].

Occupational Physical Activity

Twenty-one observational studies have examined the relationship between occupational physical activity and breast cancer risk. Two studies yielded more than one publication [110,117–120]; consequently, only the most recent report from each study has been included in Table 4.1. An association of sedentary occupations with increased risk of breast cancer has been documented in reports from three [58,64,110] of five [58,64,68,110,121] prospective cohort studies. Published reports from six [80,84,90,104,120,122] of eleven [78,80,81,84,89,90,92,93,104,120,122] population-based case-control studies and three [96,123,124] of four [96,123–125] hospital-based case-control studies also document an inverse association between occupational physical activity and breast cancer risk. Finally, one retrospective cohort study [126] documented an inverse association between high levels of occupational activity and breast cancer risk (Table 4.1).

Levels of occupational physical activity have been estimated indirectly by converting job titles using a predetermined coding schema such as the U.S. Department of Labor occupational activity codes [122,126] or by self-reported level of occupational physical activity (sedentary, light, moderate, heavy lifting) [58,68,96,121]. Generally, results across these studies have been consistent despite the different approaches for assigning intensity levels for the occupational activities.

Ten previous studies calculated a quasi-lifetime occupational physical activity score based on report of "usual lifetime" or "longest held" occupation [58,68,78,80,81,110,120,121,125,126] and eleven studies calculated occupational physical activity based on study participants reporting multiple or all jobs held throughout their lifetime [64,84,89, 90,92,93,96,104,122–124]. Studies using a composite measure of lifetime physical activity based on the reporting of multiple or all jobs held more often observed an inverse association with breast cancer risk [64,84,90, 96,104,110,122,123] than did studies that utilized usual lifetime occupation [58,80,120,126]. Using "usual occupation" to define lifetime occupational physical activity likely misclassifies and underestimates true lifetime activity levels, thus leading to a potential bias in risk estimates.

Confounding and Effect Modification

Few risk factors for breast cancer are likely to be true confounders of the relationship between physical activity and breast cancer. Moreover, lifetime or historical measures of physical activity are likely to be unaffected by adjustment for recent diet, BMI, or other baseline factors because these factors are not generally related to activity at earlier time points. In studies of recent recreational physical activity, adjustment for potential confounding factors has not had a large impact on risk estimates [61,69,70,86].

The most commonly hypothesized confounder of the relationship between physical activity and breast cancer risk is obesity; with the exception of a few studies [56,64,74,79,84], all studies of recreational physical activity adjusted for obesity using BMI. Most studies of recreational physical activity also have adjusted for other potential confounders, such as age, parity, family history, energy intake, menopausal hormone use, and alcohol intake. Studies of occupational physical activity were least likely to consider potential confounding factors [68,121,122,125–127]. However, the association between physical activity and breast cancer has not been greatly attenuated by adjustment for potential confounding factors.

Potential effect modification by various factors has been assessed in some previous studies. One may speculate that the influence of moderate levels of physical activity on hormone levels in women with a favorable estrogen profile (i.e., lower baseline levels of hormones) may be sufficient to reduce risk. Women with higher levels of baseline circulating estrogens, such as women with a positive family history of breast cancer, current menopausal hormone users, or obese women, may not experience a reduction in risk with moderate physical activity. Women with higher baseline estrogen levels may require more vigorous and frequent activity to substantiate a reduction in risk.

Results from two studies suggest that the association with physical activity may be stronger in women without a family history of breast cancer [88,91]. Two previous studies also report a greater reduction in risk with increasing physical activity among parous women compared to nulliparous women [72,101]; however, two other studies documented the opposite finding, with risk reduction greater in nulliparous women [81,105]. In four previous studies [63,69,77,85], researchers examined potential effect modification by menopausal hormone use, and one study suggests that physical activity may be more strongly associated with postmenopausal breast cancer in nonusers of menopausal hormones [69]. In four previous studies, researchers examined effect modification by adult weight gain [61,64,82,106]; one study reported a greater reduction in risk among women who had less than a 17% increase in weight [106].

Some studies documented a greater reduction in risk among leaner women compared to heavier women [58,71,81,88]. In addition to the potential role of obesity as a confounder or effect modifier, there is the possibility that obesity may be on the causal pathway between physical activity and primarily postmenopausal breast cancer development. For example, physical activity around the time of menopause may reduce postmenopausal obesity and may subsequently prevent the initiation of malignant transformation of breast cells [128]. However, most studies of physical activity and breast cancer adjusted for BMI, and an inverse association persisted; additionally, physical activity may have direct effects on circulating hormone levels independent of the impact on BMI. Thus, it is unlikely that the observed inverse association between physical activity and breast cancer risk is entirely explained by BMI. Differentiating among effects of confounding, effect modification, and factors in the causal pathway is an ongoing epidemiological challenge in examining the association between physical activity and breast cancer risk.

Discrepancies in study results may be due to underlying differences in study population characteristics, a lack of sufficient statistical power to detect a true difference between subgroups, or chance. It should also be noted that the study publications reporting no effect modification have not provided details of analyses; therefore, it is difficult to ascertain whether the failure to observe significant effect modification is due to a lack of sufficient statistical power.

CONCLUSIONS

In summary, most previous observational studies observe an inverse association between physical activity and breast cancer risk. Risk appears to be reduced among women reporting physical activity at various points throughout their lifetime. The specific amount of physical activity necessary to infer a reduction in risk is not fully understood, but many previous studies suggest that 3 to 4 or more hours per week may be necessary to see an impact on breast cancer risk. Although the exact frequency, duration, and intensity are not well established, there is sufficient evidence that promotion of physical activity is an important modifiable factor for breast cancer risk.

REFERENCES

1. McManus MJ, Welsch CW. The effects of estrogen, progesterone, and human placental lactogen on DNA synthesis on human breast ductal epithelium uaintained in athymic mice. *Cancer* 1984; 54:1920–1927.
2. Laidlaw IJ, Clarke RB, Howell A, Owen AW, Potten CS, Anderson E. The proliferation of normal human breast tissue implanted into athymic nude mice is stimulated by estrogen but not progesterone. *Endocrinology* 1995; 136:164–171.
3. Chang KJ, Lee TT, Linares–Cruz G, Fournier S, Lignieres BD. Influence of percutaneous administration of estradiol and progesterone on human breast epithelial cell *in vivo*. *Fertil Steril* 1995; 63:785–791.
4. Henderson BE, Ross RK, Judd HL, Krailo MD, Pike MC. Do regular ovulatory cycles increase breast cancer risk? *Cancer* 1985; 56:1206–1208.

5. Henderson BE, Ross RK, Bernstein L. Estrogens as a cause of human cancer: the Richard and Hinda Rosenthal Foundation award lecture. *Cancer Res* 1988; 48:246–253.
6. Warren M. The effects of exercise on pubertal progression and reproductive function in girls. *J Clin Endocrinol Metab* 1980; 51:1150–1157.
7. Frisch RE, Goetz–Welbergen AV, McArthur JW et al. Delayed menarche and amenorrhea of college athletes in relation to age at onset of training. *JAMA* 1981; 246:1559–1563.
8. Shangold M, Freeman R, Thysen B, Gatz M. The relationship between long-distance running, plasma progesterone, and luteal phase length. *Fertil Steril* 1979; 31:130–133.
9. Ellison PT, Lager C. Moderate recreational running is associated with lowered salivary progesterone profiles in women. *Am J Obstet Gynecol* 1986; 154:100–1003.
10. Bernstein L, Ross RK, Lobo RA, Hanisch R, Krailo MD, Henderson BE. The effects of moderate physical activity on menstrual cycle patterns in adolescence: implications for breast cancer prevention. *Br J Cancer* 1987; 55:681–685.
11. Bonen A, Belcastro AN, Ling WY, Simpson AA. Profiles of selected hormones during menstrual cycles of teenage athletes. *J Appl Physiol* 1981; 50:545–551.
12. Broocks A, Pirke KM, Schweeiger U et al. Cyclic ovarian function in recreational athletes. *J Appl Physiol* 1990; 68:2083–2086.
13. Cooper GS, Sandler DP, Whelan EA, Smith KR. Association of physical and behavioral characteristics with menstrual cycle patterns in women age 29–31 years. *Epidemiology* 1996; 7:624–628.
14. DeSouza MJ. Menstrual disturbances in athletes: a focus on luteal phase defects. *Med Sci Sports Exercise* 2003; 35:1553–1663.
15. Key TJA, Pike MC. The dose–effect relationship between "unopposed" estrogen and endometrial mitotic rate: its central role in explaining and predicting endometrial cancer risk. *Br J Cancer* 1988; 57:205–212.
16. Nelson ME, Meredith CN, Dawson–Hughes B, Evans WJ. Hormone and bone mineral status in endurance-trained and sedentary postmenopausal women. *J Clin Endocrinol Metab* 1988; 66:927–933.
17. Cauley JA, Gutai JP, Kuller LH, LeDonne D, Powell JG. The epidemiology of serum sex hormones in postmenopausal women. *Am J Epidemiol* 1989; 129:1120–1131.
18. Nagata C, Shimizu H, Takami R, Hayashi M, Takeda N, Yasuda K. Relations of insulin resistance and serum concentrations of estradiol and sex hormone-bonding globulin to potential breast cancer risk factors. *Jpn J Cancer Res* 2000; 91:948–953.
19. McTiernan A, Tworoger SS, Rajan KB et al. Effect of exercise on serum androgens in postmenopausal women: a 12-month randomized clinical trial. *Cancer Epidemiol Biomarkers Prev* 2004; 13:1099–1105.
20. Tymchuk CN, Tessler SB, Barnard RJ. Changes in sex hormone-binding globulin, insulin, and serum lipids in postmenopausal women on a low-fat, high-fiber diet combined with exercise. *Nutr Cancer* 2000; 38:158–162.
21. Verkasalo PK, Thomas HV, Appleby PN, Davey GK, Key TJ. Circulating levels of sex hormones and their relation to risk factors for breast cancer: a cross-sectional study in 1092 pre- and postmenopausal women (U.K.). *Cancer Causes Control* 2001; 12:47–59.
22. Newcomb PA, Klein R, Klein BEK et al. Association of dietary and life-style factors with sex hormones in postmenopausal women. *Epidemiology* 1995; 6:318–321.
23. Atkinson C, Lampe JW, Tworoger SS et al. Effects of a moderate intensity exercise intervention on estrogen metabolism in postmenopausal women. *Cancer Epidemiol Biomarkers Prev* 2004; 13:868–874.
24. Kelsey JL, Berkowitz GS. Breast cancer epidemiology. *Cancer Res* 1988; 48:5615–5623.
25. Feigelson HS, Jonas CR, Teras LR, Thun MJ, Calle EE. Weight gain, body mass index, hormone replacement therapy, and postmenopausal breast cancer in a large prospective study. *Cancer Epidemiol Biomarkers Prev* 2004; 12:220–224.
26. Endogenous Hormones and Breast Cancer Collaborative Group. Body mass index, serum sex hormones, and breast cancer risk in postmenopausal women. *J Natl Cancer Inst* 2003; 95:1218–1226.
27. Huang Z, Hankinson SE, Colditz GA et al. Dual effects of weight and weight gain on breast cancer risk. *JAMA* 1997; 278:1407–1411.
28. Morimoto LB, White E, Chen Z et al. Obesity, body size, and risk of postmenopausal breast cancer: the Women's Health Initiative (U.S.). *Cancer Causes Control* 2002; 13:741–751.

29. Thune I, Njolstad I, Lochen ML, Forde OH. Physical activity improves the metabolic risk profiles in men and women. *Arch Intern Med* 1998; 158:1633–1640.
30. Pollak MN, Schernhammer ES, Hankinson SE. Insulin-like growth factors and neoplasia. *Nat Rev* 2004; 4:505–518.
31. Nestler JE, Powers LP, Matt DW et al. A direct effect of hyperinsulinemia on serum sex hormone-binding globulin levels in obese women with the polycystic ovary syndrome. *J Clin Endocrinol Metab* 1991; 72:83–89.
32. Lawlor DA, Smith GD, Ebrahim S. Hyperinsulinaemia and increased risk of breast cancer: findings from the British Women's Heart and Health Study. *Cancer Causes Control* 2004; 15:267–275.
33. Borugian MJ, Sheps SB, Kim–Sing C et al. Insulin, macronutrient intake, and physical activity: are potential indicators of insulin resistance associated with mortality from breast cancer? *Cancer Epidemiol Biomarkers Prev* 2004; 13:1163–1172.
34. Conover CA, Lee PDK, Kanaley JA, Clarkson JT, Jensen MD. Insulin regulation of insulin-like growth factor binding protein-1 in obese and nonobese humans. *J Clin Endocrinol Metab* 1992; 74:1355–1360.
35. Jones JI, Clemmons DR. Insulin-like growth factors and their binding proteins: biological actions. *Endrocrinol Rev* 1995; 16:3–34.
36. Figueroa JA, Sharma J, Jackson JG, McDermott MJ, Hilsenbeck SG, Yee D. Recombinant insulin-like growth factor binding protein-1 inhibits IGF-1, serum, and estrogen dependent growth of MCF-7 human breast cancer cells. *J Cell Physiol* 1993; 157:229–236.
37. McGuire WL, Jackson JG, Figueroa JA, Shimasaki S, Powell DR, Yee D. Regulation of insulin-like growth factor binding protein (IGFBP) expression by breast cancer cells: use of IGFBP-1 as an inhibitor of insulin-like growth factor action. *J Natl Cancer Inst* 1992; 84:1336–1341.
38. Hankinson SE, Willett WC, Colditz GA et al. Circulating concentrations of insulin-like growth factor-I and risk of breast cancer. *Lancet* 1998; 351:1393–1396.
39. Agurs–Collins T, Adams–Campbell L, Sook K, Culten KJ. Insulin-like growth factor-I and breast cancer risk in postmenopausal African–American women [abstract]. *Proc Am Assoc Cancer Res* 1999; 40:152.
40. Sugumar A, Liu Y, Xia Q, Koh Y, Matsuo K. Insulin-like growth factor (IGF)-I and IGF-binding protein 3 and the risk of premenopausal breast cancer: a meta-analysis of the literature. *Int J Cancer* 2004; 111:293–297.
41. Helmrich SP, Ragland DR, Leung RW. Physical activity and reduced occurrence of non-insulin-dependent diabetes mellitus. *N Engl J Med* 1991; 325:147–152.
42. Kaaks R, Lukanova A. Energy balance and cancer: the role of insulin and insulin-like growth factor-I. *Proc Nutr Soc* 2001; 60:91–106.
43. Yu H, Rohan T. Role of the insulin-like growth factor family in cancer development and progression. *J Natl Cancer Inst* 2000; 92:1472–1489.
44. Pedersen BK, Tvede N, Christensen LD, Lkarlund K, Kragbak S, Halkjr–Kristensen J. Natural killer cell activity in peripheral blood of highly trained and untrained persons. *Int J Sports Med* 1989; 10:129–131.
45. Long EO. Tumor cell recognition by natural killer cells. *Semin Cancer Biol* 2002; 12:57–61.
46. Curran EM, Berghaus LJ, Vernetti NJ, Saporita AJ, Lubahn DB, Estes DM. Natural killer cells express estrogen receptor-alpha and estrogen receptor-beta and can respond via a non-estrogen receptor-alpha-mediated pathway. *Cell Immunol* 2001; 214:12–20.
47. Seaman WB, Gindhart TD. Effect of estrogen on natural killer cells. *Arthritis Rheumatol* 1979; 22:1234–1240.
48. Hanna N, Schneider M. Enhancement of tumor metastasis and suppression of natural killer cell activity by B-estradiol treatment. *J Immunol* 1983; 130:974–980.
49. Flatt JP. Dietary fat, carbohydrate balance, and weight maintenance. *Ann NY Acad Sci* 1993; 683:122–140.
50. Bruning PF, Bonfree JB, vanNoord PA, deJong–Bakker M, Nooijen WJ. Insulin resistance and breast cancer risk. *Int J Cancer* 1992; 52:511–516.
51. Ballard–Barbash R. Perspectives on integrating experimental and epidemiologic research on diet, anthropometry, and breast cancer. *J Nutr* 1997; 127 (Supp. 5).
52. Pike MC, Spicer DV, Dahmoush L, Press MF. Estrogens, progestogens, normal breast cell proliferation, and breast cancer risk. *Epidemiol Rev* 1993; 15:17–35.

53. Stallone DD. The influence of obesity and its treatment on the immune system. *Nutr Rev* 1994; 52:37–50.
54. Willett WC. Fat, energy, and cancer. *J Nutr* 1997; 127:921S–923S.
55. Blair SN. Evidence for success of exercise in weight loss and control. *Ann Intern Med* 1993; 119:702–706.
56. Dorgan JF, Brown C, Barrett M et al. Physical activity and risk of breast cancer in the Framingham Heart Study. *Am J Epidemiol* 1994; 139:662–669.
57. Fraser GE, Shavlik D. Risk factors, lifetime risk, and age at onset of breast cancer. *Ann Epidemiol* 1997; 7:375–382.
58. Thune I, Brenn T, Lund E, Gaard M. Physical activity and the risk of breast cancer. *N Engl J Med* 1997; 336:1269–1275.
59. Cerhan JR, Chiu BC, Wallace RB et al. Physical activity, physical function, and the risk of breast cancer in a prospective study among elderly women. *J Gerontol* 1998; 53A:M251–M256.
60. Sesso HD, Paffenbarger RS, Lee IM. Physical activity and breast cancer risk in the College Alumni Health Study (US). *Cancer Causes Control* 1998; 9:433–439.
61. Rockhill B, Willett WC, Hunter DJ, Manson JE, Hankinson SE, Colditz GA. A prospective study of recreational physical activity and breast cancer risk. *Arch Intern Med* 1999; 159:2290–2296.
62. Wyshak G, Frisch RE. Breast cancer among former college athletes compared to nonathletes: a 15-year follow-up. *Br J Cancer* 2000; 82:726–730.
63. Moore DB, Folsom AR, Mink PJ, Hong CP, Anderson KE, Kushi LH. Physical activity and incidence of postmenopausal breast cancer. *Epidemiology* 2000; 11:292–296.
64. Dirx MJM, Voorrips LE, Goldbohm RA, vandenBrant PA. Baseline recreational physical activity, history of sports participation, and postmenopausal breast carcinoma risk in the Netherlands Cohort Study. *Cancer* 2001; 92:1638–1649.
65. Lee IM, Rexrode KM, Cook NR, Hennekens CH, Buring JE. Physical activity and breast cancer risk: the Women's Health Study (U.S.). *Cancer Causes Control* 2001; 12:137–145.
66. Luoto R, Latikka P, Pukkala E, Hakulinen T, Vikho V. The effect of physical activity on breast cancer risk: a cohort study of 30,548 women. *Eur J Epidemiol* 2001; 16:973–980.
67. Breslow RA, Ballard–Barbash R, Munoz K, Graubard BI. Long-term recreational physical activity and breast cancer in the National Health and Nutrition Examination Survey I Epidemiologic Follow-up Study. *Cancer Epidemiol Biomarkers Prev* 2001; 10:805–808.
68. Moradi T, Adami H, Ekbom A et al. Physical activity and risk for breast cancer: a prospective cohort study among Swedish twins. *Int J Cancer* 2002; 100:76–81.
69. Patel AV, Calle EE, Bernstein L, Wu AH, Thun MJ. Recreational physical activity and risk of postmenopausal breast cancer in a large cohort of U.S. women. *Cancer Causes Control* 2003; 14:519–529.
70. Colditz GA, Feskanich D, Chen WY, Hunter DJ, Willett WC. Physical activity and risk of breast cancer in premenopausal women. *Br J Cancer* 2003; 89:847–851.
71. McTiernan A, Kooperberg C, White E et al. Recreational physical activity and the risk of breast cancer in postmenopausal women. *JAMA* 2003; 290:1331–1336.
72. Bernstein L, Henderson BE, Hanisch R, Sullivan–Halley J, Ross RK. Physical exercise and reduced risk of breast cancer in young women. *J Natl Cancer Inst* 1994; 86:1403–1408.
73. Friedenreich CM, Rohan TE. Physical activity and risk of breast cancer. *Eur J Cancer Prev* 1995; 4:145–151.
74. McTiernan A, Stanford JL, Weiss NS, Daling JR, Voigt LF. Occurrence of breast cancer in relation to recreational exercise in women age 50–64 years. *Epidemiology* 1996; 7:598–604.
75. Chen CL, White E, Malone KE, Daling JR. Leisure-time physical activity in relation to breast cancer among young women (Washington, U.S.). *Cancer Causes Control* 1997; 8:77–84.
76. Hu YH, Nagata C, Shimizu H, Kaneda N, Kashiki Y. Association of body mass index, physical activity, and reproductive histories with breast cancer: a case-control study in Gifu, Japan. *Breast Cancer Res Treat* 1997; 43:65–72.
77. Gammon MD, Schoenberg JB, Britton JA et al. Recreational physical activity and breast cancer risk among women under age 45. *Am J Epidemiol* 1998; 147:273–280.
78. Ueji M, Ueno E, Osei–Hyiaman D, Takahashi H, Kano K. Physical activity and the risk of breast cancer: a case-control study of Japanese women. *J Epidemiol* 1999; 8:116–122.

79. Marcus PM, Newman B, Moorman PG et al. Physical activity at age 12 and adult breast cancer risk (U.S.). *Cancer Causes Control* 1999; 10:293–302.
80. Verloop J, Rookus MA, Kooy KVD, Leeuwen FEV. Physical activity and breast cancer risk in women aged 20–54 years. *J Natl Cancer Inst* 2000; 92:128–135.
81. Moradi T, Nyren O, Zack M, Magnusson C, Persson I, Adami HO. Breast cancer risk and lifetime leisure-time and occupational physical activity (Sweden). *Cancer Causes Control* 2000; 11:523–531.
82. Shoff SM, Newcomb PA, Trentham–Dietz A et al. Early-life physical activity and postmenopausal breast cancer: effect of body size and weight change. *Cancer Epidemiol Biomarkers Prev* 2000; 9:591–595.
83. Adams–Campbell LL, Rosenberg L, Rao RS, Palmer JR. Strenuous physical activity and breast cancer risk in African–American women. *J Natl Med Assoc* 2001; 93:267–275.
84. Matthews CE, Shu XO, Jin F et al. Lifetime physical activity and breast cancer risk in the Shanghai Breast Cancer Study. *Br J Cancer* 2001; 84:994–1001.
85. Friedenreich CM, Courneya KS, Bryant HE. Influence of physical activity in different age and life periods on the risk of breast cancer. *Epidemiology* 2001; 12:604–612.
86. Gilliland FD, Li YF, Baumgartner K, Crumley D, Samet JM. Physical activity and breast cancer risk in Hispanic and non-Hispanic white women. *Am J Epidemiol* 2001; 154:442–450.
87. Lee IM, Cook NR, Rexrode KM, Buring JE. Lifetime physical activity and risk of breast cancer. *Br J Cancer* 2001; 85:962–965.
88. Carpenter C, Ross RK, Paganini–Hill A, Bernstein L. Effect of family history, obesity, and exercise on breast cancer risk among postmenopausal women. *Int J Cancer* 2003; 106:96–102.
89. Dorn J, Vena J, Brasure J, Freudenheim J, Graham S. Lifetime physical activity and breast cancer risk in pre- and postmenopausal women. *Med Sci Sports Exercise* 2003; 35:278–285.
90. John EM, Horn–Ross PL, Koo J. Lifetime physical activity and breast cancer risk in a multiethnic population: the San Francisco Bay Area Breast Cancer Study. *Cancer Epidemiol Biomarkers Prev* 2003; 12:1143–1152.
91. Patel AV, Press MF, Meeske K, Calle EE, Bernstein L. Lifetime recreational exercise activity and risk of breast carcinoma *in situ*. *Cancer* 2003; 98:2161–2169.
92. Steindorf K, Schmidt M, Kropp S, Chang–Claude J. Case-control study of physical activity and breast cancer risk among premenopausal women in Germany. *Am J Epidemiol* 2003; 157:121–130.
93. Yang D, Bernstein L, Wu AH. Physical activity and breast cancer risk among Asian–American women in Los Angeles. *Cancer* 2003; 97:2565–2575.
94. Taioli E, Barone J, Wynder EL. A case-control study on breast cancer and body mass. *Eur J Cancer* 1995; 31A:723–728.
95. Mezzetti M, LaVecchia C, Decarli A, Boyle P, Talamini R, Franceschi S. Population attributable risk for breast cancer: diet, nutrition, and physical exercise. *J Natl Cancer Inst* 1998; 90:389–394.
96. Levi F, Pasche C, Lucchini F, LaVecchia C. Occupational and leisure time physical activity and the risk of breast cancer. *Eur J Cancer* 1999; 35:775–778.
97. Hirose K, Hamajima N, Takezaki T, Miura S, Tajima K. Physical activity reduces risk of breast cancer in Japanese women. *Cancer Sci* 2003; 94:193–199.
98. Albanes D, Blair A, Taylor P. Physical activity and risk of cancer in the NHANES I population. *Am J Public Health* 1989; 79:744–750.
99. Steenland K, Nowlin S, Palu S. Cancer incidence in the National Health and Nutrition Survey I follow-up data: diabetes, cholesterol, pulse, and physical activity. *Cancer Epidemiol Biomarkers Prev* 1995; 4:807–811.
100. Frisch RE, Wyshak G, Albright NL et al. Lower prevalence of breast cancer and cancers of the reproductive system among former college athletes compared to nonathletes. *Br J Cancer* 1985; 52:885–891.
101. Frisch RE, Wyshak G, Albright NL et al. Lower lifetime occurrence of breast cancer and cancers of the reproductive system among former college athletes. *Am J Clin Nutr* 1987; 45:328–335.
102. Rockhill B, Willett WC, Hunter DJ et al. Physical activity and breast cancer risk in a cohort of young women. *J Natl Cancer Inst* 1998; 90:1155–1160.
103. Mittendorf R, Longnecker MP, Newcomb PA et al. Strenuous physical activity in young adulthood and risk of breast cancer (U.S.). *Cancer Causes Control* 1995; 6:347–353.

104. Friedenreich CM, Bryant HE, Courneya KS. Case-control study of lifetime physical activity and breast cancer risk. *Am J Epidemiol* 2001; 154:336–347.
105. Friedenreich CM, Courneya KS, Bryant HE. Relation between intensity of physical activity and breast cancer risk reduction. *Med Sci Sports Exercise* 2001; 33:1538–1545.
106. Carpenter CL, Ross RK, Paganini–Hill A, Bernstein L. Lifetime exercise activity and breast cancer risk among postmenopausal women. *Br J Cancer* 1999; 80:1852–1858.
107. Hirose K, Tajima K, Hamajima N et al. A large-scale, hospital-based case-control study of risk factors of breast cancer according to menopausal status. *Jpn J Cancer Res* 1995; 86:146–154.
108. Enger SM, Ross RK, Paganini–Hill A, Carpenter CL, Bernstein L. Body size, physical activity, and breast cancer hormone receptor status: results from two case-control studies. *Cancer Epidemiol Biomarkers Prev* 2000; 9:681–687.
109. King MC, Marks JH, Mandell JB, The New York Breast Cancer Study Group. Breast and ovarian cancer risks due to inherited mutations in BRCA1 and BRCA2. *Science* 2003; 302:643–646.
110. Rintala P, Pukkala E, Laara E, Vikho V. Physical activity and breast cancer risk among female physical education and language teachers: a 34-year follow-up. *Int J Cancer* 2003; 107:268–270.
111. Ainsworth BE, Sternfeld B, Slattery ML, Daguise V, Zahm SH. Physical activity and breast cancer: evaluation of physical activity assessment methods. *Cancer* (Supplement) 1998; 83:611–620.
112. Evenson KR, Rosamond WD, Cai J, Diez–Roux AV, Brancati FL. Influence of retirement on leisure-time physical activity: the Atherosclerosis Risk in Communities Study. *Am J Epidemiol* 2002; 155:692–699.
113. Alfano CM, Klesges RC, Murray DM, Beech BM, McClanahan BS. History of sport participation in relation to obesity and related health behaviors in women. *Prev Med* 2002; 34:82–89.
114. Blair SN, Dowda M, Pate RR et al. Reliability of long-term recall of participation in physical activity by middle-aged men and women. *Am J Epidemiol* 1991; 133:266–275.
115. Falkner KL, Trevisan M, McCann SE. Reliability of recall of physical activity in the distant past. *Am J Epidemiol* 1999; 150:195–205.
116. Falkner KL, McCann SE, Trevisan M. Participant characteristics and quality of recall of physical activity in the distant past. *Am J Epidemiol* 2001; 154:865–872.
117. Pukkala E, Poskiparta M, Apter D, Vihko V. Lifelong physical activity and cancer risk among Finnish female teachers. *Eur J Cancer Prev* 1993; 2:369–376.
118. Vihko V, Apter DL, Pukkala EI, Oinonen MT, Hakulinen TR, Vihko RK. Risk of breast cancer among female teachers of physical education and languages. *Acta Oncologica* 1992; 31:201–204.
119. Coogan PF, Clapp RW, Newcomb PA et al. Variation in female breast cancer risk by occupation. *Am J Ind Med* 1996; 30:430–437.
120. Coogan PF, Newcomb PA, Clapp RW, Trentham–Dietz A, Baron JA, Longnecker MP. Physical activity in usual occupation and risk of breast cancer (U.S.). *Cancer Causes Control* 1997; 8:626–631.
121. Moradi T, Adami HO, Bergstrom R et al. Occupational physical activity and risk for breast cancer in a nationwide cohort study in Sweden. *Cancer Causes Control* 1999; 10:423–430.
122. Coogan PF, Aschengrau A. Occupational physical activity and breast cancer risk in the Upper Cape Cod Cancer Incidence Study. *Am J Ind Med* 1999; 36:279–285.
123. D'Avanzo B, Nanni O, LaVecchia C et al. Physical activity and breast cancer risk. *Cancer Epidemiol Biomarkers Prev* 1996; 5:155–160.
124. Kruk J, Aboul–Enein HY. Occupational physical activity and the risk of breast cancer. *Cancer Detection Prev* 2003; 27:187–192.
125. Dosemeci M, Hayes RB, Vetter R et al. Occupational physical activity, socioeconomic status, and risks of 15 cancer sites in Turkey. *Cancer Causes Control* 1993; 4:313–321.
126. Vena JE, Graham S, Zielezny M, Brasure J, Swanson MK. Occupational exercise and risk of cancer. *Am J Clin Nutr* 1987; 45:318–327.
127. Zheng W, Shu XO, McLaughlin JK, Chow WH, Gao YT, Blot WJ. Occupational physical activity and the incidence of cancer of the breast, corpus uteri, and ovary in Shanghai. *Cancer* 1993; 71:3620–3624.
128. Williamson DF, Mandans J, Anda RF, Kleinman JC, Kahn HS, Byers T. Recreational physical activity and ten-year weight change in a U.S. national cohort. *Int J Obesity* 1993; 17:279–286.

5 Physical Activity and Colorectal Cancer

Martha L. Slattery

CONTENTS

Approximately 130,000 new cases and 55,000 deaths are attributed to colorectal cancer yearly in the U.S [1]. Worldwide, approximately 8.5% of all incident cancers are colorectal cancers [2]. A 20-fold variation in reported incidence of colorectal cancer has been noted around the world: developed countries have high incidence rates and developing countries have much lower incidence rates [2]. Furthermore, migrant populations who move from countries of low to high incidence of colon cancer adopt the rates of the host country after migration, suggesting the importance of diet and lifestyle factors in colon cancer etiology [3]. Physical inactivity is gaining in recognition as one of the lifestyle factors that may importantly contribute to the development of colon cancer.

MEASURING PHYSICAL ACTIVITY

Physical activity has many dimensions, including frequency, intensity, and time. Each of these dimensions can be linked to activity performed at work, during recreation, or around the house. The amount of and intensity with which activities are performed may influence what is being measured in physical activity. The time period during one's life when activity levels are measured may have a further impact on associations.

Early studies examining the association between physical activity and colon cancer focused on work-related activity [4,5], comparing those who were most active on the job to those who had lower levels of activity or who were sedentary. As the population transcended from one in which activity on the job was the norm to one in which it was the exception, questionnaires capturing self-reported physical activity became the primary mode of collecting physical activity data. These questionnaires usually differ in their focus on activities done at leisure, work, around the home, or pertaining to care of children and other adults — as well as in their ability to assess duration, frequency, and intensity of activities performed [6–9]. Some questionnaires have gathered detailed information about various types of activity. Others have used more general questions, asking about limited activities and sometimes ignoring intensity of activities performed, and at other times neglecting to determine time involved in specific activities [9–11].

In almost all instances, information on the benefits of continuous vs. cumulative activity and the number of days per week on which activities need to be performed to maximize protective associations have been lacking. The underlying biological mechanisms involved in the disease process and ability of questionnaires to capture these mechanisms may differ and thus influence investigator ability to detect associations with colon and rectal cancer.

In addition to issues surrounding questionnaire design is the ability of study participants to recall activities performed accurately and to assign intensity levels to activities performed that are consistent with how others view and assign their activity levels [9,11,12]. Attempts to test reliability and validity of physical activity data are limited, although activities performed at a more vigorous level of effort appear to be reported more consistently over time than activities performed at moderate levels of effort [12]. It is possible that people who perform the same activities on a regular basis may be more likely to recall their activities than those who do many different activities less frequently.

Associations between colorectal cancer and physical activity have been evaluated by metabolic equivalent tasks (METs) per week; energy expended per week; time spent in activity per week; and ranking individuals based on physical activity index scores that take all available activity data into account. Direct comparison of association between studies using the same measure of physical activity is not possible because of differences in methods used to assess and analyze physical activity. Despite this, associations between colon cancer and physical activity are remarkably consistent.

COLORECTAL CANCER SITE-SPECIFIC ASSOCIATIONS

Site-specific associations within the colorectal area have been examined, including tumors in the proximal, distal, and rectal areas. Anatomic definitions of colorectal cancer tumor sites that are often used include: proximal (cecum through transverse colon); distal (splenic flexure, descending, and sigmoid colon); and rectal (rectosigmoid junction and rectum). Differences in association by tumor site can stem from different study designs used to study associations; limited power to estimate associations when evaluating smaller subsets of data; or etiological differences in associations.

Although many studies of colon cancer and physical activity have been conducted, fewer studies have examined all tumor sites. Thus, studies generally focus on colon cancer or rectal cancer, although some studies have attempted to estimate associations between physical activity and colon and rectal cancer. In a review of the literature (Table 5.1 and Table 5.2), studies have been included that have at least 100 cases of colorectal cancer and have used questionnaires that have at least three physical activity questions. Tables are organized by date of start of data collection rather than date of publication. This was done to provide a historical reference to data collection methods.

COLON CANCER

Associations between colon cancer and physical activity have been consistent for men and women, for different study designs, and for people living in different parts of the world. Several reviews have outlined many of these studies in detail [13–15]. In a review published in 2002 [13], the inverse association was documented in 43 of 51 studies that had evaluated the association. More rigorous studies have focused on total activity, leisure time activity, intensity of activity, and, in some instances, lifetime or long-term activity [13,16–18]. Although a shift in the activity variable studied to describe the association over time has been observed, this shift most probably reflects changes in major sources of activity in the population as well as the need to better understand multiple dimensions of the physical activity and colon cancer relationship.

Potential confounding, a bias that can distort the true association between physical activity and colon and rectal cancer, has been addressed by adjusting for a variety of factors in various studies. Confounding may be an issue because physically active people are thought to have healthier lifestyles and, possibly, lower rates of colorectal cancer. Some studies (often occupational studies using census data) have adjusted only for age; however, others have adjusted for a variety of factors, including body size, diet, screening history, family history, smoking, alcohol use, and use of aspirin — all factors associated with colon and/or rectal cancer — and also may be associated with physical activity. However, studies that have adjusted for other components of a healthy lifestyle, such as not smoking cigarettes, eating a low-risk diet, and using aspirin and/or nonsteroidal anti-inflammatory drugs, still observe the inverse association observed in other studies in which not all of these factors have been taken into account [16,18–22].

Many early studies included cases of colon cancer as early as the 1950s and examined occupational activities, often comparing disease rates among individuals in agricultural or more physically active jobs to those of professionals or people who were more sedentary (Table 5.1). These early studies almost uniformly demonstrated reduced risk of colon cancer. Early studies included little information on leisure activity, often because occupational data were from census records and information on activities performed at leisure was generally lacking. Associations between colon cancer and nonoccupational activity, as well as occupational activity, were reported by Slattery and colleagues in 1988 [23]. This study was one of the first to report nonwork-related activities and to evaluate the impact of intensity of exercise on colon cancer risk. In this case-control study, participants were asked to report the number of hours spent in light, moderate, and intense activity for the 2 years prior to diagnosis or interview. Total physical activity was associated with a reduced risk of colon cancer (OR 0.7 95% CI 0.4 to 1.3 for men and 0.5 95% CI 0.3 to 0.9 for women). Associations were strongest for intense activities among men (OR 0.3 95% CI 0.1 to 0.7).

This study was one of the first to have the capability to adjust for other diet and lifestyle factors that could confound associations; associations remained after adjustment for dietary factors such as energy intake, protein, fiber, and fat. Also in 1988, Gerhardsson [24] showed the beneficial effects of leisure-time activity and that total activity had a greater influence on risk than source of activity. In 1989, Severson [25] also examined total activity and vigorous types of activities in conjunction with colon cancer in a cohort followed between 1965 and 1986; all indicators of activity were associated with reduced risk.

Since these early studies, multiple studies have replicated these early results; most studies have shown approximately a 30 to 40% reduction in risk among the most active relative to those who are sedentary [16,19,20,24–36]. Although the magnitude of the association has remained stable over time, the indicator of activity that is most importantly associated with colon cancer has varied. This change in indicator of activity associated with risk mirrors changes in activity patterns in the populations studied.

Most studies have examined activity performed as an adult to assess associations; to evaluate temporal associations, the referent period is often the year or two prior to diagnosis of cases in case-control studies [16,18,19,23,26,27,29,35,37,38]. In cohort studies, data often are collected at the baseline examination obtaining information near that time. Although some studies monitor changes in activities within the cohort, others depend on the baseline examination as the exposure and do not capture activity changes that may be associated with disease occurrence 12 to 15 years later. One study of activity performed during early adulthood did not find an association between physical activity and colon cancer [34]. In Italy, the effects of physical activity performed at various ages was examined and showed the importance of activity performed at all ages, although the greatest protective effect came from occupational activity reported before age 50 [39].

Long-term involvement in physical activity is an important discriminator of colon cancer risk [17,18] and, in some studies, the best indicator of risk [16,18,40]. This may imply that benefits come from long-term involvement in activity, although it is possible that those involved in physical activity throughout their life more accurately report their activity levels; therefore, estimates of association are less influenced by recall bias.

TABLE 5.1
Associations between Types of Physical Activity and Colon Cancer over Time

					Relative risk by activity indicator			
Study	**Dates**	**No. cases**	**Design**	**Occupation**	**Leisure**	**Total**	**V**	**Long term**
Vena 1985	1957–1965	M: 210	CC	0.5 ($p < 0.01$)				
Gerhardson 1986	1961–1979	5100	C	0.8 (0.7–0.8)				
Lee 1991	1962–1988	M: 225	C		0.9 (0.6–1.1)			0.5 (0.3–0.9)
Severson 1989	1965–1986	M: 191	C	0.7 (0.5–1.0)	0.7 (0.5–0.99)	0.7 (0.5–0.9)		
Hsing 1998b	1966–1986	M: 120	C	0.7 (0.3–1.4)				
Gerhardsson 1988	1967–1982	191	C	0.6 (0.3–1.3)	0.6 (0.4–1.0)	0.3 (0.1–0.8)		
Garabrant 1984	1972–1981	M: 2950	CC	0.55 (0.5–0.6)				
Fraser 1993	1972–1980	M: 1651	CC	0.8 (0.7–1.0)				
Thune and Lund 1996	1972–1991	M: 228	C	0.8 (0.6–1.1)	1.3 (0.9–2.0)	1.0 (0.6–1.5)		
		F: 98		0.7 (0.3–1.4)	0.8 (0.4–1.7)	0.6 (0.4–1.0)		
Vena 1987	1974–1979	M: 6459	C	PMR: 89				
		F: 604		80 ($p < 0.01$)				
Martinez 1997	1976–1992	F: 161	C		0.5 (0.3–0.9)			
Slattery 1988	1979–1983	M: 110	CC			0.7 (0.4–1.3)	0.3 (0.1–0.7)	
		F: 119				0.5 (0.3–0.9)	0.6 (0.2–1.3)	
Kato 1990	1979–1987	M: 756	CC	0.6 (0.5–0.7)				
Fredriksson 1989	1980–1983	M: 156	CC	0.8 ($p < 0.05$)				
		F: 156		0.7 ($p < 0.05$)				
Whittemore 1990	1981–1986	N. Am: M 179	CC	0.4 (0.1–0.9)	0.6 (0.4–0.9)			
		F: 114		0.8 (0.3–2.5)	0.5 (0.3–0.3)			
		China: 95		1.2 (0.5–2.5)	1.2 (0.5–2.6)			
		78		0.6 (0.2–1.7)	0.4 (0.2–1.0)			
Thun 1992	1982–1988	M: 611	C			0.6 (0.3–1.3)		
		F: 539				0.9 (0.4–2.0)		
Lee 1997a	1982–1994	M: 217	C				1.1 (0.7–1.6)	
Brownson 1989	1984–1987	M: 1211	CC	0.7 (0.5–1.0)				
Nilsen and Vatten 2001	1984–1996	M: 234	C		0.5 (0.3–0.8)			

Colbert 2001	1985–1988	M: 152	CC	0.5 (0.3–0.8)	0.8 (0.6–1.1)			
Markowitz 1992	1985–1990	M: 307	CC	0.5 (0.3–0.8)				
White 1996	1985–1989	M: 251	CC	0.8 (0.5–1.4)		0.8 (0.5–1.3)	0.6 (0.4–0.9)	
		F: 193		0.9 (0.5–1.7)		0.7 (0.4–1.3)	0.7 (0.4–1.3)	
Longnecker 1995	1986–1988	M: 163	CC	0.7 (0.3–1.5)			0.6 (0.3–0.97)	
Gerhardsson de Verdier 1990	1986–1988	452				(0.3–1.0)1990 0.6		
Giovannucci 1995	1987–1992	M: 203	C				0.5 (0.3–0.9)	
Le Marchand 1997	1987–1991	M: 467	CC	P 1.8 (p = 0.06)	0.9 (p = 0.06)		0.7 (p = 0.10)	
				D 1.3 (p = 0.26)	1.0 (p = 0.92)		0.7 (p = 0.34)	
		F: 368		P 2.1 (p = 0.05)	0.2 (p = 0.003)		0.6 (p = 0.08)	
				D1.0	1.1 (p = 0.86)		0.6 (p = 0.22)	
Marcus 1994	1990–1991	F: 536	CC			1.0 (0.8–1.3)	0.5 (0.2–1.1)	
Slattery 1997	1991–1994	M: 1099	CC	1.0 (0.8–1.2)	0.8 (0.6–1.1)	0.9 (0.7–1.2)	0.7 (0.6–0.9)	0.6 (0.5–0.8)
		F: 894		1.1 (0.9–1.4)	0.9 (0.7–1.2)	0.9 (0.7–1.2)	0.9 (0.7–1.1)	0.6 (0.5–0.8)
Tavani 1999	1991–1996	M: 688	CC	0.6 (0.4–0.9)				
		F: 537		0.5 (0.3–0.7)				
Wei 2004[a]	Extended	M: 467	C		0.7 (0.5–0.96)			
		F: 672			0.7 (0.5–1.01)			

[a]Article by Wei is an expansion of previous reports by Giovannuci and Martinez.

Notes: C = cohort; CC = case/control; risk estimates are ORs from CC studies and RR from C studies and compare highest to lowest levels of activity; M = male; F = female; P = proximal; D = distal; V = vigorous activity. Risk estimates reported are for recent activity except for long-term activity; date for cohort studies is date of baseline exam through end of follow-up.

TABLE 5.2
Associations between Types of Physical Activity and Rectal Cancer over Time[a]

Study	Dates	No. cases	Design	Relative risk by activity indicator				
				Occupation	Leisure	Total	V	Long term
Gerhardsson 1986	1961–1979	4533	C	0.9 (0.8–1.0)				
Garabrant 1984	1972–1981	1213	CC	1.0 (0.8–1.3)				
Fraser and Pearce 1993	1972–1980	M: 1046	CC	0.8 (0.7–1.0)				
Thune and Lund 1996	1972–1991	M: 170	C	1.0 (0.6–1.4)	1.0 (0.6–1.6)	1.2 (0.7–2.0)		
		F: 58		0.9 (0.3–2.4)	1.5 (0.5–4.2)	1.3 (0.6–2.7)		
Kato 1990	1979–1987	M: 753	CC	0.8 (0.6–1.0)				
Whittemore 1990	1981–1986	N Am M: 105	CC	0.6 (0.2–1.7)	0.7 (0.4–1.1)			
		F: 75		1.3 (0.5–3.3)	0.5 (0.3–1.0)			
		China M: 131		1.1 (0.6–2.5)	1.4 (0.6–3.3)			
		China F: 128		1.7 (0.6–5.0)	1.14 (0.7–3.3)			
Nilsen and Vatten 2001	1984–1986	128			0.6 (0.4–1.1)			
Colbert 2001	1985–1988	104	CC	0.5 (0.3–0.8)	0.9 (0.6–1.4)			
Markowitz 1992	1985–1990	M: 133	CC	0.6 (0.3–1.1)				
Longnecker 1995	1986–1988	M: 242	CC	1.0 (0.4–2.2)	1.2 (0.7–2.0)			
Gerhardsson de Verdier 1990a	1986–1988	268	CC	1.0 (0.8–1.3)				
LeMarchand 1997	1987–1991	M	CC	0.8 ($p = 0.49$)	1.2 (0.51)			0.5 ($p = 0.07$)
		F		1.1 ($p = 0.87$)	0.6 ($p = 0.19$)			0.8 ($p = 0.97$)
Tavani 1999	1991–1996	M: 435	CC	1.3 (0.9–2.0)				
		F: 286		0.9 (0.5–1.6)				
Levi 1999a	1992–1997	104	CC	0.5 (0.3–0.9)				
Mao 2003	1994–1997	M: 858	CC		1.2 (0.6–1.2)			

		F 587			0.9 (0.6–1.2)			
Slattery 2003	1997–2001	M	CC	1.1 (0.8–1.5)	0.6 (0.4–0.8)		0.6 (0.5–0.9)	0.6 (0.4–0.8)
		F		0.7 (0.4–0.95)	0.8 (0.5–1.2)		0.6 (0.5–0.9)	0.4 (0.3–0.7)
Wei 2004 (extended)[b]	1986 M	M: 135	C		1.0 (0.6–1.6)			
		1980 F	F 204			1.3 (0.8–2.1)		

[a]For studies of 100 or more cases of rectal cancer.

[b]Article by Wei is an expansion of previous reports by Giovannuci and Martinez.

Notes: C = cohort; CC = case/control; risk estimates are ORs from CC studies and RR from C studies and compare highest to lowest levels of activity; M = male; F = female; P = proximal; D = distal; V = vigorous activity. Risk estimates reported are for recent activity except for long-term activity; date for cohort studies is date of baseline exam through end of follow-up.

Rectal Cancer

Associations between physical activity and rectal cancer are much less consistent than those observed for colon cancer. Difference in associations could be the result of many factors, including

- Different methods used to collect physical activity data
- Power to detect significant associations
- Uncontrolled confounding because many studies of rectal cancer have examined occupational exposures
- Differences in actual mechanisms whereby physical activity works, making detection of associations more dependent on method used to ascertain physical activity

As shown in Table 5.2, eight studies report only occupational data and eight report associations from leisure activities, as well as occupational activities; two report associations only from nonwork-related activities. Of these studies, four show significantly reduced risk of rectal cancer associated with occupational activity; four show stronger associations with leisure or total activity than with occupational activity and three show reductions in risk of a similar magnitude as observed for colon cancer but with limited power to detect associations. A study of occupational activity in Italy showed protective effects for all sites within the colon, including a protective effect for tumors in the rectosigmoid junction, usually included as part of rectum, but not the rectum [39]. In that study of occupational activity by Tavini and colleagues, there was little variability in activity; most people were in the upper category of physical activity.

Perhaps most informative are studies that have assessed associations with nonwork-related activity as well as work-related activity and long-term activity patterns as they relate to rectal cancer. The study by Le Marchand and colleagues in Hawaii showed effects for rectal cancer similar to, although slightly stronger than, the protective effects from lifetime recreational activity for colon cancer [16]. One study of over 950 rectal cancer cases that used the same methods previously used in a large multicenter colon cancer study showed that the magnitude of risk reduction for rectal tumors was the same as that previously reported for colon tumors [41]. As in the companion study of colon cancer [18], the association remained after adjustment for potential confounding factors. Reduced risk was seen, for men and women, for activities performed at a vigorous level of effort among individuals who performed intense activity over a long period of their lives. However, another large case-control study of 1447 incident rectal cancer cases and 3106 controls did not detect a significantly reduced risk of rectal cancer from high levels of recreational activity (OR 0.88 95% CI 0.64 to 1.20) [42].

BIOLOGICAL MECHANISMS

Energy Balance

Energy balance has been proposed as a key mechanism through which physical activity exerts its protective effect on colon cancer because energy expenditure, along with energy intake, is a key element in determining ability to maintain energy balance [43,44]. Studies show that physical activity is associated with lower levels of obesity and abdominal obesity specifically [45–48]. Effect modification or interaction, showing differences in association by different groups within the population, is one means whereby epidemiology can obtain insight into biological mechanisms. Evaluation of the interaction between physical activity and components of energy balance, such as energy intake and obesity, has been done to gain insight into the role of energy balance and how physical activity may modulate colon cancer risk through this mechanism. Studies have shown that people at greatest risk of colon cancer are sedentary with a large BMI and that the risk is greater than would be expected from each factor independently [16,49]. Similar associations have not been observed for rectal cancer [50]. Given the role of physical activity in modifying the harmful effects of obesity on colon cancer risk, physical activity may become even more important as the prevalence of obesity increases.

It has been proposed that the influence of energy balance on risk of colon cancer may work through endogenous hormone metabolism [51]. Of particular interest is how energy balance, in general, and physical activity, specifically, relate to insulin and insulin-like growth factors (IGF) [51,52]. It has been proposed that insulin and IGF may play a central role in development and promotion of colon cancers [53–55]. Several studies have now shown that high levels of IGF-1 increase risk of colorectal cancer and that high levels of insulin-like growth factor-binding protein 3 (IGFBP-3) are associated with reduced risk of colorectal cancer [56,57].

In another study, IGF-1 and IGFBP-3 increased risk of colorectal cancer, but IGFBP-1 was associated with reduced risk of colorectal cancer; however, estimates of association were imprecise in that study [56]. Studies have shown that high levels of physical activity are associated with increased insulin sensitivity, down-regulation of IGF-1, and up-relation of IGFBP-3 [58,59]; the exact intensity of the activity at which this down-regulation occurs is not clear. Epidemiological studies also suggest interaction between physical activity and glycemic load, a dietary factor thought to be associated with insulin [60].

Genetic factors that have been proposed as being involved in an insulin-related pathway include insulin-like growth factor 1 (*IGF1*), insulin-like growth factor-binding protein 3 (*IGFBP3*), insulin receptor substrate 1 (*IRS1*), and insulin receptor substrate 2 (*IRS2*) [61]. Polymorphisms of these genes have been identified; some of these have been shown to have effects on insulin resistance and/or diabetes. High serum IGF-1 levels have been associated with an increased risk of colorectal cancer, and variation in serum IGF-1 levels has been associated with a CA repeat polymorphism 1 kb upstream of the transcription start site [62]. High levels of IGFBP-3 have been associated with a reduced risk of colorectal cancer [57]. An A/C polymorphism at nucleotide –202 is associated with different levels of IGFBP3 in a dose–response fashion, i.e., AA > AC > CC.

The AC or CC genotypes would thus be predicted to be associated with an increased risk of colorectal cancer. A Gly972Arg (*G972R*) polymorphism in the *IRS1* gene has been associated with insulin resistance and type-2 diabetes; it might be associated with an increased risk of colorectal cancer. The *G1057D IRS2* polymorphism has been associated with obesity and is therefore a plausible link to insulin resistance and colorectal cancer [63].

Evaluation of physical activity with these genes has shown a significant interaction between physical activity and *IGF1* genotype for colon cancer, a borderline ($p = 0.06$) interaction between *IRS2* and physical activity level and risk of colon cancer. Those who were most physically active with the *IGF1 192/192* genotype were at a significantly lower risk of colon cancer than those without this genotype. Low physical activity and high BMI appeared to have the greatest impact on risk in the presence of the *IGFBP3* A allele (p for interaction = 0.01) [64].

The vitamin D receptor (VDR)[4] is a nuclear receptor involved in the regulation of many physiological processes, including cell growth and differentiation and metabolic homeostasis [65]. Some studies suggest that VDR also may be involved in insulin and insulin-like growth factor-mediated disease pathways [66–68]; others suggest that it may be important as a bile acid receptor. Examination of the *Fok1 VDR* polymorphism showed that those who were least physically active were at greater risk of colon cancer if they had the *ff VDR* genotype (OR 3.46 95% CI 1.58 to 7.58; p interaction 0.05) [69].

Other Hypothesized Biological Mechanisms

Given the associations between physical activity and colon, and possibly rectal cancer, it is possible that several biological mechanisms are involved. Given the lack of association between BMI and rectal cancer and inconsistent association between physical activity and rectal cancer, it is likely that mechanisms other than energy balance are operational — if, indeed, the association between physical activity and rectal cancer is real. Findings from controlled experimental studies generate most of the support for various proposed mechanisms, although assessment of interaction in epidemiological studies can provide clues to important mechanisms.

The effect of physical activity on gastrointestinal transit time was the hypothesized mechanism put forth when the initial observation that physical activity decreased risk of colon cancer was made [70]. It has been shown that people involved in moderate-level activities, such as walking, have a decreased gastrointestinal (GI) transit time, resulting in increased propulsion of colonic contents through the colon [71]; some studies suggest that more vigorous activity is needed for stimulation of the vagus nerve responsible for increased propulsion [72,73]. Physical activity also is associated with reduced time that bile acids and other carcinogens are in contact with the GI tract. An interaction between colon cancer and fiber suggests that transit time may be an important mechanism [21,74].

Physical activity has been shown to influence immune response [73,74]. Natural killer (NK) cells and macrophages are important components of the immune system [75]. Physical exercise is known to influence the activity of these cells consistently, with a twofold increase in their circulation immediately following intense activity [78]. Regular exercise training has been shown to enhance the resting level of NK cell activity [79]. Exercise also has been shown to influence levels of cytokines, soluble immune mediators produced by various immune cells. Interleukin-1, tumor necrosis factor (TNF), and interlukin-6 are major cytokines that have been shown to vary by amount and intensity of physical activity performed in healthy individuals [76].

Prostaglandins have been associated with tumor growth in studies of animals [80]. Prostaglandin F_2 alpha inhibits tumor growth in the colon and increases gut motility; prostaglandin E_2 decreases colonic motility and increases the rate of colonic cell proliferation, especially in cancer cells [81,82]. Strenuous physical activity appears to increase levels of prostaglandin F_2 alpha and inhibit synthesis of prostaglandin E_2 [80,82]. Studies have shown that high activity was inversely associated with rectal mucosal prostaglandin E_2 [83].

TUMOR MUTATIONS AND PHYSICAL ACTIVITY

Mutations in colorectal tissue are acquired over time, ultimately leading to a tumor. Although data are limited, evaluation of physical activity with other types of mutations in colon tumors can provide clues about specific disease pathways and how physical activity relates to these factors. For colon cancer, in one study, mutations *p53*, Ki-*ras*, and microsatellite instability (MSI) have been examined with physical activity. Results suggest that *p53* and Ki-*ras* mutations may be associated with physical activity [83,84]. It appears that physical activity may be related to *p53* mutations through its association with a Western diet [83]; for Ki-*ras* mutations, the importance of physical activity may be through its modifying effect on body weight [84]. One study has examined physical activity with colorectal adenomas and has reported that more active people were more likely to have Ki-*ras*-negative than Ki-*ras*-positive tumors [85].

PUBLIC HEALTH ISSUES: DOSE–RESPONSE AND INTENSITY

Given the consistent association between physical activity and colon cancer, being physically active to reduce risk of colon, and possibly rectal, cancer is an agent of cancer prevention. In order to implement activity as a chemoprevention agent, it is important to understand how much activity is necessary, how often it should be undertaken, and how intense the activity should be to reduce risk. Most studies have not collected physical activity information that readily answers these important questions. The dose, or amount of activity needed, is often lacking, although estimates of dose can be made through examination of intensity and time, which are indicators of dose needed for protection. Dose–response has been reviewed in detail [15] and is summarized here.

Intensity of activity performed is one indicator of dose–response. More recent studies that have examined activities by intensity often show greater protection than moderate activity or total activity [16,18,19,26,33–35,86,87]. Some studies report protective effects for moderate/vigorous activities, making it difficult to determine the independent effects of each. In a study by Slattery et al. [41], activities performed at a moderate and a vigorous level of intensity were associated with reduced risk of rectal cancer. To determine the impact of exercise intensity on risk, data were modeled to evaluate the effects of moderate and vigorous levels of intensity on colon and rectal cancer risk simultaneously. Results showed that vigorous activity remained significantly protective and that the association with moderate activity disappeared after adjustment for vigorous activity.

The amount of time (in terms of frequency, duration, and whether time spent should be cumulative) needed to reduce colon cancer risk is still debated. Because studies report associations differently, it is difficult to determine the amount of activity associated with reduced risk of colon or rectal cancer for some studies. Many studies show significant protective effects at the upper tertile or quintile of activity and others have examined physical activity indices. Some report in MET minutes needed and others in hours of activity performed.

Crude estimates of frequency and duration associated with reduced risk are shown in Table 5.3. These results focus on recreational or nonwork-related activity because that activity can be altered to reduce risk; however, work activity may add to the overall activity needed or explain some of the variation in risk observed between studies. Of importance is the observation that less intense activity requires a greater amount of time to see the same protective effect observed for intense activity at less time. This is illustrated in the study by Whittemore and colleagues [27] in which the same level of risk reduction is assigned for 1 h of vigorous activity per day or 5 h of moderate activity per day.

Similarly, in the studies by Martinez and Giovannucci [19,36], calculation of MET hours per week included activities performed at a moderate to vigorous level of intensity. Activities are given an amount of time corresponding to MET h/week. For instance, running for 1 h is equivalent to roughly 10.2 MET h; playing tennis for 1 h is equivalent to roughly 6 MET h, and 1 h of walking at a moderate to brisk pace is roughly equivalent to 3.2 MET h. Again, these show that the duration during which activities should be performed depends on the intensity of the activity. For instance, for running, 2 to 4 h per week of vigorous activity would be needed to see a protective effect and, if walking at a moderate to brisk pace, 7 to 14 h of activity per week may be needed.

Taken together, recommendations based on studies in which data are available suggest that risk reduction occurs from performing somewhere around 3.5 to 4 h of vigorous activity per week; however, for moderate activity, 7 to 35 h of activity would be needed for the same risk reduction. The combination of intensity, duration, and frequency is a key element to the risk equation and therefore to any public health recommendation based on epidemiological data. A recommendation of about 3.5 to 4 h of vigorous activity per week, which translate to about 35 min of vigorous activity every day or 45 min of vigorous activity 5 days a week, may therefore be required to see a protective effect from physical activity on colon cancer risk.

SUMMARY

From existing data, it appears that sedentary people have a 60% to twofold increased risk of developing colon cancer; some evidence suggests similar associations for rectal cancer. Comparing physical inactivity to other risk factors for colon cancer, it has been have estimated that 13 to 14% of colon cancer in the population could be attributed to physical inactivity [18,88], which is comparable to estimates of 12% of colon cancer cases attributed to not using aspirin or NSAIDs and 12% of colon cancer cases attributed to eating a Western dietary pattern.

On the other hand, only 8% of colon cancer cases could be attributed to a family history of colorectal cancer. The effects of physical activity on colon cancer risk are even greater when one considers the modifying influence of physical activity on risk of colon cancer associated with other

TABLE 5.3
Physical Activity and Colon Cancer: Assessment of Dose–Response

Study	Design[1]	Sample size	RR/OR[2]	Dose for protective effect: Frequency	Level of intensity	p-Trend
Gerhardsson de Verdier et al. 1990	CC	432 cases/624 controls	0.6	>2 h leisure + active job/week	Vigorous	0.06
Martinez et al. 1997	C	161 cases	0.5	>21 MET h/wk vs. <2 MET h/wk	Moderate to vigorous	0.03
Longnecker et al. 1995	CC	163 cases (right colon)/703 controls	0.6	>2 h/week vs. none	Vigorous	0.06
White et al. 1996	CC	444 cases/427 controls	0.7	≥2 times/wk	MET value > 4.5	0.07 (M); 0.05 (F)
Slattery et al. 1997; 1999	CC	1974 cases/2405 controls	0.6	3–4 h/wk	Vigorous	<0.01
			0.8	30 to 60-min/session	Vigorous	
			0.7	>60-min/session vs. none	Vigorous	
Whittemore et al. 1990	CC	905 cases/2488 controls (includes U.S. and China)	0.6 (U.S.)	>5/day	Moderate	NA
				or >1 h/day	Vigorous	
Lee et al. 1991	C	225 cases	0.5	>2500 kcal/wk vs. <1000	Moderate–vigorous	
Giovannucci et al. 1995	C	203 cases	0.5	>46.8 MET h/wk vs. 0.9 MET h/wk	Moderate–vigorous	0.03
Thune and Lund 1996	C	236 cases	0.6 (F)	>4 h/wk	Moderate–vigorous	0.25

[1] CC = case/control; C = cohort
[2] RR = relative risk; OR = odds ratio.

Source: From Slattery, ML, *Sports Med* 2004; 34:239–252. With permission.

diet and lifestyle factors [21]. There are several possible mechanisms whereby physical activity may influence colorectal cancer risk; many of these appear to depend on frequency, duration, and intensity of the activity performed. Taken together, strong evidence indicates the importance of physical activity as a major factor in the etiology of colon, and possibly rectal, cancer. Public health policy that enhances the ability to increase physical activity patterns is warranted as a means of colon cancer prevention.

REFERENCES

1. Ries LA EM, Kosary CL, Hankey BF, Clegg K et al. SEER cancer statistics review, 1973–1998: *Natl Cancer Inst*, 2002.
2. *The World Health Report*. Geneva, Switzerland: World Health Organization, 1997.
3. Haenszel W, Kurihara M. Studies of Japanese migrants. I. Mortality from cancer and other diseases among Japanese in the United States. *J Natl Cancer Inst* 1968; 40:43–68.
4. Garabrant DH, Peters JM, Mack TM, Bernstein L. Job activity and colon cancer risk. *Am J Epidemiol* 1984; 119:1005–1014.
5. Vena JE, Graham S, Zielezny M, Swanson MK, Barnes RE, Nolan J. Lifetime occupational exercise and colon cancer. *Am J Epidemiol* 1985; 122:357–365.
6. Thune I. Assessments of physical activity and cancer risk. *Eur J Cancer Prev* 2000; 9:387–393.
7. Lamonte MJ, Ainsworth BE. Quantifying energy expenditure and physical activity in the context of dose response. *Med Sci Sports Exercise* 2001; 33:S370–378; discussion S419–420.
8. Ainsworth BE. Challenges in measuring physical activity in women. *Exercise Sport Sci Rev* 2000; 28:93–96.
9. Jacobs DR, Jr., Ainsworth BE, Hartman TJ, Leon AS. A simultaneous evaluation of 10 commonly used physical activity questionnaires. *Med Sci Sports Exercise* 1993; 25:81–91.
10. Ainsworth BE, Richardson MT, Jacobs DR, Jr., Leon AS, Sternfeld B. Accuracy of recall of occupational physical activity by questionnaire. *J Clin Epidemiol* 1999; 52:219–227.
11. Ainsworth BE, Sternfeld B, Slattery ML, Daguise V, Zahm SH. Physical activity and breast cancer: evaluation of physical activity assessment methods. *Cancer* 1998; 83:611–620.
12. Slattery ML, David R. Jacobs J. Assessment of ability to recall physical activity of several years ago. *Ann Epidemiol* 1995; 5:292–296.
13. Friedenreich CM, Orenstein MR. Physical activity and cancer prevention: etiologic evidence and biological mechanisms. *J Nutr* 2002; 132:3456S–3464S.
14. International Agency for Research on Cancer, IARC Handbook of Cancer Prevention, vol. 6, *Weight Control and Physical Activity* . Lyon, France: IARC Press, 2002.
15. Slattery ML. Physical activity and colorectal cancer. *Sports Med* 2004; 34:239–252.
16. Le Marchand L, Wilkens LR, Kolonel LN, Hankin JH, Lyu LC. Associations of sedentary lifestyle, obesity, smoking, alcohol use, and diabetes with the risk of colorectal cancer. *Cancer Res* 1997; 57:4787–4794.
17. Lee IM, Paffenbarger RS, Jr., Hsieh C. Physical activity and risk of developing colorectal cancer among college alumni. *J Natl Cancer Inst* 1991; 83:1324–1329.
18. Slattery ML, Edwards SL, Ma K-N, Friedman GD, Potter JD. Physical activity and colon cancer: a public health perspective. *Ann Epidemiol* 1997; 7:137–145.
19. Martinez ME, Giovannucci E, Spiegelman D, Hunter DJ, Willett WC, Colditz GA. Leisure-time physical activity, body size, and colon cancer in women. Nurses' Health Study Research Group. *J Natl Cancer Inst* 1997; 89:948–955.
20. Howe GR, Aronson KJ, Benito E, et al. The relationship between dietary fat intake and risk of colorectal cancer: evidence from the combined analysis of 13 case-control studies. *Cancer Causes Control* 1997; 8:215–228.
21. Slattery ML, Potter JD. Physical activity and colon cancer: confounding or interaction? *Med Sci Sports Exercise* 2002; 34:913–919.
22. Ballard–Barbash R, Schatzkin A, Albanes D, et al. Physical activity and risk of large bowel cancer in the Framingham Study. *Cancer Res* 1990; 50:3610–3613.

23. Slattery M, Schumacher M, Smith K, West D, Abd–Elghany N. Physical activity, diet, and risk of colon cancer in Utah [see comments]. *Am J Epidemiol* 1988; 128:989–999.
24. Gerhardsson M, Floderus B, Norell SE. Physical activity and colon cancer risk. *Int J Epidemiol* 1988; 17:743–746.
25. Severson RK, Nomura AMY, Grove JS, Stemmermann GN. A prospective analysis of physical activity and cancer. *Am J Epidemiol* 1989; 130:522–529.
26. White E, Jacobs EJ, Daling JR. Physical activity in relation to colon cancer in middle-aged men and women. *Am J Epidemiol* 1996; 144:42–50.
27. Whittemore AS, Wu–Williams AH, Lee M, et al. Diet, physical activity, and colorectal cancer among Chinese in North America and China. *J Natl Cancer Inst* 1990; 82:915–926.
28. Peters RK, Pike MC, Garabrant D, Mack TM. Diet and colon cancer in Los Angeles County, California. *Cancer Causes Control* 1992; 3:457–473.
29. Thune I, Lund E. Physical activity and risk of colorectal cancer in men and women. *Br J Cancer* 1996; 73:1134–40.
30. Nilsen TI, Vatten LJ. Prospective study of colorectal cancer risk and physical activity, diabetes, blood glucose and BMI: exploring the hyperinsulinaemia hypothesis. *Br J Cancer* 2001; 84:417–422.
31. Friedenreich CM. Physical activity and cancer: lessons learned from nutritional epidemiology. *Nutr Rev* 2001; 59:349–357.
32. Beitler A, Rodriguez–Bigas MA, Weber TK, Lee RJ, Cuenca R, Petrelli NJ. Complications of absorbable pelvic mesh slings following surgery for rectal carcinoma. *Dis Colon Rectum* 1997; 40:1336–1341.
33. Wu AH, Paganini–Hill A, Ross RK, Henderson BE. Alcohol, physical activity and other risk factors for colorectal cancer: a prospective study. *Br. J. Cancer* 1987; 55:687–694.
34. Marcus PM, Newcomb PA, Storer BE. Early adulthood physical activity and colon cancer risk among Wisconsin women. *Cancer Epidemiol Biomarkers Prev* 1994; 3:641–644.
35. Longnecker MP, Gerhardsson le Verdier M, Frumkin H, Carpenter C. A case-control study of physical activity in relation to risk of cancer of the right colon and rectum in men. *Int J Epidemiol* 1995; 24:42–50.
36. Giovannucci E, Ascherio A, Rimm EB, Colditz GA, Stampfer MJ, Willett WC. Physical activity, obesity, and risk for colon cancer and adenoma in men. *Ann Intern Med* 1995; 122:327–334.
37. de Verdier MG, Steineck G, Hagman U, Rieger Å, Norell SE. Physical activity and colon cancer: a case-referent study in Stockholm. *Int J Cancer* 1990; 46:985–989.
38. Kune GA, Kune S, Watson LF. Body weight and physical activity as predictors of colorectal cancer risk. *Nutr Cancer* 1990; 13:9–17.
39. Tavani A, Braga C, La Vecchia C, et al. Physical activity and risk of cancers of the colon and rectum: an Italian case-control study. *Br J Cancer* 1999; 79:1912–1916.
40. Lee IM, Paffenbarger RS, Jr. Physical activity and its relation to cancer risk: a prospective study of college alumni. *Med Sci Sports Exercise* 1994; 26:831–837.
41. Slattery ML, Edwards S, Curtin K, et al. Physical activity and colorectal cancer. *Am J Epidemiol* 2003; 158:214–224.
42. Mao Y, Pan S, Wen SW, Johnson KC. Physical inactivity, energy intake, obesity and the risk of rectal cancer in Canada. *Int J Cancer* 2003; 105:831–837.
43. Rissanen A, Fogelholm M. Physical activity in the prevention and treatment of other morbid conditions and impairments associated with obesity: current evidence and research issues. *Med Sci Sports Exercise* 1999; 31:S635–645.
44. Rogers AE. Selected recent studies of exercise, energy metabolism, body weight, and blood lipids relevant to interpretation and design of studies of exercise and cancer. *Adv Exp Med Biol* 1992; 322:239–245.
45. Saris WH, Blair SN, van Baak MA, et al. How much physical activity is enough to prevent unhealthy weight gain? Outcome of the IASO 1st Stock Conference and consensus statement. *Obesity Rev* 2003; 4:101–114.
46. Hu FB. Sedentary lifestyle and risk of obesity and type 2 diabetes. *Lipids* 2003; 38:103–108.
47. Matsuzawa Y, Shimomura I, Nakamura T, Keno Y, Kotani K, Tokunaga K. Pathophysiology and pathogenesis of visceral fat obesity. *Obesity Res* 1995; 3 Suppl 2:187S–194S.

48. McTiernan A, Ulrich C, Slate S, Potter J. Physical activity and cancer etiology: associations and mechanisms. *Cancer Causes Control* 1998; 9:487–509.
49. Slattery ML, Potter J, Caan B, et al. Energy balance and colon cancer — beyond physical activity. *Cancer Res* 1997; 57:75–80.
50. Slattery ML, Caan BJ, Benson J, Murtaugh M. Energy balance and rectal cancer: an evaluation of energy intake, energy expenditure, and body mass index. *Nutr Cancer* 2003; 46:166–171.
51. Kaaks R, Lukanova A. Energy balance and cancer: the role of insulin and insulin-like growth factor-I. *Proc Nutr Soc* 2001; 60:91–106.
52. Kaaks R. Nutrition, energy balance and colon cancer risk: the role of insulin and insulin-like growth factor-I. *IARC Sci Publ* 2002; 156:289–293.
53. McKeown–Eyssen G. Epidemiology of colorectal cancer revisited: are serum triglycerides and/or plasma glucose associated with risk. *Cancer Epidemiol Biomarkers Prev* 1994; 3:687–695.
54. Kim YI. Diet, lifestyle, and colorectal cancer: is hyperinsulinemia the missing link? *Nutr Rev* 1998; 56:275–279.
55. Giovannucci E. Insulin and colon cancer. *Cancer Causes Control* 1995; 6:164–179.
56. Kaaks R, Toniolo P, Akhmedkhanov A, et al. Serum C-peptide, insulin-like growth factor (IGF)-I, IGF-binding proteins, and colorectal cancer risk in women. *J Natl Cancer Inst* 2000; 92:1592–1600.
57. Ma J, Pollak MN, Giovannucci E, et al. Prospective study of colorectal cancer risk in men and plasma levels of insulin-like growth factor (IGF)-I and IGF-binding protein-3. *J Natl Cancer Inst* 1999; 91:620–625.
58. McCarty MF. Up-regulation of IGF binding protein-1 as an anticarcinogenic strategy: relevance to caloric restriction, exercise, and insulin sensitivity. *Med Hypotheses* 1997; 48:297–308.
59. Moore MA, Park CB, Tsuda H. Implications of the hyperinsulinaemia-diabetes-cancer link for preventive efforts. *Eur J Cancer Prev* 1998; 7:89–107.
60. Slattery ML, Benson J, Berry TD, et al. Dietary sugar and colon cancer. *Cancer Epidemiol Biomarkers Prev* 1997; 6:677–685.
61. Slattery ML, Samowitz W, Hoffman M, Ma KN, Levin TR, Neuhausen S. Aspirin, NSAIDs, and colorectal cancer: possible involvement in an insulin-related pathway. *Cancer Epidemiol Biomarkers Prev* 2004; 13:538–545.
62. Rosen CJ, Kurland ES, Vereault D, et al. Association between serum insulin growth factor-I (IGF-I) and a simple sequence repeat in IGF-I gene: implications for genetic studies of bone mineral density. *J Clin Endocrinol Metab* 1998; 83:2286–2290.
63. Lautier C, El Mkadem SA, Renard E, et al. Complex haplotypes of IRS2 gene are associated with severe obesity and reveal heterogeneity in the effect of Gly1057Asp mutation. *Hum Genet* 2003; 113:34–43.
64. Slattery ML, Murtaugh M, Caan B, Ma KN, Neuhausen S, Samowitz W. Energy balance, insulin-related genes and risk of colon and rectal cancer. *Int J Cancer* 2005; 115:148–54
65. Adachi R, Shulman AI, Yamamoto K, et al. Structural determinants for vitamin D receptor response to endocrine and xenobiotic signals. *Mol Endocrinol* 2004; 18:43–52.
66. Chokkalingam AP, McGlynn KA, Gao YT, et al. Vitamin D receptor gene polymorphisms, insulin-like growth factors, and prostate cancer risk: a population-based case-control study in China. *Cancer Res* 2001; 61:4333–4336.
67. Zeitz U, Weber K, Soegiarto DW, Wolf E, Balling R, Erben RG. Impaired insulin secretory capacity in mice lacking a functional vitamin D receptor. *FASEB J* 2003; 17:509–511.
68. Chokkalingam AP, McGlynn KA, Gao Y-T, et al. Vitamin D receptor gene polymorphisms, insulin-like growth factors, and prostate cancer risk: a population-based case-control study in China. *Cancer Res* 2001; 61:4333–4336.
69. Slattery ML, Murtaugh M, Caan B, Ma KN, Wolff R, Samowitz W. Associations between BMI, energy intake, energy expenditure, VDR genotype and colon and rectal cancers (United States). *Cancer Causes Control* 2004; 15:863-72
70. Holdstock DJ, Misiewicz JJ. Factors controlling colonic motility: colonic pressures and transit after meals in patients with total gastrectomy, pernicious anaemia or duodenal ulcer. *Gut* 1970; 11:100–110.
71. Cordain L, Latin RW, Behnke JJ. The effects of an aerobic running program on bowel transit time. *J Sports Med Phys Fitness* 1986; 26:101–104.

72. Krotkiewski M, Bjorntorp P, Holm G, et al. Effects of physical training on insulin, connecting peptide (C-peptide), gastric inhibitory polypeptide (GIP) and pancreatic polypeptide (PP) levels in obese subjects. *Int J Obesity* 1984; 8:193–199.
73. Oktedalen O, Guldvog I, Opstad PK, Berstad A, Gedde–Dahl D, Jorde R. The effect of physical stress on gastric secretion and pancreatic polypeptide levels in man. *Scand J Gastroenterol* 1984; 19:770–778.
74. Slattery ML CK, Benson J, Edwards S, Schaffer D. Plant foods, fiber, and rectal cancer. *Am J Clin Nutr* 2004; 79 (2) : 274–281.
75. Shephard RJ, Shek PN. Cancer, immune function, and physical activity. *Can J Appl Physiol* 1995; 20:1–25.
76. Shephard RJ, Rhind S, Shek PN. The impact of exercise on the immune system: NK cells, interleukins 1 and 2, and related responses. *Exercise Sport Sci Rev* 1995; 23:215–241.
77. Woods JA, Davis JM. Exercise, monocyte/macrophage function, and cancer. *Med Sci Sports Exercise* 1994; 26:147–157.
78. Nieman DC, Henson DA. Role of endurance exercise in immune senescence. *Med Sci Sports Exercise* 1994; 26:172–181.
79. Nieman DC, Nehlsen–Cannarella SL, Markoff PA, et al. The effects of moderate exercise training on natural killer cells and acute upper respiratory tract infections. *Int J Sports Med* 1990; 11:467–473.
80. Tutton PJ, Barkla DH. Influence of prostaglandin analogues on epithelial cell proliferation and xenograft growth. *Br J Cancer* 1980; 41:47–51.
81. Demers LM, Harrison TS, Halbert DR, Santen RJ. Effect of prolonged exercise on plasma prostaglandin levels. *Prostaglandins Med* 1981; 6:413–418.
82. Bennett A, Tacca MD, Stamford IF, Zebro T. Prostaglandins from tumors of human large bowel. *Br J Cancer* 1977; 35:881–884.
83. Rauramaa R, Salonen JT, Kukkonen–Harjula K, et al. Effects of mild physical exercise on serum lipoproteins and metabolites of arachidonic acid: a controlled randomised trial in middle aged men. *Br Med J* (clin res ed) 1984; 288:603–606.
84. Martinez ME, Heddens D, Earnest DL, et al. Physical activity, body mass index, and prostaglandin E2 levels in rectal mucosa. *J Natl Cancer Inst* 1999; 91:950–953.
85. Slattery ML, Curtin K, Ma K, et al. Diet activity, and lifestyle associations with p53 mutations in colon tumors. *Cancer Epidemiol Biomarkers Prev* 2002; 11:541–548.
86. Slattery ML, Anderson K, Curtin K, et al. Lifestyle factors and Ki-ras mutations in colon cancer tumors. *Mutat Res* 2001; 483:73–81.
87. Martinez ME, Maltzman T, Marshall JR, et al. Risk factors for Ki-ras protooncogene mutation in sporadic colorectal adenomas. *Cancer Res* 1999; 59:5181–5185.
88. Friedenreich CM. Physical activity and cancer prevention: from observational to intervention research. *Cancer Epidemiol Biomarkers Prev* 2001; 10:287–301.
89. Gerhardsson de Verdier M, Steineck G, Hagman U, Rieger A, Norell SE. Physical activity and colon cancer: a case-referent study in Stockholm. *Int J Cancer* 1990; 46:985–989.
90. La Vecchia C, Braga C, Franceschi S, Dal Maso L, Negri E. Population-attributable risk for colon cancer in Italy. *Nutr Cancer* 1999; 33:196–200.
91. Colbert LH, Hartman TJ, Malila N, Limburg PJ, Pietinen P, Virtamo J, Taylor PR, Albanes D. Phyiscal activity in relation to cancer of the colon and rectum in a cohort of male smokers. Cancer Epidemiol Biomarkers Prev. 2001; 10(3):265–268

6 Physical Activity and Prostate Cancer Risk

Christine M. Friedenreich

CONTENTS

INTRODUCTION

Prostate cancer incidence and mortality rates vary around the world with the highest rates observed in the U.S., Canada, and Scandinavia, and the lowest rates found in China and other Asian countries [1,2]. These differences are attributable to variability in genetic susceptibility, exposure to external risk factors, and health care and cancer registrations [2]. The incidence of prostate cancer increased rapidly in North America over the last 20 years; this was mainly attributable to the widespread use of prostate-specific antigen (PSA) tests to screen for this disease, but has recently returned to levels observed prior to the introduction of PSA testing [3,4]. Currently, prostate cancer incidence is the most common malignancy in men in the U.S. and Canada and is second only to lung cancer as a cause of cancer death among men [3,4].

Prostate cancer etiology is still relatively poorly understood, with only a few established and several postulated risk factors [2,5,6]. The main established risk factors are age, race [7], and family history [6,8,9]; possible risk factors include endogenous hormones [10,11], dietary intake [12–16], obesity [17], smoking [18,19], alcohol consumption [20–22], history of sexually transmitted diseases [23,24], vasectomy [25], and occupational exposures including cadmium, zinc, and pesticides [26,27]. There is inconsistent epidemiological evidence for these postulated risk factors.

Primary prevention strategies for prostate cancer include possible chemoprevention approaches with micronutrients (e.g., vitamins C and E, selenium, lycopene) [28–32] because some epidemiological evidence suggests that prostate cancer risk is decreased with these dietary antioxidants.

Other agents have also been proposed for pharmaceutical development, including inhibitors of cyclooxygenase-2 (COX-2) and insulin-like growth factor-1 (IGF-1) activity, because these two pathways may be involved in prostate carcinogenesis [33]. Several large-scale prostate chemoprevention trials on selenium, vitamin E, and the 5-α-reductase inhibitor, finasteride, are currently ongoing (Selenium and Vitamin E Cancer Prevention [SELECT] Trial) [34] or have recently been completed (Prostate Cancer Prevention Trial [PCPT]) [35]. The PCPT trial demonstrated a 25% reduction in prostate cancer incidence among men taking finasteride in comparison to men in the placebo group. However, important adverse side effects occurred among men in the intervention group, including an increased risk for high-grade disease; thus, the efficacy of this agent for prostate cancer chemoprevention remains uncertain.

Another modifiable lifestyle risk factor for prostate cancer that is receiving research attention is physical activity. Physical activity is an important means for the primary prevention of numerous chronic diseases, including cancers of the colon and the breast [36], and could potentially be an alternative to chemoprevention strategies for prostate cancer. The purpose of this chapter is to review the epidemiological studies on physical activity and prostate cancer risk, as well as to discuss the main biological mechanisms that may be involved in this putative association, the methodological issues that need to be considered for investigations on this topic, and future research directions in this area.

METHODS

A systematic review of the published literature through May, 2004, was conducted to identify all animal experimental and epidemiological studies that reported a measure of physical activity in relation to prostate cancer. To be included in this review, the studies needed to be examining physical activity as an etiological risk factor. No restrictions were made by language or year of publication. When multiple reports from the same study were found, the most recent and/or complete publication was chosen for inclusion into the review. The studies were categorized by type of study design and type of data collection methods and then reviewed systematically for the strength, consistency, dose–response, and coherence of the relation between physical activity and prostate cancer risk. The biological plausibility of this putative relation was examined separately by reviewing the literature on endogenous sex and metabolic hormone levels, immune function, and body size and prostate cancer risk. Methodological limitations with these studies were identified and considered as possible explanations for the differences observed across studies.

EPIDEMIOLOGIC STUDIES OF PHYSICAL ACTIVITY AND PROSTATE CANCER

A total of 38 publications of epidemiological studies and no animal experimental studies were identified that examined some aspect of the possible association between physical activity and prostate cancer risk [37–74]. Of these 38 publications, there were multiple publications from the same study. The prospective cohort study of Harvard and University of Pennsylvania students was first presented by Whittemore et al. in 1985 [38] and then updated in five subsequent publications by Paffenbarger and Lee [39,43–45,59]; only the most recent publication from this cohort is included in this review [59]. One of these updates was the paper by Paffenbarger et al. [39], which also includes two analyses from a cohort of longshoremen and is presented in this review.

Likewise, two papers describe follow-ups of different lengths of time of the cohort from the National Health and Nutrition and Examination I Survey [42,48]. Only the second publication by Steenland et al. [48] will be included. An additional analysis on energy intake and prostate cancer from the Male Health Professionals Cohort Study, originally published by Giovannucci et al. [53], was published recently by Platz et al. [62]. Because this most recent analysis [62] only examined interactions of body size and physical activity, rather than the association of physical activity and prostate cancer risk, it is not included in this review. Finally, the paper by Ilic et al. [49] was excluded because of the lack of information on the methods used in the study, including the physical activity assessment and the analytic approach. Thus, a total of 19 cohort studies [37,39,40,41,46–48,50–61] and 12 case-control studies [63–74] could be reviewed. Of the 19 cohort studies, 3 had prostate cancer mortality, rather than incidence, as the endpoint [37,39,40]. Thus far, no studies have examined the association between physical activity and prostate cancer survival. One study [50] has examined the association between physical fitness, in addition to the association with physical activity, and prostate cancer incidence and is included in this review.

Overall Results

The studies that are included here cover those conducted in different countries worldwide using wide ranging study populations, designs, endpoints, and methods for assessing physical activity and its association with prostate cancer risk (Table 6.1 and Table 6.2). Given the heterogeneity of the study methods, particularly the exposure assessment, it is not possible to provide an overall quantitative assessment of risk between physical activity and cancer risk.

There is some suggestion for an inverse relation between physical activity and prostate cancer in 16 [39,40,46,48,50,52,53,55,56,60,61,63,64,68,71,72] of the previous 31 studies reviewed here. Of these 16 studies, the risks were significantly reduced in 10 studies [40,46,50,52,56,60,61,63,64,72] for the total population and in 2 other studies [53,71] for subgroups of the study population only; in the remaining 4 studies [39,48,55,68], the risks were inverse but not statistically significant. No overall association between physical activity and prostate cancer was found in 11 studies [41,47,54,57–59,65,67,69,73,74]. An increased risk of prostate cancer among physically active men was found in four studies [37,51,66,70]. Figure 6.1 illustrates the main result for each study.

The magnitude of the overall association ranged from an 80% reduction in prostate cancer risk for the highest activity levels [72] to a 220% increased risk found in one study [70]. The overall results for 21 [37,40,41,46–48,52–55,57–59,61,63,67–69,71,73,74] of the 31 studies were distributed between a 30% reduction to a 30% increase in risk of prostate cancer for the most active men compared to inactive men, with an average risk reduction between 10 to 30%.

The potential dose–response relation of decreasing risk with increasing levels of physical activity was examined in 23 studies [41,46,47,50–55,57,59–61,63–65,67–69,71–74]. A statistically significant trend [46,52,53,61,63,64,72] or borderline statistically significant trend [55,60] of decreasing prostate cancer risk with increasing activity levels was found in nine studies, but two other studies [51,65] observed trends of increasing risk with increasing activity.

No clear pattern of risk decreases or increases by type of activity was found in these studies. Occupational activity was associated with a risk decrease in six studies [39,40,52,56,64,72] and recreational activity decreased risk in seven studies [50,52,55,60,63,74]. Only one study measured all types of physical activity, including occupational, household, and recreational activity [74]. In that study, nonsignificant risk decreases were found for occupational and recreational activity, but an increased risk was observed for household activity [74]. Five studies [46,52,56,73,74] assessed more than one type of activity and presented results for each type of activity and all activities combined. The combined activity variable demonstrated the largest risk reduction in three studies [46,52,56], but not in all studies [73,74].

Similarly, no clear patterns of consistent risk increases or decreases were found in the 14 studies that assessed current activity only [41,46,48,50–56,58–60,66] or in the 16 studies that assessed lifetime occupational activity [39,40,47,57,61,64,65,67,72,73], average recreational activity over lifetime [63], or recreational activity as measured for specific time periods in the past [37,68,69–71]. Only one of these studies has systematically measured all types of activity over an entire lifetime [74]. In that study, lifetime total activity decreased prostate cancer risk by 13% and the risk reduction was not statistically significant.

TABLE 6.1
Main Results of Epidemiological Studies of Physical Activity and Prostate Cancer Risk

Study design and population	Number and types of cases	Physical activity assessment: Definition (type of activity, time period, method of assessment)	Physical activity assessment: Frequency, intensity, duration parameters	Results	Adjustment for confounding	Author, country, year (ref.)
Cohort studies — prostate cancer mortality as endpoint						
Retrospective cohort; 8393 Harvard college students born 1860–1889, died by 1967	Not stated, fatal	Three categories of college athletic participation obtained from college records	None	Increased risk; statistical significance unknown; mortality rate: Major athletes = 3.6/100 Minor athletes=2.3/100 Nonathletes = 2.2/100 Dose–response not examined	None	Polednak et al., U.S., 1976 (37)
Retrospective cohort; 6351 San Francisco longshoreman, 22-yr follow-up	30 fatal	Occupational titles obtained from work records	Intensity	Decreased risk; statistical significance unknown RR for heavy vs. light work: 0.6 Dose–response not examined	Age	Paffenbarger et al., U.S., 1987 (39)
Retrospective cohort; occupational mortality of 430,000 males in Washington State, 1950–1979	8116 fatal	Usual lifetime occupational activity obtained from death certificate coded into five-level physical activity rating.	Intensity	Decreased risk, significant PMR for highest activity jobs vs. lowest: 93, $p \leq 0.05$ Dose–response not examined	Age	Vena et al., U.S., 1987 (40)
Cohort studies — incident prostate cancer cases as endpoint						
Prospective cohort; 8006 Japanese men living in Hawaii, 21-yr follow-up, 1965/68–1986	206 incident	Physician-administered questionnaire; 24-h physical activity index as sum of time in sleep; sitting, standing, walking; moderate and heavy activities	Intensity, duration	No effect. RR for highest vs. lowest tertile of activity: 1.1 (0.8–1.5) Highest vs. lowest tertile for resting heart rate: 1.0 (0.7–1.4) No dose–response	Age and BMI	Severson et al., U.S., 1989 (41)

Prospective cohort; three counties and two cities in Norway; 53,242 men, 16 yrs median follow-up 1972/78–1991	220 incident	Self-administered questionnaire; recreational and occupational activity in four prespecified levels	Intensity, duration	Decreased risk, borderline significant RR for occupational activity (heavy manual vs. sedentary): 0.8 (0.5–1.3); recreational activity (regular training vs. sedentary): 0.9 (0.6–1.3); combined activity (moderate/active vs. sedentary): <60 yrs: 0.9 (0.4–1.9), ≥60 yrs: 0.6 (0.4–1.0) Dose–response found	Age, geographic region, and BMI; also considered: smoking, marital status, height, blood cholesterol, triglycerides, glucose	Thune and Lund, Norway, 1994 (46)
Record linkage; Shanghai Center Registry and population census, 1980–1984	264 incident	Occupations classified into indices of sitting time and energy expended	Intensity, duration	No effect SIR for high energy expenditure: 0.9 (0.7–1.1) SIR for short sitting time: 0.9 (0.8–1.1) Borderline dose–response ($p = 0.06$)	Age	Hsing et al., China, 1994 (47)
Prospective cohort; 14,407 men and women in National Health and Nutrition Examination Survey I, 1971/75 to 1987	156 incident, fatal	Interview-administered questionnaire; two questions on current recreational (R) and nonrecreational (NR) activity	Intensity	Decreased risk, nonsignificant RR for lots vs. little nonrecreational: 0.8 (0.4–1.3) Dose–response not examined	Age, BMI, smoking, alcohol, income, diabetes, cholesterol, pulse rate, recreational activity	Steenland et al., U.S., 1995 (48) (longer follow-up of same cohort reported in Albanes et al., 1989)
Prospective cohort; 7570 men in Aerobics Centre Longitudinal Study of original cohort of 28,072 men enrolled 1971–1989 followed up to 1990	94 incident	Physical activity index based on self-reported recreational activity and cardiorespiratory fitness as assessed with Balke treadmill test	Duration, frequency, intensity	Decreased risk, significant IRR for ≥3000 vs. <1000 kcal expended per week: 0.4 (0.1–1.0) IRR for highest vs. lowest quartile of fitness: 0.3 (0.1–0.6) No dose–response	Age, BMI, smoking	Oliveria et al., U.S., 1996 (50)
Prospective cohort 1050 men from Iowa 65+ Rural Health Study, 1982–1993	71 incident	Five-item questionnaire that included household, walking, and recreational activity	Frequency	Increased risk, borderline significant RR for highly vs. inactive men: 1.9 (1.0–3.5) Dose–response found	Age, BMI, smoking	Cerhan et al., U.S., 1997 (51)

continued

TABLE 6.1 (CONTINUED)
Main Results of Epidemiological Studies of Physical Activity and Prostate Cancer Risk

		Physical activity assessment				
Study design and population	Number and types of cases	Definition (type of activity, time period, method of assessment)	Frequency, intensity, duration parameters	Results	Adjustment for confounding	Author, country, year (ref.)
Randomized controlled trial; Alpha-Tocopherol Beta-Carotene Trial; 29,133 male smokers from Finland, 1985/88–1994	317 incident	Self-administered questionnaire; current recreational and occupational activity in four prespecified levels	Intensity	Decreased risk, significant RR for occupational activity compared to sedentary workers: walkers: 0.6 (0.4–1.0); walkers/lifters: 0.8 (0.5–1.3); heavy laborers: 1.2 (0.7–2.0); RR for recreational activity compared to sedentary: moderate/heavy: 0.9 (0.7–1.1); workers: 0.7 (0.5–0.9); nonworkers: 1.1 (0.8–1.5) RR for combined activity walking occupational and moderate/heavy recreational compared to sedentary: 0.4 (0.2–0.9) Dose–response found	Age, smoking, history of benign prostatic disease, urban residence, and intervention group; also considered BMI, dietary factors, alcohol, and marital status	Hartman et al., Finland, 1998 (52)
Prospective cohort; Health Professionals Follow-up Study; 47,542 men, 12-yr follow-up, 1986–1994	1362 incident cases, including 419 advanced, and 200 metastatic cases	Self-administered questionnaire; average time per week spent engaged in recreational activity; estimated total weekly MET-h	Frequency, duration, intensity	No effect RR for total activity highest vs. lowest quintile: 0.9 (0.8–1.1) No relation with total or advanced prostate cancer for total, vigorous, and nonvigorous activity Decreased risk, significant RR for highest vs. lowest quintile for metastatic cancer: 0.5 (0.2–0.9) Dose–response found	Age, height, smoking, vasectomy, diabetes, dietary factors (fat, calcium, fructose, lycopene); also considered BMI	Giovannucci et al., U.S., 1998 (53)

Prospective cohort; Physicians' Health Study; 22,071 men, 11-yr follow-up, 1982–1995	982 incident	Self-administered questionnaire; single question on frequency (times/week) of vigorous current recreational activity performed at baseline; at 36 months, question repeated with days/week as response categories	Frequency, duration	No effect RR for 5+ vs. <1 times/week frequency of vigorous exercise: 1.1 (0.9–1.4) No dose–response found	Age, randomized treatment status, cigarette smoking, alcohol intake, height, diabetes, hypercholeste-rolemia, hypertension, multivitamin use, BMI	Liu et al., U.S., 2000 (54)
Prospective cohort; National Health Screening Service survey in one county of Norway; 22,895 men, 13-yr follow-up, 1983–1996	644 incident	Self-administered questionnaire; current recreational and occupational activity; summary index of physical activity estimated	Frequency, intensity, duration	Decreased risk, borderline significant OR for highest vs. lowest tertile of recreational activity index: 0.80 (0.6–1.0) OR for high vs. low occupational activity: 1.0 (0.8–1.3) No dose–response found	Age, smoking, alcohol, marital status, education, occupation	Lund Nilsen et al., Norway, 2000 (55)
Prospective cohort; National Health and Nutrition Examination Survey I 5377 men, up to 21-yr follow-up, 1971–1992	201 incident	Self-administered questionnaire; current recreational and nonrecreational activity	Intensity	Decreased risk, significant OR for highest vs. lowest tertile of: nonrecreational activity: 0.6 (0.4–0.9); recreational activity: 0.9 (0.6–1.3); combined activity: 0.5 (0.3–0.9) Dose–response not examined	Age, education, family history, race	Clarke and Whittemore, U.S., 2000 (56)

continued

TABLE 6.1 (CONTINUED)
Main Results of Epidemiological Studies of Physical Activity and Prostate Cancer Risk

Study design and population	Number and types of cases	Physical activity assessment: Definition (type of activity, time period, method of assessment)	Physical activity assessment: Frequency, intensity, duration parameters	Results	Adjustment for confounding	Author, country, year (ref.)
Retrospective cohort; Iowa Cancer Registry and controls aged 40–64 yrs from driver's licenses and >65 yrs from Medicare lists, 1986–1989 for original case-control study; follow-up to 1995; record linkage with SEER registry for cancer incidence in cohort of 1572 controls	101 incident	Self-administered questionnaire; frequency of moderate or strenuous recreational activity during most of the adult life; usual occupational activity	Frequency	No effect OR for very active vs. inactive recreational activity: 0.9 (0.5–1.5) OR for very active vs. inactive occupational activity: 1.0 (0.6–1.8) No dose–response found	Age	Putnam et al., U.S., 2000 (57)
Retrospective cohort; 2269 male world-class athletes from 1920–1965, followed up in cancer registry for incidence 1967–1995	23 incident	Inclusion in athletic group	Intensity	No association SIR = 1.31 (0.83–1.97)	None	Pukkala et al. Finland, 2000 (58)
Prospective cohort; Harvard Alumni Health Study, 8922 men in baseline group 1988 and 6607 of them had data on PA from 1962 or 1966; follow-up to 1993	439 incident	Self-administered questionnaire; recreational activity, blocks walked and stairs climbed; divided men into consistently active (4200 kJ/wk) vs. inactive (<4200 kJ/wk) in 1962/66, 1977, and 1988	Frequency, intensity, duration	No association Total activity, kJ/wk (1988 PA data): 12,600 vs. <4200: 1.04 (0.79–1.38) Vigorous activity (recreational activity of ≥ 6 METs): 5880 vs. none: 1.22 (0.93–1.60) No dose–response found	Age, BMI, smoking, alcohol intake, paternal history of prostate cancer	Lee et al., U.S., 2001 (59) (more recent data than Lee et al., 1992, and Lee et al., 1994)

Prospective cohort; British Regional Heart Study 7630 men ages 40–59 at baseline, mean follow-up 18.8 yrs	120 incident	Interview-administered questionnaire; recreational activity and some household activity; total physical activity score estimated	Frequency, intensity	Decreased risk, significant Most active vs. least active tertile: RR = 0.25 (0.06, 0.99) Dose–response found	Age, smoking, BMI, alcohol, social class	Wannamethee et al., U.K., 2001 (60)
Prospective cohort; Swedish nationwide censuses in 1960 and 1970; record linkage with cancer registry; 18-yr follow-up to 1989	43,836/1,348,971 (1960 cohort) 28,702/1,377,629 (1970 cohort) 19,670/1,377,629 (same occupational activity in 1960 and 1970)	Self-administered questionnaire; job title	Intensity	Decreased risk, significant OR for occupational activity (highest vs. sedentary): 1960: 0.90 (0.87–0.93); 1970: 0.91 (0.88–0.95); 1960 and 1970: 0.90 (0.85–0.95) Dose–response found	Age, calendar year of follow-up by 5-yr intervals and place of residence	Norman et al., Sweden, 2002 (61)

Notes: RR = relative risk; OR = odds ratio; SIR = standardized incidence ratio; IRR = incidence rate ratio; PMR = proportional mortality ratio; SES = socioeconomic status; BMI = body mass index; MET = metabolic equivalent; PA = physical activity; TURP = transurethral resection of the prostate; BPH = benign prostatic hyperplasia; NA = not applicable.

TABLE 6.2
Case-Control Studies of Physical Activity and Prostate Cancer Risk

Study design and population	Number and types of cases	Physical activity assessment: Definition (type of activity, time period, method of assessment)	Physical activity assessment: Frequency, intensity, duration parameters	Results	Adjustment for confounding	Author, country, year (ref.)
Hospital-based case-control; Registry of American Health Foundation (20 U.S. Hospitals), 1969–1984	1162/3124 white (W) and black (B)	Interview-administered questionnaire; average lifetime weekly frequency of recreational activity categorized into three levels	Frequency	Decreased risk, borderline significant OR for active vs. seldom exercise: W: 0.7 (0.6–1.0); B: 0.7 (0.4–1.3) Dose–response for W only	Age; considered BMI, smoking, alcohol, cholesterol, education, occupation, marital status, religion	Yu et al., U.S., 1988 (63)
Hospital-based case-control; Missouri Cancer Registry source for cases and controls, 1984–1989	2878/14,269	Occupational titles used to categorize into three levels of physical activity	Intensity	Decreased risk, significant OR for high vs. moderate (M) and low (L) activity: M: 0.9 (0.8-1.0) L: 0.7 (0.6-0.8) Dose–response found	Age and smoking	Brownson et al., U.S., 1991 (64)
Population-based case-control; Hawaii Tumor Registry, 1981–1983	452/899	Interview-administered questionnaire; complete lifetime occupational history	Intensity, duration	No effect, possible increased risk, borderline significant OR for highest vs. lowest quartile time in sedentary work throughout life: <70 yrs: 1.0 (0.6–1.7); 70 yrs: 1.6 (1.0–2.5) Dose–response found	Age, ethnicity; also considered: income, education, dietary factors (saturated fat, beta-carotene, zinc)	Le Marchand et al., U.S., 1991 (65)

Population-based case-control; Utah Cancer Registry, RDD controls, 1984–1985	358/679	Interview-administered questionnaire; time spent in moderate and vigorous activities converted to calories expended	Intensity, duration	Increased risk, nonsignificant OR for active vs. inactive: 45–67 yrs with aggressive tumors: 2.0 (0.8–5.2); no risks provided for older men Dose–response not examined	None; considered age and other factors not specifically stated	West et al., U.S., 1991 (66)
Hospital-based case-control; oncological treatment center in Istanbul source for cases and noncancer controls, 1979–1984	27/2127	Occupational titles used to estimate time-weighted average energy expenditure and sitting time during work over lifetime	Intensity, duration	No effect OR for highest vs. lowest tertile for energy expenditure: 0.3 (0.03-2.0) OR for >6 h/day vs. <2 h/day sitting time: 0.9 (0.08-10) No dose–response	Age, smoking, SES	Dosemeci et al., Turkey, 1993 (67)
Population-based case-control; Örebro county controls from population register, 1989–1992	256/252	Interview-administered questionnaire; physical activity during puberty as compared to classmates	None (physical activity relative to peers)	Decreased risk, nonsignificant OR for higher vs. lower activity in puberty: 0.7 (0.4–1.1) No dose–response	Age, grade of urbanization, farming	Andersson et al., Sweden, 1995 (68)
Multicenter population-based case-control; black (B), white (W), Japanese (J) and Chinese–(C) American cases and controls, 1989–1991	1655/1645	Interview-administered questionnaire; 24-h daily activity and occupational activity	Duration, intensity	No effect OR and p (trend) for highest vs. lowest tertiles: B: 1.2 p = 0.09; W: 0.92 p = 0.62; J: 0.84 p = 0.76; C: 0.70 p = 0.11 No dose–response	Age, energy, fat intake; also considered: region, education	Whittemore et al., U.S., Canada, 1995 (69)

continued

TABLE 6.2 (CONTINUED)
Case-Control Studies of Physical Activity and Prostate Cancer Risk

Study design and population	Number and types of cases	Physical activity assessment: Definition (type of activity, time period, method of assessment)	Physical activity assessment: Frequency, intensity, duration parameters	Results	Adjustment for confounding	Author, country, year (ref.)
Hospital-based case-control; three hospitals in Taipei source for cases and noncancer controls, 1995–1996	90/180	Interview-administered questionnaire; frequency of weekly exercise and some household activity classified into four intensity levels done 5–10 yrs before interview	Frequency, intensity, duration	Increased risk, significant OR for exercise (yes vs. no): 2.2 (1.2-3.3) Dose–response not examined	Age, BMI, education, some dietary factors; also considered: smoking, alcohol, coffee, tea, and other dietary food groups	Sung et al., Taiwan, 1999 (70)
Multicenter population-based case-control; eight provinces in Canadian National Cancer Enhanced Surveillance System project, 1994–1997	1623/1623	In seven provinces: participation in 12 recreational activities 2 yrs prediagnosis; In Ontario: participation in recreational and occupational activities for mid-teens/20s, 30s, 50s, and 2 yrs prediagnosis	Frequency, intensity, duration	No effect overall Strenuous recreational activity (non-Ontario) (yes vs. no): 1.2 (0.8–1.7); strenuous occupational and recreational activity 2 yrs before (Ontario) (yes vs. no): 0.9 (0.7–1.3) Decreased risk, significant Strenuous vs. sitting occupational activity for mid-teens/early 20s (Ontario): 0.6 (0.4–0.9) No dose–response	Age, province, race, years since quitting smoking, pack-years, BMI, diet, income, family history of cancer	Villeneuve et al., Canada, 1999 (71)

Hospital-based case-control study; eight hospitals in Quebec for cases and controls; all men referred for TURP for BPH symptoms, 1990–1992	64/546	Interview-administered questionnaire; intensity of lifetime occupational history; frequency and duration of recreational activities	Intensity, frequency, duration	Decreased risk, significant OR for highest vs. lowest quartile of occupational activity: 0.2 (0.1–0.7) OR for highest vs. lowest tertile of recreational activity: 1.1 (0.6–2.0) Dose–response found	Age, education, total energy intake, smoking, vitamin use	Bairati et al., Canada, 2000 (72)
Population-based case-control study; Shanghai Cancer Institute for cases and controls through Shanghai Resident Registry, 1993–1995	238/206 BPH controls, 471 population controls	Interview-administered questionnaire; occupational activity (main activity and job title) at ages 20–29, 40–49 and ~67 (1988); hours/day spent sleeping, sedentary, being moderately or vigorously active	Frequency, intensity, duration	No association Energy expenditure (high vs. low): ages 20–29: 1.1 (0.7–1.7); 40–49: 1.3 (0.8–1.9); ~67: 0.9 (0.5–1.8) Occupational activity: ages 20–29: 2.9 (1.1–7.5); 40–49: 2.9 (1.3–6.8); ~67: 3.2 (1.0–10.4) Moderate/vigorous activity: ages 20–29: 1.1 (0.8–1.7); 40–49: 1.2 (0.7–2.0); ~67: 1.4 (0.9–2.1) All activity: ages 20–29: 1.1 (0.7–1.8); 40–49: 1.2 (0.8–1.9); ~67: 1.4 (0.9–2.1) No dose–response found	Age, marital status, BMI, education, caloric intake, WHR	Lacey et al., Shanghai, 2001 (73)

continued

TABLE 6.2 (CONTINUED)
Case-Control Studies of Physical Activity and Prostate Cancer Risk

Study design and population	Number and types of cases	Physical activity assessment: Definition (type of activity, time period, method of assessment)	Physical activity assessment: Frequency, intensity, duration parameters	Results	Adjustment for confounding	Author, country, year (ref.)
Population-based case-control study cases identified through Alberta Cancer Registry, controls through random digit dialing, 1997–2000	988/1063	Interview-administered questionnaire using cognitive interviewing methods; lifetime occupational, household, and recreational activity	Frequency, intensity, duration	Null association OR for lifetime total activity, highest vs. lowest quartile: 0.87 (0.65–1.17) Occupational activity: 0.90 (0.66–1.22) Household activity: 1.36 (1.05–1.76) Recreational activity: 0.80 (0.61–1.04) No dose–response found except for household activity where an increased risk was observed	Age, region, education, BMI, WHR, total caloric intake, lifetime average alcohol intake, first degree family history of prostate cancer, number of PSA tests and DREs; models of each type of activity adjusted for other types of activity	Friedenreich et al., Canada, 2004 (74)

Notes: RR = relative risk; OR = odds ratio; SES = socioeconomic status; BMI = body mass index; MET = metabolic equivalent; PA = physical activity; TURP = transurethral resection of the prostate; BPH = benign prostatic hyperplasia; NA = not applicable.

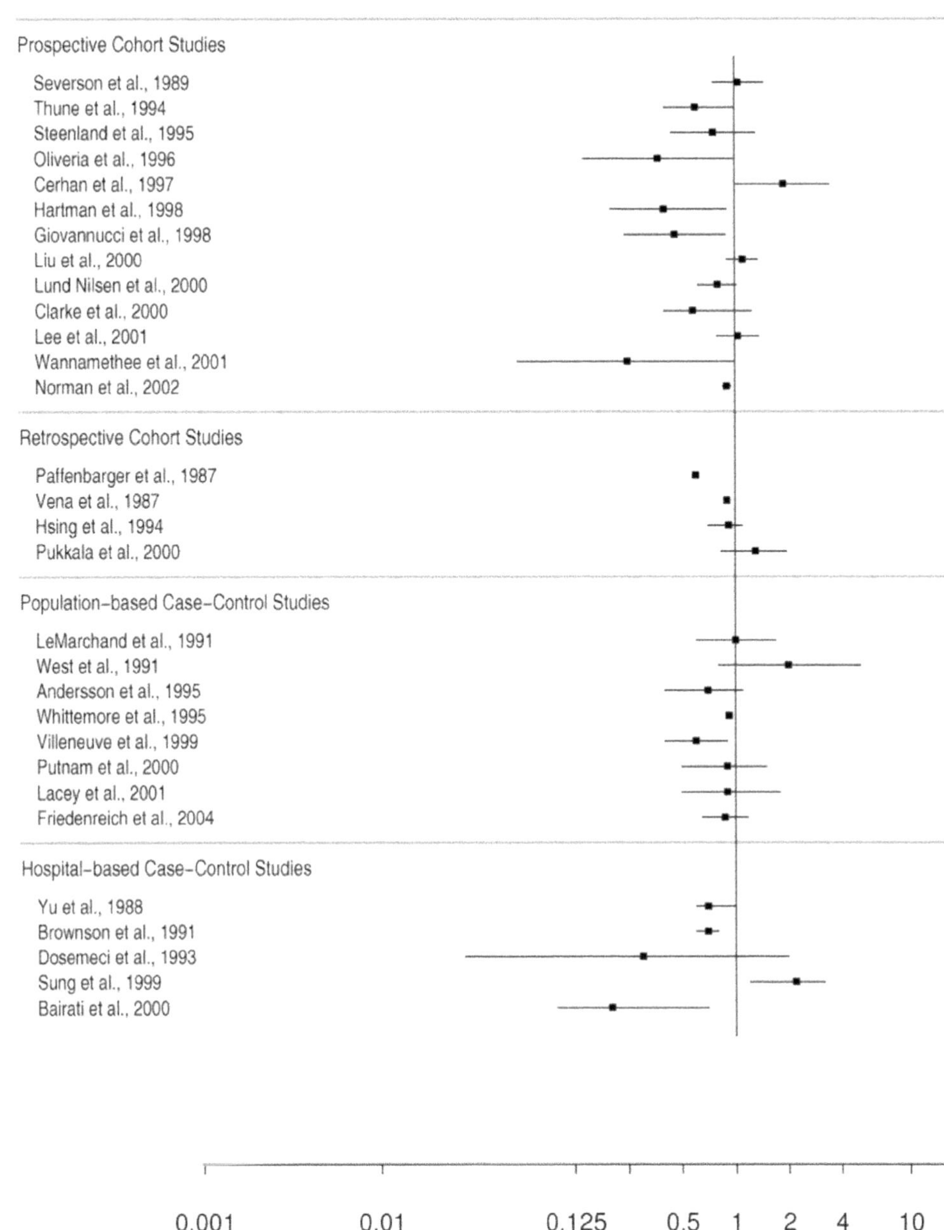

FIGURE 6.1 Main results of epidemiologic studies of physical activity and prostate cancer risk.

Population Subgroup Results

It would be of interest to know if the association between physical activity and prostate cancer varies by age at diagnosis, family history of prostate cancer, race, or other possible risk factors. Results specific to population subgroups are relevant for formulating hypotheses about the natural history of the disease and the possibility of influencing carcinogenesis during different susceptible periods, for designing and analyzing future studies, and for developing public health guidelines.

For the studies reviewed here, there appeared to be more consistent prostate cancer risk reductions among physically active men in the European studies than in the American studies. Six [46,52,55,60,61,68] of eight [46,52,55,58,60,61,67,68] studies conducted in Europe found risk decreases compared with only eight [39,40,48,50,56,63,64,72] of twenty [37,39–41,48,50,51,53,54,56,57,59,63–66,69,71,72,74] studies conducted in North America. Europeans have a wider range of recreational and occupational activities because their work is less mechanized and their lifestyles are more active than in North America. This difference in levels of physical activity is also apparent in the higher prevalence of obesity in the U.S. compared to European countries [75].

Relatively few of these previous studies have attempted any type of subgroup analysis. Nine studies have presented results stratified by different age groups [46,65,66,71,73,74], ethnic and racial groups [63,69], or stage of cancer at diagnosis [53]. No consistent subgroup effects have been delineated thus far for these factors. Giovannucci et al. [53] did find a reduction in risk for metastatic prostate cancer cases only that was not found in any other stages of cancers examined in that study. The results for age have been inconsistent because a greater risk reduction was found among older men (≥60 years) for combined occupational and recreational activity in the Norwegian cohort study [46], but the Hawaiian case-control study [65] found an increased risk of prostate cancer among older men (≥70 years) who had the highest occupational activity levels. In the one study that measured all activity from childhood to the reference period (diagnosis date or a comparable time for controls), some evidence for risk reduction for activity done in early life up to age 18 was found. The most physically active upper quartile of men experienced a 22%, nonstatistically significant decreased risk [74].

The most recently published study also examined effect modification by additional risk factors, including body mass index (BMI, kg/m^2), family history of prostate cancer, and alcohol intake [74]. In that study, the only evidence for effect modification found was for men with a family history of prostate cancer. Prostate cancer risk for men with a prostate cancer family history in the highest quartile of activity compared to the lowest was reduced by 52%; those without such a history had no risk reduction [74]. BMI was not found to be a risk factor or an effect modifier in this study [76]. Effect modification in the association of physical activity and prostate cancer risk has not yet been adequately investigated.

Physical Fitness and Prostate Cancer Risk

Only one cohort study, conducted by Oliveria et al. [50] in the Aerobics Centre Longitudinal Study, assessed the association between cardiorespiratory fitness and prostate cancer risk. In that cohort, study participants' physical fitness levels were measured at baseline using a maximal exercise treadmill test. A 74% reduction was found in the highest compared to the lowest quartile of fitness level, with clear evidence of a trend across quartiles. Physical fitness is a complex construct that combines various personal physiological and genetic factors. It is correlated with physical activity but cannot be used interchangeably as a surrogate measure for physical activity. Physical fitness is, however, an objective measure that is less likely to be subject to recall bias or recall error. Although measuring physical fitness in epidemiological studies is logistically challenging and infeasible, these preliminary findings are noteworthy and suggest that additional investigations on physical fitness and prostate cancer risk could be worthwhile.

BIOLOGICAL MECHANISMS

To understand how physical activity may be influencing prostate carcinogenesis, the natural history of prostate cancer and possible underlying biological mechanisms need to be understood. The natural history of prostate cancer is still uncertain because the disease progression is highly variable and unpredictable [77,78]. There is, however, agreement that most prostate cancers have a long, presymptomatic, nonmetastatic phase [79]. The prevalence of small prostatic carcinomas, as determined from autopsy series, is nearly 30% in men aged 30 to 40 and over 60% in men aged 60 to 70 [79]. From the PCPT [35] — the chemoprevention trial that included only men without an elevated PSA (<3 ng/ml) who were subsequently biopsied — the prevalence of prostate cancer was found to be higher than anticipated by PSA screening (24% cancer detection in placebo group vs. an expected lifetime incidence of 17%). This rate varies widely internationally because the detection of latent disease depends on the medical practices of each country. The disease course complicates treatment and assessment of etiological factors.

Although the natural history of prostate cancer is still poorly understood, several lines of evidence support a role for endogenous androgens in prostate carcinogenesis, including the following facts:

- Androgens are required for the normal growth and development of the prostate gland.
- Large doses of androgens induce prostate cancer in rodents [80].
- Prostate cancer incidence and benign prostatic hypertrophy are low in castrated men [81].
- Androgens stimulate the *in vitro* proliferation of human prostate cancer cells [82].
- Castration or estrogen therapy often causes tumor regression and is also an effective palliative treatment for metastatic prostate cancer [83,84].
- Increased levels of circulating testosterone, as well as lower levels of estradiol and sex hormone–binding globulin (SHBG), have been associated with an increased risk of prostate cancer [85] but this effect has not been consistently found [86–88].

It is hypothesized that androgens may not be involved in prostate cancer *initiation* [89] but that an altered hormone metabolism may play a role in the *progression* of prostate cancer from histological to clinically significant forms [90].

At least five biological mechanisms have been postulated for how physical activity might reduce the risk of prostate cancer. These mechanisms include alterations in endogenous hormones, energy balance, insulin-like growth factors, immune function, and antioxidant defense mechanisms. It is possible that higher levels of physical activity may affect male sex hormone metabolism by decreasing circulating testosterone. Physical activity may influence prostate carcinogenesis by suppressing dihydrotestosterone (DHT) activity via inhibition of 5-α-reductase type II, the enzyme that converts testosterone to DHT [91]. The blood level of a distal DHT metabolite, 3α-androstanediol glucuronide (3α-diol G), appears to correlate well with levels of activity of 5-α-reductase.

Several studies have shown a weak positive association between serum levels of 3α-diol G and prostate cancer risk [86,87]. Athletes have been shown to have lower basal levels of testosterone and individuals who exercise may have a temporary decrease in postexercise levels of testosterone [92–97]. However, the impact of these changes in serum androgen concentrations on the risk of prostate cancer remains unclear. At present, it can only be hypothesized that because endogenous androgens are associated with the development of prostate cancer, men who are more physically active may be at decreased risk of prostate cancer because they may have lower levels of these hormones.

Second, physical activity may affect prostate cancer risk through its influence on energy balance and prevention of obesity and weight gain. Overweight and obesity are inconsistently associated with prostate cancer risk [17]; nonetheless, several possible mechanisms whereby energy balance could influence prostate cancer risk do exist. BMI has been shown to be an important predictor of metabolically active androgen concentrations, and habitual physical activity and BMI were found to be independent predictors of serum testosterone [98]. Reducing body fat stores results in reduced conversion of androgens to estrogens and of estrogens to more potent carcinogens [99,100]. Increased fat intake has been associated with increased prostate cancer risk [101]. Physical activity may alter the metabolism of fat to decrease its carcinogenicity [102]. Low-fat, high-fiber diets have been shown to affect androgen levels by decreasing circulating testosterone [103]. Thus, physical activity, dietary intake, and endogenous hormones may have an inter-related influence on prostate carcinogenesis.

The third possible biological mechanism whereby physical activity may influence prostate cancer risk is through insulin and the insulin-like growth factor (IGF) axis. Evidence from observational epidemiological studies suggests that IGF-1 levels are associated with prostate cancer risk. This association has been observed in populations of symptomatic cases or men identified through surgical treatment for benign prostatic hyperplasia [104–107], as well as populations of screen-detected prostate cancer cases [108]. Experimental studies in humans have shown that men adopting a low-fat diet and daily exercise routine reduced their levels of serum insulin and IGF-1 while increasing their levels of IGFBP-1 and SHBG [109]. A low-fat diet and/or intensive exercise decrease serum hormones and growth factors *in vivo* that can reduce growth and induce apoptosis of LNCaP prostate cancer cells *in vitro* [110–112]. Furthermore, it appears that these effects are mediated by enhancement of the p53 gene [113]. These results suggest that prostate cancer may be another aspect of the insulin-resistance syndrome purported to be etiologically relevant in other hormone-dependent cancers [109].

The fourth plausible biological mechanism is that physical activity may enhance the immune system by improving the capacity and numbers of natural killer cells [114,115]. Although current evidence suggests that the majority of human cancers are not related to immune function, it is possible that modulation of the immune system by exercise can inhibit cancer development (through immune enhancement) and promote cancer (through immune suppression) [116]. Experimental studies have found that exercise can improve the innate immune mechanisms [117–119]. Immune function is known to decrease with aging and may account, in part, for the increased risk of cancer with aging [120]. Cross-sectional studies conducted among elderly populations have found significantly higher T-cell function among study participants who exercised regularly compared to those who were sedentary [121]. Exercise can induce changes in the activity of macrophages, natural killer cells, neutrophils, and regulating cytokines; however, further research is needed before it can be asserted that these changes have a substantial influence on cancer risk [122] because several different immune function mechanisms may contribute to the lowered cancer risk of the physically active [123]. If an association between cancer risk and immunity exists, it remains poorly understood at present and it may make a minor contribution.

Finally, physical activity may generate reactive oxygen species (i.e., free radicals) [124]. Acute exercise may promote free radical production while chronic exercise improves free radical defenses by up-regulating the activities of key free radical scavenger enzymes (i.e., superoxide dismutase and glutathione peroxidase) and levels of antioxidants (i.e., glutathione and tocopherols) [125]. Thus, the borderline between beneficial and noxious effects of physical activity depends on several factors, including the health status, age, level of training, and nutritional status of the individual [126]. Radical scavenger supplementation (e.g., antioxidant vitamins, metal ion chelators, coenzyme Q, and glutathione precursors) may improve the positive effects of exercise and provide more protection to the body against so-called oxidative stress. Antioxidants obtained from dietary sources have already been hypothesized to reduce prostate cancer risk, so a comparable causal mechanism may exist for antioxidants resulting from physical activity [127]. The extent to which these exercise-induced changes in oxidant defense influence cancer risk is still unknown.

METHODOLOGICAL ISSUES

Methodological issues to be considered when reviewing these studies on physical activity and prostate cancer risk include possible outcome misclassification, physical activity assessment methods, and the effects that confounding and effect modification may have on this relation.

Outcome Misclassification

One possible reason for the inconclusive and inconsistent results found in these studies arises from combining cases with different disease states or in combining men without disease into the case group. Only 2 [69,74] of the previous 12 case-control studies [63–74] attempted to address the issue of undetected prostate cancer in the control population and stage of cancer in the case population. The multicenter case-control study by Whittemore et al. [69] included testing of PSA levels in the controls for most of the centers involved and staging of the cases into localized vs. advanced categories. The controls were stratified in the analysis into two groups, according to PSA levels taken shortly after the interview. The population-based case-control study by Friedenreich et al. [74] included only stage T2 or greater cases in an attempt to make the comparison with the controls more valid by excluding any T1 cases that were incidentally detected.

The results of the remaining case-control studies, as well as the cohort studies, were likely influenced by some misclassification of outcome among the controls because the prevalence of undetected prostate cancer among men in the age ranges relevant for prostate cancer incidence is about 20 to 40% [128]. The effect of undetected cancer among the controls would be to bias the results towards the null. Thus, one possible explanation for the weak associations found in these studies could be the effect of differential misclassification bias.

In studies that have been conducted since PSA tests for screening were commonly introduced (late 1980s for North American countries, early 1990s for European countries and later for Asian countries), a number of lower stage prostate cancer cases could have been included in the case group because they were detected due to an elevated PSA level rather than because of clinical symptoms. Among the studies reviewed here, it was found that, on average, the more recent studies were less likely to show an effect of physical activity on prostate cancer risk than were the earlier studies.

It was previously noted that Giovannucci et al. [53] observed a risk reduction only among the metastatic cases. One explanation is that there has been outcome misclassification in recent studies that have not removed lower stage (e.g., T1) cases from the case group to ensure a more valid comparison with the controls. Because a large proportion of men have undetected, latent prostate cancer, the controls in these studies might have included cases unless some measure was taken to ensure that the controls were actually free of prostate cancer. It is also possible that men became cases solely because of elevated PSA levels detected through routine screening and that these incidental cancers would never have been clinically detected [129]. Therefore, outcome misclassification is possible in the case and control groups because of the nature of prostate carcinogenesis and the methods used for its detection.

Exposure Assessment

Some of the inconsistencies observed in these investigations are likely attributable to the differences in the physical activity assessment methods used. The main problems include crude classification systems for physical activity, incomplete measurement of all the parameters of physical activity and all time periods of life, and the lack of validated and reliable instruments.

An individual measurement of activity was made for some of the studies that measured recreational or occupational activity [41,43,50–54,63,65,66,68,70] or leisure and work activity [46,48,55–57,60,69,70–74], but not for some of the occupational studies [39,40,47,61,64,67] or recreational studies [37,58] that used a group assignment of activity. Exposure misclassification could have occurred for the studies that used the job title as a measure for physical activity rather than an individual assessment of actual occupational activity performed.

Only 9 of the 31 studies [48,50,53,55,70–74] measured the frequency, duration, and intensity of physical activity directly from the study subjects. Two other studies [39,59] combined information on frequency, intensity, and duration into a single measure of energy expenditure with intensity assigned by the investigators based on available literature. It is currently still unclear what frequency, duration, and intensity of activity are required for a prostate cancer risk reduction or what combination of these components of activity will influence risk. For example, a certain intensity level may be necessary for physical activity to have an influence on prostate cancer risk via a biological mechanism that involves androgen hormones. Friedenreich et al. [74] observed a 30% statistically significant risk reduction for vigorous intensity activity for men in the highest quartile of hours per week per year of all types of activity combined. No clear comparable pattern of risk reduction was observed when examining the association by frequency and duration only [74].

The time period in a man's life when physical activity is most etiologically relevant has only been fully addressed in one study thus far [74]. Because the prostate is a hormone-dependent organ that undergoes significant changes at different time periods in life, there may be particularly susceptible time periods when physical activity may have more influence on carcinogenesis. More studies are needed that measure activity and assess risk throughout a man's life before recommendations can be made regarding which time periods are most etiologically important for a risk reduction.

Only four studies tested the instrument for reliability and validity [41,46,53,59]. In the Hawaiian cohort study [41], a 24-hour activity grid was used that was derived from a measurement instrument developed and tested for reliability and validity in the Framingham Heart Study [130]. In the Norwegian cohort study [46], repeated assessments of activity as well as objective measures of fitness (e.g., fitness tests and heart rate measures) and metabolic risk profiles were performed to examine the reliability and validity of the instrument used [131]. The validity and reproducibility of the physical activity questionnaire used in the Health Professionals Follow-up Study [53] were investigated in a subset of the cohort [132]. In the Harvard Health Alumni study [59], university records were used to determine the approximate frequency and duration of physical activity in which study subjects engaged during their college years. Although these measurements are not subject to recall bias, because they are based on records rather than self-report they still suffer from the same limitations as the other studies because they did not measure the intensity of activity. Later measures of physical activity in this study [59] were based on a questionnaire, the validity of which had been tested against other physical activity questionnaires and physiological measures. The reliability, but not the validity, of the lifetime total physical activity questionnaire used in the Alberta case-control study was previously established [133].

Confounding and Effect Modification

Because the underlying biological model and mechanisms operative in the association between physical activity and prostate cancer are unclear, epidemiological studies need to incorporate and examine a wide range of possible confounders and effect modifiers. Possible confounding factors include diet and alcohol intake, socioeconomic status, smoking, ethnicity, family history of cancer, and, possibly, reproductive and medical factors [2,5,6]. Possible effect modifiers are anthropometric factors, endogenous hormone levels, and age. Height has been shown to be a risk factor for prostate cancer but the data are inconsistent for BMI, waist–hip ratio, and weight [17]. Height is influenced by genetic factors, but also by exposure before and during puberty to androgens that are also implicated in the normal development of the prostate gland. Physical activity may influence the level of endogenous androgens around the time of puberty through its influence on height and weight.

Residual confounding may have influenced a number of the previous studies that did not assess confounding completely. Three of the epidemiological studies reviewed here did not adjust for any confounders [38,58,66]; five adjusted for age only [39,40,47,57,63]; 16 adjusted for some prostate cancer risk factors [41,46,48,50,51,54–56,59–61,64,65,67,68,70]; and seven studies measured and controlled for most of these risk factors [52,53,69,71–74].

The main risk factor that was not measured and controlled for in the majority of the studies was dietary intake. The biological mechanism whereby dietary fat mediates an influence on prostate cancer risk is thought to be through endogenous hormones [103]. Although the interaction of steroid hormones with the development of prostate cancer is poorly understood at present, studies have found that a low-fat, high-fiber diet decreases circulating testosterone [134–136]. Physical activity may also mediate prostate cancer risk through its influence on endogenous hormones and physically active individuals may have diets that differ systematically from inactive people; therefore, dietary intake is a key factor that needs to be measured and controlled for in epidemiological studies of physical activity and prostate cancer risk.

Confounding by unmeasured and uncontrolled behavioral factors associated with being physically active may also explain, in part, the possible association between physical activity and prostate cancer risk. It is possible that individuals who are physically active are lean, generally healthier, and nonsmokers, seek medical care more readily, and generally exhibit other healthy behaviors that contribute to their observed reduction in risk of prostate cancer.

Some of the discrepancies in the study results may be attributable to underlying differences in the characteristics of the subjects included. It is therefore important that future research studies examine the modifying effects of physical activity within defined strata of other prostate cancer risk factors, particularly because such analyses may provide insights into biological mechanisms. It would be useful to examine relationships by age, body size, body fat distribution patterns, and dietary intake — to name just a few of the major risk factors. Such analyses will need to ensure that adequate power exists for meaningful interpretations of the subgroup effects.

DIRECTIONS FOR FUTURE RESEARCH

Overall, previous epidemiological studies indicate that physical activity may decrease the risk of prostate cancer; however, the association is relatively weak and considerable inconsistency exists across these studies. Given this inconsistency and the lack of understanding of the precise role of physical activity in prostate cancer etiology, numerous questions remain to be answered. Research priorities can be categorized into research on: (1) physical activity assessment methods; (2) etiological studies; and (3) biological mechanisms.

The validity of different physical activity assessment methods needs to be improved and the reliability of these methods assessed. Future studies need to measure all *types* of physical activity (occupational, recreational, household) and all *components* of physical activity (frequency, intensity and duration) across *entire lifetimes*. Direct measures of physical activity and fitness should also be included in addition to the subjective measures. New research on assessment methods should consider the underlying biological mechanisms in the design and evaluation of these tools.

Additional etiological studies on a larger scale that measure activity appropriately and include complete assessments of confounding and effect modification are needed. For future prospective studies, repeat measures of activity and any confounders that may change over time, such as dietary intake, are needed so that information pertaining to all time periods being measured is available. A full assessment of confounders will also assist in distinguishing the independent role of physical activity as an etiological risk factor for prostate cancer separate from its contribution to a healthy lifestyle. Studies within different ethnic and racial groups are also needed, as well as studies that examine the risk by different stages of prostate cancer.

Finally, additional research on the possible biological mechanisms for the role of physical activity on prostate risk is needed. At least five major mechanisms were reviewed here, including an influence of physical activity on endogenous hormones, energy balance, insulin-like growth factors, immune function, and antioxidant defenses. Experimental studies in animal and human models that examine how physical activity influences each of these biological mechanisms would provide important insights into the etiology of prostate cancer. These studies could examine how age, time of life, and the intensity, duration, and frequency of activity influence these different biological mechanisms. A better understanding of the natural history of prostate cancer would provide useful insights in the design and conduct of future etiological studies of physical activity and prostate cancer. In particular, possible surrogate endpoints that could be used as biomarkers of prostate cancer risk in future prospective etiological studies and intervention trials are also needed [137,138].

CONCLUSION

Currently, the epidemiological evidence for an etiological role of physical activity in prostate carcinogenesis remains weak and inconsistent. Although several possible biological mechanisms can be hypothesized for this putative association, additional well-designed and appropriately conducted observational studies are needed to elucidate the nature of this association more completely before intervention research on the biological mechanisms would be justified. Prostate cancer remains an important cause of cancer morbidity and mortality among men and few modifiable lifestyle risk factors appear to be strongly associated with prostate cancer; thus, physical activity as a means for the primary prevention for prostate cancer merits further research consideration.

ACKNOWLEDGMENTS

Christine M. Friedenreich was supported by a Canadian Institutes of Health Research New Investigator Award and an Alberta Heritage Foundation for Medical Research Health Scholar Award while writing this paper.

Permission has been received from Kluwer Academic Publishers to reprint parts of an earlier version of this literature review published in *Cancer Causes and Control* (2001; 12:461–475).

REFERENCES

1. Quinn M, Babb P. Patterns and trends in prostate cancer incidence, survival, prevalence, and mortality. Part I: international comparisons. *BJU Int* 2002; 90:162–173.
2. Gronberg H. Prostate cancer epidemiology. *Lancet* 2003; 361:859–864.
3. American Cancer Society. *Cancer Facts and Figures* 2003; Atlanta, GA: American Cancer Society, 2004.
4. National Cancer Institute of Canada. *Canadian Cancer Statistics* 2004; Toronto, Canada.
5. Boyle P. The epidemiology of prostate cancer. *Urol Clin N Am* 2003; 30:209–217.
6. Crawford ED. Epidemiology of prostate cancer. *Urology* 2003; 62:3–12.
7. Reddy S, Shapiro M, Morton R Jr, Brawley OW. Prostate cancer in black and white Americans. *Cancer Metast Rev* 2003; 22:83–86.
8. Lichtenstein P, Holm NV, Verkasalo PK, Iliadou A, Kaprio J, Koskenvuo M, Pukkala E, Skytthe A, Hemminki K. Environmental and heritable factors in the causation of cancer — analyses of cohorts of twins from Sweden, Denmark, and Finland. *N Engl J Med* 2000; 343:78–85.
9. Hsieh K, Albertsen PC. Populations at high risk for prostate cancer. *Urol Clin N Am* 2003; 30:669–676.
10. Bosland MC. Chapter 2: the role of steroid hormones in prostate carcinogenesis. *J Natl Cancer Inst Monogr* 2000; 27:39–66.
11. Chen C, Weiss NS, Stanczyk FZ, Lewis SK, DiTommaso D, Etzioni R, Barnett MJ, Goodman GE. Endogenous sex hormones and prostate cancer risk: a case-control study nested within the Carotene and Retinol Efficacy Trial. *Cancer Epidemiol Biomarkers Prev* 2003; 12:1410–1416.
12. Shirai T, Asamoto M, Takahashi S, Imaida K. Diet and prostate cancer. *Toxicology* 2002; 181–182; 89–94.
13. Kushi L, Giovannucci E. Dietary fat and cancer. *Am J Med* 2002; 113:63S–70S.
14. Willis MS, Wians FH Jr. The role of nutrition in preventing prostate cancer: a review of the proposed mechanism of action of various dietary substances. *Clinica Chimica Acta* 2003; 330:57–83.
15. Dagnelie PC, Schuurman AG, Goldbohm RA, van den Brandt PA. Diet, anthropometric measures and prostate cancer risk: a review of prospective cohort and intervention studies. *BJU Int* 2004; 93:1139–1150.
16. Hodge AM, English DR, McCredie MRE, Severi G, Boyle P, Hopper JL, Giles GG. Foods, nutrients and prostate cancer. *Cancer Causes Control* 2004; 15:11–20.

17. Ballard–Barbash R, Slattery M, Thune I, Friedenreich CM. Obesity, body composition and cancer risk. In: Schottenfeld D, Fraumeni JF Jr, Eds. *Cancer Epidemiology and Prevention.* 3rd ed. Oxford University Press. In press .
18. Hickey K, Do K-A, Green A. Smoking and prostate cancer. *Epidemiol Rev* 2001; 23:115–125.
19. Giovannucci E, Rimm EB, Ascherio A, Colditz GA, Spiegelman D, Stampfer MJ, Willett WC. Smoking and risk of total and fatal prostate cancer in United States health professionals. *Cancer Epidemiol Biomarkers Prev* 1999; 8:277–282.
20. Dennis LK. Meta-analyses for combining relative risks of alcohol consumption and prostate cancer. *Prostate* 2000; 42:56–66.
21. Dennis LK, Hayes RB. Alcohol and prostate cancer. *Epidemiol Rev* 2001; 23:110–114.
22. Platz EA, Leitzmann MF, Rimm EB, Willett WC, Giovannucci E. Alcohol intake, drinking patterns, and risk of prostate cancer in a large prospective cohort study. *Am J Epidemiol* 2004; 159:444–453.
23. Strickler HD, Goedert JJ. Sexual behavior and evidence for an infectious cause of prostate cancer. *Epidemiol Rev* 2001; 23:144–151.
24. Dennis LK, Dawson DV. Meta-analysis of measures of sexual activity and prostate cancer. *Epidemiology* 2002; Jan; 13:72–79.
25. Dennis LK, Dawson DV, Resnick MI. Vasectomy and the risk of prostate cancer: a meta-analysis examining vasectomy status, age at vasectomy, and time since vasectomy. *Prostate Cancer Prostatic Dis* 2002; 5:193–203.
26. Parent ME, Siemiatycki J. Occupation and prostate cancer. *Epidemiol Rev* 2001; 23:138–143.
27. Zeegers MPA, Friesema IHM, Goldbohm RA, van den Brandt PA. A prospective study of occupation and prostate cancer risk. *JOEM* 2004; 46:271–279.
28. Barqawi A, Thompson IM, Crawford ED. Prostate cancer chemoprevention: an overview of United States trials. *J Urol* 2004; 171:S5–S9.
29. Ansari MS, Gupta NP, Hemal AK. Chemoprevention of carcinoma prostate: a review. *Int Urol Nephrol* 2002; 34:207–214.
30. Leach R, Pollock B, Basler J, Troyer D, Naylor S, Thompson IM. Chemoprevention of prostate cancer. Focus on key opportunities and clinical trials. *Urol Clin N Am* 2003; 30:227–237.
31. Meuillet E, Stratton S, Cherukuri DP, Goulet A-C, Kagey J, Porterfield B, Nelson MA. Chemoprevention of prostate cancer with selenium: an update on current clinical trials and preclinical findings. *J Cell Biochem* 2004; 91:443–458.
32. Giovannucci E. Tomatoes, tomato-based products, lycopene, and cancer: review of the epidemiologic literature. *J Natl Cancer Inst* 1999; 91:317–331.
33. Mahal K, Hernandez J, Basler JW, Thompson IM. What's new in the field of prostate cancer chemoprevention? *Curr Oncol Rep* 2004; 6:237–242.
34. Klein EA, Thompson IM, Lippman SM, Goodman PJ, Albanes D, Taylor PR, Coltman C. SELECT: the selenium and vitamin E cancer prevention trial. *Urol Oncol: Sem Orig Invest* 2003; 21:59–65.
35. Thompson IM, Goodman PJ, Tangen CM, Lucia MS, Miller GJ, Ford LG, Lieber MM, Cespedes RD, Atkins JN, Lippman SM, Carlin SM, Ryan A, Szczepanek CM, Crowley JJ, Coltman CA Jr. The influence of finasteride of the development of prostate cancer. *N Engl J Med* 2003; 349:215–224.
36. Friedenreich CM, Orenstein MR. Physical activity and cancer prevention: etiological evidence and biological mechanisms. *J Nutr* 2002; 132:3456S–3464S.
37. Polednak AP. College athletics, body size, and cancer mortality. *Cancer* 1976; 38:382–387.
38. Whittemore AS, Paffenbarger RS, Anderson K, Lee JE. Early precursors of site-specific cancers in college men and women. *J Natl Cancer Inst* 1985; 74:43–51.
39. Paffenbarger RS, Hyde RT, Wing AL. Physical activity and incidence of cancer in diverse populations: a preliminary report. *Am J Clin Nutr* 1987; 45:312–317.
40. Vena JE, Graham S, Zielezny M, Brasure J, Swanson MK. Occupational exercise and risk of cancer. *Am J Clin Nutr* 1987; 45:318–327.
41. Severson RK, Nomura AMY, Grove JS, Stemmerman GN. A prospective analysis of physical activity and cancer. *Am J Epidemiol* 1989; 130:522–529.
42. Albanes D, Blair A, Taylor PR. Physical activity and risk of cancer in the NHANES I population. *Am J Public Health* 1989; 79:744–50.
43. Lee I-M, Paffenbarger RS, Hsieh C-C. Physical activity and risk of prostatic cancer among college alumni. *Am J Epidemiol* 1992; 135:169–179.

44. Paffenbarger RS Jr, Lee I-M, Wong AL. Ch. 2 The influence of physical activity on the incidence of site-specific cancers in college alumni. In: Jacobs MM, Ed. *Exercise, Fat, and Cancer.* New York: Plenum Press; 1992, pp. 7–15.
45. Lee IM, Paffenbarger RS Jr. Physical activity and its relation to cancer risk: a prospective study of college alumni. *Med Sci Sports Exercise* 1994; 26: 831–837.
46. Thune I, Lund E. Physical activity and the risk of prostate and testicular cancer: a cohort study of 53,000 Norwegian men. *Cancer Causes Control* 1994; 5:549–556.
47. Hsing AW, McLaughlin JK, Zheng W, Gao Y-T, Blot WJ. Occupation, physical activity, and risk of prostate cancer in Shanghai, People's Republic of China. *Cancer Causes Control* 1994; 5:136–140.
48. Steenland K, Nowlin S, Palu S. Cancer incidence in the National Health and Nutrition Survey I follow-up data: diabetes, cholesterol, pulse and physical activity. *Cancer Epidemiol Biomarkers Prev* 1995; 4:807–811.
49. Ilic M, Vlajinac H, Marinkovic J. Case-control study of risk factors for prostate cancer. *Br J Cancer* 1996; 74:1682–1686.
50. Oliveria SA, Kohl HW, Trichopoulos D, Blair SN. The association between cardiorespiratory fitness and prostate cancer. *Med Sci Sports Exer* 1996; 28:97–104.
51. Cerhan JR, Torner JC, Lynch CF, Rubenstein LM, Lemke JH, Cohen MB, Lubaroff DM, Wallace RB. Association of smoking, body mass, and physical activity with risk of prostate cancer in the Iowa 65+ Rural Health Study (United States). *Cancer Causes Control* 1997; 8:229–238.
52. Hartman TJ, Albanes D, Tautalahti M, Tangrea JA, Virtamo J, Stolzenberg R, Taylor PR. Physical activity and prostate cancer in the Alpha-Tocopherol, Beta-Carotene (ATBC) Cancer Prevention Study (Finland). *Cancer Causes Control* 1998; 9:11–18.
53. Giovannucci E, Leitzmann M, Spiegelman D, Rimm EB, Colditz GA, Stampfer MJ, Willett WC. A prospective study of physical activity and prostate cancer in male health professionals. *Cancer Res* 1998; 58:5117–5122.
54. Liu S, Lee I-M, Linson P, Ajani U, Buring JE, Hennekens CH. A prospective study of physical activity and risk of prostate cancer in U.S. physicians. *Int J Epidemiol* 2000; 29:29–35.
55. Lund Nilsen TI, Johnsen R, Vatten LJ. Socio-economic and lifestyle factors associated with risk of prostate cancer. *Br J Cancer* 2000; 82:1358–1363.
56. Clarke G, Whittemore AS. Prostate cancer risk in relation to anthropometry and physical activity: The National Health and Nutrition Examination Survey I Epidemiological Follow-up Study. *Cancer Epidemiol Biomarkers Prev* 2000; 9:875–881.
57. Putnam SD, Cerhan JR, Parker AS, Bianchi GD, Wallace RB, Cantor KP, Lynch CF. Lifestyle and anthropometric risk factors for prostate cancer in a cohort of Iowa men. *Ann Epidemiol* 2000; 10:361–369.
58. Pukkala E, Kaprio J, Koskenvuo M, Kujala U, Sarna S. Cancer incidence among Finnish world class male athletes. *Int J Sports Med* 2000; 21:216–20.
59. Lee I-M, Sesso HD, Paffenbarger RS Jr. A prospective cohort study of physical activity and body size in relation to prostate cancer risk (United States). *Cancer Causes Control* 2001; 12:187–193.
60. Wannamethee SG, Shaper AG, Walker M. Physical activity and risk of cancer in middle-aged men. *Br J Cancer* 2001; 85:1311–1316.
61. Norman A, Moradi T, Gridley G, Dosemeci M, Rydh B, Nyren O, Wolk A. Occupational physical activity and risk for prostate cancer in a nationwide cohort study in Sweden. *Br J Cancer* 2002; 86:70–75.
62. Platz EA, Leitzmann MF, Michaud DS, Willett WC, Giovannucci E. Interrelation of energy intake, body size, and physical activity with prostate cancer in a large prospective cohort study. *Cancer Res* 2003; 63:8542–8548.
63. Yu H, Harris RE, Wynder EL. Case-control study of prostate cancer and socioeconomic factors. *Prostate* 1988; 13:317–325.
64. Brownson RC, Chang JC, Davis JR, Smith CA. Physical activity on the job and cancer in Missouri. *Am J Public Health* 1991; 81:639–642.
65. Le Marchand L, Kolonel LN, Yoshizawa CN. Lifetime occupational physical activity and prostate cancer risk. *Am J Epidemiol* 1991; 133:103–111.

66. West DW, Slattery ML, Robison LM, French TK, Mahoney AW. Adult dietary intake and prostate cancer risk in Utah: a case-control study with special emphasis on aggressive tumors. *Cancer Causes Control* 1991; 2:85–94.
67. Dosemeci M, Hayes RB, Vetter R, Hoover RN, Tucker M, Engin K, Unsal M, Blair A. Occupational physical activity, socioeconomic status, and risks of 15 cancer sites in Turkey. *Cancer Causes Control* 1993; 4:313–321.
68. Andersson S-O, Baron J, Wolk A, Lindgren C, Bergström R, Adami H-O. Early life risk factors for prostate cancer: a population-based case-control study in Sweden. *Cancer Epidemiol Biomarkers Prev* 1995; 4:187–192.
69. Whittemore AS, Kolonel LN, Wu AH, John EM, Gallagher RP, Howe GR, Burch JD, Hankin J, Dreon DM, West DW, The C-Z, Paffenbarger RS Jr. Prostate cancer in relation to diet, physical activity, and body size in blacks, whites, and Asians in the United States and Canada. *J Natl Cancer Inst* 1995; 87:652–661.
70. Sung JFC, Lin RS, Pu Y-S, Chen Y-C, Chang HC, Lai M-K. Risk factors for prostate carcinoma in Taiwan: a case-control study in a Chinese population. *Cancer* 1999; 86:484–491.
71. Villeneuve PJ, Johnson KC, Kreiger N, Mao Y, and the Canadian Cancer Registries Epidemiology Research Group. Risk factors for prostate cancer: results from the Canadian National Enhanced Cancer Surveillance System. *Cancer Causes Control* 1999; 10:355–367.
72. Bairati I, Larouche R, Meyer F, Moore L, Fradet Y. Lifetime occupational physical activity and incidental prostate cancer. *Cancer Causes Control* 2000; 11:759–764.
73. Lacey JV Jr., Deng J, Dosemeci M, Gao Y-T, Mostofi FK, Sesterhenn IA, Xie T, Hsing AW. Prostate cancer, benign prostatic hyperplasia and physical activity in Shanghai, China. *Int J Epidemiol* 2001; 30:341–349.
74. Friedenreich CM, McGregor SE, Courneya KS, Angyalfi SJ, Elliott TG. Case-control study of lifetime total physical activity and prostate cancer risk. *Am J Epidemiol* 2004; 159:740–749.
75. World Health Organization. Obesity. Preventing and managing the global epidemic. Report of a WHO Consultation on Obesity. Geneva: World Health Organization, 1998.
76. Friedenreich CM, SE McGregor, Courneya KS, Angyalfi SJ, Elliott FG. Case-control study of anthropometric measures and prostate cancer risk. *Int J Cancer* 2004; 110:278–283.
77. Miller GJ, Torkko KC. Natural history of prostate cancer — epidemiologic considerations. *Epidemiol Rev* 2001; 23:14–18.
78. Kessler B, Albertsen P. The natural history of prostate cancer. *Urol Clin N Am* 2003; 30:219–226.
79. Sakr WA. Epidemiology of prostate cancer and its precursors. *Modern Pathol* 2004; 1–10 .
80. Noble RL. The development of prostatic adenocarcinoma in Nb rats following prolonged sex hormone administration. *Cancer Res* 1977; 37:1929–1933.
81. Wynder EL, Laakso K, Sotarauta M, Rose DP. Metabolic epidemiology of prostatic cancer. *Prostate* 1984; 5:47–53.
82. Webber MM, Bello D, Quader S. Immortalized and tumorigenic adult human prostatic epithelial cell lines: characteristics and application. Part I. Cell markers and immortalized nontumorigenic cell lines. *Prostate* 1996; 29:386–394.
83. Huggins C, Hodges CV. Studies on prostatic cancer: effect of castration, of estrogen, and of androgen injection on serum phosphases in metastatic carcinoma of the prostate. *Cancer Res* 1941; 1:293–297.
84. Coffey DS. Physiological control of prostatic growth. In: Prostate Cancer, an Overview. UICC Worshop on Prostatic Cancer. Technical Report Series, vol. 48. Geneva: International Union against Cancer; 1979. 4–23.
85. Gann PH, Hennekens CH, Ma J, Longcope C, Stampfer MJ. Prospective study of sex hormone levels and risk of prostate cancer. *J Natl Cancer Inst* 1996; 88:1118–1126.
86. Eaton NE, Reeves GK, Appleby PN, Key TJ. Endogenous sex hormones and prostate cancer: a quantitative review of prospective studies. *Br J Cancer* 1999; 80:930–934.
87. Chen C, Weiss NS, Stanczyk FZ, Lewis SK, DiTommaso D, Etzioni R, Barnett MJ, Goodman GE. Endogenous sex hormones and prostate cancer risk: a case-control study nested within the carotene and retinol efficacy trial. *Cancer Epidemiol Biomarkers Prev* 2003; 12:1410–1416.

88. Stattin P, Lumme S, Tenkanen L, Alftan H, Jellum E, Hallmans G, Thoresen S, Hakulinen T, Luostarinen T, Lehtinen M, Dillner J, Stenman U-H, Hakama M. High levels of circulating testosterone are not associated with increased prostate cancer risk: a pooled prospective study. *Int J Cancer* 2004; 108:418–424.
89. Griffiths K, Eaton CL, Davies P. Prostatic cancer: aetiology and endrocrinology. *Horm Res* 1998; 32(suppl):38–43.
90. Ross RK, Henderson BE. Do diet and androgens alter prostate cancer risk via a common etiological pathway? *J Natl Cancer Inst* 1994; 86:252–253.
91. Brawley OW, Ford LG, Thompson I, Perlman JA, Kramer BS. 5-α-reductase inhibition and prostate cancer prevention. *Cancer Epidemiol Biomarkers Prev* 1994; 3:177–182.
92. Dessypris A, Kuoppasalmi K, Adlercreutz H. Plasma cortisol, testosterone, androstenedione and luteinizing hormone (LH) in a noncompetitive marathon run. *J Steroid Biochem Mol Biol* 1997; 7:33–37.
93. Hackney AC, Sinning WE, Bruot BC. Reproductive hormonal profiles of endurance-trained and untrained males. *Med Sci Sports Exercise* 1988; 20:60–65.
94. Hackney C, Sinning WE, Bruot BC. Hypothalamic-pituitary-testicular axis function in endurance-trained males. *Int J Sports Med* 1990; 11:298–303.
95. Morville R, Pesquies PC, Guezennec CY, Serrurier BD, Guignard M. Plasma variations in testicular and adrenal androgens during prolonged physical exercise in man. *Ann Endocrinol* (Paris) 1979; 40:501–510.
96. Wheeler GD, Wall SR, Belcastro AN, Cumming DC. Reduced serum testosterone and prolactin levels in male distance runners. *JAMA* 1984; 254:514–516.
97. Hackney AC. Endurance exercise training and reproductive endocrine dysfunction in men: alterations in the hypothalamic–pituitary–testicular axis. *Curr Pharm Design* 2001; 7:261–273.
98. Mantzoros CS, Georgiadis EI. Body mass and physical activity are important predictors of serum androgen concentrations in young healthy men. *Epidemiology* 1995; 6:432–435.
99. Nelson LR, Bulun SE. Estrogen production and action. *J Am Acad Dermatol* 2001; 45:S116–124.
100. Liehr JG. Is estradiol a genotoxic mutagenic carcinogen? *Endocr Rev* 2000; 21:40–54.
101. Bosland MC, Oakley–Girvan I, Whittemore AS. Dietary fat, calories and prostate cancer risk. *J Natl Cancer Inst* 1999; 91:489–491.
102. Kiningham RB. Physical activity and the primary prevention of cancer. *Oncology* 1998; 25:515–536.
103. Adlercreutz H. Western diet and Western diseases: some hormonal and biochemical mechanisms and associations. *Scand J Clin Lab Invest* 1990; 50 (Suppl):3–23.
104. Wolk A, Mantzoros CS, Andersson SO, Bergstrom R, Signorello LB, Lagiou P, Adami HO, Trichopoulos D. Insulin-like growth factor I and prostate cancer risk: a population-based, case-control study. *J Natl Cancer Inst* 1998; 90:911–915.
105. Mantzoros CS, Tzonou A, Signorello LB, Stampfer M, Trichopoulos D, Adami HO. Insulin-like growth factor 1 in relation to prostate cancer and benign prostatic hyperplasia. *Br J Cancer* 1997; 76:1115–1118.
106. Stattin P, Bylund A, Rinaldi S, Biessy C, Dechaud H, Stenman UH, Egevad L, Riboli E, Hallmans G, Kaaks R. Plasma insulin-like growth factor-I, insulin-like growth factor-binding proteins, and prostate cancer risk: a prospective study. *J Natl Cancer Inst* 2000; 92:1910–1917.
107. Chan JM, Stampfer MJ, Giovannucci E, Ma J, Pollak M. Plasma insulin-like growth factor-I and prostate cancer risk: a prospective study. *Science* 1998; 279:563–566.
108. Oliver SE, Gunnell D, Donovan J, Peters TJ, Persad R, Gillatt D, Pearce A, Neal DE, Hamdy FC, Holly J. Screen-detected prostate cancer and the insulin-like growth factor axis: results of a population-based case-control study. *Int J Cancer* 2004; 108:887–892.
109. Barnard RJ, Aronson WJ, Tymchuk CN, Ngo TH. Prostate cancer: another aspect of the insulin-resistance syndrome? *Obesity Rev* 2002; 3:303–308.
110. Ngo TH, Barnard RJ, Leung P-S, Cohen P, Aronson WJ. Insulin-like growth factor I (IGF-I) and IGF binding protein-1 modulate prostate cancer cell growth and apoptosis: possible mediators for the effects of diet and exercise on cancer cell survival. *Endocrinology* 2003; 144:2319–2324.
111. Barnard RJ, Ngo TH, Leung P-S, Aronson WJ, Golding LA. A low-fat diet and/or strenuous exercise alters the IGF axis *in vivo* and reduces prostate tumor cell growth *in vitro*. *Prostate* 2003; 56:201–206.

112. Ngo TH, Barnard RJ, Tymchuk CN, Cohen P, Aronson WJ. Effect of diet and exercise on serum insulin, IGF-I, and IGFBP-I levels and growth of LNCaP cells *in vitro* (United States). *Cancer Causes Control* 2002; 13:929–935.
113. Leung P-S, Aronson WJ, Ngo TH, Golding LA, Barnard RJ. Exercise alters the IGF axis *in vivo* and increases p53 protein in prostate cancer cells *in vitro*. *J Appl Physiol* 2004; 96:450–454.
114. Lee IM. Exercise and physical health: cancer and immune function. *Res Q Exercise Sport* 1995; 66:286–291.
115. Shephard RJ, Shek PN. Heavy exercise, nutrition and immune function: is there a connection? *Int J Sports Med* 1995; 16:491–497.
116. Westerlind KC. Physical activity and cancer prevention — mechanisms. *Med Sci Sports Exercise* 2003; 35:1834–1840.
117. Hoffman–Goetz L. Influence of physical activity and exercise on innate immunity. *Nutr Rev* 1998; 56:S126–130.
118. Nieman DC, Pedersen BK. Exercise and immune function. Recent developments. *Sports Med* 1999; 27:73–80.
119. Woods JA, Davis MJ, Smith JA, Nieman DC. Exercise and cellular innate immune function. *Med Sci Sports Exercise* 1999; 31:57–66.
120. Mazzeo RS. Aging, immune function, and exercise: hormonal regulation. *Int J Sports Med* 2000; 21 Supplement 1: S10–S13.
121. Mazzeo RS. The influence of exercise and aging on immune function. *Med Sci Sports Exercise* 1994; 26:586–592.
122. Nieman DC. Exercise immunology: practical applications. *Int J Sports Med* 1997; 18:91–100.
123. Gleeson M, Nieman DC, Pedersen BK. Exercise, nutrition and immune function. *J Sports Sci* 2004; 22:115–125.
124. Marnett LJ. Peroxyl free radicals: potential mediators of tumor initiation and promotion. *Carcinogenesis* 1987; 9:519–526.
125. Ji LL. Exercise and oxidative stress: role of the cellular antioxidant systems. *Exercise Sport Sci Rev* 1995; 23:135–166.
126. Clinton SK. The dietary antioxidant network and prostate carcinoma. *Cancer* 1999; 86:1629–1631.
127. Giuliani A, Cestaro B. Exercise, free radical generation and vitamins. *Eur J Cancer Prev* 1997; 6:S55–S67.
128. Begg CB. Methodological issues in studies of the treatment, diagnosis and etiology of prostate cancer. *Semin Oncol* 1994; 21:569–579.
129. Frankel S, Davey Smith G, Donovan J, Neal D. Screening for prostate cancer. *Lancet* 2003; 361:1122–1128.
130. Kannel WB, Sorlie P. Some benefits of physical activity: the Framingham Study. *Arch Intern Med* 1979; 139:857–861.
131. Thune I, Njolstad I, Lochen ML, Forde OH. Physical activity improves the metabolic risk profiles in men and women: the Tromso Study. *Arch Int Med* 1998; 158:1633–1640.
132. Chasan–Taber S, Rimm EB, Stampfer MJ, Spiegelman D, Colditz GA, Giovannucci E, Ascherio A, Willett WC. Reproducibility and validity of a self-administered physical activity questionnaire for male health professionals. *Epidemiology* 1996; 7:81–86.
133. Friedenreich CM, Courneya KS, Bryant HE. The Lifetime Total Physical Activity Questionnaire: development and reliability. *Med Sci Sports Exercise* 1998; 30:266–274.
134. Hamalainen EK, Adlercreutz H, Puska P, Pietinen P. Decrease of serum total and free testosterone during a low-fat high-fiber diet. *J Steroid Biochem* 1983; 18:369–370.
135. Hamalainen E, Adlercreutz H, Puska P, Pietinen P. Diet and serum hormones in healthy men. *J Steroid Biochem* 1984; 20:459–464.
136. Dorgan JF, Judd JT, Longcope C, Brown C, Schatzkin A, Clevidence BA, Campbell WS, Nair PP, Franz C, Kahle L, Taylor PR. Effects of dietary fat and fiber on plasma and urine androgens and estrogens in men: a controlled feeding study. *Am J Clin Nutr* 1996; 64:850–855.
137. Schatzkin A, Freedman LS, Schiffman MH, Dawsey SM. Validation of intermediate end points in cancer research. *J Natl Cancer Inst* 1990; 82:1746–1752.
138. Schatzkin A, Freedman L, Schiffman M. An epidemiologic perspective on biomarkers. *J Int Med* 1993; 233:75–79.

Section III

Mechanisms Associating Physical Activity with Cancer Incidence

7 Physical Activity Effects on Sex Hormones

Anne McTiernan

CONTENTS

INTRODUCTION

One hypothesized mechanism explaining the association between increased physical activity and reduced risk for incidence of some cancers is the effect of physical activity on sex hormones [1]. This is most relevant to certain hormone-related cancers such as breast, endometrium, and possibly prostate. Women with elevated concentrations of estrogens and androgens have increased risk for breast cancer [2], and those with elevated estrogen concentrations without counterbalancing elevated progesterone concentrations are at increased risk for endometrial cancer [3]. Several cohort and nested case-control studies have examined the relationship between sex hormones and prostate cancer [4,5]. The largest of these studies, a nested case-control study with 222 cases and 390 controls from a cohort of 22,071 U.S. male physicians found that men in the highest quartile of testosterone concentration were more than two times as likely as men in the lowest quantile of testosterone levels to develop prostate cancer [6].

Events of early and late menstrual and reproductive life may be important in the induction or promotion of hormonally related cancers such as breast and endometrium. Early menarche (before 12), increased numbers of ovulatory cycles, late first birth or nulliparity, lack of lactation, and late menopause have each been found to increase risk of breast cancer from 20% to 100% [7]. Increased number of lifetime ovulatory cycles and cyclic estrogen has been proposed as a significant risk factor for breast cancer [8]. This chapter reviews the observational and clinical trial data linking physical activity to sex hormones in premenopausal women, postmenopausal women, and men.

PREMENOPAUSAL WOMEN

Observational Data

A small number of observational studies have reported on a link between physical activity and menstrual and reproductive factors including sex hormones. One reason for this lack of data is the challenge of timing of blood collection by day of menstrual cycle. This is relevant because the within-woman variability in the estrogen and progesterone concentrations over the menstrual cycle exceeds the between-woman variability of these hormones.

Girls participating in vigorous sports such as ballet dancing and running experience a high incidence of primary and secondary amenorrhea, delayed menarche, and more irregular cycles compared with nonathlete girls [9,10]. A cross-sectional study of 174 girls aged 14 to 17 years found that girls who expended 600 or more kcal energy per week (described by the authors as comparable to 2 or more hours per week in activities such as aerobic exercise classes, swimming, jogging, or tennis) were two to three times more likely than less active girls to have anovulatory menstrual cycles [7].

In a sample of 636 women aged 20 to 44 years from the European Prospective Investigation into Cancer (EPIC) study, several hormones were assayed and correlated with lifestyle and other factors [11]. Women were regularly menstruating and had a most recent menstrual cycle of less than 40 days. The day of menstrual cycle was carefully recorded, and a subsample were assayed for progesterone at day 10 to –21 and for follicle stimulating hormone and luteinizing hormone at day –6 to –21. Physical activity was assessed by questionnaire and included data on physical activity at work (sedentary occupation, standing occupation, manual work) and vigorous recreational exercise (none, 1 to 2, 3 to 4, or ≥5 hours per week). After multivariate adjustment, including day of cycle, estradiol concentrations decreased with increasing amount of vigorous recreational exercise (p-trend = 0.04). Estradiol also decreased with increasing physical activity at work (p-trend = 0.09).

Other studies suggest that recreational exercisers may have lower mean reproductive hormone levels and longer menstrual cycle lengths, although the individual effects of weight control and physical activity are difficult to discern [12–14].

Intervention Data

A handful of intervention studies have tested chronic exercise effect on menstrual factors or sex hormones in premenopausal women. Most have been very small; sample sizes ranged from 4 to 31 in five of the studies and one study randomized 132 subjects but only 57 completed the study. Thus, the information available from carefully controlled studies is scarce.

In the largest published clinical trial, Bonen et al. randomized 132 women aged 18 to 40 years to one of six jogging exercise programs for 2 or 4 months: <10 miles/week; 10 to 20 miles/week; or 20 to 30 miles/week [15]. There was no control group. Women were followed for nine menstrual cycles. Results were only presented for the 57 who completed the entire study. The researchers found no change in luteinizing hormone concentration, menstrual cycle length, or luteal phase length. Also, no trend was found toward increased change in follicle-stimulating hormone or progesterone with increasing physical activity. Body weight or percent body fat did not change, despite a significant increase in cardiovascular fitness (VO_2 max) in all study arms ($p < 0.05$). The authors concluded that recreational running of up to 30 miles/week for four menstrual cycles had no deleterious effect on menstrual cycle. This study had the benefit of a randomized design with long follow-up. The considerable dropout rate (75 out of 132), however, limits the interpretation of study results.

Investigators in Boston published two reports from a randomized clinical trial of weight loss vs. weight maintenance in 31 untrained college-aged women [16,17]. All women received the same exercise prescription of 10 miles/day running plus 3.5 hours/day of sports. All activities took place during 8 weeks at a college training camp. Food intake was carefully prescribed and controlled by camp dieticians. Overnight urine was collected daily. During the intervention, 18 women developed loss of luteneizing hormone surge (64%), 13 experienced delayed menses, and 18 developed luteal phase defects. In the weight-loss arm, 75% of the women had delayed menses vs. 8% of women in the weight-maintenance arm ($p < 0.005$). Similarly, 81% of women in the weight-loss arm experienced loss of luteneizing hormone surge vs. 42% of women in the weight-maintenance group ($p < .05$). Incidence of luteal phase defects between the two groups did not differ. All subjects were experiencing normal menstrual cycles 6 months after termination of the intervention. The authors interpret their study as suggesting that vigorous exercise, especially in conjunction with weight loss, can result in reversibly disturbed reproductive function.

In a very small study, four women aged 25 to 29 years were assigned in random order to one of three conditions of 1-week duration during the early follicular phase of the cycle: control, exercise, and exercise with energy restriction [18]. Women were followed for three menstrual cycles. Exercise alone had no effect on luteneizing hormone pulse frequency, level, or peak amplitude. However, diet plus exercise caused a decrease in luteneizing hormone pulse frequency compared with control condition and exercise alone ($p < 0.05$).

In a later study by Williams et al., 15 women were randomly assigned to one of four conditions: sedentary control, active control (jogging or cycling 45 minutes/day, 2 to 3 days/week), training during follicular phase of menstrual cycle, or training during luteal phase of the cycle [19]. The training consisted of twice daily running or cycling for five days/week. The exercise bouts consisted of running 3.2 km per exercise bout increasing by 1.2 km/bout each week. The training lasted through two menstrual cycles. Diet was controlled to maintain weight within ±2 kg of baseline weight. At the end of the intervention, almost half of the trained women showed evidence of abnormal luteal function, including short luteal defects and low urinary progesterone. None experienced loss of luteneizing hormone surge, and none had delayed menses or abnormal bleeding. The changes in luteal function were observed in both training groups, suggesting that exercise at any time in the cycle can affect menstrual function.

In the HERITAGE Family Study, parents and their adult sons and daughters completed a 20-week endurance training program (3 days/week gradually increased to 75% VO_2 max for 50 minutes) on cycle ergometers [20]. On average, sex hormone-binding globulin increased 3.4 nmol/L in the daughters (mean age 25.5) but decreased an average 7.9 nmol/L in their premenopausal mothers (mean age 48.6).

A high-intensity exercise intervention in 28 untrained college women with normal ovulation and luteal adequacy resulted in reversible abnormal luteal function in two-thirds and loss of luteinizing hormone surge in over half of the subjects [21]. The most marked disturbances were observed during the periods of most intense training and in women who had been randomized to a weight-loss (vs. weight-maintenance) group.

Although exercise effects on menarche, menstrual cycle characteristics, and endogenous sex hormones in girls and young women is often cited as a potential mechanism relating exercise to breast cancer risk, the existing evidence comes from inadequately powered intervention studies, many of which were not randomized clinical trials. Data are still lacking on the requirements to produce menstrual and hormone effects, including the amount, frequency, and type of exercise needed; the age at which a girl or woman needs to begin exercising; whether body mass and body fat must be kept low; and what type of dietary pattern is optimal. Data from primate animal models strongly suggest that negative energy balance is responsible for physical activity effects on menstrual cycle characteristics and sex hormones in reproductive years [22].

POSTMENOPAUSAL WOMEN

Observational Data

Increased physical activity measured through self-report and by movement monitors has been found to be associated with decreased serum concentrations of estradiol, estrone, and androgens after adjustment for body mass index in postmenopausal women in some [23] but not other [11] studies. Increased physical activity is also associated with increased circulating concentrations of sex hormone-binding globulin in women [24], which competitively binds to estrogens and androgens, resulting in lower amounts of free, active hormones in the circulation.

Intervention Data

The effect of a 1-year moderate intensity physical activity intervention on the endogenous sex-hormone profile of postmenopausal women was tested in a randomized controlled clinical trial in Seattle, Washington (the Physical Activity for Total Health Study) [25–28]. Women were eligible if they were aged 50 to 75 years, not using sex hormones, sedentary, nonsmokers, willing to be randomized, had no endocrine-related disease or cancer, had a body mass index greater than 24.0 and a percent body fat of 33.0 or greater. Subjects were recruited through mass mailings, supplemented with media placements.

A total of 173 women was randomized to a 1-year moderate intensity aerobic and strength training physical activity program (monitored group exercise sessions with an exercise physiologist plus home exercise) or a control program (stretching classes). The aerobic exercise intervention consisted of thrice weekly exercise sessions at a study facility and twice weekly home exercise sessions. The facility aerobic exercise sessions consisted of 45 minutes of endurance exercise (treadmill and bike) at 70 to 85% of maximal heart rate. Home exercise sessions consisted of aerobic exercises of the women's choice. All 173 women provided blood at 3-months follow-up, and 170 provided blood at 12-months follow-up. On average over the 12 months, the exercisers participated in moderate-intensity sports/recreational activity for a mean 3.7 ± 1.4 days/week for a total of 171 ± 87.9 minutes/week (vs. goal 225 minutes/week). Six (8%) exercisers dropped out of the intervention (all after 3 months) [28]. On average, cardiorespiratory fitness (VO_2 max) increased in exercisers by 12.7% and in controls by 0.8% ($p < 0.0001$).

At 3 and 12 months, women in the exercise group experienced 3.8 and 1.8% declines in estrone, respectively, compared with increases of 3.4 and 3.9% in controls (p = 0.03 and 0.13) [26]. Exercisers experienced a 7.7% decline in estradiol at 3 months, compared with a decline of just 0.6% in controls ($p = 0.07$); at 12 months, the decline in exercisers was present but attenuated. Sex hormone-binding globulin increased from baseline to 3 and 12 months in exercisers to a larger degree than controls, but the differences were of only marginal statistical significance. Exercisers had an 8.2% decrease in free estradiol from baseline to 3 months, compared with no change in controls ($p = 0.02$). At 12 months, the decline in estradiol in exercisers was slightly less than at 3 months.

Figure 7.1 to Figure 7.3 show the exercise effects on estrogens by change in body fat. Among the exercisers who lost more than 2% body fat, concentrations of estrone, estradiol, and free estradiol decreased by 11.9, 13.7, and 16.7%, respectively, at 12 months. In contrast, among the controls who lost body fat, concentrations of estradiol and free estradiol increased and estrone decreased by just 3.6%. Comparisons of these changes between exercisers and controls for those who lost body fat were statistically significant for estradiol and free estradiol.

Women in the exercise and control groups experienced similar, nonsignificant declines in testosterone, androstenedione, dehydroepiandiosterone (DHEA), and dehydroepiandiosterone-sulfate (DHEA-S) from baseline to 3 and 12 months, so the comparison of change over time between exercisers and controls was not statistically significant [27]. Exercisers experienced a 6.5% decline

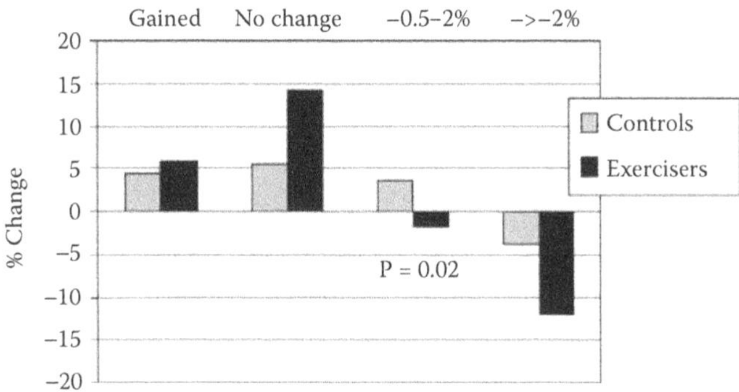

FIGURE 7.1 Percent change in estrone by percent fat change.

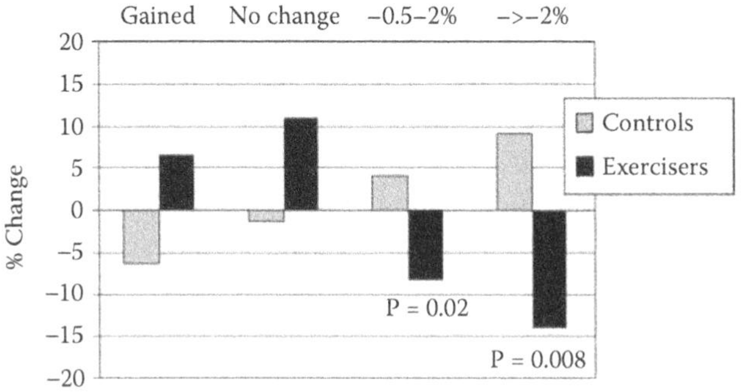

FIGURE 7.2 Percent change in estradiol by percent fat change.

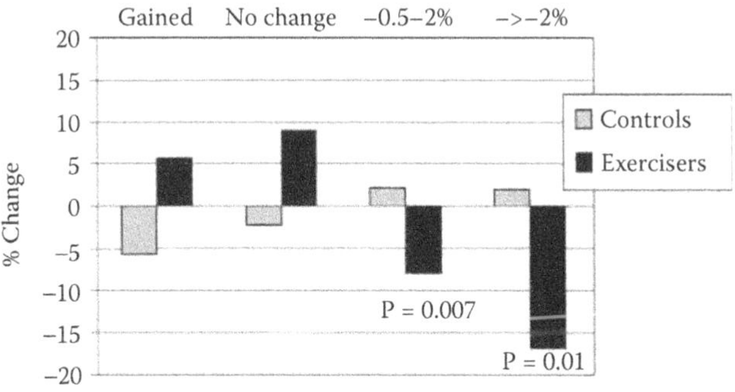

FIGURE 7.3 Percent change in free estradiol by percent fat change.

in free testosterone from baseline to 3 and 12 months, compared with a 2.1% decline in controls (p = 0.28 and 0.42, respectively).

Figure 7.4 and Figure 7.5 show the exercise effects on androgens by change in body fat. At 3 and 12 months, androgen concentrations decreased to a greater extent among exercisers who lost at least 0.5% body fat vs. exercisers who did not lose body fat. Among women who lost between 0.5 and 2% body fat, exercisers' testosterone declined by 1.5 and 4.7%, respectively, at 3 and 12 months; in controls, it did not change at 3 months and declined by only 2.8% at 12 months (p = 0.02 and 0.03, compared to exercisers, respectively). Among those who lost more than 2% body fat, exercisers' testosterone declined by 10.1 and 8.0%, respectively, at 3 and 12 months, and in controls it declined by only 1.6 and 3.6% (p = 0.005 and 0.02, compared to exercisers, respectively).

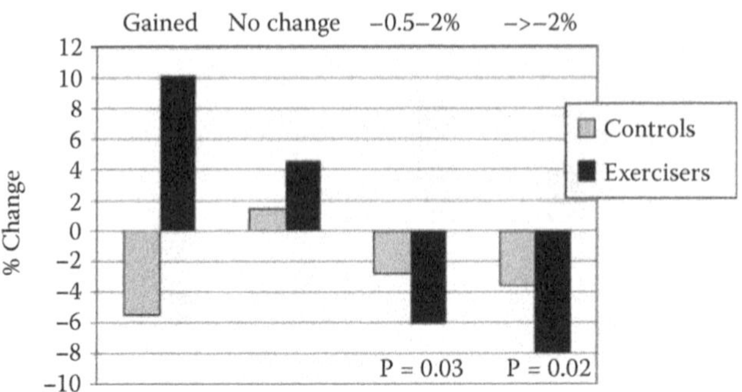

FIGURE 7.4 Percent change in testosterone by percent fat change.

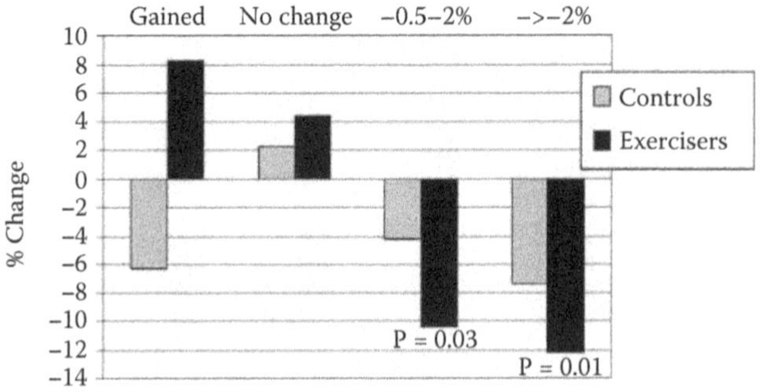

FIGURE 7.5 Percent change in free testosterone by percent fat change.

Among women who lost between 0.5 and 2% body fat, exercisers' 12-month free testosterone declined by 10.4%, but in controls it declined by only 4.3% (p = 0.03 and 0.01, respectively). Among those who lost more than 2% body fat, exercisers' 12-month free testosterone declined by 12.2% and by only 8.0% (p = 0.01 and 0.03, respectively) in controls. Although not statistically significant, exercisers vs. controls who lost more than 2% body fat had greater 12-month changes in androstenedione (–17.1 vs. –9.2%, respectively), DHEA (–20.0 vs. –8.2%, respectively), and DHEAS (–21.8 vs. +3.3%, respectively).

As previously reviewed, human estrogen metabolism is mediated primarily by cytochrome P450 enzymes [29]. Two of the major hydroxylated metabolites of estrone are 2-hydroxyestrone (2-OH E_1) and 16α-hydroxyestrone (16α-OH E_1). These metabolites are produced by competing pathways and have different properties. 2-OH E_1 is weakly estrogenic; *in vitro* studies and animal models have suggested that it is anticarcinogenic. In contrast, 16α-OH E_1 is more estrogenic, has been shown to form covalent bonds with estrogen receptors, and may be genotoxic. One hypothesis is that urinary excretion of these estrogen metabolites can be used as a risk marker for breast cancer. Some [30–33] but not all [34] epidemiologic studies have reported an increased risk of breast cancer associated with low urinary excretion of 2-OH E_1 relative to 16α-OH E_1.

In the clinical trial described earlier (the Physical Activity for Total Health Study), the effects of a 12-month moderate-intensity aerobic exercise intervention on urinary 2-OH E_1, 16α-OH E_1, and their ratio in postmenopausal women [29] were determined. Urinary 2- and 16α-OH E_1 were measured in spot urines collected at baseline, 3, and 12 months. Overall, no significant effects of the exercise intervention on 2-OH E_1, 16α-OH E_1, or their ratio ($p > 0.05$) were found.

Analyses are under way to determine the effect of various genetic polymorphisms related to hormone production and metabolism on the effect of exercise on sex hormones in the Physical Activity for Total Health Study. As described in Chapter 12, the Alpha Trial under way in Alberta, Canada (Drs. C. Friedenreich and K. Courneya, principal and coprincipal investigators respectively) is testing a similar exercise intervention to the Physical Activity for Total Health Study in over 300 postmenopausal women.

MEN

Observational Data

Few cross-sectional studies have looked at associations of physical activity levels with sex hormones in men. However, low plasma levels of free testosterone have been observed in obesity, particularly in abdominal/truncal obesity [35].

Intervention Data

Previous research in athletes suggests that exercise decreases testosterone concentrations chronically [36,37], but the effect of a moderate-intensity aerobic exercise intervention on sex hormones in previously sedentary middle-aged to older men is unknown. Exercise appears to acutely increase testosterone concentrations [38], but preliminary evidence suggests that long-term endurance exercise reduces testosterone concentrations [39]. Some researchers suggest a threshold level of physical activity needed before testosterone levels decrease significantly in men [40].

An ancillary study to a completed clinical trial (the APPEAL study; see Chapter 12) is testing the effect of a 1-year moderate-intensity aerobic exercise program vs. control on sex hormones in previously sedentary men aged 45 to 75. The hormones to be assessed are testosterone, dihydrotestosterone (DHT), and estradiol. Sex hormone-binding globulin will also be measured and free testosterone and free estradiol will be calculated [41]. Blood was collected and stored prerandomization and at months 3 and 12 of follow-up, and is available for 100 of the 102 enrolled men. Results will be available in 2005.

INTERVENTION STUDIES OF PHYSICAL ACTIVITY IN CANCER PATIENTS

Several exercise intervention studies have been conducted in cancer patients. However, the endpoints have focused on weight, physical function, and quality of life and have not provided data on effects on sex hormones. These studies are reviewed in full in the chapters in Section III of this book. In a small pilot study, an 8-week exercise–low-fat diet intervention resulted in significant reductions in weight, waist circumference, hip circumference, and percent body fat in nine breast cancer patients aged 40 to 74 years [42]. Slight, nonsignificant decreases were observed in serum concentrations of total and free estradiol, estrone sulfate, total testosterone, androstenedione, dehydroepiandrosterone, and sex hormone-binding globulin.

SUMMARY

Physical activity may affect sex hormone concentrations in women and men — directly via effects on trophic organs and indirectly via physical activity effects on adiposity, a substrate for estrogen and testosterone production. This nonsex-organ hormone production can result in excessive amounts of circulating and tissue hormone, which can affect the process of carcinogenesis in women and in men.

Because of the paucity of randomized controlled trial data, it is not yet established that change in physical activity can affect sex hormone concentrations independently of an effect of physical activity on adiposity. How much physical activity or what type would be needed to change hormones is also not clear. Additionally, the separate and combined effects of physical activity, diet patterns, and adiposity are not known. Future research should address these issues in randomized controlled trials, preferably with separate and combined physical activity and dietary interventions in a single trial. Future research should also assess the effects of physical activity on sex hormones in women and men from various races, ethnicities, ages, and geographic areas. Also, the role of genetics in modifying the effects of physical activity on sex hormone concentrations should be explored.

REFERENCES

1. McTiernan, A., Ulrich, N., Slate, S., Potter, J. Physical activity and cancer etiology: associations and mechanisms. *Cancer Causes Control* 1998; 9(5):487–509.
2. Endogenous Hormones and Breast Cancer Collaborative Group. Endogenous sex hormones and breast cancer in postmenopausal women: reanalysis of nine prospective studies. *J Natl Cancer Inst* 2002; 94:606–616.
3. Kaaks, R., Lukanova, A., Kurzer, M.S. Obesity, endogenous hormones, and endometrial cancer risk: a synthetic review. *Cancer Epidemiol Biomarkers Prev.* 2002 Dec; 11(12):1531–1543.
4. Shaneyfelt, T., Husein, R., Bubley, G., Mantzoros, C.S. Hormonal predictors of prostate cancer: a meta-analysis. *J Clin Oncol* 2000; 18:847–853.
5. Eaton, N.E., Reeves, G.K., Appleby, P.N., Key, T.J. Endogenous sex hormones and prostate cancer: a quantitative review of prospective studies. *Br J Cancer* 1999; 80:930–934.
6. Gann, P., Hennekens, C., Ma, J., Longcope, C., Stampfer, M. Prospective study of sex hormone levels and risk of prostate cancer. *JNCI Cancer Spectrum* 1996; 88:1118–1126.
7. Bernstein, L., Ross, R.K., Lobo, R.A., Hanisch, R., Krailo, M.D., Henderson, B.E. The effects of moderate physical activity of menstrual cycle patterns in adolescence: implications for breast cancer prevention. *Br. J. Cancer* 1987; 55:681–655
8. Garland, M., Hunter, D.J., Colditz, G.A., Manson, J.E., Stampfer, M.J., Spiegelman, D., Speizer, F., Willett, W.C. Menstrual cycle characteristics and history of ovulatory infertility in relation to breast cancer risk in a large cohort of U.S. women. *Am J Epidemiol* 1998 1; 147(7):636–643.
9. Frisch, R.E., Gotz–Welbergen, A.V., Mcarthur, J.W., Albright, R., Witschi, J., Bullen, B., Birnholz, J., Reed, R.B., Hermann, H. Delayed menarche and amenorrhea of college athletes in relation to age of onset of training. *JAMA* 1981; 246(14):1559–1563.
10. Frisch, R.E., Snow, R.C., Johnson, L.A., Gerard, B., Barbieri, R. and Rosen, B. Magnetic resonance imaging of overall and regional body fat, estrogen metabolism, and ovulation of athletes compared to controls. *J Clin Endocrinol Metab* 1993; 77(2):471–477.
11. Verkasalo, P.K., Thomas, H.V., Appleby, P.N., Davey, G.K., Key, T.J. Circulating levels of sex hormones and their relation to risk factors for breast cancer: a cross-sectional study in 1092 pre- and postmenopausal women (U.K.). *Cancer Causes Control* 2001; 12:47–59.
12. Ellison, P.T., Lager, C. Moderate recreational running is associated with lowered salivary progesterone profiles in women. *Am J Obstet Gynecol* 1986; 154:1000–1003.
13. Bonen, A., Belcastro, A.N., Ling, W.Y., Simpson, A.A. Profiles of selected hormones during menstrual cycles of teenage athletes. *J Appl Physiol* 1981; 50:545–551.
14. Broocks, A., Pirke, K.M., Schweiger, U., Tuschl, R.J., Laessle, R.G., Strowitzki, T., Horl, E., Horl, T., Haas, W., Jeschke, D. Cyclic ovarian function in recreational athletes. *J Appl Physiol* 1990; 68:2083–2086
15. Bonen, A. Recreational exercise does not impair menstrual cycles: a prospective study. *Int J Sports Med* 1992; 13:110–120.
16. Bullen, B.A., Skrinar, G.S., Beitins, I.Z., vonMering, G., Turnbull, B.A., McArthur, J.W. Induction of menstrual disorders by strenuous exercise in untrained women. *N Engl J Med* 1985; 312:1349–1353.

17. Beitins, I.Z., McArthur, J.W., Turnbull, B.A., Skrinar, G.S., Bullen, B.A. Exercise induces two types of human luteal dysfunction: confirmation by urinary free progesterone. *J Clin Endocrinol Metab* 1991; 72(6):1350–1358.
18. Williams, N.I., Young, J.C., McArthur, J.W., Bullen, B., Skrinar, G.S., Turnbull, B. Strenuous exercise with caloric restriction: effect on luteinizing hormone secretion. *Med Sci Sports Exercise* 1995; 27:1390–1398.
19. Williams, N.I., Bullen, B.A., McArthur, J.W., Skrinar, G.S., Turnbull, B.A. Effects of short-term strenuous endurance exercise upon corpus luteum function. *Med Sci Sports Exercise* 1999; 31(7):949–958.
20. An, P., Rice, R., Gagnon, J., Hong, Y., Leon, A.S., Skinner, J.S., Wilmore, J.H., Bouchard, C., Rao, D.C. A genetic study of sex hormone-binding globulin measured before and after a 20-week endurance exercise training program: the HERITAGE Family Study. *Metabolism* 2000; 49(8):1014–1020.
21. Bullen, B.A., Skrinar, G.S., Beitins, I.Z., Carr, D.B., Reppert, S.M., Dotson, C.O., de M. Fencl, M., Gervino, E.V., McArthur, J.W. Endurance training effects on plasma hormonal responsiveness and sex hormone excretion. *J Appl Physiol* 1984; 56:1453–1463.
22. Williams, N.I., Helmreich, D.L., Parfitt, D.B., Caston–Balderrama, A., Cameron, J.L. Evidence for a causal role of low energy availability in the induction of menstrual cycle disturbances during strenuous exercise training. *J Clin Endocrinol Metab* 2001; 86(11):5184–5193.
23. Cauley, J.A., Gutai, J.P., Kuller, L.H., LeDonne, D., Powell, J.G. The epidemiology of serum sex hormones in postmenopausal women. *Am J Epidemiol* 1989; 129:1120–1131.
24. Haffner, S.M., Newcomb, P.A., Marcus, P.M., Klein, B.E., Klein, R. Relation of sex hormones and dehydroepiandrosterone sulfate (DHSEA-SO4) to cardiovascular risk factors in postmenopausal women. *Am J Epidemiol* 1995; 142:925–934.
25. McTiernan, A., Ulrich, C.M., Yancey, D., Slate, S., Nakamura, H., Oestreicher, N., Bowen, D., Yasui, Y., Potter, J., Schwartz, R. The Physical Activity for Total Health (PATH) Study: rationale and design. *Med Sci Sports Exercise* 1999; 31:1307–1312.
26. McTiernan, A., Tworoger, S., Schwartz, R.S., Ulrich, C.M., Yasui, Y., Irwin, M., Rajan, B., Rudolph, R., Bowen, D., Stanczyk, F., Potter, J.D. Effect of exercise on serum estrogen in postmenopausal women: a 12-month randomized controlled trial. *Cancer Res* 2004; 64(8):2923–2928.
27. McTiernan, A., Tworoger, S.S., Rajan, B., Yasui, Y., Sorenson, B., Ulrich, C.M., Chubak, J., Stanczyk, F.Z., Bowen, D., Irwin, M.L., Rudolph, R.E., Potter, J.D., Schwartz, R.S. Effect of exercise on serum androgens in postmenopausal women: a 12-month randomized clinical trial. *Cancer Epidemiol Biomarkers Prev* 2004; 13(7):1–7.
28. Irwin, M., Yasui, Y., Ulrich, C.M., Bowen, D., Rudolph, R.E., Schwartz, R.S., Yukawa, M., Aiello, E., Potter, J.D., McTiernan, A. Effect of exercise on total and intra-abdominal body fat in postmenopausal women: a randomized controlled trial. *JAMA* 2003; 289:323–330.
29. Atkinson, C., Lampe, J.W., Tworoger, S.S., Ulrich, C.M., Bowen, D., Irwin, M.L., Schwartz, R.S., Rajan, B.K., Yasui, Y., Potter, J.D., McTiernan, A. Effects of a moderate intensity exercise intervention on estrogen metabolism in postmenopausal women. *Cancer Epidemiol Biomarkers Prev* 2004; 13(5):1–7.
30. Muti, P., Bradlow, H.L., Micheli, A., Krogh, V., Freudenheim, J.L., Schünemann, H.J., Stanulla, M., Yang, J., Sepkovic, D.W., Trevisan, M., Berrino, F. Estrogen metabolism and risk of breast cancer: a prospective study of the 2:16 alpha-hydroxyestrone ratio in premenopausal and postmenopausal women. *Epidemiology* 2000; 11:635–640.
31. Kabat, G.C., Chang, C.J., Sparano, J.A., Sepkovie, D.W., Hu, X.P., Khalil, A., Rosenblatt, R., Bradlow, H.L. Urinary estrogen metabolites and breast cancer: a case-control study. *Cancer Epidemiol Biomarkers Prev* 1997; 6:505–509.
32. Meilahn, E.N., De Stavola, B., Allen, D.S., Fentiman, I., Bradlow, H.L., Sepkovic, D.W., Kuller, L.H. Do urinary estrogen metabolites predict breast cancer? Guernsey III cohort follow-up. *Br J Cancer* 1998; 78:1250–1255.
33. Zheng, W., Dunning, L., Jin, F., Holtzman, J. Correspondence re: G.C. Kabat et al., urinary estrogen metabolites and breast cancer: a case-control study. *Cancer Epidemiol Biomarkers Prev* 1998; 7:85–86.
34. Ursin, G., London, S., Stanczyk, F.Z., Gentzschein, E., Paganini–Hill, A., Ross, R.K., Pike, M.C. Urinary 2-hydroxyestrone/16α-hydroxyestrone ratio and risk of breast cancer in postmenopausal women. *J Natl Cancer Inst* 1999; 91: 1067–1072.

35. Svartberg, J., von Muhlen, D., Sundsfjord, J., Jorde, R. Waist circumference and testosterone levels in community dwelling men. The TromsÃ¸ Study. *Eur J Epidemiol* 2004; 19(7):657–663.
36. Hackney, A.C. The male reproductive system and endurance exercise. *Med Sci Sports Exercise* 1996; 28:180–189.
37. Hackney, A.C., Fahrner, C.L., Gulledge, T.P. Basal reproductive hormonal profiles are altered in endurance trained men. *J Sports Med Phys Fitness* 1998; 38:138–141.
38. Willoughby, D.S. Taylor, L. Effects of sequential bouts of resistance exercise on androgen receptor expression. *Med Sci Sports Exercise* 2004; 36(9):1499–1506.
39. Hackney, A.C. Endurance exercise training and reproductive endocrine dysfunction in men: alterations in the hypothalamic–pituitary–testicular axis. *Curr Pharm Des* 2001 Mar; 7(4):261–273.
40. De Souza, M.J., Miller, B.E. The effect of endurance training on reproductive function in male runners. A "volume threshold" hypothesis. *Sports Med* 1997; 23(6):357–374.
41. Sodergard, R., Backstrom, T., Shanbhag, V., Carstensen, H. Calculation of free and bound fractions of testosterone and estradiol-17β to human plasma protein at body temperature. *J Steroid Biochem* 1982; 26:801–810.
42. McTiernan, A., Kumai, C., Bean, D., Hastings, R., Schwartz, R., Ulrich, C., Gralow, J., Potter, J. Anthropometric and hormone effects of an 8-week exercise–diet intervention in breast cancer patients: results of a feasibility pilot study. *Cancer Epidemiol Biomarkers Prev* 1998; 7, 477–481.

8 Exercise and Insulin Resistance

Laura Lewis Frank

CONTENTS

INTRODUCTION

According to the *American Cancer Society Guidelines on Diet, Nutrition, and Cancer Prevention*, it is recommended that individuals be physically active. Similar to recommendations by the American College of Sports Medicine and the Centers of Disease Control and Prevention, the American Cancer Society recommends that individuals achieve and maintain a healthy weight by being moderately active for at least 30 min on 5 or more days per week to reduce the risk for cancer, cardiovascular disease, and diabetes [1,2]. In addition, although it is not fully understood why physical activity may play an integral role in the management and survival of cancer, it has been shown that regular physical activity can reduce fatigue and anxiety in cancer patients and improve quality of life [3–5]. Exercise may also improve the lean body mass-to-fat mass ratio, increase range of motion and stability, and promote stress reduction in cancer patients and survivors.

Research in this area has shown that exercise may improve known risk factors for several chronic diseases. The focus of this chapter will be on elucidating potential underlying mechanisms by which physical activity can decrease the risk of several chronic diseases, including several cancers — namely, insulin resistance (defects in insulin action; a reduction in the rate of glucose disposal elicited by a given insulin concentration [6]) and hyperinsulinemia (elevated blood levels of insulin). Some evidence indicates that insulin resistance and hyperinsulinemia may play roles in increasing the risk of several cancers, including breast [7–12], colorectal [12,13], pancreas [14,15], endometrium [14], and stomach [12]. In addition, studies have shown elevated serum insulin concentrations in individuals with cancer but void of other diseases related to hyperinsulinemia [15–17], and impaired glucose tolerance has been found to be an independent predictor for cancer mortality [18].

Expanded molecular-based research examining the relationship between exercise and insulin resistance has been reported. Researchers have shown that physical exercise has the ability to enhance insulin sensitivity [19–25] as well as decrease levels of insulin and bioavailable insulin-like growth factor (IGF)-1, both of which enhance division of normal cells and inhibit cell death (a process known as apoptosis) [26]. There is also clear evidence that regular exercise reduces insulin resistance and hyperinsulinemia [20,21,27]. However, not all studies have shown that exercise can have a positive effect on insulin sensitivity [22–25].

PHYSICAL ACTIVITY AND CHRONIC DISEASES

Physical inactivity is associated with several chronic diseases, including obesity, coronary heart disease (CHD), type-2 diabetes mellitus, osteoporosis, and sarcopenia. Chronic disease conditions affect approximately 90 million Americans, costing the U.S. nearly two-thirds of a trillion dollars in 1990 [28]. Poor diet and physical inactivity lead to 300,000 deaths each year — second only to tobacco use [29].

Overweight and Obesity

Obesity and overweight are defined as having a body mass index (BMI) greater than or equal to 30 kg/m^2 and 25 kg/m^2, respectively [30]. Results from the 1999–2000 National Health and Nutrition Examination Survey (NHANES), using measured heights and weights, indicate that an estimated 64% of U.S. adults are overweight or obese [29]. This represents a prevalence approximately 8% higher than the age-adjusted overweight estimates obtained from the National Health and Nutrition Examination Survey (NHANES) III (1988–1994) [29]. Nearly 59 million American adults are obese, and the percentage of young people who are overweight has more than doubled in the last 20 years. Of Americans aged 6 to 19 years, 15% are overweight [31]. According to the World Health Organization, there were an estimated 200 million obese adults worldwide and another 18 million children under age 5 classified as overweight as of 1995. However, as of 2000, the number of obese adults increased to over 300 million. Crude projections, from extrapolating existing data, suggest that, by 2025, levels of obesity could be as high as 45 to 50% in the U.S.; between 30 and 40% in Australia, England, and Mauritius; and over 20% in Brazil [30].

Obesity, especially abdominal obesity, is associated with an increased risk for type-2 diabetes [32], coronary heart disease, ischemic stroke [33], and several cancers [34–37]. Epidemiological studies have shown positive associations between various measures of overweight and adiposity and a variety of cancers. The International Agency for Research of Cancer concluded that a moderate to strong association exists between increased body weight and increased risk of colon, kidney, esophagus, endometrium, thyroid, and postmenopausal breast cancer [37]. In addition, the International Agency for Research of Cancer has estimated that between one-fourth and one-third of cancer cases may be attributable to the combined effects of elevated body weight and inadequate physical exercise. Other obesity-related chronic diseases include hypertension, osteoarthritis, and gallbladder disease [38] and the number of comorbidities is highly correlated with the rise in body weight. For example, a BMI above 35 kg/m^2 is associated with a 93-fold and 42-fold increase in the risk of type-2 diabetes in women and men, respectively. With a 20% rise in body weight the risk of coronary heart disease is increased 86% in men and 360% in women [39].

An inverse association between physical activity and body weight has been reported in several cross-sectional epidemiological studies [40]. Furthermore, several large-scale prospective observational studies have shown that higher physical activity has resulted in an attenuated weight gain or lower odds of significant weight gain [41]. Evidence suggests that regular physical activity plays a greater role in attenuating age-related weight gain, rather than promoting weight loss [40]. The amount of physical activity needed to prevent weight gain or to lose weight is unknown. The American College of Sports Medicine and Centers for Disease Control and Prevention recommendations mentioned previously were originally prescribed for the prevention of cardiovascular risk factors.

Due to several variables, such as the individual's body weight, nutritional status, and principles of training such as the frequency, duration, and intensity of exercise, it is difficult to measure adequately the amount of physical activity required to promote weight loss. However, several studies have supported the role of physical activity in the promotion of weight loss and weight maintenance [42]. A meta-analysis including 28 publications concluded that aerobic exercise without dietary restriction among men caused a weight loss of 3 kg in 30 weeks compared with sedentary controls and 1.4 kg in 12 weeks among women [43]. In addition, physical activity has favorable effects on reducing insulin resistance among obese subjects [44,45].

Type-2 Diabetes Mellitus

From 1980 through 2002, the number of Americans with diabetes more than doubled (from 5.8 million to 13.3 million) [46]. This shows an increased prevalence compared to data from the NHANES III (1988–1994), which estimated that diagnosed diabetes was 5.5% for U.S. adults (≥20 years of age), or 10.2 million people when extrapolated to the 1997 U.S. population. Using the 1997 American Diabetes Association criteria, the prevalence of undiagnosed diabetes (fasting plasma glucose ≥ 126 mg/dl) was 2.7% (5.4 million) and the prevalence of impaired fasting glucose (110 to 125 mg/dl) was 6.9% (13.4 million) [47]. Using the new minimum criterion for impaired fasting glucose from 100 mg/dl to 125 mg/dl [48], the total prevalence of impaired fasting glucose using the NHANES 1999–2000 dataset would increase from 6.9 to 24.1% [49]. In addition, the worldwide prevalence of type-2 diabetes is estimated to be around 120 million people and has been predicted to almost double to 215 million people by the year 2010 [50].

The pathophysiology of type-2 diabetes involves defects in insulin action (insulin resistance) and secretion (insulin deficiency) [51] manifested by several characteristics, including impaired fasting glucose, impaired glucose tolerance, hyperinsulinemia, and hyperglycemia. In addition, the *insulin resistance syndrome* (also known as the metabolic syndrome or syndrome X) is characterized by hyperinsulinemia, hyperglycemia, hypertension, dyslipidemia [52], and, by some definitions, high urate concentrations [53]. Insulin resistance has also been correlated with several inflammatory markers such as tumor necrosis factor-alpha, interleukin-6, soluble interleukin-6 receptor, interleukin receptor agonist, and C-reactive protein [54]. Risk factors for the development of type-2 diabetes include increased age, minority ethnicity, family history, prior history of gestational diabetes [55], increased overall obesity [55–58], increased intra-abdominal fat distribution [56–62], and lifestyle factors such as physical inactivity [60], diet, and parity [59].

Several epidemiological studies have determined that regular physical exercise can reduce the risk of developing type-2 diabetes [63–66] and modest changes in diet and physical activity have been shown to decrease this risk by 58% [67,68]. In addition, a prospective study of 5159 men aged 40 to 59 years with an average follow-up period of 16.8 years found that a moderate level of physical activity was associated with a 40% reduction in the risk of hyperinsulinemia, a 30% reduction in the risk of hypertriglyceridemia, and a 25% reduction in the risk of low HDL cholesterol [69]. A single exercise bout has been found to improve insulin resistance among those with type-2 diabetes [70,71]; however, 7 consecutive days of exercise and not a single bout of exercise were needed to improve insulin resistance in some subjects [72]. According to the American College of Sports Medicine's position regarding exercise and type-2 diabetes, individuals should strive to achieve a minimum cumulative total of 1000 kcal/week from physical activities [73]. In addition, because high-intensity exercise has been shown to increase blood glucose concentrations [74] and insulin resistance [72] in some patients, low- to moderate-intensity exercise is recommended for many diabetics [73].

EXERCISE AND UNDERLYING MECHANISMS FOR IMPROVEMENT OF INSULIN RESISTANCE

The pathogenesis of insulin resistance is multifaceted. Major causes of acquired insulin resistance include aging, genetics, pregnancy, lack of physical activity, and obesity [81]. Furthermore, several hormones and regulatory factors affect insulin action and may contribute to insulin resistance, especially that observed in obesity. These include chronic hyperglycemia and increased free fatty acids [82]. Several molecular, intracellular, and systemic mechanisms of action occur during and after exercise to attenuate chronic disease risk due to hyperinsulinemia and insulin resistance. In addition, lifestyle factors, including physical activity and physical inactivity, may stimulate the expression of several genes at multiple levels (e.g., pretranslational, translational, or posttranslational); these, in turn, may affect insulin resistance [83].

Skeletal muscle is a major site of insulin resistance [84] and involves dysregulation of glucose and fatty acid metabolism [85]. In the exercising muscle, the increased need for metabolic fuel is met partially through an increase in the uptake and utilization of glucose [83]. The degree of glycogen depletion resulting from prior exercise or caloric depletion is an important factor in determining the rate and duration of the increase in muscle glucose uptake during and after exercise [86]. Glucose transport in skeletal muscle occurs primarily by facilitated diffusion utilizing glucose transporter carrier proteins. The major glucose transporter protein expressed in skeletal muscle is the glucose transporter type-4 (GLUT4). It has been shown that the insulin resistance in skeletal muscle results from alterations in the translocation, docking, or fusion of GLUT4 at the plasma membrane or the T-tubules, or potentially from changes in the specific activity of the transporters. Physical training increases muscle GLUT4 protein and mRNA in individuals with type-2 diabetes, as well as in healthy subjects [87].

Insulin receptor substrate phosphorylation is an important intermediary step in the process of GLUT4 translocation, and alterations in insulin-receptor substrate 1 or other insulin receptor substrates have been postulated to play a role in insulin resistance [88]. Animal models have shown that exercise leads to increased expression and function of several proteins involved in insulin-signal transduction and differential responses of insulin-receptor substrates 1 and 2 [89]. Normally, after stimulation by insulin, insulin-receptor substrate 1 serves as a docking protein that facilitates phosphorylation of other intracellular proteins such as phosphatidylinositol kinase [88]. Phosphatidylinositol kinase (PI 3-kinase) may be an important effector in the pathway by which GLUT4 transporters are inserted into the plasma membrane. Insulin-stimulated activation of PI 3-kinase has been shown to be impaired in skeletal muscle in humans with obesity [90] and type-2 diabetes mellitus [91].

Interestingly, several studies have shown that exercise and insulin stimulate glucose uptake through distinct mechanisms [83,86] and research has shown that insulin and exercise recruit GLUT4 from two distinct intracellular storage sites in skeletal muscle [92]. Insulin utilizes a phosphatidylinositol–kinase-dependent mechanism, whereas the exercise signal may be initiated by calcium release from the sarcoplasmic reticulum or from autocrine- or paracrine-mediated activation of glucose transport [86]. Furthermore, insulin-stimulated translocation of GLUT4 in skeletal muscle involves many proteins (including the GTP-binding protein Rab4) that are not involved in exercise-stimulated GLUT4 translocation [93].

Bierman et al. [94] first reported that plasma free fatty acids were elevated in uncontrolled diabetes mellitus, and subsequent studies have extended these findings to include nondiabetic insulin-resistant individuals, obese patients, and first-degree relatives of type-2 diabetic patients [95]. Elevated free fatty acids have been shown to produce insulin resistance in a dose-dependent manner acutely and chronically [95,96], and plasma free fatty acid concentrations correlate with the degree of hyperglycemia, skeletal muscle insulin resistance, and the risk of developing type-2 diabetes [95]. Elevated free fatty acids have been shown to alter insulin signaling [97], abolish the increase in insulin-receptor substrate 1-associated phosphatidylinositol–kinase, and decrease the concentrations of glucose-6-phosphate within the skeletal muscle, indicating direct inhibition of glucose transport/phosphorylation [96].

Exercise acts to interfere with the synthesis of fatty acids at the molecular level. More specifically, exercise, through hormonal and sympathetic nervous system control, promotes the stimulation of cyclic AMP-activated protein kinase. In turn, AMP-activated protein kinase causes the phosphorylation and inhibition of acetyl CoA carboxylase, a cytoplasmic enzyme involved in the synthesis of fatty acids. Normally, acetyl CoA carboxylase promotes the first step in the synthesis of fatty acids and generates malonyl CoA (the coenzymeA derivitive of malonic acid). Importantly, malonyl CoA is a potent inhibitor of carnitine palmitoyl transferase-1, an enzyme required for lipolysis. It has been shown that exercise decreases insulin resistance due to its ability to lower malonyl CoA concentrations within the cell [98]. In effect, therefore, exercise may divert the flow of fatty acids toward mitochondrial oxidation, leading to improved insulin signaling [99]. Furthermore, enhanced fat oxidation through physical activity has been shown to be associated with improvements in insulin sensitivity in obese individuals [85].

Several other molecular and genetic mechanisms have been proposed in the attenuation of insulin resistance due to exercise. Individuals with insulin resistance may have altered gene expression of several enzymes involved in energy homeostasis within the skeletal muscle, including hexokinase II, phosphofructokinase, and glycogen synthase [100]. Decreased muscle glucose transport/phosphorlyation, as indicated by decreased intramuscular concentrations of glucose-6-phosphate, has been shown to be lower in the offspring of individuals with type-2 diabetes [101,102]. Furthermore, decreased muscle glycogen synthase mRNA concentrations and decreased activity and activation of muscle glycogen synthase in patients with type-2 diabetes, as well as their insulin-resistant relatives, have been shown [103,104]. A single bout of exercise training has normalized glucose-6-phosphate concentrations in these subjects; however, glycogen synthase activities remained low compared to those of nontype-2 diabetic subjects [105]. In contrast, glycogen synthase activity has been shown to be increased immediately after 60 minutes of moderate-intensity cycling exercise in trained, healthy subjects, and the training effect upon glycogen synthase activity was abolished after 5 days of inactivity [106]. These results suggest differences in glycogen synthase-exercise responses between normal individuals vs. individuals with type-2 diabetes, as well as their offspring, and that increases in glycogen synthase activity may depend upon the duration and frequency of exercise training. In addition, exercise has been shown to affect signaling cascades related to glycogen synthase activity — namely, c-Jun NH2-terminal kinase and p38 kinase [107].

In summary, exercise increases insulin sensitivity through a variety of molecular pathways. Several other mechanisms have been proposed that have not been included here. For more detailed information, other resources should be sought [83,86].

THE EFFECTS OF EXERCISE TRAINING

A distinction should be made between the acute effects of exercise and genuine training effects. However, the acute and persistent effects of exercise on glucose uptake and glycogen metabolism have important implications for individuals with insulin resistance [83], and acute bouts of physical activity can favorably change abnormal blood glucose concentrations and insulin resistance [108]. The time period after exercise is characterized by increased muscle sensitivity to the actions of insulin [86]. A single bout of moderate to strenuous exercise can markedly increase rates of whole-body glucose disposal [109,110] and increase the sensitivity of skeletal muscle glucose uptake to insulin [111,112], even in individuals with type-2 diabetes mellitus [70,71]. Up to 2 h after exercise, glucose uptake is, in part, elevated due to insulin-independent mechanisms, probably involving a contraction-induced increase in the amount of GLUT4 associated with the plasma membrane and T-tubules of the skeletal muscles [86].

As reviewed earlier, acute exercise enhances insulin-stimulated GLUT4 translocation and increases muscle GLUT4 protein content, and the depletion of muscle glycogen stores with exercise plays a role in these mechanisms. Due to differences in methodology (including exercise intensity, frequency, and duration), body composition of subjects, and energy homeostasis, it is unclear how long the salutary effects on glucose homeostasis from an acute bout of exercise remain. In addition, insulin sensitivity and/or insulin responsiveness may be different after an acute exercise bout in trained vs. untrained individuals [106]; these effects may be modified by age [21].

Henriksson [21] has reported that insulin sensitivity increases with a single exercise session in the young, but that several training sessions are needed to increase insulin sensitivity in middle-aged to older subjects. This researcher also reported that these transient increases in insulin sensitivity disappeared within 3 to 6 days. In moderately trained, healthy men, improved glucose homeostatic mechanisms were observed 12 to 16 h after exercise, but these improvements disappeared within 5 days of inactivity following 5 days of moderate aerobic exercise [113]. In one study, trained subjects were compared with untrained subjects undergoing an acute bout of exercise [106] and trained subjects were compared before and after 5 days of detraining [106]; an increase in maximal insulin action on whole-body glucose uptake (insulin responsiveness) but not insulin sensitivity has been shown to be a long-term adaptation caused by endurance training.

The effects of long-term physical training seem to be beneficial in the treatment of hyperinsulinemia and impaired glucose tolerance [114]. During exercise, skeletal muscle utilizes more glucose than when at rest. However, endurance training leads to decreased glucose utilization during submaximal exercise, in spite of a large increase in the total GLUT4 content associated with training. The mechanisms involved in this reduction have not been totally elucidated, but endurance training appears to cause a decrease of the amount of GLUT4 translocated to the plasma membrane by altering the exercise-induced enhancement of glucose transport capacity. Several studies have shown that trained individuals have smaller increases in plasma insulin concentrations in response to a glucose load than do sedentary counterparts and, in spite of this lower insulin response, have unchanged or improved glucose tolerance [86]. Concentrations of amino acids, growth hormone, or catecholamines do not change for these individual which might account for the insulin decrease. Cortisol is decreased days after an acute exercise bout as well as after training, in parallel with the plasma insulin decrease. The cortisol decrease may result in changes in insulin-receptor density in tissues, leading to increased insulin sensitivity. The insulin decrease seems to be due to decreased production (to about two-thirds) and increased clearance (to about one-third) [114].

Training without compensatory increase in caloric intake leads to diminished body fat and increases in lean body mass. However, these changes are not obligatory for the plasma insulin decrease. Even studies that have controlled for these effects detect an improvement in insulin sensitivity due to exercise [86]. Therefore, exercise appears to improve insulin action independently of changes in body composition. Studies have shown improvement in insulin sensitivity with physical exercise despite no changes in body weight [115] or body composition [116] — or even increases in overall body fat [27] — when compared to nonexercising controls [27]. A meta-analytical study reviewed and quantified the effect of exercise on glycosylated hemoglobin (HbA1c) and body mass in patients with type-2 diabetes [117] and concluded that significant decreases took place in postintervention glycosylated hemoglobin with no differences in body mass between intervention and control groups.

In conclusion, the effects of exercise training could be explained, in part, by the residual effects of the last session of exercise [106], but it could also be explained by long-term up-regulation of the number and function of glucose transporters [118], capillary proliferation [119], and the number of oxidative muscle fibers, which are more insulin responsive [120]. Clearly, there is a combination of several factors whereby acute and long-term exercise can decrease hyperinsulinemia and insulin resistance. Therefore, physical training can be considered to play an important, if not essential, role in the treatment and prevention of insulin insensitivity [121].

EXERCISE, CENTRAL OBESITY, AND DISEASE RISK

Studies have shown an increased incidence of type-2 diabetes mellitus in relation to abdominal obesity [122]. Increased abdominal adiposity, even despite a normal body weight, is associated with increased cardiovascular disease and type-2 diabetes risk, in part by the concomitant increases in hyperinsulinemia and insulin resistance [123–125]. Abdominal fat, or central adiposity, is more metabolically active than peripheral adiposity and may therefore confer greater risk of some diseases than fat deposited elsewhere [76,126]. Furthermore, visceral adipose tissue has been shown to be an independent correlate of glucose disposal in obese postmenopausal women [127] and strongly influences insulin sensitivity in the early postmenopausal period [128].

Exercise has been shown to affect abdominal, or visceral, body fat preferentially [122,129,130]. Several studies have shown that decreased fasting plasma insulin, increases in insulin sensitivity, or a decrease in glucose-stimulated insulin secretion through physical exercise is mediated through improvements in adiposity [27], especially central adiposity [131,132]. Previously sedentary overweight or obese postmenopausal women were randomized to a 12-month moderate-intensity exercise intervention (goal: 45 min, 5 days per week) or a stretching control group. Exercise effects on changes in insulin concentrations were modified by changes in total fat mass ($p = 0.03$, Figure 8.1) [27]. This was primarily because of the exercise effect among women who gained total fat mass; in this group, exercisers had a smaller increase in fasting insulin concentrations than controls (1 vs. 19%, respectively). However, among exercisers, those who lost >2 kg of fat mass had a significantly larger decline in plasma insulin over the year than those who had gained fat mass. Interestingly, in this study exercise effects on changes in insulin concentrations were not modified by changes in intra-abdominal fat.

Wong et al. [133] reported that, for a given BMI, men in the high fitness group had significantly lower waist circumference ($p < 0.001$), total abdominal fat ($p < 0.001$), visceral fat ($p < 0.001$), and abdominal subcutaneous fat ($p < 0.001$) compared with men in the low fitness group. Other investigators have shown that an increase in physical activity without dietary intervention produced significant decreases in intra-abdominal fat mass [129,134–136] and that improvements in cardiovascular risk factors were related to the loss of centralized body fat rather than to improved fitness [137]. Furthermore, the relationship between the amount of exercise and the degree of exercise-induced weight, fat, and intra-abdominal fat mass loss has been shown in a dose-dependent manner [134].

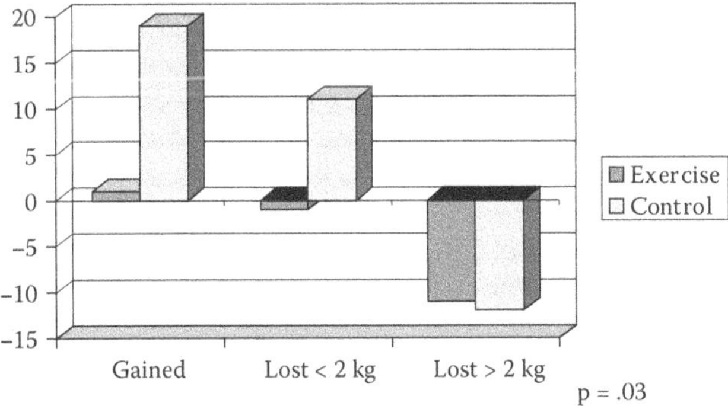

FIGURE 8.1 Percent difference in insulin by changes in total fat mass comparing those who gained total body fat vs. those who lost total body fat (kilograms). Statistical significance of the overall trend in intervention-control group differences across groups of fat mass change from baseline to 12 months: p-trend = 0.03.

ROLE OF AEROBIC EXERCISE IN GLUCOSE HOMEOSTASIS: EVIDENCE FROM CONTROLLED TRIALS

Table 8.1 presents several randomized controlled trials that include aerobic or endurance exercise interventions vs. control group on the effects of glucose homeostasis in diabetic and nondiabetic participants. Criteria used for this review included evidence-based medicine or best practice in utilizing exercise to attenuate several conditions of glucose intolerance. The table includes the basic study design, the number of subjects (*n*) completing the trial compared to the number of subjects randomized to each group (in parentheses), length of training period, and key outcomes. Studies were included if they were of at least 3 months (90 days) duration, had a sample size of at least 20 subjects, and enabled the assessment of the role of the intervention on insulin action (by an oral glucose tolerance test [OGTT], an intravenous glucose tolerance test [IVGTT], or a hyperinsulinemic, euglycemic clamp [HEC]). Although improvements in cardiorespiratory fitness measures (VO_2 max) are not discussed in detail, it must be noted that exercise promoted improvements in VO_2 max independently of losses in body weight [138,139].

Several controlled studies have shown an improvement in insulin sensitivity and a reduction in abdominal adiposity with aerobic exercise [130,140–142]. Several of these investigators observed, through subgroup analysis, that the exercise effect on insulin sensitivity or obesity biomarkers such as insulin may be modified by age, loss of body fat, or other potential biological mechanisms. Short et al. [141] evaluated the effects of 16 weeks of aerobic exercise (n = 65) vs. control (n = 37) in men and women (aged 21 to 87) on insulin sensitivity and muscle mitochondria. The exercise program was performed on a stationary bike, initiated with three sessions per week, 20-min duration, and gradually increased to four sessions per week at 80% of maximal heart rate for 40 min. Exercise increased muscle GLUT4 mRNA and protein by 30 to 52% and reduced abdominal fat by 5% and plasma triglycerides by 25%. Insulin sensitivity improved in younger (20 to 39 years) vs. older (≥60 years) participants, suggesting that the insulin sensitivity response to exercise may be modified by age.

Pratley et al. [142] tested effects of moderate-intensity aerobic exercise training on glucose-stimulated insulin responses in middle-aged and older individuals over a 9-month period. Subjects were stabilized on the step I American Heart Association diet before training, and calories were increased to prevent weight loss. The aerobic exercise training program included stationary bicycling, walking, and jogging three times per week at an exercise facility with the goal for intensity and duration of 75 to 85% heart rate reserve (HRR) for 30 to 45 min, respectively. Fasting glucose and insulin levels and glucose responses during the oral glucose tolerance test did not change, but insulin response during the oral glucose tolerance test decreased by 16% after training. Training reduced early (0 to10 min) and late (20 to 120 min) phase insulin responses by 14% (p = 0.017 and 0.042, respectively), but did not significantly change glucose disposal (+8%, p = 0.398). The authors concluded that the decrease in glucose-stimulated insulin secretion with aerobic exercise training in middle-aged and older men appears to be mediated, at least in part, by reductions in the amount of abdominal fat.

Potteiger et al. [143] examined the insulin and glucose response during an oral glucose tolerance test (OGTT) in overweight young adults (age 17 to 35 years) prior to and following exercise training in the Midwest Exercise Trial. Subjects (n = 66) were randomly assigned to nonexercise control (16 females, 13 males) or exercise (22 females, 15 males) groups. The exercise intervention comprised supervised exercise (primarily walking on motor-driven treadmills), 3 to 5 days per week in 20- to 45-min sessions at 60 to 75% of heart rate reserve for 16 months. For glucose area under the curve (determined by the oral glucose tolerance test), no significant differences were found between exercisers or controls across the 16 months of the study. Insulin area under the curve in male exercisers decreased significantly from baseline to 9 months. The authors concluded that regular exercise in healthy, previously sedentary, overweight adult males leads to improvements in VO_2 max, weight loss and a reduction in the insulin concentration required to dispose of a set

TABLE 8.1
Randomized Clinical Studies[a] of Aerobic Exercise Training and Insulin Sensitivity

Interventions	Gender (age ranges or mean age)	Measure of insulin sensitivity (IS) and glucose disposal	Main outcomes	Other outcomes, body weight (BW) (kg) and/or body composition	Authors, duration
Aerobic exercise ($n = 65$) Control ($n = 37$)	Healthy men and women (21–87 years)	IGTT	EX-induced improvement in IS for younger vs. older ($p < 0.025$)	↓ BW (kg)* ↓ BMI (kg/m2)* ↓ Total, visceral, and subcutaneous abdominal fat (cm^2)* *($p < 0.025$)	Short (2003) 16 weeks
Moderate intensity aerobic exercise ($n = 17$) Dietary control with same cohort	Middle and older men (45–75 years)	OGTT, HEC	Insulin responses during the OGTT decreased 16% ($p = 0.027$) after training Training reduced early (0–10 min) and late (20–120 min) phase insulin responses by 14% ($p = 0.017$ and 0.042, respectively), but did not change glucose disposal (+8%, $p = 0.398$)	↓ BW ($p < 0.0001$), WC ($p = 0.038$), and WHR ($p = 0.035$). ↓ WC ($r^2 = 0.68$, $p < 0.0001$) and % body fat ($r^2 = 0.08$, $p = 0.049$) were independent predictors of the reductions in the late phase insulin responses with EX training	Pratley (2000) 9 months
Aerobic exercise ($n = 37$) Control ($n = 29$)	Overweight young adults (17–35 years)	OGTT	No difference in glu AUC between EX or CON across the 16 months ↓ For male EX from baseline to 9 months in insulin AUC	EX males had ↓ from baseline to 9 months in weight, and % fat with no further changes at 16 months* CON females had ↑ in weight and % fat from baseline to 16 months* * ($p \leq 0.05$)	Potteiger (2003) 16 months
Exercise only ($n = 21$) Exercise + Weight Loss (WL) ($n = 21$) Control ($n = 11$)	Men and women (29 years or older)	OGTT	Post-treatment 2-h insulin conc. ↓ in the EX + WL group ($p < 0.001$) and the EX-only group ($p = 0.003$). Those with largest amount of WL had most robust improvements in abnormal insulin responses (EX + WL group, 47% reduction; EX-only group, 27% reduction)	EX-only ↓ BW and BMI compared to CON* EX + WL ↓ BW and BMI compared to CON and EX-only group* *($p < 0.05$)	Watkins (2003) 6 months

TABLE 8.1 (CONTINUED)
Randomized Clinical Studies of Aerobic Exercise Training and Insulin Sensitivity

Interventions	Gender (age ranges or mean age)	Measure of insulin sensitivity (IS) and glucose disposal	Main outcomes	Other outcomes, body weight (BW) (kg) and/or body composition	Authors, duration
Weekly behavioral modification (BM)/weight loss (WL) (n = 14) Three times/week aerobic exercise (n = 10) Aerobic exercise + WL (n = 14) Control (n = 9)	Nondiabetic sedentary men (mean age 57.6 ± 7.5 years)	OGTT, HEC	EX + WL ↓ fasting insulin responses over other groups* Glu AUC ↓ in EX + WL and WL groups compared to CON and EX groups* Insulin AUC ↓ in WL and EX groups over CON*, and in EX + WL group over all other groups* *($p < 0.05$)	EX + WL and WL groups = ↓ BW and % fat that were greater than those in the CON and EX groups* EX + WL and WL ↓ WHR compared to CON and EX groups* *($p < 0.05$)	Dengel (1996) 10 months
Diet-induced WL (n = 15) Exercise-induced WL (n = 17) Exercise without WL (n = 12) Control (n = 10)	Obese premenopausal females (36–42 years)	OGTT, HEC	↑ Glu disposal in the EX-induced WL groups vs. CON ($p < 0.0001$). Δ In OGTT insulin AUC in EX-induced WL vs. CON ($p < 0.008$)	Total fat loss was greater in both WL groups vs. CON ($p < 0.001$) Average ↓ in total fat was greater in EX-induced WL group vs. diet-induced WL group ($p < 0.001$) ↓ WC within both WL groups was greater vs. CON ($p < 0.001$) but did not differ from each other ($p > 0.05$) ↓ WC within EX-without WL was greater vs. CON ($p < 0.001$), was less than ex-induced WL group but not different from the diet-induced WL group ($p > 0.01$) Average ↓ in total abdominal fat within the EX-induced WL group was greater than all other groups ($p < 0.001$) ↓ Visceral fat in all treatment groups vs. CON ($p < 0.008$)	Ross (2004) 14 weeks

Diet-induced WL (n = 14) Exercise-induced WL (n = 16) Exercise without WL (n = 14) Control	Healthy obese men (43–56 years)	OGTT, HEC	Average improvement in Glu disposal was similar in the diet-induced and EX-induced WL groups ($p < 0.02$), and both were significantly greater than CON ($p < 0.01$). EX-induced WL group showed greater improvements in Glu disposal than EX without WL group ($p = 0.01$). Improvement did not differ between EX-induced WL and CON ($p = 0.09$). ↑ Glu tolerance and insulin AUCs in EX-induced WL vs. EX without WL ($p = 0.01$)	BW ↓ in both WL groups but not EX without WL vs. CON ($p < 0.05$) Total fat ↓ in both WL groups ($p < 0.001$). Mean ↓ was 1.3 kg (95% CI: 0.3 to 2.3 kg) greater in the EX-induced WL group than in the diet-induced WL group ($p = 0.03$). ↓ In abdominal, subcutaneous, visceral, and visceral fat-to-subcutaneous fat ratios were observed in both WL groups ($p < 0.001$). ↓ Abdominal fat in the EX without WL group was greater than CON ($p < 0.001$) but significantly less than both WL groups ($p < 0.001$). ↓ Visceral fat shown in all treatment groups vs. CON ($p < 0.001$) but greater decreases were observed in WL groups vs. EX without WL group ($p < 0.001$)	Ross (2000) 3 months
Diet-induced WL (n = 44) Exercise-program (n = 49) Control (n = 18)	Obese men (mean age 61 ± 1 year)	OGTT	Diet-induced WL ↓ fasting Glu conc by 2%, insulin by 18%, and Glu and insulin AUCs during OGTT by 8 and 26%, respectively ($p < 0.01$). EX-induced ↓ in insulin AUCs by 17% ($p < 0.001$)	Diet-induced ↓ in BW ($p < 0.001$) but EX and CON groups did not change BW ($p > 0.05$).	Katzel (1995) 9 months
Diet advice (n = 40) Exercise (n = 39) Diet + exercise (n = 39) Control (n = 39)	Overweight men (mean age 46 years)	OGTT	Insulin AUC ↓ in EX group ($p < 0.05$), and diet + EX group ($p < 0.01$). Glu AUC ↓ in diet + EX group only ($p = 0.06$)	Significant diet-induced ↓ in BW ($P < 0.001$). EX and CON groups did not change BW ($p > 0.05$).	Hellenius (1995) 6 months

.[a]Randomized clinical trials published in the last 10 years.

Notes: Abbreviations: IGTT: intravenous glucose tolerance test; OGTT: oral glucose tolerance test; HEC: hyperinsulinemic euglycemic clamps; AUCs: areas under the curve; TG: triglycerides; EX: exercise; CON: control; BW: body weight; WC: waist circumference; Glu: glucose; WL: weight loss glucose load. In females, improvement in VO_2 max without weight loss did not lead to improvement in insulin sensitivity. These results suggest that gender may modify the changes in insulin sensitivity from the exercise-induced changes in cardiorespiratory fitness and weight loss, at least for young adults.

Watkins et al. [144] evaluated the effects of a 6-month intervention involving aerobic exercise training alone (exercise only) or exercise combined with a structured weight loss program (exercise plus weight loss) on coronary heart disease risk factors associated with metabolic syndrome. Participants exercised three to four times per week for 26 weeks at a level of 70 to 85% of their initial HRR by walking, jogging, or cycling at a supervised facility. Hyperinsulinemic responses to glucose challenge were significantly reduced in the exercise plus weight loss group and the exercise-only group. Participants with the greatest amount of weight loss showed the most robust improvements in abnormal insulin responses. The authors concluded that the addition of a structured weight loss program to an exercise intervention produces a larger degree of improvement in insulin response compared to exercise alone. However, they stressed that although these results reaffirmed the importance of weight loss in improving hyperinsulinemia, weight loss in this study was achieved in the context of an exercise intervention.

Dengel et al. [138] studied the independent and combined effects of aerobic exercise training and weight loss on glucose metabolism in 47 nondiabetic sedentary older men. There were 14 men in a weekly behavioral modification/weight loss program, 10 in a three times per week aerobic exercise program, 14 in an aerobic exercise plus weight loss program, and 9 in the control group. Exercise training consisted of stationary cycling and walking or jogging on a treadmill at an exercise facility with intensity and duration goals of 75 to 85% heart rate reserve for 40 min, respectively. Oral glucose tolerance tests showed significant reductions in insulin responses in all intervention groups, with the decrease in insulin response in the aerobic exercise plus weight loss group significantly greater than that in the other three groups. The glucose area under the curve decreased significantly in the weight loss and in the aerobic exercise plus weight loss groups, but did not change in the control or in the aerobic exercise-alone groups. Insulin-mediated glucose disposal rates, as measured by the hyperinsulinemic euglycemic clamps, increased significantly in the aerobic exercise and aerobic exercise plus weight loss groups; they were significantly greater than those in the weight loss and control groups. These data suggest that aerobic exercise and weight loss improve glucose metabolism through different mechanisms and that the combined intervention of aerobic exercise plus weight loss may be necessary to improve glucose tolerance and insulin sensitivity in older men.

Despite evidence that exercise appears to improve insulin action independently of changes in body composition, research is ongoing in order to compare the efficacy of diet-induced vs. exercise-induced improvements in body composition, insulin sensitivity, and other chronic disease risk factors. For more studies examining the diet-induced decreases in weight and adiposity, the reader is encouraged to see the *Clinical Guidelines on the Identification, Evaluation, and Treatment of Overweight and Obesity in Adults, the Evidence Report,* from the National Heart Blood and Lung Institute [42].

Ross et al. [140] determined the effects of equivalent diet- or exercise-induced weight loss and exercise without weight loss on subcutaneous fat, visceral fat, and insulin sensitivity in obese women. Premenopausal women (n = 54) with abdominal obesity (waist circumference 110.1 ± 5.8 cm and BMI 31.3 ± 2.0 kg/m^2) were randomly assigned to one of four groups: diet weight loss (n = 15), exercise weight loss (n = 17), exercise without weight loss (n = 12), and a weight-stable control group (n = 10). Subjects in both exercise groups performed daily exercise (brisk walking, or light jogging on a motorized treadmill) at approximately 80% of their maximal heart rate and in order to expend 500 kcal for the duration of the 14-week trial.

Body weight decreased by approximately 6.5% within both weight loss groups and was unchanged in the exercise without weight loss and control groups. Reduction in total, abdominal, and abdominal subcutaneous fat within the exercise weight loss group was greater ($p < 0.001$) than within all other groups. The reduction in total and abdominal fat within the diet weight loss and exercise without weight loss groups was greater than within controls ($p < 0.001$) but not different from each other ($p > 0.05$). Visceral fat decreased within all treatment groups, and these changes were not different from each other. In comparison with the control group, insulin sensitivity improved within the exercise weight loss group alone ($p < 0.001$) and, in comparison with controls, cardiorespiratory fitness improved within the exercise groups only ($p < 0.01$). This study underscores the importance of exercise, even without weight loss, to reduce substantially total fat, abdominal fat, visceral fat, and to improve insulin resistance in obese women.

Ross et al. [130] determined the effects of equivalent diet- or exercise-induced weight loss and exercise without weight loss on subcutaneous fat, visceral fat skeletal muscle mass, and insulin sensitivity in 52 obese men with a mean waist circumference of 110.1 ± 5.8 cm. Participants were randomly assigned to one of four study groups (diet-induced weight loss, exercise-induced weight loss, exercise without weight loss, and control) and were observed for 3 months. The intervention included daily exercise (brisk walking or light jogging on a motorized treadmill) at an intensity of ≤70% of their initial VO_2 max or approximately 80% of maximal heart rate for the time it took to expend 700 kcal. Similar reductions in abdominal subcutaneous, visceral, and visceral fat to subcutaneous fat ratios were observed in the weight loss groups. Plasma glucose and insulin values (fasting and oral glucose challenge) did not change in the treatment groups compared with controls. However, the average improvement in glucose disposal was similar in both weight loss groups. Of note is that weight loss induced by increased daily physical activity without caloric restriction substantially reduced obesity (particularly abdominal obesity) and insulin resistance in men.

Katzel et al. [139] compared the effects of weight loss from a hypocaloric diet vs. aerobic exercise training on coronary artery disease risk factors in healthy, sedentary, obese middle-aged and older men. Diet-induced weight loss decreased fasting glucose and insulin concentrations and glucose and insulin areas during the oral glucose tolerance test (OGTT). By contrast, aerobic exercise did not improve fasting glucose or insulin concentrations or glucose responses during the oral glucose tolerance test, but it decreased insulin areas. In an analysis of variance, the decrement in fasting glucose and insulin levels and glucose areas with intervention differed between weight loss and aerobic exercise when compared with the control group ($p < 0.05$). In multiple regression analyses, the improvement in glucose metabolism was related primarily to the reduction in obesity. These authors concluded that weight loss — not aerobic fitness — is the preferred treatment to improve coronary artery disease risk factors in overweight middle-aged and older men.

Hellenius et al. [145] studied 157 normoglycemic healthy men (age range of 35 to 60 years) with moderately elevated cardiovascular risk factors and randomly assigned them to one of four groups: diet advice ($n = 40$), exercise advice ($n = 39$), a combination of both ($n = 39$), and a control group ($n = 39$). Participants in the exercise group were asked to engage in regular aerobic exercise (walking, jogging, etc.) two to three times per week at an intensity of 60 to 80% of maximal heart rate for a duration of 30 to 45 min. Results showed that the number of pathological oral glucose tolerance tests in the intervention groups decreased from 42/118 to 33/118 compared to no change in the control group. Fasting insulin levels decreased in the exercise and the combined diet + exercise groups ($p < 0.01$) as well as insulin areas under the oral glucose tolerance test curve. Significant increases in IGFBP-1 were observed for all three intervention groups, especially the combined diet + exercise group ($p < 0.001$). The marked changes in IGFBP-1 suggested a decrease in insulin secretion and enhanced insulin sensitivity. The researchers concluded that a combination of increased exercise and improved diet, as well as increased exercise alone, improved glucose and insulin homeostasis in middle-aged men with moderately elevated cardiovascular risk factors.

Serum insulin levels have been used as an estimate of insulin sensitivity and a significant independent relationship between hyperinsulinemia and chronic disease risk has been reported from several large epidemiological studies [146–148]. Exercise has been shown to lower insulin concentrations with and without weight loss [27,144,149]. Furthermore, intermittent exercise for 18 months (walking briskly at approximately 50 to 65% heart rate reserve, two times per day, 15 min per session, 5 days per week) [149] or continuous exercise (≥45 min of moderate-intensity aerobic activity 5 days per week) for 12 months [127] has been shown to improve serum or plasma insulin concentrations in obese females. However, interestingly, Donnelly et al. [149] showed that intermittent exercise did not affect body weight, percent body fat, and fat mass from baseline to 18 months; however, continuous exercise resulted in significant differences in body weight, total body fat, intra-abdominal fat, and subcutaneous body fat from baseline to 12 months [129]. They suggested that insulin concentrations are affected by intermittent and continuous exercise with or without concomitant weight loss or changes in body composition. Furthermore, short-term (8-week) exercise training in overweight males has been shown to improve insulin resistance [150] by using the homeostasis model assessment (HOMA) score, a surrogate measure of whole-body insulin sensitivity [151,152].

Previously sedentary overweight or obese postmenopausal women randomized to a 12-month study examining the effects of moderate-intensity exercise (n = 87) vs. stretching control (n = 86) showed short-term (3 months) and long-term (12 months) improvements in HOMA scores [27]. Compared with baseline, exercisers had a 7 and 2% decline in HOMA scores, whereas controls had a 10 and 14% increase in HOMA scores, at 3 (p = 0.0024) and 12 months (p = 0.0005), respectively (Figure 8.2). Glycemic control through improvements in glycosylated hemoglobin has also been shown to improve after 12 weeks of walking 1 h per day, 5 days per week in diabetic postmenopausal as well as in normoglycemic postmenopausal women [137]. In conclusion, there appears to be sufficient evidence that aerobic exercise can improve insulin sensitivity as measured by more sophisticated methods (e.g., hyperinsulinemic euglycemic clamps) or by using less sensitive measures (e.g., HOMA) and/or blood biomarkers (e.g., changes in serum or plasma insulin concentrations).

ROLE OF RESISTANCE EXERCISE IN GLUCOSE HOMEOSTASIS: EVIDENCE FROM RANDOMIZED-CONTROLLED TRIALS

Several limitations are present when reviewing the literature regarding the effects of resistance training on insulin resistance, including small sample sizes, inconsistent protocols, and lack of longer term (e.g., 12-month) studies. For randomized clinical studies that have been published within the last 10 years, four studies used a nonexercising control group [153–156], two compared aerobic training vs. resistance training [155,157], and four observed the effects of aerobic-plus-resistance training on insulin sensitivity [153,154,158,159]. Few studies included normal vs. impaired glucose-tolerant or diabetic participants [160,161]. Other studies had no control group,

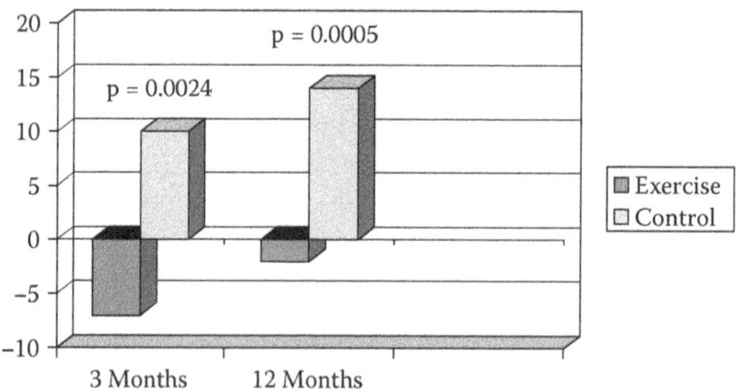

FIGURE 8.2 Percent difference in HOMA scores at 3 and 12 months. HOMA was used as a surrogate measure of whole-body insulin sensitivity and was calculated as fasting glucose (mmol/l) × fasting insulin (μ U/ml) /22.5). Significant differences in percent change in HOMA scores at 3 and 12 months postrandomization of overweight/obese previously sedentary postmenopausal women.

per se; however, they observed pre–post training differences [162] or randomized participants to resistance training vs. resistance training plus diet-induced weight loss groups [163,164].

Although most studies were at least 6 weeks in duration, three studies examined insulin sensitivity after a single bout of resistance exercise [160,165,166]. Chapman et al. [165] examined healthy, postmenopausal women before and after a session of three sets of ten repetitions performed at 50, 75, and 100% of a ten-repetition-maximum for seven different exercises. They found that insulin sensitivity was unaltered by a single session of resistance exercise in postmenopausal women. In contrast, Fluckey et al. [166] showed that a single bout of resistance training (a warm-up set of 10 to 12 repetitions followed by a repitition maximum (1-RM) using several Nautilus exercise machines) improved insulin area under the curves in male and female young (mean age 27.1 ± 1.24 years) and type-2 diabetic subjects, but not in older, nondiabetic subjects (mean age 50.7 ± 1.9 years). In agreement with these findings, Fenicchia et al. [160] reported that the glucose area under the curve improved significantly after an acute bout of resistance training (3-RM strength test for eight exercises), but was not improved with chronic resistance training in type-2 diabetic women or age-matched controls. Therefore, several biological mechanisms may modify the effects of insulin sensitivity to a single resistance-training bout, including age or glucose intolerance. More research is needed in order to explain these differences.

Consistent among these studies, however, was the significant increase in strength that accompanied long-term resistance exercise training (>6-week duration) [155,156,158,160–164]. Furthermore, recent studies have demonstrated that improvement in insulin sensitivity was highly correlated with increased muscle mass [167]. Therefore, it is not surprising that resistance training resulted in improvements in insulin action in several [153,155,156,157,161–163], but not all [164], of the previously listed trials.

Comparison of the effects of endurance vs. resistance training on glucose tolerance has been studied [155,157]. Eriksson et al. [157] randomized 14 subjects with impaired glucose tolerance into an aerobic-trained group (three times per week for 6 months; three males, four females) vs. a nonexercising control group (four males, three females) (mean age 60 ± 5 years) and compared the effects on body composition and insulin sensitivity (as measured by an euglycemic clamp) in eight male subjects (mean age 40 ± 3 years) randomized to a progressive circuit-type resistance program (three times per week for 3 months). No significant differences were found between the aerobic-exercise intervention and the control group for any of the parameters assessed. However, a significant ($p < 0.05$) 23% improvement in total body glucose disposal was observed in the circuit-trained group. The authors attributed this improvement in glucose disposal to a 27% (nonsignificant) increase in nonoxidative glucose disposal.

In contrast, Smutok et al. [155] studied 26 untrained men (mean age 54 ± 9 years) with type-2 diabetes ($n = 8$) or impaired glucose tolerance ($n = 12$) randomly assigned to a strength-training group ($n = 8$), aerobic training group ($n = 8$), or no exercise control group ($n = 10$) for 20 weeks and found that both intervention groups improved plasma glucose responses to an oral glucose tolerance test compared to controls. No significant differences in insulin sensitivity between the two intervention groups were found. A 12% reduction ($p < 0.05$) in total glucose area under the curve was found in the strength-training group compared to a 16% reduction ($p < 0.01$) in the aerobic-trained group. Fasting insulin levels were reduced in the strength-training group ($p < 0.05$) but not in the aerobic-trained group. Total insulin area under the curve was decreased by 22% ($p < 0.05$) following the strength-training program and 21% following the aerobic-trained program. Glucose tolerance was normalized for impaired glucose tolerant subjects following either intervention program; however, subjects with type-2 diabetes did not obtain oral glucose tolerance tests, which fell out of the diagnostic range for diabetes, despite improvements in glucose tolerance.

The effects of endurance and resistance training on insulin sensitivity and hyperinsulinemia have also been studied. Cuff et al. [153] studied 28 obese postmenopausal women with type-2 diabetes randomly assigned to one of three 16-week treatments: control, aerobic only training, or aerobic plus resistance training. Glucose infusion rates increased significantly ($p < 0.05$) in the aerobic-plus-resistance training group. In addition, the aerobic-plus-resistance training group exhibited a significantly greater increase in muscle density than the aerobic-only training group. Improved glucose disposal was independently associated with changes in subcutaneous adipose tissue, visceral adipose tissue, and muscle density. Furthermore, muscle density retained a relationship with glucose disposal after controlling for abdominal adipose tissue.

Wallace et al. [158] studied sedentary adult males with hyperinsulinemia randomly assigned to an endurance-only group (exercised by a continuous cycle exercise or walking for 30 min, 3 days/week^{-1} at 60 to 70% heart rate reserve, $n = 8$) or a cross-training group (performed endurance and resistance exercise; eight exercises, four sets per exercise, 8 to 12 repetitions per set, $n = 8$) in a single session). The changes induced by cross-training were significantly greater than those from endurance training alone in percent fat ($p < 0.01$), insulin concentration ($p < 0.05$), and glucose levels ($p < 0.01$).

Ferrara et al. [159] examined the effects of 4 months of resistance exercise to an existing aerobic exercise program ($n = 7$) compared to a "maintenance" aerobic exercise program ($n = 8$) in overweight, older men. The subjects in this study had recently completed a 6-month aerobic exercise program (treadmill walking, 45 min/day, 2 days/week). The aerobic-plus-resistance trained group added six exercises on upper- and lower-body pneumatic-resistance machines (two sets, 15 repetitions each, 2 days/week) to an aerobic-only exercise program at ≥70% heart rate reserve for 30 to 40 min, 2 days/week on a treadmill. The aerobic-trained group continued the same maintenance treadmill program. No baseline differences in body weight, VO_2 max, or glucose metabolism were found between groups. The aerobic-plus-resistance trained group increased upper- and lower-extremity strength ($p < 0.05$), despite a 9% decrease in VO_2 max ($p < 0.05$); VO_2 max did not change in the aerobic-only trained group. The insulin responses decreased by 25 ± 4% in the aerobic-plus-resistance trained group ($p < 0.01$), but did not change in the aerobic trained only group. However, no changes occurred in fasting glucose or insulin levels or the 3-h glucose responses to an oral glucose load in either group.

These results suggest an additive benefit of resistance training and aerobic training compared to aerobic training alone to improve insulin sensitivity, especially when such training results in loss of abdominal, subcutaneous, and visceral adipose tissue as well as increased muscle density. Poehlman et al. [154] showed that endurance and resistance training improved insulin sensitivity but that, when the glucose disposal rate was expressed per kilogram of fat-free mass, the improved insulin sensitivity persisted in endurance-trained women only. These results suggest that the combined endurance- and resistance-training effect on insulin sensitivity may be modified by gender; however, additional studies are needed to confirm these findings.

Resistance training has also been shown to improve markers of glycemic control — namely, glycosylated hemoglobin [168,169] — as well as body composition [170,171]. In addition, 10 weeks of resistance training ($n = 8$) resulted in significantly lower total body fat ($p < 0.05$) compared to aerobic training ($n = 11$) in untrained males. Furthermore, the effect of a 25-week resistance training program (two sets of ten repetitions at 65 to 80% of 1-RM, three times each week) on intra-abdominal adipose tissue in older women and men showed that despite similar decreases in fat mass, women lost significant amounts of intra-abdominal fat and subcutaneous fat compared to men [171]. These results suggest that the resistance-training changes in adiposity may be modified by gender.

LIFESTYLE INTERVENTIONS (DIET PLUS EXERCISE) AND GLUCOSE HOMEOSTASIS

Although not exhaustive, several studies have examined the effects of diet plus aerobic exercise [85,172–180] or resistance exercise [175,177,180,181] on glucose homeostasis and insulin resistance. However, the primary aim of these trials was to induce weight loss and, secondarily, to observe the effects on insulin resistance. Goodpaster et al. [85] showed improvements in insulin sensitivity after combined exercise- and diet-induced weight loss in obese subjects and that the weight loss was likely due to increased fat oxidation during fasting conditions. Exercise training at moderate intensity can induce a higher capacity for, and reliance upon, fat oxidation during the exercise session [182], and chronic effects of exercise, such as increased activity of oxidative enzymes and increased capillary density, facilitate fatty acid utilization at rest and during physical activity [85]. Thus, it is likely that the enhanced fat oxidation during fasting is due to exercise and not caloric restriction. In addition, unlike diet-induced negative energy balance, in which muscle plays a passive role, exercise-induced negative energy balance has been shown to be associated with concomitant muscle consumption of glycogen and triglyceride [183,184].

Several large randomized controlled trials ($n \geq 100$) [172,173,185–188] have examined a lifestyle intervention (diet plus exercise) on improving insulin resistance. Most of these studies have shown that insulin resistance was improved in the intervention group, but not independently from changes in weight or body composition. In addition, clinical evidence from multicenter trials has suggested that a lifestyle intervention of diet and increased physical activity can decrease the incidence of type-2 diabetes mellitus [189]. Therefore, physical activity should be an adjuvant to diet-induced weight loss strategies and clinicians should stress the importance of exercise in the lifestyle management of chronic disease.

SUMMARY

Insulin resistance and hyperinsulinemia are risk factors for several chronic diseases, including cardiovascular disease, type-2 diabetes mellitus, and several cancers. Cancer research has shown that high levels of plasma insulin as well as insulin-like growth factors can stimulate cell growth and inhibit apoptosis (death of the cell). Physical exercise has been shown to be an important adjunct to the treatment of hyperinsulinemia and insulin resistance because exercise training has been associated with increases in skeletal muscle insulin action and reduction in adipose tissue. Through multifaceted molecular and intracellular systems, exercise can attenuate and abolish increases in insulin concentrations, even in individuals who gain body fat. Complete elucidation of the exercise-induced molecular and intracellular signaling pathways responsible for the amelioration of several chronic diseases will be a worthwhile goal for the improvement of public health. Additional exercise intervention trials in cancer prevention research, with protocol methodologies including validated measures of insulin sensitivity, are recommended to better understand the associations between exercise and insulin resistance.

REFERENCES

1. American Cancer Society. Advisory Committee on Diet, Nutrition, and Cancer Prevention. Guidelines on diet, nutrition, and cancer prevention: reducing the risk of cancer with healthy food choices and physical activity. *Calif Cancer J Clin*. 1996; 46:325–342.
2. Pate R et al., Physical activity and public health: a recommendation from the Centers of Disease Control and Prevention and the American College of Sports Medicine. *JAMA*. 1995; 273:402–407.
3. American Cancer Society Workgroup on Nutrition and Physical Activity for Cancer Survivors. Nutrition after cancer: a guide for informed choices. *Calif Cancer J Clin*. 2001; 51:153–187.
4. Courneya K, Friedenreich C. Physical exercise and quality of life following cancer diagnosis: a literature review. *Ann Behav Med*. 1999; 127:61–69.
5. Burnham TR, Wilcox A. Effects of exercise on physiological and psychological variables in cancer survivors. *Med Sci Sports Exercise*. 2002; 34(12):1863–1867.
6. Ryan AS. Insulin resistance with aging: effects of diet and exercise. *Sports Med*. 2000; 30(5):327–346.
7. Malin A et al. Evaluation of the synergistic effect of insulin resistance and insulin-like growth factors on the risk of breast carcinoma. *Cancer*. 2004;100(4):694–700.

8. Schairer C et al. Serum concentrations of IGF-I, IGFBP-3 and c-peptide and risk of hyperplasia and cancer of the breast in postmenopausal women. *Int J Cancer.* 2004; 108(5):773–779.
9. Hirose K et al. Insulin, insulin-like growth factor-I and breast cancer risk in Japanese women. *Asian Pac J Cancer Prev.* 2003; 4(3):239–246.
10. Brunning PF, Banfer JMG, van Noord PAH. Insulin resistance and breast cancer risk. *Int J Cancer.* 1992; 52: 511–516.
11. Yang G et al. Population-based, case-control study of blood C-peptide level and breast cancer risk. *Cancer Epidemiol Biomarkers Prev.* 2001; 10(11):1207–1211.
12. Yam D, Fink A, Mashiah A, Ben–Hur E. Hyperinsulinemia in colon, stomach and breast cancer patients. *Cancer Lett.* 1996; 104(2):129–32.
13. Saydah SH et al. Association of markers of insulin and glucose control with subsequent colorectal cancer risk. *Cancer Epidemiol Biomarkers Prev.* 2003; 12(5):412–418.
14. Kaaks R, Lukanova A. Energy balance and cancer: the role of insulin and insulin-like growth factor-I. *Proc Nutr Soc.* 2001; Feb; 60(1):91–106.
15. Jee SH et al. Fasting serum glucose level and cancer risk in Korean men and women. *JAMA.* 2005; 293:194–202.
16. Del Guidice ME et al. Insulin and related factors in premenopausal breast cancer risk. *Breast Cancer Res Treat.* 1998; 47:111–120.
17. Lawlor DA, Smith GD, Ebrahim S. Hyperinsulinaemia and increased risk of breast cancer: findings from the British Women's Heart and Health Study. *Cancer Causes Control.* 2004;(3):267–275.
18. Saydah SH, Loria CM, Eberhardt MS, Brancati FL. Abnormal glucose tolerance and the risk of cancer death in the United States. *Am J Epidemiol.* 2003; 157(12):1092–1100.
19. Ardies CM. Exercise, cachexia, and cancer therapy: a molecular rationale. *Nutr Cancer.* 2002; 42(2):143–157.
20. Koivisto VA, Yki–Jarvinen H, DeFronzo RA. Physical training and insulin sensitivity. *Diabetes Metab Rev.* 1988; 1:445–481.
21. Henriksson J. Influence of exercise on insulin sensitivity. *J Cardiovasc Risk.* 1995; 2:303–309.
22. Segal KR et al. Effect of exercise training on insulin sensitivity and glucose metabolism in lean, obese, and diabetic men. *J Appl Physiol.* 1991; 71(6):2402–2411.
23. Mikines KJ et al. Effect of training on the dose–response relationship for insulin action in men. *J Appl Physiol.* 1989;66(2):695–703.
24. Ligtenberg PC et al. Effects of physical training on metabolic control in elderly type 2 diabetes mellitus patients. *Clin Sci (Lond).* 1997;93(2):127–135.
25. Tudor–Locke C et al. Controlled outcome evaluation of the First Step Program: a daily physical activity intervention for individuals with type II diabetes. *Int J Obesity Relat Metab Disord.* 2004;28(1):113–119.
26. Friedenreich CM, Orenstein MR. Physical activity and cancer prevention: etiologic evidence and biological mechanisms. *J Nutr.* 2002; 132(11 Suppl):3456S–3464S.
27. Frank LL et al. Effects of physical activity on metabolic risk variables in overweight postmenopausal women. A randomized clinical trial. *Obesity Res.* 2005; 13(3):615–625.
28. Hoffman C, Rice D, Sung H-Y. Persons with chronic conditions. *JAMA.* 1996; 276(18):1473–1479.
29. Prevalence of overweight and obesity among adults: United States, 1999–2000. National Center of Health Statistics. Centers for Disease Control and Prevention.
30. World Health Organization (WHO). *Obesity: Preventing and Managing the Global Epidemic.* World Health Organization, Geneva, 1998.
31. *Improving Nutrition and Increasing Physical Activity.* National Center of Health Statistics. Centers of Disease Control and Prevention. http://www.cdc.gov/nccdphp/bb_nutrition/htm.
32. Colditz G et al. Weight gain as a risk factor for clinical diabetes mellitus in women. *Ann Intern Med.* 1995; 122:481–486.
33. Rexrode K, Buring J, Manson J. Abdominal and total adiposity and risk of coronary heart disease in men. *Int J Obesity Relat Metab Disord.* 2001; 25(7):1047–1056.
34. Carroll K et al. Obesity as a risk factor for certain types of cancer. *Lipids.* 1998; 33(11):1055–1059.
35. Giovannucci E et al. Physical activity, obesity, and risk of colorectal adenoma in women (United States). *Cancer Causes Control.* 1996; 7(2):253–263.

36. Morimoto L et al., Obesity, body size, and risk of postmenopausal breast cancer: the Women's Health Initiative (United States). *Cancer Causes Control.* 2002; 13:741–751.
37. IARC Working Group. *IARC Handbook of Cancer Prevention.* 2002; vol. 6: *Weight Control and Physical Activity.* IARC, Lyon.
38. Must A et al. The disease burden associated with overweight and obesity. *JAMA.* 1999; 282:1523–1529.
39. Jung RT. Obesity as a disease. *Br Med Bull.* 1997; 53:307–321.
40. DiPietro L. Physical activity, body weight, and adiposity: an epidemiologic perspective. *Exercise Sports Sci Rev.* 1995; 23:275–303.
41. French SA et al. Predictors of weight change over 2 years among a population of working adults: the Healthy Worker Project. *Int J Obesity.* 1994; 22:55–62.
42. National Heart Blood Lung Institute. Clinical guidelines on the identification, evaluation, and treatment of overweight and obesity in adults. The evidence report. 1998; NIH publication No. 98–4083.
43. Garrow JS, Summerbell CD. Meta-analysis: effect of exercise, with or without dieting, on the body composition of overweight subjects. *Eur J Clin Nutr.* 1995; 49(1):1–10.
44. Kelley DE, Goodpastor BH. Effects of physical activity on insulin action and glucose tolerance in obesity. *Med Sci Sports Exercise.* 1999; 31:S619–S623.
45. Kang HS et al. Physical training improves insulin resistance syndrome markers in obese adolescents. *Med Sci Sports Exercise.* 2002; 34(12):1920–1927.
46. CDC-prevalence and trend of DM. http://www.cdc.gov/diabetes/statistics/prev/national/figpersons.htm. Last accessed June 2004.
47. Harris MI et al. Prevalence of Diabetes, Impaired fasting glucose, and impaired glucose tolerance in U.S. Adults. *Diabetes Care.* 1998; 21(4): 518–524.
48. The Expert Committee on the Diagnosis and Classification of Diabetes Mellitus. Follow-up report on the diagnosis of diabetes mellitus. *Diabetes Care.* 2003; 26(11):3160–3167.
49. Davidson MB, Landsman PB, Alexander CM. Lowering the criterion for impaired fasting glucose will not provide clinical benefit. *Diabetes Care.* 2003; 26(12):3329–3330.
50. British Nutrition Information. http://www.nutrition.org.uk/information/dietandhealth/diabetes.htm. Last accessed June 2004.
51. Reaven GM. Syndrome X. *Clin Diabetes.* 1994; 12(4):32–36.
52. Ford ES, Giles WH, Dietz WH. Prevalence of the metabolic syndrome among U.S. adults: findings from the third National Health and Nutrition Examination Survey. *JAMA.* 2002; 287(3):356–359.
53. Liese AD, Mayer–Davis EJ, Haffner SM. Development of multiple metabolic syndrome: an epidemiological perspective. *Epidemiol Rev.* 1998; 42:172–179.
54. Abbatecola AM et al. Diverse effect of inflammatory markers on insulin resistance and insulin-resistance syndrome in the elderly. *J Am Geriatr Soc.* 2004; 52(3):339–404.
55. CDC Diabetes Fact Sheet. http://www.cdc.gov/omh/AMH/factsheets/diabetes.htm. Last accessed June 2004.
56. Carey VJ et al. Body fat distribution and risk of non-insulin-dependent diabetes mellitus in women. The Nurse's Health Study. *Am J Epidemiol.* 1997; 145(7):614–619.
57. Chan JM et al. Obesity, fat distribution, and weight gain as risk factors for clinical diabetes in men. *Diabetes Care.* 1994; 17(9):961–969.
58. Haffner SM et al. Role of obesity and fat distribution in non-insulin-dependent diabetes mellitus in Mexican Americans and non-Hispanic whites. *Diabetes Care.* 1986; Mar–Apr; 9(2):153–161.
59. Shaten BJ, Smith GD, Kuller LH, Neaton JD. Risk factors for the development of type II diabetes among men enrolled in the usual care group of the Multiple Risk Factor Intervention Trial. *Diabetes Care.* 1993; 16(10):1331–1339.
60. Dowse GK et al. Abdominal obesity and physical inactivity as risk factors for NIDDM and impaired glucose tolerance in Indian, Creole, and Chinese Mauritians. *Diabetes Care.* 1991; Apr; 14(4):271–282.
61. Kissebah AH, Peiris AN. Biology of regional body fat distribution: relationship to non-insulin-dependent diabetes mellitus. *Diabetes Metab Rev.* 1989; 5(2):83–109.
62. Ohlson LO et al. The influence of body fat distribution on the incidence of diabetes mellitus. 13.5 years of follow-up of the participants in the study of men born in 1913. *Diabetes.* 1985; 34(10):1055–1058.

63. Manson JE et al. Physical activity and incidence of non insulin dependent diabetes mellitus in women. *Lancet.* 1991; 338:774–778.
64. Manson JE et al. A prospective study of exercise and incidence of diabetes among U.S. male physicians. *JAMA.* 1992; 268:63–67.
65. Helmrich SP, Ragland DR, Leung RW, Paffenbarger RS. Physical actvitiy and reduced occurrence of non-insulin dependent diabetes mellitus. *N Engl J Med.* 1991; 325:147–152.
66. Burchfiel CM et al. Physical activity and diabetes: the Honolulu Heart Program. *Am J Epidemiol.* 1995; 141:360–368.
67. Lindstrom J et al. Finnish Diabetes Prevention Study Group. The Finnish Diabetes Prevention Study (DPS): Lifestyle intervention and 3-year results on diet and physical activity. *Diabetes Care.* 2003; 26(12):3230–3236.
68. The Diabetes Prevention Program Research Group: Reduction in the incidence of type-2 diabetes with lifestyle intervention or metformin. *N Engl J Med.* 2002; 346:393–403.
69. Wannamethee SG, Shaper AG, Alberti GMM. Physical activity, metabolic factors, and the incidence of coronary heart disease and type 2 diabetes. *Arch Intern Med.* 2000; 160:2108–2116.
70. Burstein R et al. Effect of an acute bout of exercise on glucose disposal in human obesity. *J Appl Physiol.* 1990; 69(1):299–304.
71. Devlin JT, Hirshman M, Horton ED, Horton ES. Enhanced peripheral and splanchnic insulin sensitivity in NIDDM men after single bout of exercise. Diabetes. 1987; 36(4):434–439.
72. Rogers MA et al. Improvement in glucose tolerance after 1 wk of exercise in patients with mild NIDDM. *Diabetes Care.* 1988; 11(8):613–618.
73. Albright A et al. American College of Sports Medicine position stand. Exercise and type-2 diabetes. *Med Sci Sports Exercise.* 2000; 32(7):1345–1360.
74. Kjaer M et al. Glucoregulation and hormonal responses to maximal exercise in non-insulin-dependent diabetes. *J Appl Physiol.* 1990; 68(5):2067–2074.
75. Westerlind KC. Physical activity and cancer prevention — mechanisms. *Med Sci Sports Exercise.* 2003; 35(11):1834–1840.
76. McTiernan A, Ulrich C, Slate S, Potter J. Physical activity and cancer etiology: associations and mechanisms. *Cancer Causes Control* 1998; 9: 487–509.
77. McTiernan A. Intervention studies in exercise and cancer prevention. *Med Sci Sports Exercise.* 2003; 35(11):1841–1845.
78. Calle EE, Rodriguez C, Walker–Thurmond K, Thun MJ. Overweight, obesity, and mortality from cancer in a prospectively studied cohort of U.S. adults. *N Engl J Med.* 2003; 348(17):1625–1638.
79. Bianchini F, Kaaks R, Vainio H. Weight control and physical activity in cancer prevention. *Obesity Rev.* 2002; 3(1):5–8.
80. Nagata C et al. Relations of insulin resistance and serum concentrations of estradiol and sex hormone-binding globulin to potential breast cancer risk factors. *Jpn J Cancer Res.* 2000; 1(9):948–953.
81. Boden G. Pathogenesis of type-2 diabetes. Insulin resistance. *Endocrinol Metab Clin North Am.* 2001; 30(4): 801–815.
82. Randle PJ, Garland PB, Hales CN, Newsholme EA. The glucose-fatty acid cycle. Its role in insulin sensitivity and the metabolic disturbances of diabetes mellitus. *Lancet.* 1963; 785–789.
83. Hayashi T, Wojtaszweski JFP, Goodyear LJ. Exercise regulation of glucose transport. *Am J Physiol Endocrinol Metab.* 1997; 36: E1039–E1051.
84. Perez–Martin A, Raynaud E, Mercier J. Insulin resistance and associated metabolic abnormalities in muscle: effects of exercise. *Obesity Rev.* 2001; 2(1):47–59.
85. Goodpaster BH, Katsiaras A, Kelley DE. Enhanced fat oxidation through physical activity is associated with improvements in insulin sensitivity in obesity. *Diabetes.* 2003; 52(9):2191–2197.
86. Goodyear LJ, Kahn BB. Exercise, glucose transport, and insulin sensitivity. *Annu Rev* Med. 1998; 49:235–261.
87. Dela F et al. Physical training increases muscle GLUT4 protein and mRNA in patients with NIDDM. *Diabetes.* 1994; 43(7):862–865.
88. Kahn BB. Type-2 diabetes: insulin secretion fails to compensate for insulin resistance. *Cell.* 1998; 92: 593–596.

89. Chibalin AV et al. Exercise-induced changes in expression and activity of proteins involved in insulin signal transduction in skeletal muscle: differential effects on insulin-receptor substrates 1 and 2. *Proc Natl Acad Sci USA*. 2000; 97(1):38–43.
90. Goodyear LJ et al. Insulin receptor phosphorylation, insulin receptor substrate-1 phosphorylation, and phosphatidylinositol 3-kinase activity are decreased in intact skeletal muscle strips from obese subjects. *J Clin Invest*. 1995; 95(5):2195–2204.
91. Bjornholm M, Kawano Y, Lehtihet M, Zierath JR. Insulin receptor substrate-1 phosphorylation and phosphatidylinositol 3-kinase activity in skeletal muscle from NIDDM subjects after in vivo insulin stimulation. *Diabetes*. 1997; 46(3):524–527.
92. Coderre L, Kandror KV, Vallega G, Pilch PF. Identification and characterization of an exercise-sensitive pool of glucose transporters in skeletal muscle. *J Biol Chem*. 1995; 270(46):27584–27588.
93. Sherman LA et al. Differential effects of insulin and exercise on Rab4 distribution in rat skeletal muscle. *Endocrinology*. 1996; 137(1):266–73.
94. Bierman EL, Doyle VP, Roberts TN. An abnormality of nonesterfied fatty acid metabolism in diabetes mellitus. *Diabetes* 1957; 6:475–479.
95. Roden M. Noninvasive studies of glycogen metabolism in human skeletal muscle using nuclear magnetic resonance spectroscopy. *Curr Opin Clin Nutr Metab Care*. 2001; 4(4):261–266.
96. Roden M. How free fatty acids inhibit glucose utilization in human skeletal muscle. *News Physiol Sci*. 2004; 19: 93–96.
97. Dresner A et al. Effects of free fatty acids on glucose transport and IRS-1-associated phosphatidylinositol 3-kinase activity. *J Clin Invest*. 1999; 103(2):253–259.
98. Ruderman NB, Dean D. Malonyl CoA, long chain fatty acyl CoA and insulin resistance in skeletal muscle. *J Basic Clin Physiol Pharmacol*. 1998; 9(2–4):295–308.
99. Shulman GI. Cellular mechanisms of insulin resistance. *J Clin Invest*. 2000; 106:171–176.
100. Vestergaard H. Studies of gene expression and activity of hexokinase, phosphofructokinase, and glucogen synthase in human skeletal muscle in states of altered insulin-stimulated glucose metabolism. *Dan Med Bull*. 1999; 46(1):13–34.
101. Rothman DL, Shulman RG, Shulman GI. 31P nuclear magnetic resonance measurements of muscle glucose-6-phosphate. Evidence for reduced insulin-dependent muscle glucose transport or phosphorylation activity in non-insulin-dependent diabetes mellitus. *J Clin Invest*. 1992; 89(4):1069–1075.
102. Rothman DL et al. Decreased muscle glucose transport/phosphorylation is an early defect in the pathogenesis of non-insulin-dependent diabetes mellitus. *Proc Natl Acad Sci USA*. 1995; 92(4):983–987.
103. Schalin–Jantti C, Harkonen M, Groop LC. Impaired activation of glycogen synthase in people at increased risk for developing NIDDM. *Diabetes*. 1992; 41(5):598–604.
104. Vaag A, Henriksen JE, Beck–Nielsen H. Decreased insulin activation of glycogen synthase in skeletal muscles in young nonobese Caucasian first-degree relatives of patients with non-insulin-dependent diabetes mellitus. *J Clin Invest*. 1992; 89(3):782–788.
105. Perseghin G et al. Increased glucose transport-phosphorylation and muscle glycogen synthesis after exercise training in insulin-resistant subjects. *N Engl J Med*. 1996; 335(18):1357–1362.
106. Mikines KJ, Sonne B, Tronier B, Galbo H. Effects of acute exercise and detraining on insulin action in trained men. *J Appl Physiol*. 1989; 66(2):704–711.
107. Goodyear LJ et al. Effects of exercise and insulin on mitogen-activated protein kinase signaling pathways in rat skeletal muscle. *Am J Physiol*. 1996; 271(2 Pt 1):E403–408.
108. Laws A, Reaven GM. Physical activity, glucose tolerance, and diabetes in older adults. *Ann Behav Med*. 1991; 13:125–131.
109. Pruett ED, Oseid S. Effect of exercise on glucose and insulin response to glucose infusion. *Scand J Clin Lab Invest*. 1970; 26(3):277–285.
110. Bogardus C et al. Effect of muscle glycogen depletion on *in vivo* insulin action in man. *J Clin Invest*. 1983; 72(5):1605–1610.
111. Richter EA, Mikines KJ, Galbo H, Kiens B. Effect of exercise on insulin action in human skeletal muscle. *J Appl Physiol*. 1989; 66(2):876–885.
112. King DS et al. Insulin action and secretion in endurance-trained and untrained humans. *J Appl Physiol*. 1987; 63(6):2247–2252.

113. King DS et al. Time course for exercise-induced alterations in insulin action and glucose tolerance in middle-aged people. *J Appl Physiol.* 1995; 78(1):17–22.
114. Holm G, Bjorntorp P. Metabolic effects of physical training. *Acta Paediatr Scand Suppl.* 1980; 283:9–14.
115. Duncan GE et al. Exercise training, without weight loss, increases insulin sensitivity and postheparin plasma lipase activity in previously sedentary adults. *Diabetes Care.* 2003; 26(3):557–562.
116. DiPietro L et al. Moderate-intensity aerobic training improves glucose tolerance in aging independent of abdominal adiposity. *J Am Geriatr Soc.* 1998; 46(7):875–879.
117. Boule NG et al. Effects of exercise on glycemic control and body mass in type 2 diabetes mellitus: a meta-analysis of controlled clinical trials. *JAMA.* 2001; 286(10):1218–1227.
118. Goodyear LJ, Hirshman MF, Valyou PM, Horton ES. Glucose transporter number, function, and subcellular distribution in rat skeletal muscle after exercise training. *Diabetes.* 1992; 41(9):1091–1099.
119. Andersen P, Henriksson J. Capillary supply of the quadriceps femoris muscle of man: adaptive response to exercise. *J Physiol.* 1977; 270(3):677–690.
120. Ebeling P et al. Mechanism of enhanced insulin sensitivity in athletes. Increased blood flow, muscle glucose transport protein (GLUT-4) concentration, and glycogen synthase activity. *J Clin Invest.* 1993; 92(4):1623–1631.
121. Borghouts LB, Keizer HA. Exercise and insulin sensitivity: a review. *Int J Sports Med.* 2000; 21(1):1–12.
122. Kaye SA et al. Increased incidence of diabetes mellitus in relation to abdominal adiposity in older women. *J Clin Epidemiol.* 1991; 44(3):329–334.
123. Goodpaster BH et al. Association between regional adipose tissue distribution and both type-2 diabetes and impaired glucose tolerance in elderly men and women. *Diabetes Care.* 2003; 26(2):372–379.
124. Despres JP, Tremblay A, Nadeau A, Bouchard C. Physical training and changes in regional adipose tissue distribution. *Acta Med Scand Suppl.* 1988; 723:205–212.
125. Hernandez–Ono A et al. Association of visceral fat with coronary risk factors in a population-based sample of postmenopausal women. *Int J Obesity Relat Metab Disord.* 2002; 26(1):33–39.
126. Matsuzawa Y et al. Pathophysiology and pathpogenesis of visceral fat obesity. *Obesity Res* 1995; 3(suppl 2):187S–194S.
127. Brochu M et al. Visceral adipose tissue is an independent correlate of glucose disposal in older obese postmenopausal women. *J Clin Endocrinol Metab.* 2000; 85(7):2378–2384.
128. Rendell M et al. Relationship between abdominal fat compartments and glucose and lipid metabolism in early postmenopausal women. *J Clin Endocrinol Metab.* 2001; 86(2):744–749.
129. Irwin ML et al. Effect of exercise on total and intra-abdominal body fat in postmenopausal women: a randomized controlled trial. *JAMA.* 2003; 289(3):323–330.
130. Ross R et al. Reduction in obesity and related comorbid conditions after diet-induced weight loss or exercise-induced weight loss in men. A randomized, controlled trial. *Ann Intern Med.* 2000; 133(2):92–103.
131. Boudou P et al. Absence of exercise-induced variations in adiponectin levels despite decreased abdominal adiposity and improved insulin sensitivity in type-2 diabetic men. *Eur J Endocrinol.* 2003; 149(5):421–424.
132. Miyatake N et al. Daily walking reduces visceral adipose tissue areas and improves insulin resistance in Japanese obese subjects. *Diabetes Res Clin Pract.* 2002; 58(2):101–107.
133. Wong SL et al. Cardiorespiratory fitness is associated with lower abdominal fat independent of body mass index. *Med Sci Sports Exercise.* 2004; 36(2):286–291.
134. Slentz CA et al. Effects of the amount of exercise on body weight, body composition, and measures of central obesity: STRRIDE — a randomized controlled study. *Arch Intern Med.* 2004; 164(1):31–39.
135. Lehmann R et al. Loss of abdominal fat and improvement of the cardiovascular risk profile by regular moderate exercise training in patients with NIDDM. *Diabetologia.* 1995; 38(11):1313–1319.
136. Mourier A et al. Mobilization of visceral adipose tissue related to the improvement in insulin sensitivity in response to physical training in NIDDM. Effects of branched-chain amino acid supplements. *Diabetes Care.* 1997; 20(3):385–391.
137. Walker KZ et al. Effects of regular walking on cardiovascular risk factors and body composition in normoglycemic women and women with type-2 diabetes. *Diabetes Care.* 1999; 22(4):555–561.

138. Dengel DR et al. Distinct effects of aerobic exercise training and weight loss on glucose homeostasis in obese sedentary men. *J Appl Physiol.* 1996; 81(1):318–325.
139. Katzel LI et al. Effects of weight loss vs. aerobic exercise training on risk factors for coronary disease in healthy, obese, middle-aged and older men. A randomized controlled trial. *JAMA.* 1995; 274(24):1915–1921.
140. Ross R et al. Exercise-induced reduction in obesity and insulin resistance in women: a randomized controlled trial. *Obesity Res.* 2004; 12(5):789–798.
141. Short KR et al. Impact of aerobic exercise training on age-related changes in insulin sensitivity and muscle oxidative capacity. *Diabetes.* 2003; 52(8):1888–1896.
142. Pratley RE et al. Aerobic exercise training-induced reductions in abdominal fat and glucose-stimulated insulin responses in middle-aged and older men. *J Am Geriatr Soc.* 2000; 48(9):1055–1061.
143. Potteiger JA, Jacobsen DJ, Donnelly JE, Hill JO. Glucose and insulin responses following 16 months of exercise training in overweight adults: the Midwest Exercise Trial. *Metabolism.* 2003; 52(9):1175–1181.
144. Watkins LL et al. Effects of exercise and weight loss on cardiac risk factors associated with syndrome X. *Arch Intern Med.* 2003; 163(16):1889–1895.
145. Hellenius ML, Brismar KE, Berglund BH, de Faire UH. Effects on glucose tolerance, insulin secretion, insulin-like growth factor 1 and its binding protein, IGFBP-1, in a randomized controlled diet and exercise study in healthy, middle-aged men. *J Intern Med.* 1995; 238(2):121–130.
146. Zimmet PZ et al. Is hyperinsulinaemia a central characteristic of a chronic cardiovascular risk factor clustering syndrome? Mixed findings in Asian Indian, Creole and Chinese Mauritians. Mauritius Noncommunicable Disease Study Group. *Diabet Med.* 1994; 11(4):388–396.
147. Fontbonne A et al. Hyperinsulinaemia as a predictor of coronary heart disease mortality in a healthy population: the Paris Prospective Study, 15-year follow-up. *Diabetologia.* 1991; 34(5):356–361.
148. Pyorala M, Miettinen H, Laakso M, Pyorala K. Plasma insulin and all-cause, cardiovascular, and noncardiovascular mortality: the 22-year follow-up results of the Helsinki Policemen Study. *Diabetes Care.* 2000; 23(8):1097–1102.
149. Donnelly JE et al. The effects of 18 months of intermittent vs. continuous exercise on aerobic capacity, body weight and composition, and metabolic fitness in previously sedentary, moderately obese females. *Int J Obesity.* 2000; 24: 566–572.
150. Dumortier M et al. Low intensity endurance exercise targeted for lipid oxidation improves body composition and insulin sensitivity in patients with the metabolic syndrome. *Diabetes Metab.* 2003; 29(5):509–518.
151. Mathews D et al. Homestasis model assessment: insulin resistance and beta-cell function from fasting plasma glucose and insulin concentrations in man. *Diabetologia.* 1985; 28:412–419.
152. Bonora E et al. Homeostasis model assessment closely mirrors the glucose clamp technique in the assessment of insulin sensitivity: studies in subjects in subjects with various degrees of glucose tolerance and insulin sensitivity. *Diabetes Care.* 2000; 23:57–63.
153. Cuff DJ et al. Effective exercise modality to reduce insulin resistance in women with type-2 diabetes. *Diabetes Care.* 2003; 26(11):2977–2982.
154. Poehlman ET et al. Effects of resistance training and endurance training on insulin sensitivity in nonobese, young women: a controlled randomized trial. *J Clin Endocrinol Metab.* 2000; 85(7):2463–2468.
155. Smutok MA et al. Effects of exercise training modality on glucose tolerance in men with abnormal glucose regulation. *Int J Sports Med.* 1994; 15(6):283–289.
156. Dunstan DW et al. Effects of a short-term circuit weight training program on glycaemic control in NIDDM. *Diabetes Res Clin Pract.* 1998; 40(1):53–61.
157. Eriksson J et al. Aerobic endurance exercise or circuit-type resistance training for individuals with impaired glucose tolerance? *Horm Metab Res.* 1998; 30(1):37–41.
158. Wallace MB, Mills BD, Browning CL. Effects of cross-training on markers of insulin resistance/hyperinsulinemia. *Med Sci Sports Exercise.* 1997; 29(9):1170–1175.
159. Ferrara CM, McCrone SH, Brendle D, Ryan AS, Goldberg AP. Metabolic effects of the addition of resistive to aerobic exercise in older men. *Int J Sport Nutr Exercise Metab.* 2004; 14(1):73–80.
160. Fenicchia LM et al. Influence of resistance exercise training on glucose control in women with type-2 diabetes. *Metabolism.* 2004; 53(3):284–289.

161. Ryan AS et al. Insulin action after resistive training in insulin resistant older men and women. *J Am Geriatr Soc.* 2001; 49(3):247–253.
162. Miller JP et al. Strength training increases insulin action in healthy 50- to 65-year-old men. *J Appl Physiol.* 1994; 77(3):1122–1127.
163. Ryan AS, Pratley RE, Goldberg AP, Elahi D. Resistive training increases insulin action in postmenopausal women. *J Gerontol A Biol Sci Med Sci.* 1996; 51(5):M199–205.
164. Joseph LJ et al. Short-term moderate weight loss and resistance training do not affect insulin-stimulated glucose disposal in postmenopausal women. *Diabetes Care.* 2001; 24(11):1863–1869.
165. Chapman J, Garvin AW, Ward A, Cartee GD. Unaltered insulin sensitivity after resistance exercise bout by postmenopausal women. *Med Sci Sports Exercise.* 2002; 34(6):936–941.
166. Fluckey JD et al. Effects of resistance exercise on glucose tolerance in normal and glucose-intolerant subjects. *J Appl Physiol.* 1994; 77(3):1087–1092.
167. Pereira LO, Lancha AH Jr. Effect of insulin and contraction up on glucose transport in skeletal muscle. *Prog Biophys Mol Biol.* 2004; 84(1):1–27.
168. Castaneda C et al. A randomized controlled trial of resistance exercise training to improve glycemic control in older adults with type-2 diabetes. *Diabetes Care.* 2002; 25(12):2335–2341.
169. Durak EP, Jovanovic–Peterson L, Peterson CM. Randomized crossover study of effect of resistance training on glycemic control, muscular strength, and cholesterol in type I diabetic men. *Diabetes Care.* 1990; 13(10):1039–1043
170. Banz WL et al. Effects of resistance versus aerobic training on coronary artery disease risk factors. *Exp Biol Med.* 2003; 228:434–440.
171. Hunter GR et al. Resistance training and intra-abdominal adipose tissue in older men and women. *Med Sci Sports Exercise.* 2002; 34(6):1023–1028.
172. Esposito K et al. Effect of weight loss and lifestyle changes on vascular inflammatory markers in obese women: a randomized trial. *JAMA.* 2003; 289(14):1799–1804.
173. Mensink M et al. Lifestyle intervention according to general recommendations improves glucose tolerance. *Obesity Res.* 2003; 11(12):1588–1596.
174. McAuley KA et al. Intensive lifestyle changes are necessary to improve insulin sensitivity: a randomized controlled trial. *Diabetes Care.* 2002; 25(3):445–452.
175. Janssen I, Fortier A, Hudson R, Ross R. Effects of an energy-restrictive diet with or without exercise on abdominal fat, intermuscular fat, and metabolic risk factors in obese women. *Diabetes Care.* 2002; 25(3):431–438.
176. Racette SB et al. Modest lifestyle intervention and glucose tolerance in obese African Americans. *Obesity Res.* 2001; 9(6):348–355.
177. Weinstock RS, Dai H, Wadden TA. Diet and exercise in the treatment of obesity: effects of three interventions on insulin resistance. *Arch Intern Med.* 1998; 158(22):2477–2483.
178. Yamanouchi K et al. Daily walking combined with diet therapy is a useful means for obese NIDDM patients not only to reduce body weight but also to improve insulin sensitivity. *Diabetes Care.* 1995; 18(6):775–778.
179. Nilsson PM, Lindholm LH, Schersten BF. Life style changes improve insulin resistance in hyperinsulinaemic subjects: a 1-year intervention study of hypertensives and normotensives in Dalby. *J Hypertension.* 1992; 10(9):1071–1078.
180. Rice B, Janssen I, Hudson R, Ross R. Effects of aerobic or resistance exercise and/or diet on glucose tolerance and plasma insulin levels in obese men. *Diabetes Care.* 1999; 22(5):684–691.
181. Joseph LJ et al. Short-term moderate weight loss and resistance training do not affect insulin-stimulated glucose disposal in postmenopausal women. *Diabetes Care.* 2001; 24(11):1863–1869.
182. Bergman BC et al. Evaluation of exercise and training on muscle lipid metabolism. *Am J Physiol.* 1999; 276(1 Pt 1):E106–117.
183. Goodpaster BH, Wolfe RR, Kelley DE. Effects of obesity on substrate utilization during exercise. *Obesity Res.* 2002; 10(7):575–584.
184. Romijn JA et al. Regulation of endogenous fat and carbohydrate metabolism in relation to exercise intensity and duration. *Am J Physiol.* 1993; 265(3 Pt 1):E380–391.
185. Hellenius ML, Brismar KE, Berglund BH, de Faire UH. Effects on glucose tolerance, insulin secretion, insulin-like growth factor 1 and its binding protein, IGFBP-1, in a randomized controlled diet and exercise study in healthy, middle-aged men. *J Intern Med.* 1995; 238(2):121–130.

186. Torjesen PA et al. Lifestyle changes may reverse development of the insulin resistance syndrome. The Oslo Diet and Exercise Study: a randomized trial. *Diabetes Care.* 1997; 20(1):26–31.
187. Eriksson J et al. Prevention of type II diabetes in subjects with impaired glucose tolerance: the Diabetes Prevention Study (DPS) in Finland. Study design and 1-year interim report on the feasibility of the lifestyle intervention program. *Diabetologia.* 1999; 42(7):793–801.
188. Tuomilehto J et al. Finnish Diabetes Prevention Study Group. Prevention of type-2 diabetes mellitus by changes in lifestyle among subjects with impaired glucose tolerance. *N Engl J Med.* 2001; 344(18):1343–1350.
189. Ryan DH. Diabetes Prevention Program Research Group. Diet and exercise in the prevention of diabetes. *Int J Clin Pract Suppl.* 2003; (134):28–35. Review.

9 Mechanisms Associating Physical Activity with Cancer Incidence: Exercise and Immune Function

Catherine M. Wetmore and Cornelia M. Ulrich

CONTENTS

INTRODUCTION

There is mounting evidence that the benefits of physical activity go above and beyond those of weight loss and cardiovascular fitness. Numerous cross-sectional studies and a growing body of exercise intervention studies (the majority of them randomized trials) suggest that habitual physical activity may enhance immune function. In addition to the observed decreased incidence of respiratory infections among moderate-intensity exercisers,[1–6] exercise may induce augmentation of immune function through enhanced natural killer cell cytotoxicity, increases in CD4 and CD8 cell counts, and increases in concentrations of circulating antibodies (IgA, IgG, and IgM). Thus, the immunomodulatory effects of regular exercise may also protect against other infections, may contribute to enhanced wound healing, and may contribute to the observed decreased incidence of certain types of cancers among physically active individuals.[7–10] (See Chapter 4 and Chapter 6.)

Regular physical activity may also be associated with improved cancer prognosis, at least in the early stages of the disease, and reduced mortality rates for certain types of cancers.[7,8] (See Chapter 4 through Chapter 6 and Chapter 24 through Chapter 26.) Although the data are still relatively sparse and inconsistent, the potential immunomodulatory impact of moderate intensity physical activity may have profound public health implications. This review will summarize the findings of a growing body of literature exploring the effects of moderate-intensity exercise on the immune system.

OVERVIEW OF THE IMMUNE SYSTEM

Comprising a complex network of organs, tissues, cells, and soluble factors, the immune system guards the body from bacterial, viral, parasitic, and fungal infections. The immune system is also capable of recognizing and eliminating cells that have become cancerous.[11] Many of the components of this multifaceted system have specialized functions; some are designed to elicit a nonspecific (or innate) response, and others produce a specific (or acquired) response.

Major components of the nonspecific immune response include phagocytes, such as neutrophils and macrophages, which attract, adhere to, engulf, and ingest extracellular pathogens such as bacteria. In addition to nonspecific phagocytosis, macrophages also secrete enzymes, coagulation factors, and several cytokines (regulatory molecules), such as interleukin-6 (IL-6), interleukin-1 (IL-1), and tumor necrosis factor-α (TNF-α). These secreted cytokines induce hepatic transcription factors to upregulate expression of nonspecific acute-phase proteins such as C-reactive protein (CRP) and serum amyloid A (SAA), which are markers of inflammatory processes.[11–14] Natural killer (NK) cells another major component of the nonspecific immune response, lyse cells that have become abnormal or virus infected. The complement system, a complex-triggered enzyme plasma system that coats microbes with molecules and makes them more susceptible to engulfment by phagocytes, is yet another component of the nonspecific immune response; it is the major effector of the humoral (antibody-based) immune response.[11]

The major components of the specific immune response, T-lymphocytes and B-lymphocytes, are derived from stem cells in the bone marrow. T-lymphocytes, which form the basis of acquired immune recognition (cell-mediated immunity), mature in the thymus and secrete cytokines, such as interleukins and interferons, which regulate the complex interactions among lymphocytes and other components of the immune system. These soluble signaling proteins have the potential to influence a variety of downstream parameters of immune function. T-lymphocytes are also capable of attacking other cells directly, through the action of lymphotoxins, which are secreted by cytotoxic T-cells (CD8+) and can induce lysis of infected or abnormal cells. Additionally, lymphokines secreted by helper/inducer T-cells (CD4+) stimulate proliferation of cytotoxic T-cells, induce B-cells to produce antibodies, attract neutrophils, and enhance the ability of macrophages to engulf and destroy microbes. B-lymphocytes primarily function as mediators of humoral immunity via secretion of proteins called antibodies or immunoglobulins (Ig). Antibodies, each of which has a unique molecular structure corresponding to a specific antigen, bind to and neutralize pathogens so that they may be destroyed by phagocytes. Long-lived memory B-cells are programmed to recognize and respond quickly and efficiently to subsequent invasions by pathogens that have previously been targeted.[11]

With its complex yet efficient network of interacting components, the immune system has the ability to protect the body from foreign organisms and from cancer development. Research has shown that aging or lifestyle factors such as smoking, alcohol consumption, and stress can inhibit optimal immune response, impeding the immune system from fulfilling its mission.

IMMUNE FUNCTION AND CANCER DEVELOPMENT

As mentioned earlier, in addition to protecting against bacterial, viral, parasitic, and fungal infections, the immune system is also thought to play a role in protecting against carcinogenesis by recognizing and eliminating abnormal cells.[11,15] Additionally, immunodeficiency of any origin, whether it is congenital, therapeutic (e.g., following organ transplantation), or acquired via infection, has been observed to increase the risk of certain types of cancer, specifically those etiologically associated with viral infections.[15,16] AIDS patients, who have T-cell deficiencies, not only have an increased risk of AIDS-defining malignancies (e.g., Kaposi's sarcoma), but also show in cohort studies an increased risk of several types of solid tumors, including lung and, probably, colon cancer.[17,18]

Data from a large, population-based cohort study in Japan suggest that differences in immunological host defense — specifically, natural killer (NK) cell cytotoxic activity — among apparently healthy individuals may influence stomach, lung, and intestine cancer risk.[19] This study followed approximately 3500 adults (mostly older than 40) for 11 years, recorded more than 150 incident cancer cases during follow-up, and found that men in the lowest tertile for natural killer cell activity were at an estimated 40 to 60% increased risk of developing cancer compared to those with medium or high NK cell activity (adjusting for age, relative body weight, cigarette smoking, alcohol consumption, and intake of green vegetables); women in the lowest tertile were at approximately 70 to 90% increased risk (after adjustment for the same confounders).[19]

Studies have detected elevated levels of CRP in patients with advanced breast cancer and suggest that CRP concentrations increase as the disease progresses to more advanced stages.[20–22] Although it is likely that these elevated concentrations merely signal the presence of an inflammatory response to the breast tumor, recent findings by Erlinger and colleagues support the notion of inflammation as an actual risk factor for colorectal cancer.[23] Data from their prospective, nested case-control study of a cohort of almost 23,000 adults followed for approximately 11 years indicate that baseline plasma CRP concentrations were significantly higher among those who subsequently developed colorectal cancer compared to controls (median CRP, 2.44 vs. 1.94 mg/L; $p = 0.01$). These findings suggest that even modestly elevated levels of CRP are associated with an increased risk of colorectal cancer. Furthermore, convincing evidence indicates that use of nonsteroidal anti-inflammatory drugs (NSAIDs), including aspirin, is associated with a decreased risk of colon cancer and colorectal adenomas, other cancers of the digestive tract, and, possibly, breast or lung cancer.[24–34]

MEASURES OF IMMUNE FUNCTION

Several *in vivo* and *in vitro* techniques have been developed to measure immune function. Many assays have been designed to enumerate specific classes of immune cells or simply to measure the presence of signaling molecules or antibodies; however, several assays have been designed to measure specific cellular functions (e.g., lymphocyte proliferation, NK cell cytotoxicity, or cytotoxic T-cell activity). Determining the clinical significance of "altered immunity" as measured by any of the available *in vivo* or *in vitro* assays is a challenge.[35] Many of the advantages and limitations of the wide variety of immune function assays employed in the literature have been reviewed by Vedhara et al.[35] and Mitchell et al.[36] and deserve some consideration here.

Enumeration and phenotyping of immune cells by flow cytometry is a commonly employed assay for the measurement of immune function. This technique involves the identification of cell types using color-labeled antibodies that recognize cell type-specific markers. This method has high reproducibility and allows for the comparison of cell ratios and the analysis of cell counts. Enumerative assays may be limited by a lack of correspondence between cell number and cell activity[37]; however, in combination with functional assays, it is possible to ascertain whether observed alterations in enumerative assays are of functional relevance.

Another method for assaying immune function involves measuring the concentration of circulating cytokines, or cytokines secreted *in vitro*. As mentioned earlier, cytokines are signaling molecules that regulate the complex interactions among lymphocytes and other components of the immune system; therefore, the concentration of these signaling molecules may mediate the up- or down-regulation of the immune response. Assays have been designed to measure concentrations of a variety of major cytokines, including IL-1, which affects T-cell activation, and IL-2, which is produced by T-helper cells and induces T-cell proliferation. Unfortunately, assessment of serum cytokine levels, although useful for determining the presence or degree of inflammation, does not necessarily provide a good measure of normal function of the immune response due to the usually low concentrations of circulating cytokines detected in the plasma of healthy individuals. Thus, polyclonal mitogen stimulation is a commonly employed technique for measuring cytokine levels produced by proliferating lymphocytes *in vitro*.

Antibody assays such as the enzyme-linked immunosorbent assay (ELISA) are a simple, robust, and sensitive means of measuring the efficacy of humoral immune response by quantifying the amount of antibody secreted by B-cells following exposure to antigens. However, total antibody levels are a poor indicator of specific antibody response. Therefore, antigen-specific antibody assays, which may have greater clinical relevance, are preferred over measurement of total antibody levels, which may obscure true relationships between physical activity and a specific antibody response.

Assays that target cell function such as proliferation or cytotoxicity, may provide a more meaningful assessment of immune function. Lymphocyte proliferation occurs naturally in the presence of pathogens and serves to increase the number of immune cells available to fight an infection. The effectiveness of T-lymphocyte proliferation can be measured *in vitro* by culturing T-cells in the presence of common mitogens or specific antigens, although this method does not always accurately reflect the *in vivo* response of the cells.

Cytotoxicity assays (for T-cells and NK cells) assess the cytotoxic potential of cytotoxic T-cells and NK cells critical in the defense against infections and tumors. These assays measure the ability to lyse target tumor cells *in vitro*.[36,38] However, these techniques cannot identify the mechanism associated with observed reduced cytotoxicity. For example, cytotoxicity may be impaired due to a variety of defects in the immune response, including: antigen presentation, cytokine secretion, defects in the release or function of perforin (a protein secreted by cytotoxic cells that causes lysis of target cells on contact), or decreased proliferation of effector cells. Additionally, in most cases, it is not possible to attribute the cytotoxic effects exclusively to natural killer cells or other lymphocyte subsets. Although the mechanisms underlying potential deficiencies cannot be readily delineated, the interplay of multiple cell types does more accurately reflect *in vivo* immune function.[35,36,39]

Because each of these techniques for measuring immune function has advantages and limitations,[35,36] most studies rely on a combination of assays to assess immune function.

IMMUNOMODULATORY EFFECTS OF REGULAR MODERATE-INTENSITY PHYSICAL ACTIVITY

The past decade has seen tremendous growth in published epidemiological data in the field of exercise immunology. For example, evidence now supports the proposed J-shaped dose–response relationship that has been used to describe the effects of varying intensities of physical activity on immune function.[40–42] At one end of the spectrum, athletes under tremendous physical stress during periods of intense training or competitions are more susceptible to some illnesses (e.g., upper respiratory tract infections).[42] At the same time, accumulating evidence suggests that regular moderate exercise can reduce susceptibility to illnesses such as the common cold.[1–6,42] This and other advances in our understanding of the immunomodulatory effects of regular moderate-intensity physical activity will be discussed later.

Strengths and limitations of the various epidemiological study designs employed to explore the associations between a variety of measures of immune function and regular physical activity have been summarized in Table 9.1. Although numerous cross-sectional comparisons have investigated this relationship (summarized in Table 9.2) the immunological effects of moderate-intensity physical activity, the focus of this review, can best be delineated through large, well-designed randomized exercise intervention studies.

Table 9.3 presents a summary of findings from published exercise intervention studies conducted in the last two decades. It has been organized into broad categories of immunological parameters:

- Functional assays
- Enumeration and phenotyping of immune cells

TABLE 9.1
Summary of Strengths and Limitations for Exercise Immunology Study Designs

Study design	Strengths	Limitations
Randomized-controlled trial	Strongest design to establish causal relationship Can study multiple outcomes Random assignment prevents bias/avoids confounding (can balance known and unknown potential confounding factors) Blinding prevents measurement bias Can use run-in period to demonstrate compliance Provides firm basis for statistical hypothesis testing (p-values, confidence intervals)	Expensive Not always possible or ethical Inefficient for rare or long-delayed outcomes Usually limited to shorter interventions (e.g., up to 1 year)
Prospective cohort study	Good design to support a causal relationship Can study multiple outcomes Prospective nature minimizes recall bias Can reflect effects of long-term patterns of exercise	Susceptible to bias due to confounding Inefficient for rare or long-delayed outcomes Can be expensive and time consuming Requires continued effort for follow-up Cannot establish causation
Cross-sectional comparison	Can be quick and inexpensive Easier to obtain large sample size Can reflect effects of long-term patterns of exercise	Susceptible to bias due to confounding Cannot determine temporal sequence Susceptible to recall bias Cannot establish causation

- Concentrations of acute phase proteins and cytokines that indicate the presence of inflammation
- Concentrations of other cytokines
- Antibody concentrations
- Clinical manifestations (incidence of upper respiratory tract infection)

The findings of well-conducted intervention studies (bold) that employed a randomized design, had ten or more individuals in the intervention and in the control groups, and had a retention of 85% or greater are discussed in detail. Findings from randomized studies that suffered from small sample size or high dropout rates are only mentioned briefly. Nonrandomized studies or studies that lacked baseline samples are not described further here.

EXERCISE EFFECTS ON NATURAL KILLER CELL ACTIVITY AND LYMPHOCYTE PROLIFERATION

In cross-sectional studies, exercisers show consistently higher NK cell cytotoxicity than sedentary individuals do (Table 9.2). Yet, several intervention studies have investigated the effects of physical activity on NK cell cytotoxicity and have yielded inconsistent results (Table 9.3). The strongest data on the effects of exercise on NK cell cytotoxicity, coming from well-designed, large randomized studies, suggest that exercise has no statistically significant effect on NK cell cytotoxicity.[3,4,43]

Nieman et al. randomized 32 healthy elderly Caucasian women (mean age, 73 years) to supervised brisk walking for 30 to 40 minutes, five times per week at 60% heart rate reserve, or a nonexercise stretching control group.[3] The 12-week intervention was completed by 30 women, with

TABLE 9.2
Summary of Observations from Cross-Sectional Studies: Exercisers Compared to Sedentary or Less Active Individuals[a]

Measure of immune function	Increased ↑ (ref.)	Decreased ↓ (ref.)	No statistically significant difference (ref.)
Functional assays			
NK cell cytotoxicity	3, 94		95, 96
Lymphocyte proliferation	3, 95, 97, 98		
Neutrophilic phagocytosis	96[a]		
Cell counts and percentages			
NK cells	96		3
Total leukocytes		**73, 74, 76, 78**	3, 96, 99
Total lymphocytes			3
Neutrophils			3
CD3 (T-cells)			3, 96
CD4 (T-helper/inducer)		96[d]	3
CD8 (T-cytotoxic/suppressor)	96[b]		3
CD4:CD8 ratio		96[e]	
CD20 (B-cells)		96	3
Activated T-lymphocytes %	97[c]		97[c]
Markers of inflammation			
C-reactive protein		69, **71, 72, 73, 74, 75**[f], **76**, 77[g], **78, 79**, 81,	62, 99, **100**
Serum amyloid A		81, **101**[h], **102**	**78**[i]
Interleukin-6		**72**, 81[f], **100**	**79**

(continued)

TABLE 9.2 (CONTINUED)
Summary of Observations from Cross-Sectional Studies: Exercisers Compared to Sedentary or Less Active Individuals[a]

Measure of immune function	Increased ↑ (ref.)	Decreased ↓ (ref.)	No statistically significant difference (ref.)
Other cytokines			
Interleukin-1			95
Interleukin-2	95		
Clinical manifestations			
URTI incidence		3, 5, **6**	**103**

[a] Age-associated decline in neutrophilic phagocytosis was attenuated among exercisers.
[b] Exercisers did not exhibit the age-associated decrease in CD8 counts observed in the sedentary group.
[c] Significantly higher in trained young (mean age 27, n = 10) compared to sedentary young (mean age 26, n = 10); no difference between trained elderly (mean age 68, n = 10) and sedentary elderly (mean age 72, n = 10).
[d] Exercisers did not exhibit the age-associated increase in CD4 counts observed in the sedentary group.
[e] Exercisers did not exhibit the same age-associated increase in CD4:CD8 ratio; CD4:CD8 ratio significantly lower among elderly exercisers compared to sedentary exercisers.
[f] Quintiles of cardiorespiratory fitness, assessed with a maximal treadmill test; significantly decreasing level with increasing level of fitness.
[g] Fitness level assessed with maximal treadmill test; no difference observed among African–American women.
[h] Significantly lower levels with increasing level of physical activity (frequent exercise ≥12 times per month; infrequent 1 to 11 times per month; sedentary) for most types of activity measured but not lower for cycling or gardening.
[i] Nonsignificantly lower among exercisers (p = 0.059).
[j] Only significantly lower for exercisers not taking hormone therapy (nonsignificantly lower levels among exercisers taking hormone therapy), compared to sedentary controls.
Note: Well-designed studies with ≥10 subjects per group and <15% dropout are in bold.

no statistically significant difference in NK cell cytotoxicity observed, despite significant improvements in cardiorespiratory fitness in the walking group, relative to the control group.

A larger study conducted by Nieman et al. yielded similar results.[4] The 102 obese women (mean age, 46 years) in the trial were randomized to one of four arms: brisk walking for 45 minutes, five times per week at 60 to 80% maximum heart rate; energy restriction (1200 to 1300 kcal/day); exercise and diet; and control. Again, the exercise intervention had no statistically significant effect on NK cell cytotoxicity among the 21 women who completed the 12-week study, as compared to the 22 controls.

Sagiv and colleagues[43] randomized 25 men (mean age, 46 years) with coronary artery disease who were being treated with atenolol (a β-adrenergic blocking agent) to an exercise intervention consisting of aerobic walking or running for 45 minutes, three to four times per week, at 65 to 70% of the maximal work capacity of each subject. Although the generalizability of the study results may be limited due to the health condition and use of concomitant medication of study subjects, all men completed the 12-week study, and the exercise intervention appeared to have no statistically significant effect on natural killer cell cytotoxicity.[43] Two small 8-week randomized-controlled trials (n = 18, n = 16) also reported no statistically significant effect.[44,45]

On the other hand, several studies detected significant increases in NK cell cytotoxicity associated with exercise interventions. Unfortunately, many of these studies lacked a control group or baseline samples.[46–49] However in one well-conducted randomized trial, Fahlman et al. did detect significantly higher NK cell cytotoxicity (on a per-cell basis) among 15 elderly nuns (mean age,

TABLE 9.3
Summary of Effects of Exercise Intervention Studies: Immunological Changes in Exercisers, Usually Compared to Nonexercise Controls

Measure of immune function	Increased ↑ (ref.)	Decreased ↓ (ref.)	No statistically significant effect (ref.)
Functional assays			
NK cell cytotoxicity	RCT: 1[b,c], 46[a], **50**	RCT: 57[f]	RCTs: **3**, **4**, **43**, 44, 45, 51[d], 105[g,h]
	non-RCT: 47, 48[d], 49[d,e]	non-RCT: 104[d]	non-RCT: 55
Lymphocyte proliferation	non-RCT: 104[d]	RCT: **4** non-RCT: 82[d]	RCTs: **3**, 44, **50**, **51**, 52, **53** non-RCTs: 54, 55, 56
Phagocytotic activity of monocytes	non-RCT: 47, 48[d]		
Monocyte and granulocyte phagocytosis and oxidative burst			RCT: **4**
Cell counts and percentages			
NK cells (e.g., CD16 or CD56)	non-RCT: 54, 55	RCT: **50**	RCTs: 1, **3**, **43**[j], 44, 45, 57, **51**, 105[g] non-RCTs: 47, 48[d], 82[d]
Total leukocytes			RCTs: **3**, **43**[j], 44, 45, **51**, 52, **58** non-RCTs: 47, 48[d], 54, 55
Total lymphocytes		RCT: 52 non-RCTs: 47, 48	RCTs: **3**, **43**[j], 45, **51**, **53**, **58**
			non-RCTs: 44, 54, 56[k], 60, 82[d]
Granulocytes	non-RCTs: 47 (%), 48[d] (%)		non-RCTs: 47 (count), 48[d] (count), 54
Monocytes		non-RCTs: 47 (%), 48[d] (%)	RCT: **51** non-RCTs: 47 (count), 48[d] (count), 54
Neutrophils			RCTs: **3**, **43**[j], 44, 45, **51**
Eosinophils			RCTs: **43**[j], **51**
Basophils			RCT: **51**
CD2 (T-cells, NK cells)	RCT: 59		
CD3 (T-cells)	non-RCT: 104[d]		RCTs: **3**, 44, 45, **50**, **51** non-RCTs: 49[d,e], 54, 55[l], 56[k], 60
CD5 (T-cells)		RCT: 52[b]	
CD4 (T-helper/inducer)	RCTs: **43**[j], 59	non-RCT: 60	RCTs: **3**, 44, **50**, **51**, 52
	non-RCT: 49[d,e]		non-RCTs: 54, 55, 56[k]

-- continued

TABLE 9.3 (CONTINUED)
Summary of Effects of Exercise Intervention Studies: Immunological Changes in Exercisers, Usually Compared to Nonexercise Controls

Measure of immune function	Increased ↑ (ref.)	Decreased ↓ (ref.)	No statistically significant effect (ref.)
CD8 (T-cytotoxic/ suppressor)	RCTs: **43**[j], 59 non-RCT: 60	RCT: **50**[m]	RCTs: **3**, 44, **51**, 52 non-RCTs: 49[d,e], 54, 55, 56[k]
CD4:CD8 ratio	non-RCT: 49[d,e]	RCT: **43**[j]	RCTs: 44, 52 non-RCTs: 54, 56[k], 60
CD 14 (myelomonocytic cells)			RCT: 44
CD19 or CD20 (B-cells)	RCT: 59	non-RCTs: 54, 55	RCTs: **3**, 44, 52 non-RCT: 49[e,q]
CD122 (IL-2rβ chain lymphocytes)	non-RCT: 54		
Naïve CD45RA+	RCT: 59		
Activated T-lymphocytes (e.g., CD25)			non-RCTs: 49[d,e], 54, 55
Markers of inflammation			
C-reactive protein		RCT: 93[n] non-RCTs: 90, 91, 92	RCTs: 44, **58**, **88**[q], **89**[r] non-RCTs: 82[d,o], 87[d,p]
Serum amyloid A		non-RCT: 90[d]	
Interleukin-6 (IL-6)		RCTs: **84**[s], **86**[p,t], 93	RCTs: 44, **84**[s], **86**[p,t], **88**[q] non-RCTs: 83[p], 85[p], 87[d,p], 90[d]
Tumor necrosis factor-α		RCTs: **84**[s], **86**[p,f] non-RCTs: 82[d], 83[p], 106	RCTs: **84**[s], **86**[p,t], **88**[q] non-RCTs: 85[p], 87[d,p]
Other Cytokines			
Interleukin-1		RCT: **86**[p,t] non-RCT: 82[d]	RCTs: 44, **86**[p,t] 86[p,t] (RCT)
sIL-2R	non-RCT: 54		
Antibody assays			
IgA, IgG, IgM	RCT: 52		RCT: **53**
IgG, IgM	non-RCT: 49[d,e]		
IgA			non-RCT: 49[d,e]
Salivary IgA concentration	non-RCT: 107[d]		
Clinical manifestations			
URTI incidence		RCTs: 1, **3**, **4**[u] non-RCT: 2[d]	RCT: **50**

-(continued)

TABLE 9.3 (CONTINUED)
Summary of Effects of Exercise Intervention Studies: Immunological Changes in Exercisers, Usually Compared to Nonexercise Controls

[a]No baseline samples.
[b]Significant at week 6 but not at week 15.
[c]Nieman (1990) and Nehlsen–Cannarella (1991) use same data, present same results for NK cytotoxicity.
[d]No nonexercise controls.
[e]Subjects are transplant patients.
[f]Despite transient exercise-induced increase.
[g]Subjects are on 950 kcal/day diet.
[h]Despite significant decrease in NK cytotoxicity among nonexercising dieters.
[i]Performed only on a subset of 19; nonsignificant increase, $p < 0.10$.
[j]Subjects are coronary artery disease patients being treated with β-blockers.
[k]Subjects are cancer patients who received high-dose chemotherapy followed by peripheral blood stem cell transplants.
[l]Subjects are moderate trainers; among subset of light trainers a transient exercise-induced increase was followed by significant decrease.
[m]Concurrent with significant increase in NK cell counts among nonexercising controls.
[n]Intervention also included low-calorie Mediterranean-style diet and weight loss advice.
[o]Nonsignificant decrease (35%), $p = 0.12$.
[p]Subjects have stable chronic heart failure.
[q]Subjects are overweight or obese and have knee osteoarthritis.
[r]Nonsignificantly lower among subjects randomized to exercise, $p > 0.2$.
[s]Decrease seen only in subset of exercisers with moderate to severe chronic heart failure ($n = 24$); no decrease in healthy subjects ($n = 20$).
[t]Decrease in local skeletal muscle expression; no significant effect on serum concentrations.
[u]Analysis includes data from 30 nonobese physically active women from a cross-sectional comparison group.
Note: Well-designed randomized-controlled studies with ≥10 subjects per group and <15% dropout are in bold.

77 years), randomized to 20 to 50 minutes of brisk walking three times per week at 70% of their heart rate reserve for 10 weeks, compared to 14 nonexercise controls with whom they lived.[50]

In addition, NK cell cytotoxicity was also assessed for a subset of the elderly participants ($n = 19$; mean age, 65 years) in a 6-month randomized-controlled trial conducted by Woods and colleagues and was found to be nonsignificantly higher ($p < 0.10$) among those randomized to the exercise intervention compared to stretchers in the control group.[51] It is possible that the size of the subset selected for this assay was simply too small to detect any statistically significant intervention effects. Another small randomized study among 50 mildly obese women (intervention group mean age, 36 years; control group mean age, 33 years), of whom only 36 completed the 3-month trial, detected significantly increased NK cell cytotoxicity 6 weeks into the intervention, but not at week 15.[1]

Although the data are not conclusive, most evidence from randomized-controlled trials to date suggests that exercise has no statistically significant effect on NK cell cytotoxicity. However, the assigned exercise interventions may have been too shortin duration (generally 10 to 15 weeks) to show effects. Certainly, the implications for enhanced NK cell function associated with habitual moderate intensity physical activity would be profound, especially in light of findings from epidemiological studies, which noted increased cancer incidence with depressed natural killer cell cytotoxicity .[19]

Similarly, most evidence from randomized-controlled trials (Table 9.3) suggests that moderate-intensity exercise has no statistically significant effect on lymphocyte proliferation.[3,44,50–56] Details of two of these studies with null findings, conducted by Nieman et al. and Fahlman et al., have been described earlier in this chapter.[3,50] Mitchell et al. assessed lymphocyte proliferation in 21 male college students (intervention group mean age, 23 years; control group mean age, 20 years) who completed a 12-week randomized exercise intervention, consisting of 30 minutes on a stationary bike three times per week, at 75% of their VO_2 peak.[53] It is possible that this study was unable to detect any significant exercise effects because young people generally have better immune function regardless of exercise tendencies.

Woods et al. randomized 33 otherwise healthy elderly individuals (mean age, 65 years) to 15 to 40 minutes of supervised brisk walking or stretching three times per week.[51] For the 29 subjects who completed the 6-month intervention, no statistically significant difference in lymphocyte proliferation was observed, despite a significant ($p < 0.05$) increase in VO_2 max among the exercisers. In fact, both groups exhibited increased lymphocyte proliferation, which was somewhat, though nonsignificantly, greater among the exercisers. A large ($n = 50$) randomized-controlled study among mildly obese women also found no statistically significant effect of exercise on lymphocyte proliferation[52]; however, this study did suffer from a 28% dropout rate, which could have biased the results. A small ($n = 18$) 8-week randomized-controlled trial among middle-aged individuals with rheumatoid arthritis also reported no statistically significant effect.[44]

Finally, in the large four-arm exercise and diet study conducted by Nieman et al. (described earlier), a significant decrease in lymphocyte proliferation was detected among those randomized to exercise only.[4] This study also assessed monocyte and granulocyte phagocytosis and oxidative burst and did not detect any significant effect associated with the exercise intervention.

EXERCISE AND ENUMERATION AND PHENOTYPING OF IMMUNE CELLS

Cross-sectional analyses of specific cell counts among exercisers and nonexercisers have been largely inconsistent (Table 9.2). For example, some studies report reduced total leukocyte counts among exercisers[73,74,76,78] whereas several others did not.[3,96,99]

As was the case with NK cell cytotoxicity, the majority of the well-conducted intervention studies assessing NK cell count were unable to detect any significant effect associated with physical activity [1,3,43–45,51,57] (Table 9.3). However, two nonrandomized studies have reported increased[54,55] NK cell counts associated with exercise interventions and although Fahlman et al. detected increased NK cell cytotoxicity (on a per-cell basis) among 15 elderly nuns randomized to the exercise intervention, they found decreased NK cell counts among these exercisers concurrent with increased NK cell counts among nonexercising controls.[50]

All of the exercise intervention studies published in the last two decades indicate that exercise has no statistically significant effect on total leukocyte counts.[3,43–45,51,52,58] With the exception of one randomized-controlled study that suffered from 28% dropout rate,[52] the literature to date also suggests no statistically significant effect of exercise on total lymphocyte counts.[3,43–45,51,53,58]

Although the data are less consistent with respect to CD4 (T-helper/inducer) and CD8 (T-cytotoxic/suppressor) counts, the majority of the studies that have investigated the effects of exercise on either of these measures of immune function were unable to detect any significant effect.[3,44,51,52] However, two randomized-controlled trials did report significant increases in CD4 and CD8 counts among subjects randomized to exercise, but no effect on CD4 counts among exercisers[43,59] and one randomized-controlled trial detected a significant decrease in CD8 counts.[50]

Though the majority of the studies (including two randomized trials[44,52]) that have investigated the impact of exercise on the CD4:CD8 ratio found no significant effect,[44,52,54,56,60] the largest randomized study to present data on this measure of immune function reports a significant decrease among male coronary artery disease patients (mean age, 46 years) being treated with atenolol; they were randomized to aerobic walking or running for 45 minutes, three to four times per week, at 65 to 70% of the maximal work capacity of each subject.[43]

EXERCISE EFFECTS ON MARKERS OF INFLAMMATION

Concentrations of markers of inflammation, such as C-reactive protein (CRP) and serum amyloid A (SAA), are often elevated among overweight or obese individuals — an association most likely related to the upstream role of adipose tissue-secreted cytokines (e.g., IL-6) in the production of these acute phase proteins. In fact, elevated levels of C-reactive protein and serum amyloid A have been associated with body fatness[61–70] and sedentary lifestyles[61,69,71–81] in cross-sectional surveys. Despite a strong suggestion of an association between lower concentrations of circulating inflammatory markers such as C-reactive protein, serum amyloid A, IL-6, and TNF-α with increasing level of physical activity observed in these cross-sectional studies (Table 9.2), the best designed intervention studies actually support the absence of a significant association between exercise and these markers of inflammation (Table 9.3).

For example, three large, well-designed randomized-controlled trials have yielded results indicating that physical activity interventions have no significant effect on serum concentrations of CRP.[58,88,89] Specifically, de Jong and colleagues were unable to detect a significant association between C-reactive protein levels and exercise intervention among 217 frail elderly individuals (mean age, 78 years) randomized to an exercise intervention (strength, endurance, coordination, and flexibility training), micronutrient-supplemented diet, exercise and diet, or control group.[58] Although only 145 subjects completed the 17-week intervention, the authors indicate that the high (24%) dropout rate was mainly due to health problems (frequent among this study population of frail elderly individuals) and not related to the assigned intervention.

In a more recent four-armed randomized-controlled trial investigating the effects of exercise, diet-induced weight loss, or the combination of exercise and diet-induced weight loss on markers of inflammation, Nicklas and colleagues also found that exercise had no significant effect on circulating concentrations of C-reactive protein among the 252 older (mean age, 69 years), obese individuals with knee osteoarthritis who completed the 18-month trial.[88] Although this study had only 80% retention, the authors report that concentrations of inflammatory markers from the baseline blood draws were not statistically significantly different for subjects who completed, dropped out, or failed to provide follow-up blood samples. They suggested that individuals for whom change in concentration of inflammatory markers could not be assessed were similar to those who completed the 18 months, with respect to baseline inflammatory markers.

Additionally, Rauramaa et al. conducted an impressive 6-year randomized-controlled study, in which 140 middle-aged men (mean age, 57 years) were randomized to exercise (walking, jogging, swimming, and/or cycling) for 30 to 60 minutes, three to five times per week.[89] The C-reactive protein concentrations of the 125 men who completed the study were analyzed on an intent-to-treat basis. At the end of the 6-year intervention, circulating C-reactive protein levels were lower among those randomized to exercise; however, despite the large sample size, the difference was not statistically significant ($p > 0.2$). Finally, a small 8-week randomized trial similarly found no significant effect on C-reactive protein among rheumatoid arthritis patients randomized to bicycle training four to five times per week at 80% of the subjects' VO_2 max.[44]

Of the four intervention studies that reported a decrease in C-reactive protein levels associated with physical activity, three were nonrandomized[90–92] (one of which also lacked a nonexercise control group[90]). The one randomized study to date that has reported a decrease in C-reactive protein associated with an intervention was primarily focused on weight loss through a low-energy Mediterranean-style diet among 120 obese premenopausal women.[93] Participants randomized to the intervention arm also received information about the importance of physical activity, mainly through walking, and attended monthly or bimonthly sessions with an exercise trainer. No structured exercise regimen was established for participants randomized to the intervention arm in this study, and evidence of change in physical activity level in study subjects was assessed only through self-report. Nonetheless, women randomized to the intervention group reportedly increased from 64 to 175 minutes of physical activity per week, compared to women in the control group who increased from 71 to only 102 minutes per week ($p = 0.009$). At the end of the 24-month trial, women randomized to the intervention had experienced significant reductions in BMI and serum concentrations of C-reactive protein, although the effect of the modest exercise aspect of the intervention of this randomized-controlled trial could not be isolated from that of the effects of the diet-induced weight loss.

Likewise, the majority of findings from studies investigating the effects of exercise on levels of IL-6, a precursor in the production of C-reactive protein and serum amyloid A, are similarly most convincing for no effect,[44,83–89,90] with a handful of studies reporting a significant decrease.[84,86,93] Interestingly, Adamopoulos et al. observed a significant decrease in IL-6 among exercisers with chronic heart failure, but not among healthy exercisers.[84] Gielen et al. observed a significant decrease in IL-6 expression in local skeletal muscle (*vastus lateralis*) but no effect on serum concentrations of the proinflammatory molecule.[86] Finally, while some studies have also shown that consistent exercise significantly lowers levels of other cytokines implicated in the production of C-reactive protein and serum amyloid A such as IL-1α, IL-1β, and TNF-α,[82–84,86,106] others have not.[44,84–88]

EXERCISE EFFECTS ON ANTIBODY CONCENTRATIONS

Very few studies have investigated the effects of exercise interventions on circulating concentrations of antibodies (immunoglobulins). Although the study by Nehlsen–Cannarella et al. (described earlier) suffered from a high (28%) dropout rate, they did report significantly higher concentrations of IgA, IgG, and IgM among the premenopausal women randomized to 45 minutes of supervised brisk walking five times per week.[52] Mitchell and colleagues' randomized study (described earlier) of male college students found no significant effect on immunoglobulin concentrations associated with the exercise intervention.[53] However, it is possible that the small study size ($n = 21$) and the generally high baseline immune function of study participants impeded the ability to detect significant effects after only 12 weeks.

EXERCISE EFFECTS ON CLINICAL MANIFESTATIONS OF IMMUNE FUNCTION

Perhaps the most convincing line of evidence suggesting that regular, moderate-intensity physical activity has positive immunomodulatory effects can be seen with respect to incidence or duration of upper respiratory tract infections.[1,3,4] Specifically, in two 12-week randomized studies, Nieman and colleagues demonstrated a significantly lower incidence of upper respiratory tract infections among elderly women (mean age, 73 years) randomized to walking compared to those randomized to calisthenics[3] and significantly fewer upper respiratory tract infections symptomatic days among female exercisers (mean age, 46 years) compared to nonexercisers.[4] Unfortunately, assessing the incidence of upper respiratory tract infections as a clinical manifestation of immune function may be limited by differential self-reporting of events among exercisers compared to nonexercisers.

CONCLUSION

From the large body of exercise immunology literature that has accumulated, it is difficult to distill a single take-home message regarding the effects of regular moderate-intensity exercise on immune function. The benefits of physical activity may in fact go above and beyond those of weight loss and cardiovascular fitness; however, the inconsistencies in existing data make it difficult to draw firm conclusions about the immunomodulatory effects of exercise.

Many factors may have contributed to some of the seemingly contradictory findings summarized earlier, including

- Widely diverse study populations
- The type, intensity, duration, and frequency of the exercise prescribed
- Incorporation of unmonitored exercise sessions in conjunction with supervised training sessions
- The lack of a "true" nonexercise control group in some instances (or any control group, for many studies)
- Lack of baseline samples
- Varying time of sample collection

Additionally, for many of the intervention studies, small sample sizes (frequently less than ten subjects per trial arm), in conjunction with the wide variability inherent in most measures of immune function, limited the ability to detect significant associations when, in fact, they may have existed and potentially contributed to the increased risk of biased or chance findings. In many instances, we cannot be sure whether the null findings truly reflect the absence of an intervention effect or whether the studies are simply too underpowered to detect even modest effects that may still be clinically significant. It is also important to acknowledge that studies with null or contrary findings may have a lower likelihood of publication (this may be an issue in particular with observational studies).

Associations that were detected cross-sectionally (Table 9.2) in many instances are not apparent in the randomized data (Table 9.3). In the observational studies, physically active individuals likely differed from their sedentary counterparts by more than just the amount of time they devoted to exercise each week; other health habits associated with physical activity, such as use of nutritional supplements, may have confounded the observed associations. Furthermore, the observational studies may reflect the impact of a lifelong pattern of physical activity, whereas the intervention studies can usually measure only the impact of several months of activity. It is possible that long-term moderate exercise training is needed to reveal a positive impact of physical activity on immune function measures.

Determining the clinical relevance of the *in vitro* measures of immune function is another challenge inherent in the exploration of this scientific question. Due to the complex nature of the immune system, quantifying the absolute impact that physical activity might have on an individual's overall immune function is a difficult task. *In vitro* measures of immune function, the endpoint considered in the majority of the studies reviewed in this chapter, may only have limited clinical relevance. Thus, although a great deal of the *in vitro* measures were not significantly associated with physical activity, perhaps we should focus our attention on the convincing evidence suggesting that incidence and intensity of upper respiratory tract infections, which are clinical manifestations of immune function, can be modulated with exercise interventions.

Despite a large quantity of null findings, a suggestion that regular moderate-intensity physical activity is beneficial for host immune defense persists, mostly with respect to markers of inflammation and incidence of respiratory tract infections. It is imperative that additional large, well-conducted, randomized-controlled exercise intervention studies are undertaken to further substantiate that claim. These studies should combine the measurement of *in vitro* immune function markers and relevant clinical outcomes.

REFERENCES

1. Nieman DC, Nehlsen–Cannarella SL, Markoff PA, et al. The effects of moderate exercise training on natural killer cells and acute upper respiratory tract infections. *Int J Sports Med.* 1990; 11(6):467–473.
2. Karper WB, Boschen MB. Effects of exercise on acute respiratory tract infections and related symptoms. Moderate exercise may boast an elder's natural defenses against common illnesses. *Geriatric Nursing.* 1993; 14(1):15–18.

3. Nieman DC, Henson DA, Gusewitch G, et al. Physical activity and immune function in elderly women. *Med Sci Sports Exercise.* 1993; 25(7):823–831.
4. Nieman DC, Nehlsen–Cannarella SL, Henson DA, et al. Immune response to exercise training and/or energy restriction in obese women. *Med Sci Sports Exercise.* 1998; 30(5):679–686.
5. Kostka T, Berthouze SE, Lacour J, Bonnefoy M. The symptomatology of upper respiratory tract infections and exercise in elderly people. *Med Sci Sports Exercise.* 2000; 32(1):46–51.
6. Matthews CE, Ockene IS, Freedson PS, Rosal MC, Merriam PA, Hebert JR. Moderate to vigorous physical activity and risk of upper-respiratory tract infection. *Med Sci Sports Exercise.* 2002; 34(8):1242–1248.
7. Shephard RJ, Shek PN. Cancer, immune function, and physical activity. *Can J Appl Physiol.* 1995; 20(1):1–25.
8. Woods JA. Exercise and resistance to neoplasia. *Can J Physiol Pharmacol.* May 1998; 76(5):581–588.
9. Lee IM. Physical activity and cancer prevention — data from epidemiologic studies. *Med Sci Sports Exercise.* Nov 2003; 35(11):1823–1827.
10. Quadrilatero J, Hoffman–Goetz L. Physical activity and colon cancer. A systematic review of potential mechanisms. *J Sports Med Phys Fitness.* Jun 2003; 43(2):121–138.
11. Janeway CA, Travers P, Walport MJ, Capra JD. *Immunobiology: the Immune System in Health and Disease.* 4th ed. New York: Elsevier Science Ltd/Garland Publishing; 1999.
12. Doggen CJ, Berckmans RJ, Sturk A, Manger Cats V, Rosendaal FR. C-reactive protein, cardiovascular risk factors and the association with myocardial infarction in men. *J Intern Med.* Nov 2000; 248(5):406–414.
13. Ridker PM. Connecting the role of C-reactive protein and statins in cardiovascular disease. *Clin Cardiol.* Apr 2003; 26(4 Suppl 3):III39–44.
14. Backes JM, Howard PA, Moriarty PM. Role of C-reactive protein in cardiovascular disease. *Ann Pharmacother.* Jan 2004; 38(1):110–118.
15. Jakobisiak M, Lasek W, Golab J. Natural mechanisms protecting against cancer. *Immunol Lett.* 2003/12/15 2003; 90(2–3):103–122.
16. Beral V, Newton R. Overview of the epidemiology of immunodeficiency-associated cancers. *J Natl Cancer Inst Monogr.* 1998(23):1–6.
17. Bonnet F, Lewden C, May T, et al. Malignancy-related causes of death in human immunodeficiency virus-infected patients in the era of highly active antiretroviral therapy. *Cancer.* Jul 15 2004; 101(2):317–324.
18. Herida M, Mary–Krause M, Kaphan R, et al. Incidence of non-AIDS-defining cancers before and during the highly active antiretroviral therapy era in a cohort of human immunodeficiency virus-infected patients. *J Clin Oncol.* Sep 15 2003; 21(18):3447–3453.
19. Imai K, Matsuyama S, Miyake S, Suga K, Nakachi K. Natural cytotoxic activity of peripheral-blood lymphocytes and cancer incidence: an 11-year follow-up study of a general population. *Lancet.* 2000; 356(9244):1795–1799.
20. Mahmoud FA, Rivera NI. The role of C-reactive protein as a prognostic indicator in advanced cancer. *Curr Oncol Rep.* May 2002; 4(3):250–255.
21. O'Hanlon DM, Lynch J, Cormican M, Given HF. The acute phase response in breast carcinoma. *Anticancer Res.* Mar–Apr 2002; 22(2B):1289–1293.
22. Blann AD, Byrne GJ, Baildam AD. Increased soluble intercellular adhesion molecule-1, breast cancer and the acute phase response. *Blood Coagul Fibrinolysis.* Mar 2002; 13(2):165–168.
23. Erlinger TP, Platz EA, Rifai N, Helzlsouer KJ. C-reactive protein and the risk of incident colorectal cancer. *JAMA.* Feb 4 2004; 291(5):585–590.
24. Schreinemachers DM, Everson RB. Aspirin use and lung, colon, and breast cancer incidence in a prospective study (see comments). *Epidemiology.* 1994; 5(2):138–146.
25. Thun MJ, Henley SJ, Patrono C. Nonsteroidal anti-inflammatory drugs as anticancer agents: mechanistic, pharmacologic, and clinical issues. *J Natl Cancer Inst.* 2002; 94(4):252–266.
26. Sandler RS, Halabi S, Baron JA, et al. A randomized trial of aspirin to prevent colorectal adenomas in patients with previous colorectal cancer. *N Engl J Med.* 2003; 348(10):883–890.
27. Baron JA, Cole BF, Sandler RS, et al. A randomized trial of aspirin to prevent colorectal adenomas. *N Engl J Med.* 2003; 348(10):891–899.

28. Farrow DC, Vaughan TL, Hansten PD, et al. Use of aspirin and other nonsteroidal anti-inflammatory drugs and risk of esophageal and gastric cancer. *Cancer Epidemiol Biomarkers Prev.* Feb 1998; 7(2):97–102.
29. Akre K, Ekstrom AM, Signorello LB, Hansson LE, Nyren O. Aspirin and risk for gastric cancer: a population-based case-control study in Sweden. *Br J Cancer.* Apr 6 2001; 84(7):965–968.
30. Cotterchio M, Kreiger N, Sloan M, Steingart A. Nonsteroidal anti-inflammatory drug use and breast cancer risk. *Cancer Epidemiol Biomarkers Prev.* 2001; 10(11):1213–1217.
31. Khuder SA, Mutgi AB. Breast cancer and NSAID use: a meta-analysis. *Br J Cancer.* May 4 2001; 84(9):1188–1192.
32. Corley DA, Kerlikowske K, Verma R, Buffler P. Protective association of aspirin/NSAIDs and esophageal cancer: a systematic review and meta-analysis. *Gastroenterology.* Jan 2003; 124(1):47–56.
33. Harris RE, Chlebowski RT, Jackson RD, et al. Breast cancer and nonsteroidal anti-inflammatory drugs: prospective results from the Women's Health Initiative. *Cancer Res.* Sep 15 2003; 63(18):6096–6101.
34. Muscat JE, Chen SQ, Richie JP, Jr., et al. Risk of lung carcinoma among users of nonsteroidal antiinflammatory drugs. *Cancer.* Apr 1 2003; 97(7):1732–1736.
35. Vedhara K, Fox JD, Wang EC. The measurement of stress-related immune dysfunction in psychoneuroimmunology. *Neurosci Biobehav Rev.* 1999; 23(5):699–715.
36. Mitchell BL, Ulrich CM, McTiernan A. Supplementation with vitamins or minerals and immune function: can the elderly benefit? *Nutr Res.* 2003; 23(8):1117–1139.
37. Villas BH. Flow cytometry: an overview. *Cell Vis.* Jan–Feb 1998; 5(1):56–61.
38. Whiteside TL, Bryant J, Day R, Herberman RB. Natural killer cytotoxicity in the diagnosis of immune dysfunction: criteria for a reproducible assay. *J Clin Lab Anal.* 1990; 4(2):102–114.
39. Whiteside TL, Herberman RB. Role of human natural killer cells in health and disease. *Clin Diagnc Lab Immunol.* 1994; 1(2):125–133.
40. Nieman DC. Exercise, upper respiratory tract infection, and the immune system. *Med Sci Sports Exercise.* 1994; 26(2):128–139.
41. Shephard R. *Physical Activity, Training and the Immune Response.* Carmel, IN: Cooper; 1997.
42. Mackinnon LT. *Advances in Exercise Immunology.* Champaign, IL: Human Kinetics; 1999.
43. Sagiv M, Ben–Sira D, Goldhammer E. Beta-blockers, exercise, and the immune system in men with coronary artery disease. *Med Sci Sports Exercise.* 2002; 34(4):587–591.
44. Baslund B, Lyngberg K, Andersen V, et al. Effect of 8 wk of bicycle training on the immune system of patients with rheumatoid arthritis. *J Appl Physiol.* 1993; 75(4):1691–1695.
45. Nieman DC, Cook VD, Henson DA, et al. Moderate exercise training and natural killer cell cytotoxic activity in breast cancer patients. *Int J Sports Med.* 1995; 16(5):334–337.
46. Crist DM, Mackinnon LT, Thompson RF, Atterbom HA, Egan PA. Physical exercise increases natural cellular-mediated tumor cytotoxicity in elderly women. *Gerontology.* 1989; 35(2–3):66–71.
47. Peters C, Lotzerich H, Niemeier B, Schule K, Uhlenbruck G. Influence of a moderate exercise training on natural killer cytotoxicity and personality traits in cancer patients. *Anticancer Res.* 1994; 14(3A):1033–1036.
48. Peters C, Lotzerich H, Niemeir B, Schule K, Uhlenbruck G. Exercise, cancer and the immune response of monocytes. *Anticancer Res.* 1995; 15(1):175–179.
49. Surgit O, Ersoz G, Gursel Y, Ersoz S. Effects of exercise training on specific immune parameters in transplant recipients. *Transplantation Proc.* 2001; 33(7–8):3298.
50. Fahlman M, Boardley D, Flynn MG, Braun WA, Lambert CP, Bouillon LE. Effects of endurance training on selected parameters of immune function in elderly women. *Gerontology.* 2000; 46(2):97–104.
51. Woods JA, Ceddia MA, Wolters BW, Evans JK, Lu Q, McAuley E. Effects of 6 months of moderate aerobic exercise training on immune function in the elderly. *Mechanisms Ageing Dev.* 1999; 109(1):1–19.
52. Nehlsen–Cannarella SL, Nieman DC, Balk–Lamberton AJ, et al. The effects of moderate exercise training on immune response. *Med Sci Sports Exercise.* 1991; 23(1):64–70.
53. Mitchell JB, Paquet AJ, Pizza FX, Starling RD, Holtz RW, Grandjean PW. The effect of moderate aerobic training on lymphocyte proliferation. *Int J Sports Med.* 1996; 17(5):384–389.

54. Rhind SG, Shek PN, Shinkai S, Shephard RJ. Effects of moderate endurance exercise and training on *in vitro* lymphocyte proliferation, interleukin-2 (IL-2) production, and IL-2 receptor expression. *Eur J ApplPhysiol Occup Physiol.* 1996; 74(4):348–360.
55. Shore S, Shinkai S, Rhind S, Shephard RJ. Immune responses to training: how critical is training volume? *J Sports Med Phys Fitness.* 1999; 39(1):1–11.
56. Hayes SC, Rowbottom D, Davies PS, Parker TW, Bashford J. Immunological changes after cancer treatment and participation in an exercise program. *Med Sci Sports Exercise.* 2003; 35(1):2–9.
57. Rincon HG, Solomon GF, Benton D, Rubenstein LZ. Exercise in frail elderly men decreases natural killer cell activity. *Aging* (Milano). 1996; 8(2):109–112.
58. de Jong N, Chin APMJ, de Groot LC, de Graaf C, Kok FJ, van Staveren WA. Functional biochemical and nutrient indices in frail elderly people are partly affected by dietary supplements but not by exercise. *J Nutr.* 1999; 129(11):2028–2036.
59. LaPerriere A, Antoni MH, Ironson G, et al. Effects of aerobic exercise training on lymphocyte subpopulations. *Int J Sports Med.* 1994; 15(Suppl 3):S127–130.
60. Kawada E, Kubota K, Kurabayashi H, Tamura K, Tamura J, Shirakura T. Effects of long-term running on lymphocyte subpopulations. *Tohoku J Expl Med.* 1992; 167(4):273–277.
61. Danesh J, Whincup P, Walker M, et al. Low grade inflammation and coronary heart disease: prospective study and updated meta-analyses. *Br Med J.* Jul 22 2000; 321(7255):199–204.
62. Rawson ES, Freedson PS, Osganian SK, Matthews CE, Reed G, Ockene IS. Body mass index, but not physical activity, is associated with C-reactive protein. *Med Sci Sports Exercise.* 2003; 35(7):1160–1166.
63. Visser M, Bouter LM, McQuillan GM, Wener MH, Harris TB. Elevated C-reactive protein levels in overweight and obese adults (see comments). *JAMA.* 1999; 282(22):2131–2135.
64. Yudkin JS, Stehouwer CD, Emeis JJ, Coppack SW. C-reactive protein in healthy subjects: associations with obesity, insulin resistance, and endothelial dysfunction: a potential role for cytokines originating from adipose tissue? *Arteriosclerosis, Thrombosis Vasc Biol.* Apr 1999; 19(4):972–978.
65. Ford ES. Body mass index, diabetes, and C-reactive protein among U.S. adults. *Diabetes Care.* Dec 1999; 22(12):1971–1977.
66. Hak AE, Stehouwer CD, Bots ML, et al. Associations of C-reactive protein with measures of obesity, insulin resistance, and subclinical atherosclerosis in healthy, middle-aged women. *Arteriosclerosis, Thrombosis Vasc Biol.* Aug 1999; 19(8):1986–1991.
67. Barinas–Mitchell E, Cushman M, Meilahn EN, Tracy RP, Kuller LH. Serum levels of C-reactive protein are associated with obesity, weight gain, and hormone replacement therapy in healthy postmenopausal women. *Am J Epidemiol.* Jun 1 2001; 153(11):1094–1101.
68. Tchernof A, Nolan A, Sites CK, Ades PA, Poehlman ET. Weight loss reduces C-reactive protein levels in obese postmenopausal women. *Circulation.* Feb 5 2002; 105(5):564–569.
69. Manns PJ, Williams DP, Snow CM, Wander RC. Physical activity, body fat, and serum C-reactive protein in postmenopausal women with and without hormone replacement. *Am J Hum Biol.* Jan–Feb 2003; 15(1):91–100.
70. Aronson D, Bartha P, Zinder O, et al. Obesity is the major determinant of elevated C-reactive protein in subjects with the metabolic syndrome. *Int J Obesity Relat Metab Disord.* May 2004; 28(5):674–679.
71. Rohde LE, Hennekens CH, Ridker PM. Survey of C-reactive protein and cardiovascular risk factors in apparently healthy men. *Am J Cardiol.* 1999; 84(9):1018–1022.
72. Taaffe DR, Harris TB, Ferrucci L, Rowe J, Seeman TE. Cross-sectional and prospective relationships of interleukin-6 and C-reactive protein with physical performance in elderly persons: MacArthur studies of successful aging (comment). *J Gerontol Ser A-Biol Sci Med Sci.* 2000; 55(12):M709–715.
73. Geffken DF, Cushman M, Burke GL, Polak JF, Sakkinen PA, Tracy RP. Association between physical activity and markers of inflammation in a healthy elderly population. *Am J Epidemiol.* 2001; 153(3):242–250.
74. Abramson JL, Vaccarino V. Relationship between physical activity and inflammation among apparently healthy middle-aged and older U.S. adults. *Arch Intern Med.* 2002; 162(11):1286–1292.
75. Church TS, Barlow CE, Earnest CP, Kampert JB, Priest EL, Blair SN. Associations between cardiorespiratory fitness and C-reactive protein in men. *Arteriosclerosis, Thrombosis Vasc Biol.* 2002; 22(11):1869–1876.

76. Ford ES. Does exercise reduce inflammation? Physical activity and C-reactive protein among U.S. adults. *Epidemiology*. 2002; 13(5):561–568.
77. LaMonte MJ, Durstine JL, Yanowitz FG, et al. Cardiorespiratory fitness and C-reactive protein among a tri-ethnic sample of women. *Circulation*. 2002; 106(4):403–406.
78. Pitsavos C, Chrysohoou C, Panagiotakos DB, et al. Association of leisure-time physical activity on inflammation markers (C-reactive protein, white cell blood count, serum amyloid A, and fibrinogen) in healthy subjects (from the ATTICA study). *Am J Cardiol*. 2003; 91(3):368–370.
79. Reuben DB, Judd–Hamilton L, Harris TB, Seeman TE. The associations between physical activity and inflammatory markers in high-functioning older persons: MacArthur Studies of Successful Aging. *J Am Geriatr Soc*. 2003; 51(8):1125–1130.
80. Rothenbacher D, Hoffmeister A, Brenner H, Koenig W. Physical activity, coronary heart disease, and inflammatory response. *Arch Intern Med*. May 26 2003; 163(10):1200–1205.
81. Stauffer BL, Hoetzer GL, Smith DT, DeSouza CA. Plasma C-reactive protein is not elevated in physically active postmenopausal women taking hormone replacement therapy. *J Appl Physiol*. Jan 2004; 96(1):143–148.
82. Smith JK, Dykes R, Douglas JE, Krishnaswamy G, Berk S. Long-term exercise and atherogenic activity of blood mononuclear cells in persons at risk of developing ischemic heart disease. *JAMA*. 1999; 281(18):1722–1727.
83. Larsen AI, Aukrust P, Aarsland T, Dickstein K. Effect of aerobic exercise training on plasma levels of tumor necrosis factor alpha in patients with heart failure. *Am J Cardiol*. 2001; 88(7):805–808.
84. Adamopoulos S, Parissis J, Karatzas D, et al. Physical training modulates proinflammatory cytokines and the soluble Fas/soluble Fas ligand system in patients with chronic heart failure. *J Am Coll Cardiol*. 2002; 39(4):653–663.
85. Conraads VM, Beckers P, Bosmans J, et al. Combined endurance/resistance training reduces plasma TNF-alpha receptor levels in patients with chronic heart failure and coronary artery disease. (comment). *Eur Heart J*. 2002; 23(23):1854–1860.
86. Gielen S, Adams V, Mobius–Winkler S, et al. Anti-inflammatory effects of exercise training in the skeletal muscle of patients with chronic heart failure (comment). *J Am Coll Cardiol*. 2003; 42(5):861–868.
87. LeMaitre JP, Harris S, Fox KA, Denvir M. Change in circulating cytokines after 2 forms of exercise training in chronic stable heart failure. *Am Heart J*. Jan 2004; 147(1):100–105.
88. Nicklas BJ, Ambrosius W, Messier SP, et al. Diet-induced weight loss, exercise, and chronic inflammation in older, obese adults: a randomized controlled clinical trial. *Am J Clin Nutr*. Apr 2004; 79(4):544–551.
89. Rauramaa R, Halonen P, Vaisanen SB, et al. Effects of aerobic physical exercise on inflammation and atherosclerosis in men: the DNASCO Study: a 6-year randomized, controlled trial. *Ann Intern Med*. Jun 15 2004; 140(12):1007–1014.
90. Wegge JK, Roberts CK, Ngo TH, Barnard RJ. Effect of diet and exercise intervention on inflammatory and adhesion molecules in postmenopausal women on hormone replacement therapy and at risk for coronary artery disease. *Metabolism*. Mar 2004; 53(3):377–381.
91. Mattusch F, Dufaux B, Heine O, Mertens I, Rost R. Reduction of the plasma concentration of C-reactive protein following nine months of endurance training. *Int J Sports Med*. 2000; 21(1):21–24.
92. Milani RV, Lavie CJ, Mehra MR. Reduction in C-reactive protein through cardiac rehabilitation and exercise training. *J Am Coll Cardiol*. Mar 17 2004; 43(6):1056–1061.
93. Esposito K, Pontillo A, Di Palo C, et al. Effect of weight loss and lifestyle changes on vascular inflammatory markers in obese women: a randomized trial. *JAMA*. 2003; 289(14):1799–1804.
94. Kusaka Y, Kondou H, Morimoto K. Healthy lifestyles are associated with higher natural killer cell activity. *Prev Med*. 1992; 21(5):602–615.
95. Shinkai S, Kohno H, Kimura K, et al. Physical activity and immune senescence in men. *Med Sci Sports Exercise*. 1995; 27(11):1516–1526.
96. Yan H, Kuroiwa A, Tanaka H, Shindo M, Kiyonaga A, Nagayama A. Effect of moderate exercise on immune senescence in men. *Eur J Appl Physiol*. 2001; 86(2):105–111.
97. Di Pietro R, Alba Rana R, Sciscio A, Centurione L, Centurione MA, Mazzotti G. Age- and training-related events in active T-subpopulation. Changes in polyphosphoinositide metabolism during mitogenic stimulation. *Mechanisms Ageing Dev*. 1996; 90(2):103–109.

98. Gueldner SH, Poon LW, La Via M, et al. Long-term exercise patterns and immune function in healthy older women. A report of preliminary findings. *Mechanisms Ageing Dev.* 1997; 93(1–3):215–222.
99. Lippi G, Bassi A, Guidi G, Zatti M. Relation between regular aerobic physical exercise and inflammatory markers. *Am J Cardiol.* 2002; 90(7):820.
100. Bermudez EA, Rifai N, Buring J, Manson JE, Ridker PM. Interrelationships among circulating interleukin-6, C-reactive protein, and traditional cardiovascular risk factors in women. *Arteriosclerosis, Thrombosis Vasc Biol.* Oct 1 2002; 22(10):1668–1673.
101. King DE, Carek P, Mainous AG, 3rd, Pearson WS. Inflammatory markers and exercise: differences related to exercise type. *Med Sci Sports Exercise.* Apr 2003; 35(4):575–581.
102. Albert MA, Glynn RJ, Ridker PM. Effect of physical activity on serum C-reactive protein. *Am J Cardiol.* Jan 15 2004; 93(2):221–225.
103. Hemila H, Virtamo J, Albanes D, Kaprio J. Physical activity and the common cold in men administered vitamin E and beta-carotene. *Med Sci Sports Exercise.* 2003; 35(11):1815–1820.
104. Watson RR, Moriguchi S, Jackson JC, Werner L, Wilmore JH, Freund BJ. Modification of cellular immune functions in humans by endurance exercise training during beta-adrenergic blockade with atenolol or propranolol. *Med Sci Sports Exercise.* 1986; 18(1):95–100.
105. Scanga CB, Verde TJ, Paolone AM, Andersen RE, Wadden TA. Effects of weight loss and exercise training on natural killer cell activity in obese women. *Med Sci Sports Exercise.* 1998; 30(12):1666–1671.
106. Tsukui S, Kanda T, Nara M, Nishino M, Kondo T, Kobayashi I. Moderate-intensity regular exercise decreases serum tumor necrosis factor-alpha and HbA1c levels in healthy women. *Int J Obes Relat Metab Disord.* Sep 2000; 24(9):1207–1211.
107. Akimoto T, Kumai Y, Akama T, et al. Effects of 12 months of exercise training on salivary secretory IgA levels in elderly subjects. *Br J Sports Med.* 2003; 37(1):76–79.

10 Mechanisms Associating Physical Activity with Cancer Incidence: Exercise and Prostaglandins

María Elena Martínez

CONTENTS

PHYSICAL ACTIVITY AND COLON CANCER

As reviewed in Chapter 5, despite the imperfect measurement of physical activity, results of epidemiological studies indicate that a higher activity level is associated with a 50% reduction in risk of colon cancer [1,2]. These results are consistent across various populations, study designs (prospective and retrospective), and types of activities (leisure and occupational). Perhaps the only debatable issue is whether strenuous and nonstrenuous activities are equally protective. However, little is known about the biological mechanisms of action responsible for the association between higher physical activity and lower risk of colon cancer.

Proposed biological mechanisms for the effect of physical activity on colon carcinogenesis include a decrease in bowel transit time, alteration of immune function, decreased bile acid metabolism, and insulin resistance [3–6]. Alternatively, given the evidence linking higher prostaglandin production (particularly of the E series) to the development of colorectal cancer, it is plausible that physical activity may protect against colon cancer through its effect on mucosal prostaglandin levels.

PROSTAGLANDINS AND COLON CANCER

Prostaglandins are the primary cellular metabolites from the action of the cyclooxygenases on arachidonic acid and exert various physiological actions in the gastrointestinal tract, including maintenance of mucosal integrity, regulation of secretion, and motility [7]. Previous research has suggested that prostaglandins play a role in the development of colon cancer given that tumor cells produce higher amounts of prostaglandins than normal cells. Increased prostaglandin production, particularly of the E series, has been reported in colonic tumor cells in humans and in experimental models [8–11]. It has also been shown that individuals with colorectal polyps or cancer have higher levels of colonic mucosal prostaglandin (PG)E_2 than control individuals do [12].

The mechanism by which prostaglandins contribute to colon carcinogenesis remains uncertain. Prostaglandins may modulate the development of colorectal neoplasia through the stimulation of cell proliferation and differentiation [13] or the inhibition of apoptosis [14]. Furthermore, prostaglandins are known to regulate growth and spread of tumors [15,16]. It is also possible that the effect of prostaglandins is mediated by nuclear receptors such as peroxisome proliferator activated receptors (PPARs), which have been shown to alter colon carcinogenesis [17–19]. Because PGI_2 has been found to act as a ligand for PPARδ [20], and PPARγ is activated by fatty acids and other arachidonic acid metabolites, it is possible that prostaglandins alter colon carcinogenesis through this receptor.

Support for the role of prostaglandins on colorectal neoplasia is derived from animal and human studies in which aspirin and other nonsteroidal anti-inflammatory drugs — inhibitors of prostaglandin synthesis — reduce risk of colorectal cancer and adenomas [21]. The biological mechanism is thought to be through the effect of these agents on arachidonic acid metabolism by inhibiting cycooxygenases, key enzymes involved in the synthesis of prostaglandins from arachidonic acid [22]. At least two isoforms of cycooxygenase (prostaglandin synthetase, COX) exist in humans. COX-1 is constitutively expressed in most tissues. Conversely, COX-2 is induced by agents such as cytokines and growth factors. However, whether COX-2 directly modulates the function of tumor cells is still unclear, so it is possible that prostaglandins produced by COX-2 are responsible for tumor promotion.

STUDIES LINKING PHYSICAL ACTIVITY, PGE_2, AND COLON CANCER

Given the consistent epidemiological findings for the protective effect of physical activity on colon cancer, as well as the strong link between prostaglandin synthesis and colorectal neoplasia, an observational cross-sectional study was conducted to test the hypothesis that physical activity mediates colon cancer risk through its effect on PGE_2 synthesis [23]. Analyses were conducted among 41 men and 22 women, 42 to 78 years of age and with a history of polyps, who participated in a clinical trial testing the effects of piroxicam on rectal mucosal PGE_2 levels. Only nonusers of aspirin or other nonsteroidal anti-inflammatory medications were eligible for the trial. A study schema is shown in Figure 10.1.

For the cross-sectional studies, PGE_2 concentration was measured in rectal mucosal biopsies collected during the run-in period at visits one and two prior to randomization. A self-administered questionnaire collected at baseline was used to assess leisure-time activity and to calculate a commonly used energy expenditure score (MET-hours per week) from the activities reported. Results showed that a higher level of leisure-time physical activity was significantly inversely related to PGE_2 concentration in rectal mucosa ($p < 0.03$). Based on the results of the statistical

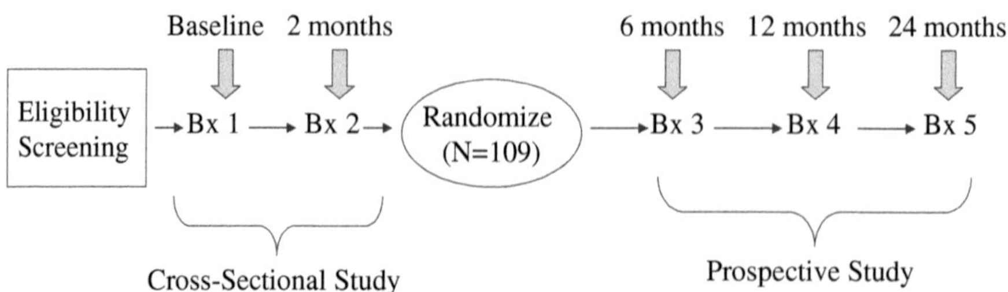

FIGURE 10.1 Piroxicam study schema. Biopsies (Bx) 1 and 2 were used for cross-sectional study and biopsies 3, 4, and 5 were used for prospective study (placebo group only).

model, an increase in activity level from 5.2 to 27.7 MET-hours/week was associated with a 28% decrease in levels of PGE_2. This change in activity is approximately equal to 1 hour of walking or 30 minutes of jogging or other aerobic exercise per day. The results were consistent when total time per week spent in leisure-time activities was used instead of MET-hours/week, further strengthening the findings.

In addition, a positive association between body mass index (BMI), a measure of obesity, and PGE_2 levels was shown ($p < 0.001$). In this setting, it is possible that BMI is merely a marker for physical activity because active individuals tend to be leaner than inactive ones [23]. However, when physical activity and BMI were included in the same statistical model, the results for each variable were unchanged, suggesting an independent effect of each factor on PGE_2 levels.

Our published study comprised cross-sectional analyses, so it was not possible to assess temporality of the association. Therefore prospective analyses of these data were conducted after the trial results were published. Because of the beneficial effects of the piroxicam intervention on PGE_2 levels [24], analyses were limited to the control group ($n = 29$). As shown in Figure 10.1, three biopsy samples were taken after randomization. As was done in the cross-sectional analyses, PGE_2 concentration at the three time points was modeled using a maximum-likelihood repeated measures model. Results of these analyses showed that a higher level of leisure-time physical activity was significantly inversely related to PGE_2 concentration ($p < 0.01$), indicating that an increase in activity level from 5.2 to 27.7 MET-hours/week was associated with an 18% decrease in levels of PGE_2. Although a positive association between BMI and PGE_2 was observed, this was not statistically significant ($p = 0.17$). The prospective data support the cross-sectional analyses, indicating that higher physical activity levels are significantly associated with lower PGE_2 concentrations in rectal mucosa.

The overall significance of rectal mucosal PGE_2 to colorectal cancer risk is unknown; no evidence to date directly links rectal mucosal PGE_2 levels to the development of colon cancer development. Furthermore, although one study showed that PGE_2 levels in the upper rectum are correlated with those in the remainder of the colon [12], this requires further study. Nonetheless, given the current knowledge of increased prostaglandin production in human colonic tumor cells, these data support the potential for PGE_2 playing a role in the protective mechanism of physical activity on risk of colon cancer. Whether this is a direct role of prostaglandins is unknown.

It is also possible that this effect is linked to production of insulin or the regulation of insulin-like growth factors because it has been shown that prostaglandins of the E series are capable of stimulating insulin secretion [25,26] and that insulin-like growth factor 1 (IGF-1) synthesis is regulated by PGE_2 as well as other agents that stimulate cAMP [27–29]. Also, as noted earlier, the study population comprised nonusers of nonsteroidal anti-inflammatory medications; therefore, it is not known whether these findings are applicable to users of these drugs.

It was hoped that these findings would stimulate further work in this area. However, to our knowledge, these results have not been replicated. At least one intervention study testing the effect of exercise on colon and rectal cell markers, including prostaglandins, has been conducted — the APPEAL (A Program Promoting Exercise and an Active Lifestyle) Study [2]. Details of this study are found in Chapter 12. Briefly, 102 men and 100 women were randomized to an intervention or a control group. The intervention comprised a 1-year period of moderate- to vigorous-intensity aerobic exercise intervention, with a goal of 60 minutes per day, 6 days per week. Adherence to this intensive program was excellent, with 85% of participants meeting 80% or more of their goals. The control group was given the opportunity to participant in exercise classes for 2 months at the end of the 1-year period. Final results pertaining to the PGE_2 findings are expected to be available in 2006.

Strenuous exercise has been shown to produce acute increase in prostaglandin levels [30], including PGE_2 [31]. In a study involving trained runners, participants were placed on 15, 30, or 40% energy from fat for 4 weeks [32] and were exposed to running to exhaustion at 80% of their VO_2 max in the last week of the dietary regimen. A series of markers, including PGE_2, were measured in plasma before and after the run. It was hypothesized that a low-fat diet would result in higher PGE_2 prior to and after the endurance run compared to the high-fat diets.

Results of the study showed that pre-exercise plasma PGE_2 levels of participants in the 40% diet were significantly lower than those in the lower fat diets. Furthermore, PGE_2 levels were significantly higher after the endurance run compared to levels before the run among all participants, regardless of dietary regimen; thus, fat intake had no effect on the plasma postexercise PGE_2 levels. Furthermore, the postexercise PGE_2 level was significantly lower on the 40% fat diet compared to the 15% diet, which led the investigators to conclude that dietary fat helps reduce stress caused by exercise and has few adverse effects in well-trained athletes. The overall relevance of these acute responses in prostaglandin concentrations to risk of colorectal cancer, however, is unknown.

SUMMARY AND FUTURE DIRECTIONS

In conclusion, the results of a single cross-sectional study show a significant reduction in rectal mucosal PGE_2 concentration associated with a higher level of leisure-time physical activity and a lower BMI. Furthermore, follow-up prospective analyses of this study also support the inverse association between physical activity and PGE_2 levels. To our knowledge, these findings have not been replicated; however, results of the APPEAL intervention study should provide stronger evidence for the direct effect of physical activity on a variety of markers in rectal mucosa, including prostaglandins.

As can be appreciated, much work is needed in this important area of colon cancer prevention research. Studies linking levels of PGE_2 and other prostanoids in various tissues, including rectal mucosa, to the development of colorectal cancer are needed to validate these biomarkers. If they are successful, concentrations of these markers could be used to assess biologically plausible mechanistic effects of various lifestyle factors. Furthermore, these surrogate biomarkers can be useful to assess drug dosage and compliance in prevention trials of nonsteroidal anti-inflammatory medications and other agents, including those such as the APPEAL study, whose mechanism of action is exerted via prostaglandins.

REFERENCES

1. Thune, I. and E. Lung, Physical activity and risk of colorectal cancer in men and women. *Br J Cancer*, 1996. 73:1134–1140.
2. McTiernan, A., Intervention studies in exercise and cancer prevention. *Med Sci Sports Exercise*, 2003. 35(11):1841–1845.
3. Bartram, H.P. and E.L. Wynder, Physical activity and colon cancer risk? Physiological considerations. *Am J Gastroenterol*, 1989. 84:109–112.
4. Giovannucci, E., Insulin and colon cancer. *Cancer Causes Control*, 1995. 6:164–179.
5. McTiernan, A. et al., Physical activity and cancer etiology: associations and mechanisms. *Cancer Causes Control*, 1998. 9(5):487–509.
6. Sternfeld, B., Cancer and the protective effect of physical activity: the epidemiological evidence. *Med Sci Sports Exercise*, 1992. 24(11):1195–1209.
7. Levy, G.N., Prostaglandin H synthases, nonsteroidal anti-inflammatory drugs, and colon cancer. *FASEB J*, 1997. 11(4):234–247.
8. Karmali, R.A., Prostaglandins and cancer. *Calif Cancer J Clin*, 1983. 33:322–332.
9. Bennett, A. and M. Del Tacca, Prostaglandins in human colonic carcinoma. *Gut*, 1975. 16:409.
10. Bennett, A. et al., Prostaglandins from tumors of human large bowel. *Br J Cancer*, 1977. 35:881–884.
11. Jaffe, B.M., C.W. Parker, and G.W. Philpott, Immunochemical measurement of prostaglandin or prostaglandin-like activity from normal and neoplastic cultured tissue. *Surgical Forum*, 1971. 22:90–92.

12. Pugh, S. and G.A.O. Thomas, Patients with adenomatous polyps and carcinomas have increased colonic mucosal prostaglandin E2. *Gut*, 1994. 35:675–678.
13. Hubbard, A.L. et al., N-acetyl transferase: two polymorphisms in coding sequence identified in colorectal cancer patients. *Br J Cancer*, 1998. 77:913–916.
14. Sheng, H. et al., Modulation of apoptosis and Bcl-2 expression by prostaglandin E2 in human colon cancer cells. *Cancer Res*, 1998. 58(2):362–366.
15. Fulton, A.M., Ineractions of natural effector cells and prostaglandins in the control of metastasis. *J Natl Cancer Inst*, 1987. 78:735–741.
16. Furuta, Y. et al., Prostaglandin production by murine tumors as a predictor for therapeutic response to indomethacin. *Cancer Res*, 1988. 48:3002–3007.
17. Saez, E. et al., Activators of the nuclear receptor PPAR-gamma enhance colon polyp formation. *Nat Med*, 1998. 4(9):1058–1061.
18. Kitamura, S., Peroxisome proliferator-activated receptor-gamma induces growth arrest and differentiation markers of human colon cancer cells. *Jpn J Cancer Res*, 1999. 99(335):36–45.
19. Serraf, P., Loss-of-function mutations in PPAR gamma associated with human colon cancer. *Mol Cell*, 1999(3):799–804.
20. Lim, H. et al., Cyclo-oxygenase-2-derived prostacyclin mediates embryo implantation in the mouse via PPAR-delta. *Genes Dev*, 1999. 13(12):1561–1574.
21. Thun, M.J., S.J. Henley, and C. Patrono, Nonsteroidal anti-inflammatory drugs as anticancer agents: mechanistic, pharmacologic, and clinical issues. *J Natl Cancer Inst*, 2002. 94:252–266.
22. Shiff, S.J. and B. Rigas, Nonsteroidal anti-inflammatory drugs and colorectal cancer: evolving concepts of their chemopreventive actions. *Gastroenterology*, 1997. 113:1992–1998.
23. Martinez, M.E. et al., Physical activity, body mass index, and PGE_2 levels in rectal mucosa. *J Natl Cancer Inst*, 1999. 91:950–953.
24. Calaluce, R. et al., Effects of piroxicam on prostaglandin E2 levels in rectal mucosa of adenomatous polyp patients: a randomized phase IIb trial. *Cancer Epidemiol Biomarkers Prev*, 2000. 9(12):1287–1292.
25. Johnson, D.F., W.F. Fujimoto, and R.H. Williams, Enhanced release of insulin by prostaglandins in isolated pancreatic islets. *Diabetes*, 1973. 22:302–308.
26. Pek, S. et al., Stimulation by prostaglandin E2 of glucagon and insulin release from isolated rat pancreas. *Prostaglandins*, 1975. 10:493–502.
27. McCarthy, T.L. et al., Promoter-dependent and -independent activation of insulin like growth factor binding protein-5 gene expression by prostaglandin E2 in primary rat osteoblasts. *J Biological Chem*, 1996. 271:6666–6671.
28. Pash, J.M. et al., Regulation of insulin-like growth factor 1 transcription by prostaglandin E2 in osteoblast cells. *Endocrinology*, 1995. 136:33–38.
29. Fournier, T. et al., Divergence in macrophage insulin-like growth factor-I (IGF-I) synthesis induced by TNF-alpha and prostaglandin E2. *J Immunol*, 1995. 155:2123–2133.
30. Rauramaa, R. et al., Inhibition of platelet aggregability by moderate-intensity physical exercise: a randomized clinical trial in overweight men. *Circulation*, 1986. 74(5):939–944.
31. Smith, L.L. et al., Increases in plasma prostaglandin E2 after eccentric exercise. A preliminary report. *Horm Metab Res*, 1993. 25(8):451–452.
32. Venkatraman, J.T., X. Feng, and D. Pendergast, Effects of dietary fat and endurance exercise on plasma cortisol, prostaglandin E2, interferon-gamma and lipid peroxides in runners. *J Am Coll Nutr*, 2001. 20(5):529–536.

11 Mechanisms Associating Physical Activity with Cancer Incidence: Animal Models

Lisa H. Colbert

CONTENTS

INTRODUCTION

Studies of the effects of exercise on carcinogenesis have used a variety of animal models, including chemically induced tumors, transplantable tumors, spontaneous tumor models, and transgenic and induced-mutant mice, in addition to experimental metastasis models [1]. Many of the studies have identified some form of protective effect of voluntary or involuntary exercise on carcinogenesis, although more recent studies have been less consistent (reviewed in Shephard and Futcher [2] and Woods [3]). To the detriment of the field, the number of studies has not increased dramatically over the years and, perhaps more importantly, few studies have really focused on potential mechanisms that might explain the exercise effects.

Mechanisms most commonly cited as potential mediators include enhanced antioxidant defense, reductions in body fat, decreases in reproductive hormones, enhanced immunity, or a change in insulin-like growth factor-1 (IGF-1) and its related binding proteins, some of which could be acting through similar pathways (Figure 11.1). There are also site-specific mechanisms for various cancers, such as a decreased colonic transit time in relation to colon cancer. Many of the mechanisms that have received more attention in humans (e.g., estrogen, IGF-1) have not received much focus in exercised animal models and vice versa (e.g., immunity in animal models). Some of the more intriguing proposed mechanisms will be examined here.

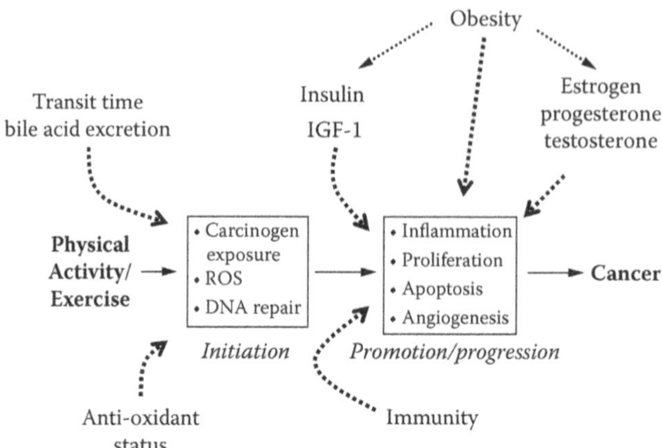

FIGURE 11.1 Commonly cited potential mechanisms for the effects of physical activity and exercise on carcinogenesis. Factors may work in the initial or promotion/progression phases of the disease, and they may act directly or through other intermediates.

FRAMEWORK FOR IDENTIFYING MECHANISMS

Animal models have the benefit of a short time for the development of cancer, so training the animal until the development of the disease is feasible. Unfortunately, few studies that have used a training approach have also examined potential mechanisms within that same study or model. Therefore, evidence for the potential mechanisms, as with studies in humans, largely comes from a synthesis of data from studies in which exercise training's effects on biomarkers or potential risk factors are examined separately from studies looking at the association between the marker or mediator and a cancer endpoint. When examined in this fashion, the strength of the association between exercise and the mechanistic factor, as well as that between the mechanistic factor and disease, is important (Figure 11.2).

The evidence to be addressed in this review will focus largely on the first types of studies, if available (option A), and then on studies that have looked at associations between exercise and the potential mediator (option B). We will largely not consider the strength of the evidence for associations between the mediator and the cancer outcome. An additional caveat to this review is

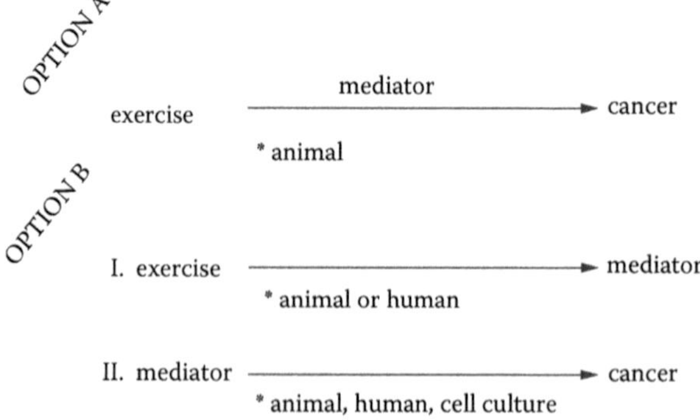

FIGURE 11.2 Conceptual framework for how a mechanism can be evaluated. In option A, which is currently limited to animal models, one can examine mechanisms in the context of a cancer endpoint. In option B, which can use animal, human, or cell culture experiments, the links between exercise and the mediator, and the mediator and the cancer outcome, are examined independently. The strength of the proposed mechanism depends on both relationships in this type of approach.

that effects of chronic exercise training will be considered rather than the effects of acute bouts of exercise. Although the latter may have some effect on carcinogenesis, the effects of regular, chronic activity or exercise on basal levels of the mediators may be more relevant when considering the carcinogenic process.

OXIDATIVE STRESS

Reactive oxygen species can play a significant role in carcinogenesis via their ability to produce DNA damage as well as damage to other cellular components that interact with DNA [4]. The idea that endogenous sources of these reactive oxygen species may play a bigger role in carcinogenesis than exogenous sources (e.g., environmental carcinogens) is particularly relevant to exercise research because the increased metabolism associated with acute exercise can be a significant source of free radical generation [4,5]. Fortunately, the body has a battery of antioxidant enzymes as well as nonenzymatic repair systems that work to prevent and/or repair the damage induced by reactive oxygen species, and chronic exercise training may be an important stimulus to upregulate these systems [5–7].

To date, few studies have examined reactive oxygen species-related damage or relevant antioxidant enzymes in the context of exercise in a cancer model. One study has examined wheel running in a tumor-bearing rat model and its effects on coenzymes Q_9 and Q_{10} in skeletal muscle because exercise in this same model had been found to delay cancer-induced cachexia [8]. Both enzymes appeared to be upregulated in anterior tibialis muscle, and Q_9 also in the soleus. We have just completed our first studies of urinary 8-hydroxydeoxyguanosine (8-OHdG) and the 8-epi-prostaglandin F2α (8-PGF2α) isoprostane in a transgenic mouse model of mammary cancer and have found largely unchanged values. The exception is a decrease in excreted 8-PGF2α in wheel-run compared to sedentary mice coupled with no effect of the wheel running on tumor-specific survival (unpublished data).

Exercise studies to date have largely focused on tissues relevant to exercise (e.g., skeletal muscle, heart) and not necessarily those tissues relevant to common human cancers (e.g., mammary, colon, lung). One group, however, examined antioxidant defense mechanisms in relevant tissues following a 10-week treadmill training program in rats; they found that superoxide dismutase and catalase were upregulated with exercise in the lung, and UDP-glucuronosyl transferase was upregulated in liver and lung [9]. Radak et al. also reported a decrease in reactive oxygen species production in the liver following 8 weeks of treadmill training in Fischer 344 rats [10].

Given the wide array of relevant enzymes such as superoxide dismutase, catalase, and glutathione peroxidase; relevant nonenzymatic proteins such as the heat shock proteins and hemoxygenase-1; the various techniques and measures used to evaluate antioxidant status and/or DNA damage; and the variety of animal models and exercise protocols, it will clearly be difficult to draw firm conclusions regarding this factor as an anticancer mechanism for exercise until many more studies have been conducted. Despite this, evidence is accumulating to suggest that chronic exercise training promotes beneficial effects in many animal antioxidant systems [6].

BODY WEIGHT/OBESITY/ENERGY BALANCE

One frequently cited mechanism for the association between activity and cancer prevention in humans is a decrease in body weight or obesity as a result of exercise, which would subsequently work through further "downstream" targets such as estrogen metabolism, inflammation, or insulin sensitivity. In animals, calorie restriction has long been known to have significant effects on body size and carcinogenesis [11]. Consequently, a reasonable hypothesis is that loss of body mass through exercise might also result in a reduction or delay in carcinogenesis. Few studies have actually examined body composition; however, body weights have frequently been recorded with training. Whether weight loss and/or body fat reductions are achieved can depend largely on the training protocol used, diet consumed, and the animal model and sex of the animal used. Table 11.1 is a summary of studies addressing the effects of exercise in various cancer models in which body weight and/or composition was also assessed. Mammary tumor studies have dominated the literature in this area, with the majority of studies cited using chemically induced carcinogenesis.

Only one group to date has used voluntary wheel running in mammary models; in each of the studies, all the animals were placed on high-fat diets (20 to 23%) [12–14]. In the studies using 1-methyl 1-nitrosurea (MNU) in F344 rats, body weight in the exercised animals was increased compared to that of sedentary rats [12,13]; however, in a study of 7,12-dimethylbenz(a)anthracene (DMBA) in Sprague–Dawley rats, the voluntary exercise resulted in lower body weights [14]. In all three studies, the trend was for lower body fat with the exercise. Despite the differences in body weight, the exercise beneficially affected carcinogenesis in all of the studies. Time to tumor formation was delayed in both models, adenocarcinoma incidence was decreased in the MNU-treated F344 rats [12,13], and total tumor number was decreased in the DMBA-treated Sprague–Dawley rats [14].

Among the studies using treadmill exercise, results are quite variable concerning the effects of exercise on carcinogenesis as well as on body weight and composition. Increases in body weight with treadmill exercise have led to increased incidence of tumors [15,16]. In one of these studies, in which a high-fat diet was given, body fat was increased with the exercise [15]; however, in the other study, body fat was not different from that of the sedentary rats [16]. Studies in which exercise had no effect on body weight have had varied results: decreased tumor multiplicity or incidence [17,18], no effect on tumor incidence or multiplicity [19–21], increase in the tumor growth rate [20], or decrease in the tumor growth rate [21]. Perhaps the most important point to be derived from a review of these studies is that no consistent relationship between the effects of exercise on body weight/composition and its effect on carcinogenesis has been found.

In terms of intestinal cancers in rodents, Thorling et al. found that a substantial volume of exercise resulted in lower body weight and body fat along with a decreased incidence of adenomas, but not carcinomas [22]. Reddy et al., on the other hand, saw no effect of voluntary wheel running on body weight in rats, but a significant decreased incidence of colonic adenocarcinomas, but not adenomas [23]. We have looked at polyp development following treadmill exercise in the Min mouse, an induced mutant mouse in which an APC tumor suppressor gene mutation results in multiple intestinal polyps [24]. In *ad libitum* fed animals, body weights were unchanged by exercise, and polyp development was not significantly affected [25].

In a follow-up experiment, exercised mice were pair-fed with the sedentary control mice in order to produce a negative energy balance due solely to the exercise. Body weights in the exercised mice were significantly lower in the last few weeks of the study compared to control mice, and body fat was significantly lower in female exercised mice compared to female controls [26]. Despite the negative energy balance, total polyp number was not affected in males or females by exercise, and there was only a suggestion of a decrease in jejunal polyps with exercise in the male mice. Therefore, although limited in number, studies of exercise effects on intestinal tumors have not been consistent in regard to body weight or fatness as a mediating effect of exercise.

So far, the data on body weight with exercise in pancreatic cancer models suggest that this factor may be somewhat important. In the three studies identified to date, exercise appeared ineffective in only one of the studies, which also showed a lack of change in body weight [27]. For liver cancer models, however, all three identified studies found that exercise decreased tumor incidence or burden [28–30], with a decrease in body weight only found in one study [30].

To date, the various models of exercise and carcinogenesis suggest that the negative energy balance created by exercise is not a likely mechanism of cancer prevention in these animals, with the possible exception of pancreatic cancer. This is consistent with studies of caloric restriction and exercise effects on aging. Holloszy demonstrated that, although voluntary exercise in Long–Evans rats increased average lifespan, it did not increase maximal lifespan as calorie restric-

TABLE 11.1
Studies of Exercise and Carcinogenesis Including Examinations of Body Weight or Fatness

Animals	Age at treatment (wks)	N	Cancer model	Exercise/diet	Body wgt/body fat effects	Tumor effects	Study (ref.)
F344 rats	7 — MNU; 7 — Ex	30–36/group	MNU 37.5 mg/kg body wgt	Voluntary wheel running for ~20 weeks; high-fat (20%) diet *ad libitum*	Ex ↑ body wgt vs Sed; trend towards ↓ body fat in Ex	Ex ↓ palpable adenocarcinoma incidence, ↑ time to tumor	Cohen et al., 1988, 1991 (12,13)
Sprague–Dawley rats	7 — DMBA; 9 — Ex	28–35/group	DMBA 5 mg	Treadmill; 20 m/min, 1° incline, 15 min/d, 5 d/wk for 18 wks; high-fat (25%) diet *ad libitum*	Ex ↑ body wgt vs Sed; no diff in body fat	Ex ↑ incidence, and tumor multiplicity, ↓ time to tumor formation	Thompson et al., 1988 (15)
Sprague–Dawley rats	7 — DMBA; 9 — Ex	~30/group	DMBA 5 mg	Treadmill; MOD: 20 m/min, LOW: 2 m/min, 1° incline, 15 min/d, 5 d/wk for 20 wks; low-fat (5%) corn-oil and high-fat (25%) diets: corn oil group and palm/corn group *ad libitum*	MOD ↑ body wgt vs LOW; no diff in body fat	MOD ↑ incidence vs LOW on all diets; MOD ↑ tumor multiplicity and ↓ time to tumor vs LOW in corn-oil fed rats	Thompson et al., 1989 (16)
Sprague–Dawley rats	7 — DMBA; 7 — Ex	30/group	DMBA low dose = 5 mg; high dose = 10 mg	Voluntary wheel running for ~11 wks (high dose) or ~19 wks (low dose); high-fat (23%) diet *ad libitum*	EX ↓ body wgt vs Sed in low-, not high-dose group; trend towards ↓ body fat in Ex at high dose	Ex ↓ total tumors but not incidence at both doses; Ex delayed time to tumor formation in low dose and tumor multiplicity at high dose	Cohen et al., 1993 (14)
F344 rats	7 — MNU; 9 — Ex	28–30/group	MNU 50 mg/kg body wgt	Treadmill exercise at 15% grade, 5 d/wk at low (35%) or high (70%) intensity with short (20 min) or long (40 min) durations for 3 mos; AIN76A diet *ad libitum*	No differences in body wgt	Incidence and tumor multiplicity ↓ with intensity, not duration	Thompson et al., 1995 (17)
Sprague–Dawley rats	3–7 — Ex; 7 — MNU	26–29/group	MNU 50 mg/kg body wgt	Treadmill exercise at 15% grade, 5 d/wk, 18 m/min, 60 min/d; sacrificed at 24 wks postcarcinogen; rodent diet 5001 *ad libitum*	No differences in body wgt	Ex ↓ total tumor number and multiplicity, but not incidence or time to tumor development	Whittal and Parkhouse, 1996 (18)
F344 rats	7 — MNU; 9 — Ex	30–32/group	MNU 50 mg/kg body wgt	Treadmill exercise at 15% grade, 5 d/wk, 20 m/min, 30 min/d, with or without 20% CR of AIN76A diet for 20.5 wks	Ex alone did not affect body wgt; Ex, not CR, resulted in ↓ body fat	Ex had no effect on incidence or multiplicity, even combined with CR; CR alone ↓ both measures	Gillette et al., 1997 (19)

(continued)

TABLE 11.1 (CONTINUED)
Studies of Exercise and Carcinogenesis Including Examinations of Body Weight or Fatness

Animals	Age at treatment (wks)	N	Cancer model	Exercise/diet	Body wgt/body fat effects	Tumor effects	Study (ref.)
Sprague–Dawley rats	3–7 — Ex; 7 — MNU	26–40/group	MNU 37.5 mg/kg body wgt	Treadmill exercise at 15% grade, 5 d/wk, 18 m/min, 60 min/d; sacrificed at 22 weeks postcarcinogen; rodent diet 5001 *ad libitum*	No differences in body wgt	Exercise had no effect on incidence multiplicity, or time to tumor; Ex ↑ the tumor growth rate and wgt	Whittal–Strange et al., 1998 (20)
Sprague–Dawley rats	3 —MNU; 4 — Ex	10–30/group	MNU 50 or 25 mg/kg body wgt	Treadmill exercise at 15% grade, 5 d/wk, 23–25 m/min, 30 min/d for 2, 4, 6, or 8 wks; AIN93G diet *ad libitum*	No differences in body wgt	Ex delayed time to tumor development and ↓ tumor growth rate with no effect on incidence or multiplicity	Westerlind et al., 2003 (21)
Intestinal/colorectal							
Male F344 rats	7 — AOM; 10 — Ex	27/group	AOM 15 mg/kg body wgt	Wheel running for 38 wks; AIN-76A *ad libitum*	No diff in body wgt with Ex	Ex ↓ colon adenocarcinoma incidence and multiplicity; no effect on adenomas	Reddy et al., 1988 (23)
Male Fischer rats	5 — AOM; 6 — Ex	32/group	AOM 15 mg/kg body wgt	Treadmill; 7 m/min, 5 h/d, 5 d/wk for 38 wks; standard chow *ad libitum*	Ex ↓ body wgt vs Sed; Ex ↓ body fat (torso) vs. Sed	Ex ↓ tumor incidence (adenomas not carcinomas)	Thorling et al., 1993 (22)
Male and female Min mice	3	6–11/group	APC_{min}-induced mutation in APC gene	Treadmill; 18-21 m/min, 5% grade, 60 min/d, 5 d/wk for 7 wks; standard chow *ad libitum*	No differences in body weight	No differences in polyp numbers	Colbert et al., 2000 (25)
Male and female Min mice	6	27–30/group	APC_{min}-induced mutation in APC gene	Voluntary wheel running for 3 wks; treadmill, 20 m/min, 5% grade, 45 min/d, 5 d/wk for 5 wks — total of 8 wks of running; AIN76A with Ex restricted to Sed consumption	Ex ↓ body wgt vs Sed in males and females; Ex ↓ total body fat in females, not significant in males	No differences in total polyp numbers; fewer jejeunal polyps in male EX vs. male SED	Colbert et al., 2003 (26)
Pancreatic							
Male Lewis and female F344 rats	2 — azaserine; 3–4 — Ex	10-24/group	Azaserine 30 mg/kg body wgt — males; 90 mg/kg body wgt — females	Voluntary wheel running for 2 or 4 months	Male rats had ↓ body wgt and perirenal fat pad wgt at 4, not 2 months; no differences in females	No diff in no. of preneoplastic foci; Ex ↓ foci size in males and females	Roebuck et al., 1990 (79)

Male Lewis rats	2 — azaserine; 4 — Ex	7-10/group	Azaserine 90 mg/kg body wgt	Voluntary wheel running for 21 wks; with or without food restriction (10–33%) from ages 6–14	No differences in body wgt; perirenal fat pad ↓ in Ex vs Sed	No significant reduction in preneoplastic foci with Ex; trend towards decreased foci volume ($p = 0.054$)	Giles and Roebuck, 1992 (80)
Female Syrian hamsters	4 — Ex 8 — BOP	25-30/group	BOP 20 mg/kg body wgt	Voluntary wheel running with 10 g/day low-fat (4.5%) or high-fat (24.6%) diet for 44 wks	Ex mice were heavier at weeks 8–24	No effect of exercise on the cancer burden	Kazakoff et al., 1996 (27)
	Liver						
Male and female Sprague–Dawley rats	Age not reported; Wks on study: 0 — Ex 3 — tumor implant	8–16/group	Subcutaneous injection of Morris hepatoma 7777	Swimming: progressive increase in min/d up to 120 min/d for 3 wks preimplant and 3 wks postimplant	No diff in carcass wgt	Ex ↓ tumor weight vs SED	Baracos, 1989 (28)
Male F344 rats	7 — AOM; 8 — Ex	27/group	AOM 15 mg/kg/body wgt	Voluntary wheel running for 38 wks	No diff in body wgt	Ex ↓ foci area and density; no effect on incidence	Sugie et al., 1992 (29)
Male Jc1:Wistar rats	10 — Ex 27 —DAB	17–19/group	DAB 0.0177 g/d/kg body wgt throughout study	Voluntary wheel running until 62 wks of age; restricted feeding begun at 17 wks	Ex ↓ body wgt from 57–61 wks of age; Ex ↓ epididymal fat pad wgt	Ex significant ↓ incidence of hepatoma	Ikuyama et al., 1993 (30)

Notes: MNU = 1-methyl 1-nitrosurea; Ex = exercise; Sed = sedentary; CR = calorie restriction; DMBA = 7,12-dimethylbenz(a)anthracene; wgt = weight; BOP, N-nitrosobis-(2 oxopropyl)amine; DAB = 3′-methyl-4-dimethylaminoazobenzene; d = day; wk = week; mos = months.

tion did [31]. Additionally, the combination of exercise and calorie restriction extended lifespan to the same degree that calorie restriction alone did. Holloszy concluded that those results, as well as results from a prior study [32], suggested that caloric restriction acts, at least on aging, through some other consequence of caloric restriction aside from the energy deficit that it creates.

A recent statistical analysis of caloric restriction on longevity in Wistar rats concluded that changes in body weight could only account for ~11% of the effects of caloric restriction on longevity [33]. Similarly, it is quite possible that the effects of exercise on carcinogenesis are largely independent of its effects on energy balance. Unfortunately, the limited evidence to date in animal models of exercise is not yet conclusive; few studies have attempted to control both sides of the energy balance equation. Additionally, many of the studies of mammary cancer have used young animals, which may not be relevant as models of the exercise effects in postmenopausal women because mice and rats cease cycling around ~12 and ~19 months of age, respectively [34]. Clearly, more studies are needed in which energy expenditure and energy intake are manipulated in young and older animals to examine the resultant outcomes definitively in terms of body weight, body composition, and carcinogenesis.

REPRODUCTIVE HORMONES

Changes in steroid hormone levels — estrogen and testosterone in particular — are perhaps the most consistently cited potential mechanism for the association of physical activity with breast and prostate cancer. Relatively few studies have been conducted in rodents, perhaps due to the difficulties in measuring these hormones at specific times in the considerably shorter reproductive cycle in rodents, which averages ~4 to 6 days [34]. Nonetheless, results suggest that, in younger rodents, exercise training must be of a considerable volume and/or intensity in order to disrupt regular cycling and estrogen levels.

A 12-week treadmill training program in 8-week-old Harlan Sprague–Dawley rats resulted in lower estradiol levels and an anestrous state in 5 of 16 exercised animals compared to no changes in the 16 sedentary rats [35]. Through this progressive training protocol, animals were running 4 h/day, 7 days/week, at 30 to 38 m/min, up a 10 to 15% grade by the end of the program. It cannot be discerned, in this case, whether the disruptions were a result of the volume of training or its intensity, although the *ad libitum* fed exercised animals did not differ in weight at the end of the protocol compared to the controls. Eight weeks of 5 days/week, 2.5-h swims combined with access to running wheels resulted in a decrease in estradiol levels and disruption of regular cycling in CD-strain rats; this was accompanied by lower body weights as well as weights of the ovarian fat pads [36].

In contrast, 8 weeks of a more moderate exercise training did not alter body weight or estradiol levels in 8-week-old Sprague–Dawley rats [37], although mesenteric and subcutaneous levels of body fat were lower in the trained vs. untrained rats [38]. Similarly, a 12-week moderate treadmill training program in 4-week-old Sprague–Dawley rats had no effect on estradiol or progesterone [39]. This latter study is the only one to examine hormones in the context of a model used to study exercise effects on tumorigenesis. This same treadmill training program was repeated in a separate study in which rats of the same age received low or high doses of the carcinogen MNU [40]. Although exercise had no effect on tumor-free survival time, incidence, or tumor multiplicity, it did result in lower tumor weights and growth rates.

Results are not as consistent in older or ovariectomized animals. Moderate treadmill training for 8 weeks in 26-week-old Wistar rats resulted in significantly lower estradiol and progesterone levels [41]. Body weights also appeared lower vs. control animals, although the significance of the difference was not reported. In ovariectomized Sprague–Dawley rats of the same age and exercised in a similar training program to the previous study, the training had no effect on estradiol levels or body weight [37]. Voluntary wheel running for 3 weeks had no effect on body weight or estrogen in 8-month-old B6DF1 mice [42], but increased progesterone in 2-month-old ovariectomized mice of the same strain [43].

One primate study was identified that was consistent with the suggestion of a high training volume necessary for disturbance of the reproductive hormones. Adult cytomolgous monkeys were progressively trained on a treadmill until they were running approximately 12 km/day (2 h/day), 7 days/week [44]. All eight of the exercised monkeys became amenorrheic but none of the eight control monkeys did. The time to develop the amenorrhea varied considerably, with a range of 7 to 24 months. Lutenizing hormone and progesterone were lower during the amenorrhea as well as during the month preceding it; estradiol was only significantly lower during the amenorrhea. Surprisingly, despite this large volume of running, the body weights of the monkeys were reported not to change, although food intake was reported to remain constant.

Collectively, these studies appear reasonably consistent in demonstrating a need for high volumes or intensities of activity in order to disrupt luteal function. Although body weights were reported, few attempts were made to disentangle the effects of exercise from those of energy balance in general. This has been shown to be important in humans, in whom it appears that negative energy balance and not physical activity per se can alter reproductive hormones in young women [45].

One of the mechanisms suggested for the potentially decreased risk of prostate cancer with activity is a reduction in testosterone levels. To date, no studies of exercise in an animal model of prostate cancer have been published. In rodent models in general, evidence is quite inconsistent in terms of exercise effects on testosterone levels. With varying exercise training protocols and rodent species, basal testosterone levels have been found to increase [46,47], decrease [48], or remain unchanged after the training program; however, the changes may depend on how many weeks into the training the hormone is assayed [49].

IMMUNE FUNCTION

Along with body composition and energy balance, immune function has been the area most studied in relation to the potential affects of exercise on cancer outcomes. Most tumor-related models to date have looked at immunity in models of metastasis or implanted tumors. This review will focus on studies that have examined immunity in the context of a cancer model or immunity to cancer cells *in vitro*. Excellent reviews have already been produced on the effects of acute and chronic exercise on potentially relevant immune markers such as natural killer cells, other lymphocytes, and macrophages [50,51].

Several studies have examined exercise effects on immune function in the context of implanted tumors. In only one case did moderate exercise training reduce the growth of the tumor and, in this case, the survival of the rats [52]. Lymphocyte proliferative responses were also increased in the trained rats. In other studies, final tumor weights or volumes were unaffected by the various exercise regimens despite increases in various immune functions such as splenocyte mitogen response and phagocytic activity of macrophages [53–55]. One study examined the growth and regression of allogeneic EL-4 lymphoma cells and found that repeated strenuous exercise delayed the time to peak tumor volume and resulted in a quicker regression of the tumor [55]. This latter study found fewer inflammatory cells within the tumors as well as a decrease in angiogenesis [55].

Many studies have examined exercise effects on experimental tumor metastasis models in association with innate immune cell activity. An acute bout of exhaustive exercise and 6 days of hour-long bouts of higher intensity exercise have been found to decrease the number of lung tumor foci following intravenous injection of B16 melanoma cells [56,57]. In both studies, the same exercise was found to increase macrophage cytotoxicity against the same tumor *in vitro*. Additionally, studies with other models of exercise have found that chronic and short-term repeated bouts of acute exercise can increase macrophage antitumoral cytotoxicity *in vitro* [58–60]. Collectively, the studies demonstrate a beneficial effect of many types of exercise on macrophage function and, in the two cases examined, on experimental lung tumor metastasis.

Studies looking at natural killer cell activity in relation to tumor retention have been less consistent in terms of the tumor outcome relating to the *in vitro* cell function. Several studies have identified a beneficial effect of exercise training on splenic natural killer cell cytotoxicity [61,62] or on lymphokine-activated killer cell activity [63]. Additionally, tumor cell retention in the lungs following intravenous injection — considered by some to be a marker of natural killer cell activity — has frequently been found to be reduced with exercise training [61,62], although this effect may depend on the aggressiveness of the tumor used in the assay [64].

Unfortunately, these apparently beneficial effects on immunity have not translated into a reduction in lung tumor metastasis [62–65]. These results may not agree for a number of reasons, including differences in the tumor cell lines, the comparison of splenic natural killer activity to metastasis at another organ site, or the assumption that lung retention of tumors is a marker of natural killer activity. It is more likely, however, that any effect of exercise on the complex process of lung tumor metastasis will likely involve more than one immune cell as well as other processes not directly related to innate immune cell cytotoxicity, such as cell adhesion, inflammation, and angiogenesis.

Nonetheless, the data in animals are promising in the sense that exercise of many types and intensities appears to have beneficial effects on innate immunity that may be important in cancer prevention. Prior studies have primarily used transplanted tumors and intravenous injection of tumor cells as a model of metastasis. What are needed are more studies of exercise training-induced changes in immunity in the context of different cancer models including spontaneous, chemically induced, or genetically modified carcinogenesis.

IGF-1

Within the past several years, insulin-like growth factor-1 and its related binding proteins have received considerable attention as potential mediators of the protective effects of physical activity on cancer incidence. Although the evidence that IGF-1 is relevant to carcinogenesis is convincing (reviewed in Yu and Rohan [66] and Kaaks and Lukanova [67]), the link between physical activity and IGF-1 is quite inconsistent and, in the case of animals, quite limited. One group has nicely demonstrated with liver-specific IGF-1-deficient transgenic mice that circulating IGF-1 is important in colon and mammary carcinogenesis [68,69]. Additionally, another group has shown in various models that a decrease in circulating IGF-1 mediates, in part, the effect of caloric restriction on carcinogenesis [70].

It is overly simplistic to assume that because caloric restriction and exercise can result in a negative energy balance, exercise may also act on carcinogenesis via a lowering of IGF-1. In fact, given that IGF-1 functions in protein synthesis and is associated with the development of lean mass [71,72], one would expect that IGF-1 might be increased early in exercise training in order to increase lean mass. Unfortunately, the variety of exercise protocols, heterogeneity of subjects, and timing and type of IGF-1 measurements have resulted in an unclear association even in humans [73]. As previously mentioned, data in animals are much more limited, particularly in regard to exercise training and circulating IGF-1.

In a model of carcinogen-induced pancreatic cancer, Syrian hamsters with access to running wheels had IGF-1 levels that were no different than those of controls at three time points across the experiment [27]. In this study, insulin levels were also examined and found to be lower in the exercised mice that were also on a high-fat (25%) corn-oil diet compared to their high-fat diet controls. Neither in high- or low-fat (5%) fed animals, however, did the wheel running affect the incidence or multiplicity of tumors. This is consistent with a study we have recently completed that examined moderate- and vigorous-intensity treadmill running as well as wheel running in a transgenic mouse model of mammary tumorigenesis. We measured IGF-1 at two to three timepoints during the study and found no differences in IGF-1 by group (unpublished data). Similar to the pancreatic cancer study, no beneficial effect of the exercise on tumor outcomes was found. In the limited studies to date, therefore, a lack of exercise effect on IGF-1 has paralleled a lack of effect on tumor outcomes; although interesting, this clearly does not aid in identifying IGF-1 as a potential mechanism.

In one other study, rats were run on a treadmill with and without added weight for 5 weeks to examine the effect on various bone growth factors. No difference was found between the exercise and control conditions on circulating IGF-1 measured at the end of the 5 weeks [74]. Collectively, these experiments suggest that exercise training does not appear to affect basal levels of IGF-1 in various rodent models, although clearly the evidence in this area is limited.

TISSUE SIZE/MORPHOLOGY

Proliferation, apoptosis, and structure of organs can all determine susceptibility to and/or the progression of cancer. It was hypothesized in the late 1980s that total cell number and cellular proliferation could be risk factors for cancer; some of the underlying evidence was the increased cancer risk associated with body weight and height and the decreased risk with calorie restriction [75]. Indeed, the balance between cellular proliferation and programmed cell death, or apoptosis, plays a role in the carcinogenic process [76]. In terms of breast cancer, in particular, mammographic density, which is indicative of the relative amount of stroma and epithelium compared to fat tissue in the breast, is considered an important marker of breast cancer risk [77].

Westerlind et al. proposed that the beneficial effects of exercise on mammary carcinogenesis in rats may be to alter the glands during the critical window between sexual maturity and first pregnancy [39]. In particular, the study examined the terminal end buds that are the mammary structures most susceptible to carcinogens [78]. Moderate exercise training begun at 28 days of age in Sprague–Dawley rats had no effect on body weight or growth, age at sexual maturation (average age = 36 days), or the number of terminal end buds. Cellular proliferation in the mammary gland, as measured by proliferating cell nuclear antigen (PCNA) immunohistochemistry, was higher at 42 through 70 days of age in the exercising animals. Apoptosis, assessed by counting apoptotic cells in stained gland sections, was also higher in the exercised rats at 70 days of age and, nonsignificantly, at 84 days of age.

In a similar study, 21-day-old Sprague–Dawley rats underwent moderate treadmill exercise training until 50 days of age, at which time some were sacrificed for the examination of mammary development and proliferation. The rest received a 50-mg/kg dose of NMU and were followed for 24 more weeks [18]. The exercise training did not alter body weight, mammary gland development, or cellular proliferation. Although exercise did not affect tumor incidence, it did result in a reduction in total tumor number as well as the number of tumors per rat. In a repeat experiment with a lower dose of NMU (37.5 mg/kg), exercise still did not affect incidence, no longer had an effect on tumor multiplicity, and actually increased the growth rate of the tumors [20].

SUMMARY

To date, few studies have examined potential mechanisms of an exercise-induced decrease in carcinogenesis within the same experiment or model system. Although body size and fatness have received the most attention, the evidence is largely unsupportive of an energy balance–mediated reduction in cancer risk with exercise. One possible exception is pancreatic cancer, although only three studies have evaluated this. Rodent studies suggest an enhancement of antioxidant defense systems with chronic, moderate training, although few studies have looked at tissues that may be most relevant to carcinogenesis.

Similar to the findings in studies in younger women, it appears that high-volume or high-intensity exercise training is necessary to lower estrogen levels in animals or to disrupt cycling. It is not completely clear whether these effects are due to a reduction in total energy reserves or to the exercise. Innate immunity appears to be enhanced with exercise training in rodent models; however, frequently, this enhanced immunity has not coincided with a reduction in tumor burden or metastasis. There is very little evidence to date to evaluate the potential role of IGF-1 in the exercise and cancer relationship. Finally, studies have not found an influence on mammary gland development, which could be relevant to breast cancer, although it appears that some changes with cellular proliferation take place.

REFERENCES

1. Hoffman–Goetz L. Physical activity and cancer prevention: animal-tumor models. *Med Sci Sports Exercise* 2003; 35:1828–1833.
2. Shephard RJ, Futcher R. Physical activity and cancer: how may protection be maximized? *Crit Rev Oncogenesis* 1997; 8:219–272.
3. Woods J. Exercise and resistance to neoplasia. *Can J Physiol Pharmacol* 1998; 76:581–588.
4. Marnett L. Oxyradicals and DNA damage. *Carcinogenesis* 2000; 21:361–370.
5. Ji L. Antioxidants and oxidative stress in exercise. *Proc Soc Exp Biol Med* 1999; 222:283–292.
6. Radak Z et al. Adaptation to exercise-induced oxidative stress: from muscle to brain. *Exercise Immunol Rev* 2001; 7:90–107.
7. Fehrenbach E, Northoff H. Free radicals, exercise, apoptosis, and heat shock proteins. *Exercise Immunol Rev* 2001; 7:66–89.
8. Daneryd P et al. Coenzymes Q9 and Q10 in skeletal and cardiac muscle in tumor-bearing exercising rats. *Eur J Cancer* 1995; 31A:760–765.
9. Duncan K, Harris S, Ardies C. Running exercise may reduce risk for lung and liver cancer by inducing activity of antioxidant and phase II enzymes. *Cancer Lett* 1997; 116:151–158.
10. Radák Z et al. Age-associated increases in oxidative stress and nuclear transcription factor κB activation are attenuated in rat liver by regular exercise. *FASEB J* 2004; 18:749–750.
11. Weindruch R, Walford R. *The Retardation of Aging and Disease by Dietary Restriction.* Springfield: Charles C. Thomas, 1988.
12. Cohen LA, Choi KW, Wang C. Influence of dietary fat, caloric restriction, and voluntary exercise on n-nitrosomethylurea-induced mammary tumorigenesis in rats. *Cancer Res* 1988; 48:4276–4283.
13. Cohen LA et al. Modulation of N-nitrosomethylurea induced mammary tumorigenesis by dietary fat and voluntary exercise. *In Vivo* 1991; 5:333–344.
14. Cohen LA et al. Inhibition of rat mammary tumorigenesis by voluntary exercise. *In Vivo* 1993; 7:151–158.
15. Thompson HJ et al. Effect of exercise on the induction of mammary carcinogenesis. *Cancer Res* 1988; 48:2720–2723.
16. Thompson HJ et al. Effect of type and amount of dietary fat on the enhancement of rat mammary tumorigenesis by exercise. *Cancer Res* 1989; 49:1904–1908.
17. Thompson HJ et al. Exercise intensity dependent inhibition of 1-methyl-1-nitrosurea induced mammary carcinogenesis in female F-344 rats. *Carcinogenesis* 1995; 16:1783–1786.
18. Whittal K, Parkhouse W. Exercise during adolescence and its effects on mammary gland development, proliferation, and nitrosomethylurea (NMU) induced tumorigenesis in rats. *Breast Cancer Res Treat* 1996; 37:21–27.
19. Gillette C et al. Energy availability and mammary carcinogenesis: effects of calorie restriction and exercise. *Carcinogenesis* 1997; 18:1183–1188.
20. Whittal–Strange K, Chadau S, Parkhouse W. Exercise during puberty and NMU induced mammary tumorigenesis in rats. *Breast Cancer Res Treat* 1998; 47:1–8.
21. Westerlind K et al. Moderate exercise training slows mammary tumor growth in adolescent rats. *Eur J Cancer Prev* 2003; 12:281–287.
22. Thorling E, Jacobsen N, Overvad K. Effect of exercise on intestinal tumor development in the male Fischer rat after exposure to azoxymethane. *Eur J Cancer Prev* 1993; 2:77–82.
23. Reddy BS, Sugie S, Lowenfels A. Effect of voluntary exercise on azoxymethane-induced colon carcinogenesis in male F344 rats. *Cancer Res* 1988; 48:7079–7081.

24. Moser AR, Pitot HC, Dove WF. A dominant mutation that predisposes to multiple intestinal neoplasia in the mouse. *Science* 1990; 247:322–324.
25. Colbert L et al. Exercise and tumor development in a mouse predisposed to multiple intestinal adenomas. *Med Sci Sports Exerc* 2000; 32:1704–1708.
26. Colbert L et al. Exercise and intestinal polyp development in APCMin mice. *Med Sci Sports Exerc* 2003; 35:1662–1669.
27. Kazakoff K et al. Effects of voluntary physical exercise on high-fat diet-promoted pancreatic carcinogenesis in the hamster model. *Nutr Cancer* 1996; 26:265–279.
28. Baracos VE. Exercise inhibits progressive growth of the Morris hepatoma 7777 in male and female rats. *Can J Physiol Pharmacol* 1989; 67:864–870.
29. Sugie S et al. Effect of voluntary exercise on azoxymethane-induced hepatocarcinogenesis in male F344 rats. *Cancer Lett* 1992; 63:67–72.
30. Ikuyama T et al. Effect of voluntary exercise on 3′-methyl-4-dimethylaminoazobenzene-induced hepatomas in male Jc1:Wistar rats. *Proc Soc Exp Biol Med* 1993; 204:211–215.
31. Holloszy J. Mortality rate and longevity of food-restricted exercising male rats: a reevaluation. *J Appl Physiol* 1997; 82:399–403.
32. Holloszy J, Schechtman K. Interaction between exercise and food restriction: effects on longevity of male rats. *J Appl Physiol* 1991; 70:1529–1535.
33. Wang C et al. Caloric restriction and body weight independently affect longevity in Wistar rats. *Int J Obesity* 2004; 28:357–362.
34. Davis B, Travlos G, McShane T. Reproductive endocrinology and toxicological pathology over the life span of the female rodent. *Toxicol Pathol* 2001; 29:77–83.
35. Caston A, Farrell P, Deaver D. Exercise training-induced changes in anterior pituitary gonadotrope of the female rat. *J Appl Physiol* 1995; 79:194–201.
36. Axelson J. Forced swimming alters vaginal estrous cycles, body composition, and steroid levels without disrupting lordosis behavior or fertility in rats. *Physiol Behav* 1987; 41:471–479.
37. Latour M, Shinoda M, Lavoie J-M. Metabolic effects of physical training in ovariectomized and hyperestrogenic rats. *J Appl Physiol* 2001; 90:235–241.
38. Shinoda M, Latour M, Lavoie J-M. Effects of physical training on body composition and organ weights in ovariectomized and hyperestrogenic rats. *Int J Obesity* 2002; 26:335–343.
39. Westerlind K et al. Effect of exercise on the rat mammary gland: implications for carcinogenesis. *Acta Physiol Scand* 2002; 175:147–156.
40. Westerlind K. Physical activity and cancer prevention — mechanisms. *Med Sci Sports Exercise* 2003; 35:1834–1840.
41. Sakakura Y et al. Effects of running exercise on the mandible and tibia of ovariectomized rats. *J Bone Miner Metab* 2001; 19:159–167.
42. Hoffman-Goetz L et al. Effect of 17β-estradiol and voluntary exercise on lymphocyte apoptosis in mice. *Physiol Behav* 2001; 74:653–658.
43. Hoffman-Goetz L, Fietsch C. Lymphocyte apoptosis in ovariectomized mice given progesterone and voluntary exercise. *J Sport Med Phys Fitness* 2002; 42:481–487.
44. Williams N et al. Longitudinal changes in reproductive hormones and menstrual cyclicity in cynomolgus monkeys during strenuous exercise training: abrupt transition to exercise-induced amenorrhea. *Endocrinology* 2001; 142:2381–2389.
45. Loucks A, Verdun M, Heath E. Low energy availability, not stress of exercise, alters LH pulsatility in exercising women. *J Appl Physiol* 1998; 84:37–46.
46. Pieper D et al. Voluntary exercise increases gonadotropin secretion in male Golden hamsters. *Am J Physiol* 1995; 269:R179–R185.
47. Pieper D et al. Dehydroepiandrosterone and exercise in Golden hamsters. *Physiol Behav* 1999; 67:607–610.
48. Hu Y et al. Relationship between serum testosterone and activities of testicular enzymes after continuous and intermittent training in male rats. *Int J Sports Med* 2004; 25:99–102.
49. Hu Y et al. Serum testosterone responses to continuous and intermittent exercise training in male rats. *Int J Sports Med* 1999; 20:12–16.
50. Shephard RJ, Shek PN. Cancer, immune function, and physical activity. *Can J Appl Physiol* 1995; 20:1–25.

51. Woods J et al. Exercise and cellular innate immune function. *Med Sci Sports Exercise* 1999; 1–57.
52. Bacurau R et al. Effect of a moderate intensity exercise training protocol on the metabolism of macrophages and lymphocytes of tumor-bearing rats. *Cell Biochem Funct* 2000; 18:249–258.
53. Woods JA et al. Effects of exercise on the immune response to cancer. *Med Sci Sports Exercise* 1994; 26:1–7.
54. Shewchuk L, Baracos V, Field C. Dietary L-glutamine supplementation reduces the growth of the Morris hepatoma 7777 in exercise-trained and sedentary rats. *J Nutr* 1997; 127:158–166.
55. Zielinski M et al. Exercise delays allogeneic tumor growth and reduces intratumoral inflammation and vascularization. *J Appl Physiol* 2004; 96:2249–2256.
56. Davis JM et al. Exercise effects on lung tumor metastases and *in vitro* alveolar macrophage antitumor cytotoxicity. *Am J Appl Physiol* 1997; 274:R1454–R1459.
57. Murphy E et al. Effects of moderate exercise and oat b-glucan on lung tumor metastases and macrophage antitumor cytotoxicity. *J Appl Physiol* 2004; 97:955–959.
58. Woods JA et al. Exercise increases inflammatory macrophage antitumor cytotoxicity. *J Appl Physiol* 1993; 75:879–886.
59. Woods JA et al. Effects of exercise on macrophage activation for antitumor cytotoxicity. *J Appl Physiol* 1994; 76:2177–2185.
60. Lu Q et al. Chronic exercise increases macrophage-mediated tumor cytolysis in young and old mice. *Am J Physiol* 1999; 276:R482–R489.
61. MacNeil B, Hoffman–Goetz L. Chronic exercise enhances *in vivo* and *in vitro* cytotoxic mechanisms of natural immunity in mice. *J Appl Physiol* 1993; 74:388–395.
62. MacNeil B, Hoffman–Goetz L. Effect of exercise on natural cytotoxicity and pulmonary tumor metastases in mice. *Med Sci Sports Exercise* 1993; 25:922–928.
63. Hoffman–Goetz L, May KM, Arumugam Y. Exercise training and mouse mammary tumor metastasis. *Anticancer Res* 1994; 14:2627–2632.
64. Jadeski L, Hoffman–Goetz L. Exercise and *in vivo* natural cytotoxicity against tumor cells of varying metastatic capacity. *Clin Exp Metastasis* 1996; 14:138–144.
65. Hoffman–Goetz L et al. Differential effects of exercise and housing condition on murine natural killer cell activity and tumor growth. *Int J Sports Med* 1992; 13:167–71.
66. Yu H, Rohan T. Role of insulin-like growth factor family in cancer development and progression. *J Natl Cancer Inst* 2000; 92:1472–1489.
67. Kaaks R, Lukanova A. Energy balance and cancer: the role of insulin and insulin-like growth factor-1. *Proc Nutr Soc* 2001; 60:91–106.
68. Wu Y et al. Circulating insulin-like growth factor-1 levels regulate colon cancer growth and metastasis. *Cancer Res* 2002; 62:1030–1035.
69. Wu Y et al. Reduced circulating insulin-like growth factor 1 levels delay the onset of chemically and genetically induced mammary tumors. *Cancer Res* 2003; 63:4384–4388.
70. Kari F et al. Roles for insulin-like growth factor-1 in mediating the anticarcinogenic effects of caloric restriction. *J Nutr Health Aging* 1999; 3:92–101.
71. Russell–Jones D et al. Use of a leucine clamp to demonstrate that IGF-1 actively stimulates protein synthesis in normal humans. *Am J Physiol* 1994; 267:E591–E598.
72. Adams G, McCue S. Localized infusion of IGF-1 results in skeletal muscle hypertrophy in rats. *J Appl Physiol* 1998; 84:1716–1722.
73. Consitt L, Copeland J, Tremblay M. Endogenous anabolic hormone responses to endurance versus resistance exercise and training in women. *Sports Med* 2002; 32:1–22.
74. Bravenboer N et al. The effect of exercise on systemic and bone concentrations of growth factors in rats. *J Orthopaed Res* 2001; 19:945–949.
75. Albanes D, Winick M. Are cell number and cell proliferation risk factors for cancer? *J Natl Cancer Inst* 1988; 80:772–775.
76. Hursting S et al. Mechanism-based cancer prevention approaches: targets, examples, and the use of transgenic mice. *J Natl Cancer Inst* 1999; 91:215–225.
77. Boyd N et al. Mammographic densities as a marker of human breast cancer risk and their use in chemoprevention. *Curr Oncol Rep* 2001; 3:321.
78. Russo J, Russo I. Biological and molecular bases of mammary carcinogenesis. Lab Invest 1987; 57:112–37.

79. Roebuck B, McCaffrey J, Baumgartner K. Protective effects of voluntary exercise during the postinitiation phase of pancreatic carcinogenesis in the rat. *Cancer Res* 1990; 50:6811–6816.
80. Giles T, Roebuck B. Effects of voluntary exercise and/or food restriction on pancreatic tumorigenesis in male rats. In: Jacobs M, Ed. *Exercise, Calories, Fat, and Cancer.* New York: Plenum Press, 1992:17–27.

12 Physical Activity Intervention Studies in Humans

Anne McTiernan

CONTENTS

INTRODUCTION

As described in Chapter 4 through Chapter 6, epidemiological studies have shown that increased physical activity is associated with decreased risk for several cancers. Yet, the amount, type, and intensity of physical activity needed are unknown. Furthermore, the effect of an increase in activity levels in previously sedentary persons is unknown. Finally, the mechanisms through which exercise might reduce cancer risk are unproven in humans.

Intervention studies can help to answer some of these open questions in cancer prevention [1]. Through intervention studies, researchers can test the effect of one or more specific exercise prescriptions on disease biomarkers or disease. In monitored interventions (e.g., in a study facility with supervising staff), the researcher can be assured that the individual actually performed the exercise, and the length and intensity of the exercise can be accurately measured. It is easier to control the effects of confounding factors such as other health behaviors in intervention studies, which makes such studies a useful addition to other human research such as epidemiological observational studies.

With intervention studies, researchers can assess the effect of increase in exercise on risk factors for cancer; this is very difficult to assess in observational studies because the population trend is for people to decrease physical activity over time rather than to increase it. Furthermore, intervention studies designed to study cancer risks can include exercise programs that are likely to be most relevant to cancer, such as aerobic exercise and colon cancer risk, conditioning for cancer patients, etc. Selected populations, such as persons at high risk for cancer, of different age groups, or of different racial or ethnic backgrounds, can be studied to determine exercise effects on the biology in different settings.

Finally, intervention studies can focus on cancer patients and survivors, whose physical abilities and needs are different from most other patient and healthy population groups. Such intervention studies can focus on rehabilitation for such individuals, biological effects relevant to survival, or both.

This chapter reviews the exercise intervention studies that have been designed and conducted to focus on cancer prevention–related endpoints. It does not include the trials conducted in cancer patients — those will be covered in Chapter 25 through Chapter 28. A number of trials have been focused on exercise effects on endpoints related to diabetes, cardiovascular disease, or aging. These are not covered in depth in this chapter, but may be included in other chapters dealing with specific factors such as exercise effect on insulin or sex hormones.

UNIQUE ASPECTS OF PHYSICAL ACTIVITY INTERVENTION STUDIES PERTAINING TO CANCER PREVENTION

Exercise intervention studies related to cardiovascular disease, diabetes, and other chronic diseases have a rich history; however, very few such studies related to cancer have been conducted. Intervention studies focused on cancer can concentrate on the exercise type, dose, and frequency most relevant to cancer. These studies can focus on persons at high risk for cancer (e.g., those with a family history of cancer, a personal history of benign precursors, particular genetic polymorphisms, etc.). Exercise intervention studies can assess exercise effects on biological endpoints most relevant to cancer etiology and prevention.

This is not to dismiss the important knowledge that can be gained from intervention studies originally focused on other diseases. For example, several studies point to etiological roles for insulin, insulin-like growth factors (IGF) and their binding proteins, and risk for cancer. Many exercise intervention studies have addressed the effects of various types of exercise on insulin levels in various age, gender, race/ethnic, and other demographic groups. A smaller number of studies have assessed exercise effects on various IGFs and their binding proteins (IGFBPs). The information from these studies can be applied to the cancer prevention field, although studies will still be needed to confirm these associations in persons at elevated risk for cancer and in persons who already have a diagnosis of cancer.

PREVIOUS EXERCISE INTERVENTION STUDIES RELEVANT TO CANCER

Several studies have looked at exercise training effects on ovulatory and menstrual patterns in girls and young women [2–5]. Some [3,4] but not all [2] of these studies have found that exercise increases menstrual cycle length, suppresses ovulation, and lowers estrogen and progesterone levels. One found that weight loss was necessary to cause changes in reproductive factors in young women [5]. These reproductive effects are relevant to etiology of several cancers — most notably breast and endometrium — because lowered numbers of ovulatory menstrual cycles and lowered levels of estrogen are associated with lower risk of developing these cancers.

Several clinical trials have assessed exercise effects on insulin as a biomarker of diabetes and cardiovascular disease risk in relation to exercise [6]. Other trials have assessed the effect of exercise interventions on IGF-1 and IGFBP-3 as possible mechanisms linking exercise effects on the aging process with variable results [7–10]. One recently published randomized clinical trial assessed the effect of a 10-month strength-training program on IGF and IGFBP in 54 women aged 30 to 50 years and found that, after 15 weeks, the subjects randomized to the strength-training program experienced a decrease in IGF-1 of –30.47 ng/mL vs. an increase of 5.86 ng/mL in controls ($p = 0.02$) [10]. After 10 months, IGF-1 returned to baseline levels in the treatment group, but remained 15% lower in treatment compared to control participants. The study found no effect of the strength-training program on IGFBP-1 and -3.

A 6-month endurance exercise trial in 21 older women did not change IGF-1 concentrations in exercisers when compared with controls [11]. A small trial found that an 8-week endurance exercise program produced a small, nonsignificant increase in IGF-1 concentrations in older women [12]. As summarized in an excellent review by Orenstein and Friedenreich, little evidence of an effect of exercise on insulin-like growth factors has been found [13].

There is a growing literature of small intervention studies that have assessed the effect of exercise on immune function [14,15], with varied effects. The role of immune function in cancer etiology is unclear, but certainly several cancers have immune components, including lymphoma, Kaposi's sarcoma, cervical cancer, and other cancers caused by infectious agents. The effect of exercise on immune function and inflammatory markers is covered in depth in Chapter 9.

HUMAN EXERCISE INTERVENTION STUDIES FOCUSED ON RELEVANCE TO CANCER PREVENTION

Two clinical trials of exercise effects on cancer prevention mechanisms have been completed at the Fred Hutchinson Cancer Research Center in Seattle, Washington:

- The Physical Activity for Total Health Study tested the effect of a 12-month moderate-intensity exercise program on serum estrogens and other breast cancer biomarkers in postmenopausal, sedentary overweight women.
- The APPEAL (A Program Promoting Exercise and an Active Lifestyle) trial tested the effect of a 12-month moderate-intensity exercise program on colorectal cell proliferation, apoptosis, and prostaglandin levels in men and women at increased risk for colon cancer.

Exercise Effect on Sex Hormones in Postmenopausal Women (Physical Activity for Total Health Study)

The Physical Activity for Total Health Study design has been described in detail elsewhere (A. McTiernan, Principal Investigator) [16]. The aims of the study were to examine, in postmenopausal women, the effect of moderate-intensity exercise on: serum sex hormones (estrogens, androgens, sex hormone binding globulin); metabolic hormones (insulin, IGF-1, IGFBP-3); weight and adipose tissue stores; and immune function. The study was a randomized controlled clinical trial testing a 12-month moderate-intensity aerobic exercise intervention. Exercise participants were asked to exercise for at least 45 minutes per session, 5 days per week. The intervention was a combination of facility-based and home-based exercise. During the first 3 months, participants came three times per week to a study facility where they exercised in small groups using treadmills and stationary bicycles. They also exercised 2 days per week on their own, doing exercise of their choosing. The control participants met weekly for a 1-hour nonaerobic stretching class.

To be eligible for the study, women needed to be postmenopausal, between the ages of 50 and 75 years, and in good health (no serious chronic disease such as cancer, diabetes, coronary artery disease, etc.). They had to be overweight (body mass index [BMI] of 25 kg/m^2 or more, or BMI between 24.0 and 24.9 with percent body fat greater than 33%). Women had to be sedentary (no more than 60 minutes per week of moderate-intensity or greater exercise). They could not be taking hormone replacement therapy in the past 3 months. They had to be nonsmokers and consume less than two alcohol drinks per day on average. Women were recruited to the study by a variety of methods, including mass mailings and media, as described in detail elsewhere [17].

Primary study data were collected at study baseline, and at 3 and 12 months. We used several methods to measure and monitor adherence to the exercise intervention, including facility class attendance, daily activity logs, heart rate monitors, physical activity questionnaires, pedometers, and fitness testing (VO_2 max treadmill tests).

A total of 173 women were randomized, and exercise and control groups were virtually identical at baseline for age, body mass index, education, and other demographic variables. Adherence and retention were excellent. Only three women refused their 12-month endpoint collection, and six women dropped the exercise intervention (all after 3 months). We therefore had complete outcome data for 3 months and nearly complete for 12 months. Exercisers on average increased their VO_2 max by 12.7%; controls increased by just 0.8% ($p < 0.0001$ for exercise vs. control change from baseline to 12 months) [18]. Women randomized to the exercise group ($n = 87$) participated in moderate-intensity sports/recreational physical activity on 3.7 ± 1.4 days/week (79% of the prescribed 5 days/week) for 171 ± 88 minutes/week (87% of the prescribed 225 minutes/week) over the yearlong trial period [19]. Of the exercisers, 68% had a yearlong average physical activity level exceeding the national recommendation of 150 minutes/week.

Several endpoints were assessed, including:

- Sex hormones (estrone, free and total estradiol, SHBG [18])
- Free and total testosterone, androstenedione, dehydroepiandrosterone (DHEA), dehydroepiandrosterone sulfate (DHEAS) [20]
- Adiposity and body composition [21]
- Urine estrogen metabolites [22]
- Insulin and leptin [23]
- Insulin-like growth hormone 1 (IGF-1) and insulin-like growth hormone binding protein 3 (IGFBP-3) [24]
- Ghrelin [25]
- Immune function (natural killer cell numbers and activity, cytokines, immunoglobulins, lymphocyte proliferation)
- Mammogram densities
- Quality of life including menopause symptoms [26]
- Sleep [27]

Compared with controls, exercisers experienced significant declines in adiposity, including weight, BMI, percent body fat measured by DEXA scan, and intra-abdominal fat measured by abdominal CT scan [21]. We found that the exercise intervention resulted in a significant decrease in estradiol, estrone, and free estradiol from baseline to 3 months, with an attenuation of effect at 12 months [18]. Among women who lost body fat, however, the exercise intervention resulted in statistically significant reductions in these estrogens at both time points. Similarly, among women who lost body fat, testosterone and free testosterone decreased significantly more in exercisers than in controls [20]. Urinary estrogen metabolites did not change with the exercise intervention, however [22], nor did IGF-1 or IGFBP-3 [24].

We found that some markers of quality of life change with exercise. Women who exercised in the morning, for example, had improved sleep quality compared with night-time exercisers, and women who were assigned to a stretching control group also experienced improvements in sleep [27]. The prevalence and severity of menopausal symptoms, on the other hand, were little changed by exercise [26].

Additional exploratory analyses have provided intriguing information regarding the genetic control of weight and its association with sex hormones. For example, we found that exercisers carrying the CYP19 (the gene controlling aromatase activity) 8r allele had a smaller decrease than did noncarriers in percent fat (–0.3 vs. –1.5%, respectively, $p = 0.05$) [28]. Exercisers with two vs. no CYP19 11r alleles had a larger decrease in BMI (–1.0 vs. 0.1 kg/m^2, respectively, $p = 0.02$), total fat (–3.0 vs. –0.4 kg, respectively, $p = 0.01$), and percent body fat (–2.4 vs. –0.5%, respectively, $p < 0.001$). Additional analyses are under way to assess the role of genetic polymorphisms on exercise effect on cancer biomarkers.

Exercise Effect on Colorectal Cell Proliferation and Apoptosis (The APPEAL Study)

The APPEAL (A Program Promoting Exercise and an Active Lifestyle) Study is testing the effect of a moderate intensity exercise program on colon and rectal cell proliferation, apoptosis, and prostaglandins in men and women (A. McTiernan, Principal Investigator). Other study endpoints include metabolic hormones (insulin, IGF-1, IGFBP-3), weight, and adipose tissue stores (percent body fat measured via DEXA scan, intra-abdominal and subcutaneous abdominal fat measured by one-slice CT scan).

The APPEAL study is a randomized controlled clinical trial. A total of 102 men and 100 women between the ages of 40 and 75 years were randomized. To be eligible, men and women must have had a colonoscopy within the previous 3 years. The sample is over-representative of persons with a history of adenomatous colon polyps (a colon cancer precursor) and persons with a first-degree family history of colorectal cancer (which increases risk for colon cancer). Participants must also have been physically inactive (engaging in less than 60 minutes per week of moderate- or vigorous-intensity exercise), drink less than two alcohol drinks per day, nondiabetic, and with no personal history of invasive cancer.

Participants were recruited to the APPEAL study through several methods. The primary recruitment method was through gastroenterologists' practices, in which persons who had had a colonoscopy in the past 3 years were identified and sent an invitation letter from their physician with an enclosed Interest Survey to complete and return. Additional recruitment methods included media placements, flyers, a study website, and referrals.

From the 9828 letters mailed to gastroenterology practice patients, 2033 (21%) responded with interest in joining the study and, of these, 956 (47%) were potentially eligible. These 956 persons were interviewed by phone regarding eligibility requirements and 240 (25%) were preliminarily eligible. In addition, 1328 calls were made to the study line in response to media placements, of which 1092 interviews were completed and 107 were preliminarily eligible. The major reasons for ineligibility were because a respondent was not interested in being randomly assigned to exercise or control groups, was too physically active, or did not have time available to attend classes (such as working excessive hours). After extensive screening, 102 men and 100 women were enrolled in the trial and randomized to exercise or control (delayed exercise).

The intervention was a 1-year, moderate-to-vigorous intensity aerobic exercise program. The goal was 60 minutes per day, 6 days per week. The intervention included both gym-based and home-based exercise programs. Participants met in classes to exercise with an exercise specialist in attendance 3 days per week. Four facilities were available to participants (one located at the Fred Hutchison Cancer Research Center Prevention Center, A. McTiernan, director) and three private health clubs (participant membership paid by the study).

At the facilities, participants performed aerobic exercise for 45 minutes per session on machines (primarily treadmills and stationary bikes, supplemented with rowing machines and elliptical machines). They also performed some limited weight-training exercises, which were personalized according to the participants' needs and interests. (If they chose to do weight training, it was in addition to the 60-minute aerobic exercise session.) Warm-up, cool-down, and stretching exercise completed the exercise sessions.

Participants also were asked to exercise at home 3 days per week. Some of the study facilities provided the opportunity for participants to work out during any open hours, so some participants did their home exercise as unsupervised gym workouts using various machines. Other participants chose outdoor walking or jogging as their primary home exercise. An additional part of the intervention was a series of monthly behavior change classes in which participants met individually or in a group with an exercise physiologist trained in behavior change techniques. In these meetings, participants discussed issues and challenges to exercise adherence and came up with strategies to overcome challenges.

Several strategies were used to increase and maintain adherence to the exercise program. The exercise specialists met individually with participants every month to review progress and to address any particular adherence problems with that participant. Graphs showing study goals and individual performance were shared with the participant, and discrepancies between the two were discussed. Participant adherence was monitored by the study staff and principal investigator (PI) weekly through automated reports from weekly downloads of participants' daily exercise log data (data were entered weekly). Participants with adherence problems were discussed in depth, and strategies for improvement were discussed. Quarterly newsletters were sent to participants with tips on exercise and news on study progress. Small incentives were included, such as giving participants pedometers or water bottles after certain goals were met. Finally, group activities such as hikes and snowshoeing were arranged.

Several methods were used to measure and monitor adherence, including facility class attendance (entered on facility logs), home exercise logs, quarterly total physical activity questionnaires, VO_2 max treadmill tests (baseline and 12 months), and pedometers recording daily steps (done quarterly for 1 week).

Adherence to the program was excellent, with 80% of participants meeting 80% or more of their goal of 360 exercise minutes per week. On average, the participants met 91% of their goal minutes per week of exercise. Only seven individuals (two men and five women) dropped out of the exercise program. The control group was given the opportunity to participate in exercise classes for 2 months (with the same progression as that offered to the exercise-arm participants during months 1 and 2 of intervention) at the end of the 1-year period.

Analyses of study specimens for proliferation, apoptosis, and prostaglandins are under way. Final primary results should be available in 2005. Several ancillary studies are in place or under consideration, including an ongoing study to assess the effect of exercise on subjective and objective sleep measures, a study measuring exercise effect on proteomics, a study of exercise effect on mammogram density in women, and a study of exercise effect on testosterone and other sex hormones in men. In addition, blood and biopsy specimens are being stored for potential future uses.

The ALPHA Trial

The ALPHA Trial (Alberta Physical Activity and Breast Cancer Prevention Trial) is a randomized controlled trial examining how a 1-year aerobic exercise intervention, as compared to a usual sedentary lifestyle, influences specific biological mechanisms hypothesized to be operative in the association between physical activity and breast cancer risk (C. Friedenreich, Principal Investigator). Proposed biological mechanisms include an effect on endogenous sex hormones, obesity and central adiposity, mammographic density, insulin and insulin-like growth factors, and immune function. The ALPHA Trial is examining the effect of physical activity on several biological mechanisms in a controlled trial setting. The ALPHA Trial is the first such study in Canada and only the second worldwide.

A two-centered, two-armed randomized controlled trial of exercise and intermediate endpoints for breast cancer is being conducted. The study is recruiting 334 postmenopausal, sedentary women from the provincial breast screening program in Alberta. Participants are randomized to an exercise intervention or a control group. The intervention group will undertake 60-minute exercise sessions five times/week for 12 months; the control group will be asked not to change their usual level of activity. No change in dietary intake will be made for either group.

Baseline and 12-month assessments will be made of changes in serum sex hormones, obesity and adiposity, mammographic density, insulin-like growth factors, insulin resistance, aerobic capacity, psychosocial health measures, and potential covariates. These assessments will combine questionnaire data with direct biological and physical testing. Adherence to the exercise intervention is enhanced by several measures, including individual, ongoing counseling with on-site trainers who design an exercise program appropriate for the fitness level of the participant that interests her.

Intention-to-treat analyses will be performed to determine how physical activity changes these intermediate endpoints for breast cancer. The ultimate goal of this research is to provide evidence-based data for guidelines on physical activity for breast cancer risk reduction.

The Nutrition and Exercise for Women (NEW) Trial

The NEW Trial is testing the effects of dietary and exercise-induced weight loss on breast cancer biomarkers in 503 overweight, sedentary postmenopausal women from the Seattle area (A. McTiernan, Principal Investigator). The design is a 12-month randomized controlled trial with four study arms: dietary weight loss alone, exercise alone, dietary weight loss plus exercise, and control. The exercise intervention consists of combined facility and home exercise: 45 minutes of aerobic activity, five times/week. The diet is a modification of the Diabetes Prevention Program diet [29], with goals of <25% calories from fat, a caloric deficit of about 500 kcal/day, and a 7% loss of initial body weight.

FUTURE RESEARCH NEEDS

More exercise intervention clinical trials are needed to provide much needed information. Future exercise intervention studies should test different types of exercise, various intensities of exercise, different frequencies of activity, and intermittent vs. continuous exercise effects. Different populations and age groups should be studied because the effects of exercise may vary by age, gender, race, ethnicity, geography, and culture. Persons at varying risks of developing cancer should be studied because exercise may have different types and magnitudes of effects in persons at high vs. low risk of cancer. Finally, novel biomarkers of cancer risk should be studied.

The clinical trials and other intervention studies reviewed in this chapter make the assumption that the biomarker endpoints lie in the causal pathway between physical activity and cancer development. If, in fact, the pathways diverge, then assessing the exercise effect on such biomarkers will give an inaccurate picture of the physical activity–cancer picture. The optimal study would be a large-scale randomized clinical trial testing the effect of exercise on disease endpoints, such as that being done to test the effect of a low-fat dietary pattern on incidence of breast cancer [6]. Such a trial would be expensive and time-consuming, but could be done more efficiently if several disease endpoints were studied (e.g., cardiovascular, diabetes, etc.), and its results would have great public health implications.

SUMMARY

Intervention studies, particularly randomized clinical trials, can provide important information to the knowledge base on the association between physical activity and cancer risk and prognosis. Relatively few such studies have been conducted and more are needed.

Previous intervention studies suggest that several hormonal mechanisms might explain the associations between increased physical activity and reduced risk for several types of cancers. These hormones include estrogens, androgens, SHBG, insulin, IGF, and IGFBP. Future advances in this area can be made as novel hormonal cancer biomarkers are identified. A small number of past and ongoing exercise intervention studies suggest that exercise can improve immune function (as reviewed in Chapter 9), which could in part explain the exercise–cancer association.

Ongoing exercise randomized clinical trials can provide some important information on these and other biomarkers, but more studies are needed to assess different exercise programs in different populations with different biomarkers and other endpoints.

REFERENCES

1. McTiernan, A., Schwartz, R.S., Potter, J., and Bowen, D. Exercise clinical trials in cancer prevention research: a call to action. *Cancer Epidemiol Biomarkers Prev.* 8:201–207, 1999.
2. Bonen, A. Recreational exercise does not impair menstrual cycles: a prospective study. *Int J Sports Med.* 13:110–120, 1992.
3. Bullen, B.A., Skrinar, G.S., Beitins, I.Z., von Mering, G., Turnbull, B.A., and McArthur, J.W. Induction of menstrual disorders by strenuous exercise in untrained women. *N Engl J Med.* 312:1349–1353, 1985.
4. Williams, N.I., Bullen, B.A., McArthur, J.W., Skrinar, G.S., and Turnbull, B.A. Effects of short-term strenuous endurance exercise upon corpus luteum function. *Med Sci Sports Exercise.* 31:949–958, 1999.
5. Williams, N.I., Young, J.C., McArthur, J.W., Bullen, B., Skrinar, G.S., and Turnbull, B. Strenuous exercise with caloric restriction: effect on luteinizing hormone secretion. *Med Sci Sports Exercise.* 27:1390–1398, 1995.
6. Boule, N.G., Haddad, E., Kenny, G.P., Wells, G.A., and Sigal, R.J. Effects of exercise on glycemic control and body mass in type 2 diabetes mellitus: a meta-analysis of controlled clinical trials. *JAMA.* 286:1218–1227, 2001.
7. Bermon, S., Ferrari, P. Bernard, P., Altare, S., and Dolisi, C. Responses of total and free insulin-like growth factor-I and insulin-like growth factor binding protein-3 after resistance exercise and training in elderly subjects. *Acta Physiol Scand.* 165:51–56, 1999.
8. Eliakim, A., Brasel, J.A., Mohan, S., Wong, W.L., and Cooper, D.M. Increased physical activity and the growth hormone-IGF-I axis in adolescent males. *Am J Physiol.* 275:R308–314, 1998.
9. Maddalozzo, G.F. and Snow, C.M. High-intensity resistance training: effects on bone in older men and women. *Calcif Tissue Int.* 66:399–404, 2000.
10. Schmitz, K.H., Ahmed, R.L., and Yee, D. Effects of a 9-month strength training intervention on insulin, IGF-1, IGFBP1, and IGFBP-3 in 30- to 50-year-old women. *Cancer Epidemiol Biomarkers Prev.* 11:1597–1604, 2002.
11. Vitiello, M.V., Wilkinson, C.W., Merriam, G.R., Moe, K.E., Prinz, P.N., Ralph, D.D., Colasurdo, E.A., and Schwartz, R.S. Successful 6-month endurance training does not alter insulin-like growth factor-I in healthy older men and women. *J Gerontol A Biol Sci Med Sci.* 52:M149–M154, 1997.
12. Poehlman, E.T., Rosen, C.J., and Copeland, K.C. The influence of endurance training on insulin-like growth factor-1 in older individuals. *Metabolism.* 43:1401–1405, 1994.
13. Orenstein, M.R. and Friedenreich, C.M. Review of physical activity and the IGF family. *J Phys Activity Health.* 1(4):291–320, 2004.
14. Nieman, D.C., Nehlsen–Cannarella, S.L., Henson, D.A., et al. Immune response to exercise training and/or energy restriction in obese women. *Med Sci Sports Exercise.* 30:679–686, 1998.
15. Woods, J.A., Lowder, T.W., and Keylock, K.T. Can exercise training improve immune function in the aged? *Ann NY Acad Sci.* 959:117–127, 2002
16. McTiernan, A., Ulrich, C.M., Yancey, D., et al. The Physical Activity for Total Health (PATH) Study: rationale and design. *Med Sci Sports Exercise.* 31:1307–1312, 1999.
17. Tworoger, S.S., Yasui, Y., Ulrich, C.M., et al. Mailing strategies and recruitment into an intervention trial of the exercise effect on breast cancer biomarkers. *Cancer Epidemiol Biomarkers Prev.* 11:73–77, 2002.
18. McTiernan, A., Tworoger, S., Schwartz, R.S., Ulrich, C.M., Yasui, Y., Irwin, M., Rajan, B., Rudolph, R., Bowen, D., Stanczyk, F., and Potter, J.D. Effect of exercise on serum estrogen in postmenopausal women: a 12-month randomized controlled trial. *Cancer Res.* April 64(8):2923–2928, 2004.
19. Irwin, M.L., Tworoger, S.S., Yasui, Y., Rajan, K., McVarish, L., LaCroix, K., Ulrich, C., Bowen, D., Shwartz, R.S., Potter, J., and McTiernan, A. Adherence to a yearlong moderate-intensity exercise trial in postmenopausal women. *Prev Med.* 39(6):1080–1086, 2004.
20. McTiernan, A., Tworoger, S.S., Rajan, B., Yasui, Y., Ulrich, C.M., Chubak, J., Stanczyk, F.Z., Bowen, D., Irwin, M.L., Sorensen, B., Rudolph, R.E., Potter, J.D., and Schwartz, R.S. Effect of exercise on serum androgens in postmenopausal women: a 12-month randomized clinical trial. *Cancer Epidemiol Biomarkers Prev.* 13(7):1–7, 2004.

21. Irwin, M., Yasui, Y., Ulrich, C.M., Bowen, D., Rudolph, R.E., Schwartz, R.S., Yukawa, M., Aiello, E., Potter, J.D., and McTiernan, A. Effect of exercise on total and intra-abdominal body fat in postmenopausal women: a randomized controlled trial. *JAMA*. 289: 323–330, 2003.
22. Atkinson, C., Lampe, J.W., Tworoger, S.S., Ulrich, C.M., Bowen, D., Irwin, M.L., Schwartz, R.S., Rajan, B.K., Yasui, Y., Potter, J.D., and McTiernan, A. Effects of a moderate-intensity exercise intervention on estrogen metabolism in postmenopausal women. *Cancer Epidemiol Biomarkers Prev.* 13(5):1–7, 2004.
23. Frank, L.L., Rajan, K.B., Yasui, Y., Tworoger, S.S., Ulrich, C.M., and McTiernan, A. Effects of physical activity on metabolic risk variables in overweight postmenopausal women. A randomized clinical trial. *Obesity Res.* 13:615–625, 2005.
24. McTiernan, A., Sorensen, B., Yasui, Y., Tworoger, S.S., Ulrich, C.M., Irwin, M.L., Rudolph, R.E., Stanczyk, F.Z., Schwartz, R.S., and Potter, J.D. Effect of exercise on insulin-like growth factor 1 and insulin-like growth factor binding protein 3 in postmenopausal women: a 12-month randomized clinical trial. *CEBP.* 14(4):1020–1021, 2005.
25. Foster–Schubert, K.E., McTiernan, A., Frayo, R.S., Schwartz, R.S., Rajan, K.B., Yasui, Y., Tworoger, S.S., and Cummings, D.E. Exercise-induced weight loss increases human plasma ghrelin levels. *J Clin Endoc Metab.* 90(2):820–825, 2004.
26. Aiello, E.J., Yasui, Y., Tworoger, S.S., Ulrich, C.M., Irwin, M., Bowen, D., Schwartz, R.S., Kumai, C., Potter, J.D., and McTiernan, A. Effect of a yearlong moderate-intensity exercise intervention on the occurrence and severity of menopausal symptoms in postmenopausal women. *Menopause: J North Am. Menopause Soc.* 11(4):382–388, 2004.
27. Tworoger, S., Yasui, Y., Ulrich, C.M., Vitiello, M., Bowen, D., Irwin, M., Aiello, E.J., Schwartz, R.S., Potter, J., and McTiernan, A. Effect of a yearlong moderate to vigorous intensity exercise or low intensity stretching intervention on self-reported sleep quality measures in postmenopausal women. *Sleep.* 26(7):830–836, 2003.
28. Tworoger, S.S., Chubak, J., Aiello, E.J., Yasui, Y., Ulrich, C.M., Farin, F.M., Stapleton, P.L., Irwin, M.L., Potter, J.D., Schwartz, R.S., and McTiernan, A. The effect of CYP19 and COMT polymorphisms on exercise-induced fat loss in postmenopausal women. *Obesity Res.* 12(6):972–981, 2004.
29. Knowler, W.C., Barrett–Connor, E., Fowler, S.C., Hamman, R.F., Lachin, J.M., Walker, E.A., et al. Reduction in the incidence of type 2 diabetes with lifestyle intervention or metformin. *N Engl J Med.* 346:393–403, 2002.

13 Genetics, Physical Activity, and Cancer

Tuomo Rankinen

CONTENTS

INTRODUCTION

The favorable effects of endurance training and physically active lifestyle on the risk of several chronic diseases and their risk factors have been well documented. As presented elsewhere in the book, regular physical activity seems to protect also against several types of cancer. The effects of exercise training and regular physical activity are usually reported and interpreted in terms of group means and these trends are then generalized in the whole population. However, over the last two decades, it has become evident that there are marked interindividual differences in the adaptation to exercise training, even when the exercise stimulus is identical across the subjects. Consequently, a concept of individualized exercise prescription has gained popularity. The purpose of this chapter is to introduce the concept of interindividual differences in the adaptation to exercise, summarize the contribution of genetic factors to the person-to-person variability, and review the available data regarding the genotype–physical activity interactions on cancer.

INTERINDIVIDUAL DIFFERENCES IN RESPONSIVENESS TO EXERCISE TRAINING

As evidenced by several consensus meetings and expert panel recommendations [1–5], the body of scientific evidence regarding physical activity and sedentarism and their effects on risk factors, health outcomes and mortality rates is already impressive and is growing. However, the effects of exercise and physical activity have been almost always tested and reported in terms of main effects and mean group differences. Consequently, the interpretations and conclusions have been based on the average effects observed in groups of subjects. Although means and main effects are effective and convenient ways to summarize large amounts of data, it tends to be forgotten that not all members of the group follow the pattern reflected by the group mean. In fact, considerable individual differences are present in the risk factor responses to regular physical activity, even when all subjects are exposed to the same volume of exercise, adjusted for their tolerance levels [6].

The concept of heterogeneity in responsiveness to standardized exercise programs was first introduced in the early 1980s [7]. In a series of carefully controlled and standardized exercise training studies in young and healthy volunteers, it was shown that the individual differences in training-induced changes in several physical performance and health-related fitness phenotypes are large, with low and high responders showing 8- to 13-fold differences [7–11]. The most extensive data on the individual differences in trainability come from the HERITAGE Family Study, in which 742 healthy, but sedentary, subjects followed a highly standardized, well-controlled endurance-training program for 20 weeks. The average increase in maximal oxygen consumption (VO_2 max), a measure of cardiorespiratory fitness, was 384 mL O_2 with an SD of 202. However, the training responses varied from no change to increases of more than 1000 mL O_2 per minute [6,12].

A similar pattern of variation in training responses was observed for several other phenotypes, such as plasma lipid levels and submaximal exercise heart rate and blood pressure [6,13,14]. For example, systolic and diastolic blood pressure measured during steady-state submaximal (50 W) exercise decreased on average by 7 and 3.5 mmHg, respectively, in response to exercise training [14]. However, the responses varied from marked decreases (systolic blood pressure > 25 mmHg and diastolic blood pressure > 12 mmHg) to no changes or, in some cases, even to slight increases [6,14].

This kind of variation is an example of normal biological diversity, is observed in most populations, is generally beyond measurement error, and is potentially very informative in terms of the adaptive mechanisms involved [6,15]. However, only now are the factors contributing to these interindividual differences beginning to be understood.

GENETICS AND HETEROGENEITY IN EXERCISE RESPONSIVENESS

The available studies on the interindividual differences in adaptation to regular physical activity have shown that the phenomenon is independent of age, sex, and ethnic background of the subjects [6,8]. The contribution of the pretraining levels of the response phenotype seems to vary depending on the trait. For example, in the HERITAGE Family Study cohort, baseline VO_2 max and HDL cholesterol levels explained only about 1% of the variance in the respective training responses. On the other hand, contribution of the pretraining values was much greater for the training-induced changes in submaximal exercise blood pressure, heart rate, and stroke volume, with R^2-values ranging from 30 to 40% [6].

A common feature for most of the training response phenotypes is that they show significant familial aggregation, i.e., individuals within the same family tend to be more alike in terms of trait values than those from different families. Familial aggregation and maximal heritability of a trait, i.e., the combined effect of genes and shared environment on a phenotype, can be estimated using data from family and twin studies. The heritability estimates are based on comparisons of phenotypic similarities between pairs of relatives with different level of biological relatedness. For example, biological siblings, who share about 50% of their genes identical by descent, should be phenotypically more similar than their parents (biologically unrelated individuals) if genetic factors contribute to the trait of interest. Likewise, a greater phenotypic resemblance between identical twins (100% of genes identical by descent) than between dizygotic twins (50% of genes identical by descent) indicates genetic effect on the phenotype.

In pairs of monozygotic twins, the between-identical-twin-pairs variance in response to regular exercise has been reported to be from two to nine times larger than the within-pairs variance for cardiorespiratory fitness, hemodynamic, and metabolic phenotypes [9,16,17]. Thus, gains in absolute VO_2 max were much more heterogeneous between pairs of twins than within pairs of twins. In the HERITAGE Family Study, the increase in VO_2 max in 481 individuals from 99 two-generation families of Caucasian descent showed 2.6 times more variance between families than within families. Maximum likelihood estimation of familial correlations (spouse, four parent–offspring, and three sibling correlations) revealed a maximal heritability estimate of 47% [18].

In addition to VO_2 max, the heritability of training-induced changes in several other phenotypes, such as submaximal aerobic performance [19]; resting and submaximal exercise blood pressure, heart rate, stroke volume, and cardiac output [20–23]; body composition and body fat distribution [24,25]; and plasma lipid, lipoprotein, and apolipoprotein levels [26], have been investigated in the HERITAGE Family Study. The maximal heritabilities for these traits ranged from 25 to 55% — further confirming the contribution of familial factors to the person-to-person variation in responsiveness to endurance training.

MOLECULAR GENETICS

The evidence from the genetic epidemiology studies suggests that a genetically determined component affects exercise-related phenotypes. However, because these traits are complex and multifactorial in nature, the search for genes and mutations responsible for the genetic regulation must not only target several families of phenotypes, but also consider the phenotypes in the sedentary state and in response to exercise training.

It is also obvious that the research on molecular genetics of exercise-related phenotypes is still in its infancy. For example, the 2003 update of the Human Gene Map for Performance and Health-Related Fitness phenotypes map included 109 gene entries and quantitative trait loci on the autosomes and two on the X chromosome for physical performance (cardiorespiratory endurance, elite endurance athlete status, muscle strength, other muscle performance traits, and exercise intolerance) and health-related fitness (hemodynamic traits, anthropometry, and body composition; insulin and glucose metabolism; blood lipids and lipoproteins; and hemostatic factors) phenotypes [27]. As a comparison, the latest version of a similar map for obesity-related phenotypes included more than 330 loci [28].

These numbers demonstrate that relatively little has been accomplished to date. For instance, no gene contributing to human variation in endurance performance has been identified yet as a result of studies based on model organisms. Now that the era in which large fractions of the human, mouse, and rat genomic sequences are available is here, the field of exercise science and sports medicine will need to devote more attention to molecular and genetic research.

CANDIDATE GENE STUDIES

The majority of the exercise-related molecular genetic studies published so far have utilized a candidate gene approach, i.e., a gene has been targeted based on its potential physiological and metabolic relevance to the trait of interest. Statistical tests for an association are based on the comparison of allele and genotype frequencies of genetic markers between two groups of subjects: one with the phenotype of interest (e.g., high VO_2 max or endurance athletes — i.e., the "cases") and the other one without (the "controls"). However, with continuous traits, the test is done by comparing mean phenotypic values across genotype groups or between carriers and noncarriers of a specific allele.

The genetic data hold great promise to help in understanding why some individuals respond favorably to exercise training in terms of reduction of chronic disease risk factor levels and others do not. The major problem of the candidate gene association studies with multifactorial traits is the lack of repeatability of the positive findings across different populations. For example, in the 2003 update of the Human Performance and Health-Related Fitness Gene Map, all the genes associated with body composition, plasma lipid, and hemostatic phenotype training responses were based on a single study [27].

However, with hemodynamic phenotypes, some candidate gene findings have been replicated in at least two studies. For example, an association between blood pressure training response and the angiotensinogen (AGT) M235T polymorphism has been reported in the HERITAGE Family Study and the DNASCO study [29,30]. In white HERITAGE males, the angiotensinogen M235M homozygotes showed the greatest reduction in submaximal exercise diastolic blood pressure following a 20-week endurance training program [29]. In middle-aged Eastern Finnish men, the M235M homozygotes had the most favorable changes in resting systolic blood pressure and diastolic blood pressure during a 6-year exercise intervention trial [30].

Similarly, an association between the ACE I/D polymorphism and training-induced left ventricular growth has been reported in two studies [31,32]. In 1997, Montgomery and coworkers reported that the ACE D-allele is associated with greater increases in left ventricular mass, and septal and posterior wall thickness after 10 weeks of physical training in British Army recruits [32]. In 2001, the same group reported a new study using a similar training paradigm in British Army recruits [31]. The cohort included 62 ACE I/I and 79 ACE D/D homozygotes, and the training-induced increase in left ventricular mass was 2.7 times greater in the D/D genotype compared to the I/I homozygotes. Interestingly, the association between the ACE genotype and left ventricular mass response was not affected by angiotensin II type 1 receptor inhibitor (Losartan) treatment [31].

GENOTYPE–PHYSICAL ACTIVITY INTERACTIONS

So far this chapter has dealt with the genetics of heterogeneity of responsiveness to physical activity in terms of interindividual differences in training-induced changes in risk factors. However, a similar phenomenon can be described in observational studies in terms of genotype–physical activity interactions on health-related traits. Akin to the variability in training responses, epidemiologists have also faced the fact that, despite the general inverse relationship between physical activity level and the risk of chronic diseases, some physically active individuals still develop the disease and some of their sedentary counterparts may remain healthy until advanced age. Already, a considerable amount of evidence shows that [33]

- Genetic and environmental factors contribute to the risk of chronic diseases and to the variability of their risk factor levels
- The etiology of these multifactorial traits is characterized by complex interactions between genetic and environmental factors

The interactions between genetic and environmental factors can manifest themselves in several ways. One possible scenario for the interactions between genotype and physical activity and obesity is presented in Figure 13.1. The lowest risk of disease is in subjects who lack the genetic risk factor and are physically active or have normal weight. In subjects with increased genetic risk, being active or maintaining normal body weight can potentially prevent or delay the onset of the disease, prevent the complications of the disease, or increase the subject's responsiveness to treatment. On the other hand, sedentary and/or obese persons may have an increased risk of morbidity in general; however, with a genetic predisposition, the disease may manifest at an earlier age, have more severe complications, and be more resistant to treatment. These examples underline the idea that a behavior or a state, such as physical activity or lack of obesity, can potentially compensate a genetic predisposition to a disease.

The following three cases will provide examples of the genotype–physical activity and genotype–obesity interactions documented in the epidemiological studies:

- In the ECTIM Study cohort of 648 male myocardial infarction survivors and 760 population-based controls, a Lys198Asn polymorphism of the endothelin-1 gene was not associated with blood pressure in the whole cohort [34]. However, the genotype and

		Genetic predisposition: No	Genetic predisposition: Yes
Sedentary / obese	No	- No disease, or late onset - No complications - Good response to treatment	- Average or late onset - Minor complications - Good response to treatment
	Yes	- Average or early onset - Moderate to severe complications - Impaired or normal response to treatment	- Early onset - Severe complications - Resistant to treatment

FIGURE 13.1 A schematic presentation of possible genotype–physical activity interaction effects on a risk of multifactorial disease.

body mass index (BMI, kg/m^2) showed a significant interaction effect on resting systolic blood pressure. The increase in systolic blood pressure as a function of BMI was steeper in the carriers of the Asn198 allele than in the Lys198 homozygotes.

- A similar interaction effect was also observed in the Glasgow Heart Scan Study cohort: the obese subjects who carried at least one copy of the Asn198 allele showed significantly higher maximum systolic blood pressure measured during a treadmill exercise test than the obese Lys198 homozygotes [34]. However, no difference in maximum systolic blood pressure between the genotype groups among the normal weight subjects was found.
- A similar example of genotype–physical activity interactions comes from another French study, in which strong associations between a β2-adrenoceptor gene polymorphism and BMI and body fat distribution phenotypes were reported in sedentary men but not in those who were physically active [35].

In the San Luis Valley Diabetes Study, 397 Hispanics and 569 non-Hispanic whites were followed for 14 years. During the follow-up, 91 coronary heart disease events were recorded. The frequency of the T/T genotype of the C–480T polymorphism in the hepatic lipase gene locus was higher among the coronary heart disease cases; the coronary heart disease-free survival during the follow-up among the T/T homozygotes was significantly worse than in the C/C homozygotes and the C/T heterozygotes. A multivariate analysis revealed a significant interaction between the hepatic lipase C-480T genotype and physical activity level on the coronary heart disease risk. The increased coronary heart disease risk associated with the T/T genotype was observed in the sedentary or moderately active subjects, but not in subjects who participated in vigorous physical activities [36].

GENE–PHYSICAL ACTIVITY INTERACTIONS AND CANCER

Data on the genotype-by-physical activity interactions on the risk of cancer are still scarce. However, the first study supporting the idea that physical activity may modify the outcome of breast cancer even among the women with verified genetic predisposition to the disease was published in 2003. King and coworkers investigated the risk of breast and ovarian cancer associated with the mutations in the *BRCA1* and *BRCA2* genes in Ashkenazi Jewish women [37]. Although mutations in both genes significantly increase the risk of breast cancer, the results suggested that physical activity and body weight might modify the penetration of the disease.

Mutation carriers who were physically active as teenagers were diagnosed with breast cancer significantly later in life (i.e., older age of onset) than those who were sedentary. In the sedentary group, 60 and 95% of the women were diagnosed with breast cancer by the age of 45 and 55 years, respectively; the corresponding ages in the physically active women were 53 and 73 years [37]. Similarly, women who were overweight at menarche and were heavier at age 21 had an earlier age of breast cancer onset among the carriers of *BRCA1* and *BRCA2* mutations.

CONCLUSIONS

The past decade has witnessed remarkable progress in human genetics. The availability of the almost complete DNA sequence of the human genome has changed our ability to study the genetic basis of complex multifactorial traits and to develop novel treatments for several chronic diseases. The recent advances in molecular genetics are starting to have an impact on physical activity research and exercise physiology. Although the research on molecular genetics of physical performance and health-related fitness is still in its infancy, understanding the effects of DNA sequence variation on interindividual differences in responsiveness to acute exercise and regular physical activity holds great promise. Such data would ultimately help to utilize physical activity more efficiently in the prevention and treatment of chronic diseases.

REFERENCES

1. Physical activity and cardiovascular health. NIH Consensus Development Panel on Physical Activity and Cardiovascular Health. *JAMA* 1996; 276(3):241–246.
2. Bouchard C. Physical activity and health: introduction to the dose–response symposium. *Med Sci Sports Exercise* 2001; 33(6 Suppl):S347–350.
3. Bouchard C, Blair SN. Introductory comments for the consensus on physical activity and obesity. *Med Sci Sports Exercise* 1999; 31(11 Suppl):S498–501.
4. Leon A, Ed. *Physical Activity and Cardiovascular Health: a National Consensus*. Champaign, IL: Human Kinetics Publishers, 1997.
5. U.S. Department of Health and Human Services. *Physical Activity and Health: a Report of the Surgeon General*. Atlanta: US Dept of Health and Human Services, Centers for Disease Control and Prevention, National Center for Chronic Disease Prevention and Health Promotion; 1996.
6. Bouchard C, Rankinen T. Individual differences in response to regular physical activity. *Med Sci Sports Exercise* 2001; 33:S446–S451.
7. Bouchard C. Human adaptability may have a genetic basis. In: Landry F, Ed. *Risk Reduction and Health Promotion. Proceedings of the 18th annual meeting of the Society of Prospective Medicine*. Ottawa: Canadian Public Health Association; 1983. 463–476.
8. Bouchard C. Individual differences in the response to regular exercise. *Int J Obesity Relat Metab Disord* 1995; 19(Suppl 4):S5–8.
9. Bouchard C, Dionne FT, Simoneau JA, Boulay MR. Genetics of aerobic and anaerobic performances. *Exercise Sport Sci Rev* 1992; 20:27–58.
10. Lortie G, Simoneau JA, Hamel P, Boulay MR, Landry F, Bouchard C. Responses of maximal aerobic power and capacity to aerobic training. *Int J Sports Med* 1984; 5:232–236.
11. Simoneau JA, Lortie G, Boulay MR, Marcotte M, Thibault MC, Bouchard C. Inheritance of human skeletal muscle and anaerobic capacity adaptation to high-intensity intermittent training. *Int J Sports Med* 1986; 7(3):167–171.
12. Skinner JS, Wilmore KM, Krasnoff JB, Jaskolski A, Jaskolska A, Gagnon J, et al. Adaptation to a standardized training program and changes in fitness in a large, heterogeneous population: the HERITAGE Family Study. *Med Sci Sports Exercise* 2000; 32(1):157–161.
13. Leon AS, Rice T, Mandel S, Despres JP, Bergeron J, Gagnon J, et al. Blood lipid response to 20 weeks of supervised exercise in a large biracial population: the HERITAGE Family Study. *Metabolism* 2000; 49(4):513–520.
14. Wilmore JH, Stanforth PR, Gagnon J, Rice T, Mandel S, Leon AS, et al. Heart rate and blood pressure changes with endurance training: the HERITAGE Family Study. *Med Sci Sports Exercise* 2001; 33:107–116.
15. Shephard RJ, Rankinen T, Bouchard C. Test-retest errors and the apparent heterogeneity of training response. *Eur J Appl Physiol* 2004; 91(2–3):199–203.
16. Prud'homme D, Bouchard C, Leblanc C, Landry F, Fontaine E. Sensitivity of maximal aerobic power to training is genotype dependent. *Med Sci Sports Exercise* 1984; 16(5):489–493.
17. Hamel P, Simoneau JA, Lortie G, Boulay MR, Bouchard C. Heredity and muscle adaptation to endurance training. *Med Sci Sports Exercise* 1986; 18(6):690–696.

18. Bouchard C, An P, Rice T, Skinner JS, Wilmore JH, Gagnon J, et al. Familial aggregation of VO_2 max response to exercise training: results from the HERITAGE Family Study. *J Appl Physiol* 1999; 87(3):1003–1008.
19. Perusse L, Gagnon J, Province MA, Rao DC, Wilmore JH, Leon AS, et al. Familial aggregation of submaximal aerobic performance in the HERITAGE Family study. *Med Sci Sports Exercise* 2001; 33(4):597–604.
20. An P, Rice T, Perusse L, Borecki I, Gagnon J, Leon A, et al. Complex segregation analysis of blood pressure and heart rate measured before and after a 20-week endurance exercise training program: The HERITAGE Family Study. *Am J Hypertension* 2000; 13:488–497.
21. An P, Perusse L, Rankinen T, Borecki IB, Gagnon J, Leon AS, et al. Familial aggregation of exercise heart rate and blood pressure in response to 20 weeks of endurance training: the HERITAGE Family Study. *Int J Sports Med* 2003; 24(1):57–62.
22. An P, Rice T, Gagnon J, Leon AS, Skinner JS, Bouchard C, et al. Familial aggregation of stroke volume and cardiac output during submaximal exercise: the HERITAGE Family Study. *Int J Sports Med* 2000; 21:566–572.
23. Rice T, An P, Gagnon J, Leon A, Skinner J, Wilmore J, et al. Heritability of HR and BP response to exercise training in the HERITAGE Family Study. *Med Sci Sports Exercise* 2002; 34:972–979.
24. Rice T, Hong Y, Perusse L, Despres JP, Gagnon J, Leon AS, et al. Total body fat and abdominal visceral fat response to exercise training in the HERITAGE Family Study: evidence for major locus but no multifactorial effects. *Metabolism* 1999; 48(10):1278–1286.
25. Perusse L, Rice T, Province MA, Gagnon J, Leon AS, Skinner JS, et al. Familial aggregation of amount and distribution of subcutaneous fat and their responses to exercise training in the HERITAGE family study. *Obesity Res* 2000; 8(2):140–150.
26. Rice T, Despres JP, Perusse L, Hong Y, Province MA, Bergeron J, et al. Familial aggregation of blood lipid response to exercise training in the Health, Risk Factors, Exercise Training, and Genetics (HERITAGE) Family Study. *Circulation* 2002; 105(16):1904–1908.
27. Rankinen T, Perusse L, Rauramaa R, Rivera MA, Wolfarth B, Bouchard C. The Human Gene Map for Performance and Health-Related Fitness phenotypes: the 2003 update. *Med Sci Sports Exercise* 2004; 36(9):1451–1469.
28. Snyder EE, Walts B, Perusse L, Chagnon YC, Weisnagel SJ, Rankinen T, et al. The human obesity gene map: the 2003 update. *Obesity Res* 2004; 12(3):369–439.
29. Rankinen T, Gagnon J, Perusse L, Chagnon Y, Rice T, Leon A, et al. AGT M235T and ACE ID polymorphisms and exercise blood pressure in the HERITAGE Family Study. *Am J Physiol: Heart Circulatory Physiol* 2000; 279(1):H368–374.
30. Rauramaa R, Kuhanen R, Lakka TA, Vaisanen SB, Halonen P, Alen M, et al. Physical exercise and blood pressure with reference to the angiotensinogen M235T polymorphism. *Physiological Genomics* 2002; 10:71–77.
31. Myerson SG, Montgomery HE, Whittingham M, Jubb M, World MJ, Humphries SE, et al. Left ventricular hypertrophy with exercise and ACE gene insertion/deletion polymorphism: a randomized controlled trial with Losartan. *Circulation* 2001; 103(2):226–230.
32. Montgomery HE, Clarkson P, Dollery CM, Prasad K, Losi MA, Hemingway H, et al. Association of angiotensin-converting enzyme gene I/D polymorphism with change in left ventricular mass in response to physical training. *Circulation* 1997; 96(3):741–747.
33. Tiret L. Gene–environment interaction: a central concept in multifactorial diseases. *Proc Nutr Soc* 2002; 61(4):457–463.
34. Tiret L, Poirier O, Hallet V, McDonagh TA, Morrison C, McMurray JJ, et al. The Lys198Asn polymorphism in the endothelin-1 gene is associated with blood pressure in overweight people. *Hypertension* 1999; 33(5):1169–1174.
35. Meirhaeghe A, Helbecque N, Cottel D, Amouyel P. Beta2-adrenoceptor gene polymorphism, body weight, and physical activity. *Lancet* 1999; 353(9156):896.
36. Hokanson JE, Kamboh MI, Scarboro S, Eckel RH, Hamman RF. Effects of the hepatic lipase gene and physical activity on coronary heart disease risk. *Am J Epidemiol* 2003; 158(9):836–843.
37. King MC, Marks JH, Mandell JB. Breast and ovarian cancer risks due to inherited mutations in BRCA1 and BRCA2. *Science* 2003; 302(5645):643–646.

Section IV

Overweight/Obesity and Cancer Incidence

14 Obesity, Weight Change, and Breast Cancer Incidence

Rachel Ballard-Barbash

CONTENTS

INTRODUCTION

The association between overweight or obesity and breast cancer incidence has been an area of extensive epidemiological research, beginning with studies in the 1970s that demonstrated that heavier women were at increased risk of breast cancer [1]. Such extensive research has been needed in part because the association of diverse measures of weight and body fat mass with breast cancer varies by a number of different characteristics of women. For example, the epidemiological evidence on weight or body mass index (BMI — a measure of weight adjusted for height, most commonly weight in kilograms divided by height in meters squared) and breast cancer risk varies by menopausal status (Table 14.1), age at diagnosis, hormone receptor status of the breast cancer, and exposure to exogenous estrogens. In addition, the associations observed vary by time period during the life cycle when weight or BMI is measured.

This chapter will summarize the epidemiological evidence on overweight and obesity and breast cancer risk over three major periods in the life cycle: birth and early childhood, adolescence, and adulthood. The most informative studies have distinguished between pre- and postmenopausal breast cancer; examined the effect of weight or BMI, weight gain, and central body fat; and examined the differential effects of exposure to endogenous and exogenous estrogens. With the recognition of the potential role of insulin-related peptides and possible interactions between these peptides and estrogen, recent studies have also begun to explore the potential interactions of insulin-related peptides with body size. Because studies of breast cancer have used so many different BMI cutpoints that are not consistent with current World Health Organization (WHO) criteria of overweight and obesity, the term "heavier women" is used to describe the upper BMI groups rather than the terms "overweight" and "obese."

TABLE 14.1
Summary of Measures of Body Size and Fat Distribution Examined Relative to Breast Cancer Incidence among Pre- and Postmenopausal Women

	Predominant direction of association	
Measures examined	**Premenopausal women**	**Postmenopausal women**
Birth weight	Variable, most often positive	Variable, most often null
Young adult weight or BMI	Inverse	Inverse
Measures during adult life		
Adult weight or BMI	Inverse	Positive
Weight change	Inverse	Positive
Fat distribution		
Waist-to-hip ratio	Variable, most often null	Variable, most often positive
Waist circumference	Variable, most often null	Positive
Hip circumference	Variable, most often null	Positive

Investigators have increasingly begun to examine the risk for many chronic diseases by standard WHO BMI categories: underweight as BMI of less than 18.50, normal weight as BMI of 18.50 to 24.99, and overweight as BMI of 25.00 or higher. This latter overweight category is further subdivided into four categories: preobese 25.00 to 29.99, obese class I 30.00 to 34.99, obese class II 35.00 to 39.99, and obese class III ≥ 40.00 [2]. More recent meta-analyses have the ability to examine risk by these broad weight categories; however, analyses should not be limited to these categories because risk may vary within them, depending on the chronic diseases and the populations examined.

BIRTH AND EARLY CHILDHOOD MEASURES

A limited number of studies have examined weight or BMI at birth, during childhood, and early in adulthood relative to breast cancer. The data on birth weight and breast cancer are limited by a very small number of cases; most studies have fewer than 100 cases. Some studies find no association [3,4] or a nonsignificant increased risk [5,6]; others find an increase in risk with increasing birth weight for premenopausal but not postmenopausal breast cancer [7–11] or a stronger increase in risk for premenopausal compared to postmenopausal breast cancer [12,13]. One study that examined the association of measured birth weight with early onset premenopausal breast cancer (before age 40) found a significant relative risk of 1.25 for birth weights over 4000 g as well as a significant relative risk of 1.59 for low-birth weight of below 2500 g [14] compared with birth weights in the middle range. Some studies have found an association between birth weight and adult BMI [15,16], suggesting that women with a high birth weight may also have a high adult BMI, which is also associated with an increased risk of postmenopausal breast cancer.

YOUNG ADULT MEASURES

The association of young adult weight, BMI, or other measures of relative weight adjusted for height has been examined in over 35 case-control studies and at least seven cohort studies and was well summarized in a review by Okasha et al. in 2003 [17]. In most of these studies, weight and height are based on self-report during midlife in which women are asked to recall their weight and height at age 18 or 20, but have included self-report of weight and height at various ages from age 12 to 25. In most case-control studies, heavier weight or BMI during teenage and young adulthood is associated with a 10 to 30% decrease in breast cancer risk for pre- and postmenopausal breast cancer.

However, this decreased risk is most often not statistically significant [18–41]. In one cohort study that examined changes in risk by 5-year intervals from age 30 to 69 for relative weight based on measured weight and height [42], the relative risk associated with BMI was less than 1 up to age 55 (comparing the highest to the lowest BMI quintiles) and gradually increased to 1.22 by ages 65 to 69. Few studies have measured heights and weights at younger ages and, with the exception of a study by Le Marchand et al. [26], most have limited numbers of breast cancer cases and therefore are difficult to interpret [17].

ADULTHOOD MEASURES

WEIGHT OR BMI MEASURES

Most studies find that heavier women have a decreased risk of premenopausal breast cancer [18,22–27,29,33,35–37,39,42–51]. Other studies find no association between BMI and premenopausal breast cancer [52–54]. Relative risks of approximately 0.6 to 0.7 have been reported whether weight or BMI is assessed at the time of diagnosis or at earlier times during childhood, adolescence, or adulthood [18,25,27,55]. Early studies suggested that the protective effect among heavier women was limited to early stage disease due to poorer detection of small tumors [43,44]. However, subsequent studies in these same groups suggest that detection bias does not explain the increased risk for breast cancer observed among lean premenopausal women [18,27,49].

A large case-control study of 1588 cases found that risk was increased about twofold among women who were tall and thin compared with women who were heavy and short [49]. A meta-analysis of seven cohorts comprising 723 incident cases of invasive breast cancer in premenopausal women found an inverse association between BMI and premenopausal breast cancer, with a relative risk of 0.54 for women with a BMI higher than 31 compared to women with a BMI less than 21 [56]. This estimate is consistent with the reduction in risk of 0.6 to 0.7 observed in many studies and does not appear to be present for BMIs less than 28.

Conversely, most studies have found that heavier women are at increased risk of postmenopausal breast cancer [1,19–22,24–26,29,30,33,34,37,40–42,46,50–52,54,55,57–75]. A meta-analysis of seven cohorts comprising 3208 cases of invasive postmenopausal breast cancer found gradual increases in risk to a BMI of 28 after which risk did not increase further; the relative risk for a BMI of 28 compared with a BMI of less than 21 was 1.26 [56]. The majority of studies on BMI and breast cancer risk have adjusted for major breast cancer risk factors, including reproductive factors. Few studies have examined in detail the effect of confounding or interactions with diet and physical activity.

Breast density has recently emerged as an important breast cancer risk factor. However, studies on obesity and breast cancer have not generally had information on breast density and thus have not examined the effect of any possible interactions between obesity and breast density. Only one study in Vermont that had data on breast density from screening mammograms has controlled for the effect of breast density [71]. Because BMI is inversely related to breast density, adjustment for breast density resulted in an increase in the risk estimations at all levels of BMI; the odd ratio increased from 1.9 to 2.5 after adjustment for breast density among obese women.

When examined, risk estimates for the association between obesity and breast cancer vary by age at diagnosis, history of hormone replacement therapy, estrogen receptor status of the tumor, and, possibly, family history of breast cancer. Risk has been found to increase with age at diagnosis in some studies that include a substantial number of postmenopausal women older than 65 years [51,56,66,71]. In one study, risk estimates increased from 1.1 among women younger than 60 years to 1.8 among women older than 65 years [66].

The effect of exogenous estrogen or estrogen receptor status of tumors has been examined with stratified analyses in more recent studies (Table 14.2). In these studies, obesity-related risk has been higher among women who have never used hormone replacement therapy (HRT) as shown in Table 14.2 [23,41,51,71,74,75]. Huang et al. were the first to report this finding in a large cohort study in the U.S. They found a statistically significant BMI and estrogen replacement interaction, with no increase in risk (RR of 1.1) among all women, but an increase in risk (RR of 1.6) among heavier women who had not used HRT [23]. The Women's Health Initiative cohort in the U.S., which had measured height and weight, found an even larger increase in risk among obese postmenopausal women who had never used HRT (RR of 2.52 among women with a BMI of over 31.1 kg/m^2), but no increase in risk in similarly obese women who had ever used HRT [41].

At least three studies have examined risk by BMI and estrogen receptor status of the breast tumor [37,52,73]. In one U.S. study, risk for a BMI of 27 compared to a BMI of 22 was 2.4 for tumors that were estrogen- and progesterone receptor-positive [37]. In another study, risk estimates were 2.0 and 2.2 for a BMI of 30.7 compared to a BMI of 23 for estrogen receptor-positive and progesterone-positive tumors, respectively [73]. In both of these studies, obesity-related risk was not increased for estrogen- and progesterone receptor-negative tumors. In one Japanese study, risk did not vary by estrogen or progesterone status of the tumor [52]. However, the women in this study were lean; the upper quartile of BMI of 22 in this study is lower than the lowest quartile of BMI in most U.S. studies.

Data are very limited on variation in BMI-related risk for postmenopausal breast cancer by family history. In several studies from the Iowa Women's Health Study, heavier postmenopausal women with a family history of breast cancer have a greater risk of developing breast cancer than do heavier women without a family history [30,73]. In one study in Japan, no differences were observed in associations of weight, BMI, or change in BMI by family history for premenopausal breast cancer, although somewhat stronger associations were seen for weight and change in BMI and postmenopausal breast cancer among postmenopausal women with a family history of breast cancer; this confirmed earlier results by Sellers and colleagues [73]. Only one study has examined variation in BMI-related risk for premenopausal breast cancer by family history of breast cancer [76]. In that study, the inverse association commonly observed between BMI and breast cancer risk was only observed in women without a family history of breast cancer.

Waist Circumference or Other Measures of Body Fat Distribution

Data on central adiposity and premenopausal breast cancer do not suggest a consistent association between measures, such as waist circumference or waist-to-hip ratio, and breast cancer risk [22,49–51,54,77–81]. Only five of these studies observed statistically significant increases in risk [50,54,77,78,81]. Increases in central adiposity, assessed by waist circumference or the ratio of waist to hip circumference, have been associated with a 1.3- to 2.0-fold increase in breast cancer risk among postmenopausal women in most studies [21,30,41,51,54,77–80,82–85]. However, not all studies show this association [74,81,86,87].

The association in postmenopausal women may be modified by a family history of breast cancer and ovarian cancer. In the Iowa Women's Health Study, among women with elevated waist-to-hip ratio, only women with a positive family history of breast cancer were at increased risk. The combination of a high wasit-to-hip ratio with a family history of breast and ovarian cancer was associated with a more than fourfold increase in risk of breast cancer [21,88]. Several studies have also reported on the association of hip circumference with breast cancer; most show no association among premenopausal women [79,80,89]. Among postmenopausal women, variable increases in risk with increasing hip circumference have been found in some [41,51,74,80] but not all [21,79,89] studies. In the few studies that have examined risk stratified by HRT use, risk for increases in waist and hip circumference were increased among women who had never used HRT but were not increased among women who had ever used HRT [41,51,74].

TABLE 14.2
Summary of Breast Cancer Relative Risks for BMI Stratified by Use of Hormone Replacement Therapy in Studies of Postmenopausal Women

		Relative risks (95% CI) postmenopausal women				
No. cases, design	**BMI categories**[a]	**Overall**	**Women ever used HRT**[b]	**Women never used HRT**	**Adjustment for confounding**	**Author, date, location**
1517, Cohort	Top (≥31) vs. bottom decile (≤20)	113 (0.87–1.46)	Stated as null	1.59 (1.09–2.32)[c]	Age, history of benign breast disease, family history, reproductive factors	Huang et al., 1997. U.S.
529, Case/control	<22.0	1.0	1.0	1.0	Breast density	Lam et al., 2000, U.S.
	22.0–24.9	1.4 (0.7–3.0)	1.5 (0.7–3.0)	1.1 (0.7–3.0)		
	25.0–27.4	1.6 (0.9–2.7)	1.4 (0.6–3.0)	2.5 (0.6–3.0)		
	27.5–29.9	1.6 (0.9–2.7)	1.2 (0.5–2.9)	1.9 (0.9–4.1)		
	≥30	2.5 (1.6–4.1)	1.8 (0.8–3.9)	3.6 (1.8–7.9)[d]		
771, Case/control	<23.1	1.0	1.0	1.0	Age, calories, physical activity, education, history of benign breast disease, family history, alcohol, smoking	Friedenreich et al., 2002, Canada
	23.1–25.7	0.93 (0.69–1.24)	1.06 (1.71–1.56)	0.79 (0.50–1.25)		
	25.7–29.2	0.94 (0.70–1.26)	0.83 (0.56–1.24)	1.12 (0.72–1.75)		
	≥29.2	0.99 (0.74–1.32)	0.85 (0.57–1.26)	1.18 (0.76–1.85)		
1030, Cohort	<22.6	Not stated	1.0	1.0	Age, education, age at menopause, parity, age at first birth, family history, smoking, age at menarche, race, alcohol, physical activity, dietary energy	Morimoto et al., 2002, U.S.[e]
	22.6–24.9		0.89 (0.70–1.13)	1.52 (0.95–2.42)		
	24.9–27.4		0.86 (0.68–1.11)	1.40 (0.87–2.23)		
	27.4–31.1		0.92 (0.72–1.19)	1.70 (1.98–2.68)		
	>31.1		0.96 (0.73–1.27)	2.52 (1.62–3.93)		
246, Cohort	<22.0	1.0	Stated as nonsignificant	1.0	Age, occupation, marital status, smoking, alcohol, reproductive factors	Lahmann et al., 2003, Sweden
	22.0–23.8	1.05 (0.67–1.62)		0.79 (0.43–1.45)		
	23.9–25.7	1.20 (0.78–1.85)		1.43 (0.85–2.41)		
	25.8–28.5	1.31 (0.86–2.01)		1.52 (0.91–2.55)		
	>28.5	1.54 (1.01–2.35)		1.68 (1.01–2.80)[d]		
1405, Cohort	<25.0	Not stated	1.0	1.0	Study center, age, education, smoking, alcohol, reproductive factors	Lahmann et al., 2004, Europe
	25.0–29.9		0.94 (0.76–1.15)	1.30 (1.12–1.51)		
	>30.0		0.66 (0.45–0.98)	1.31 (1.08–1.59)[c]		

[a] BMI defined as kilograms per square meters.
[b] HRT = hormone replacement therapy.
[c] P for interaction < 0.003.
[d] P for interaction was nonsignificant.
[e] P for interaction < 0.001.

Adult Weight Gain

The most consistent body size predictor of postmenopausal breast cancer risk is adult weight gain [4,18,21,23,34,37,40,51,53,54,59,65,67,70,72,74,75,90–94]. This association has been found in cohort studies that found no association between BMI at baseline and subsequent development of breast cancer and that also adjusted for baseline BMI [21,23,82]. Findings from one of the largest cohort studies suggest that a doubling of risk occurred with a weight gain of more than 20 kg after the age of 18 years, but only among women who had never used postmenopausal HRT [23]. Other studies have also observed similar results, with increases in risk limited to or much larger among women who have gained more weight and who have never used HRT compared to current users [24,34,51,72,74,75].

Consistent with findings for BMI and premenopausal breast cancer, weight gain appears to be associated with a reduced or no significantly increased risk of premenopausal breast cancer in most studies [18,23,26,27,35,36,39,40,51,53,54]. However, a study by Wenten et al. in New Mexico found differences in risk for Hispanic compared to non-Hispanic white women [40]. In that study, no association was found between weight gain and risk of premenopausal breast cancer among non-Hispanic white women; in contrast, a nonstatistically significant but nearly twofold increased risk was observed with more than 14 kg of weight gain among Hispanic white women.

The only study that has examined the effect of percent body fat measured by bioelectric impedance as well as several other measures of body size, fat mass, and distribution found the strongest association for percent body fat, with a doubling of risk for women with a percent body fat of over 36% compared to women with a percent body fat of less than 27%. Similar to results reported for BMI and weight gain, risk for percent body fat was stronger among women who had never used HRT. Among women with a percent body fat of more than 36%, the risk estimate among women who did not use HRT was 3.4 compared to 1.0 among women using HRT [74].

Other Modifying Factors

Race/Ethnicity

The majority of research on the association of obesity with breast cancer incidence has been based on white populations from Europe, Canada, and the U.S. A limited number of studies in other racial or ethnic groups suggest there may be some differences in observed associations among Hispanic and African American women; observed associations in Asian populations have been similar to those among white women. Among the major racial/ethnic groups in the U.S., African American women have the highest prevalence of obesity. Several studies have estimated that the high rates of severe obesity may account for some of the later stage at diagnosis observed for African American women in comparison to white women [95,96]. However, few studies have examined the association of BMI or regional adiposity with breast cancer in African American women.

In the Carolina Breast Cancer Study, similar patterns of an inverse association between BMI and premenopausal breast cancer were observed for African American and white women. In contrast to other studies, BMI was not associated with an increased risk for postmenopausal breast cancer in African American or white women. Curiously, an increased waist-to-hip ratio, a measure of central adiposity, was associated with an increased risk of pre- and postmenopausal breast cancer, although the increased risk estimates were only statistically significant among premenopausal women. A small case-control study in Nigeria found an increased risk (RR = 1.82, 955 CI = 0.78 to 4.31) for breast cancer for women with a BMI of 30 or more; however, the risk estimate was not statistically significant due to small numbers (only 104 breast cancer cases) [97].

National data also indicate that Hispanic women in the U.S. have higher rates of obesity. Studies on the association of BMI and other measures of obesity and breast cancer incidence among Hispanic women are very limited. One study in New Mexico that included Hispanic white and non-Hispanic white women found that usual BMI and weight change during adult life increased risk for premenopausal as well as postmenopausal breast cancer among both groups of women. However, none of the relative risk estimates in this analysis stratified by menopausal status and ethnicity were statistically significant because of limited sample size. One small study in Brazil found an inverse association between BMI and premenopausal breast cancer and a positive association between BMI and postmenopausal breast cancer.

Larger studies are needed in these populations in the U.S. to better define how obesity in these populations is associated with breast cancer. In contrast, a number of studies among Asian populations in the U.S., Japan, and China have found similar associations between obesity and breast cancer risk as those observed among white populations.

Physical Activity

As summarized by Bernstein and Patel in Chapter 4 of this book and in other recent reviews [98–100], the evidence that physical activity is associated with reduced risk of pre- and postmenopausal breast cancer is increasing. A limited number of studies on physical activity and breast cancer risk have had sufficient numbers of cases to examine the effect of physical activity stratified by BMI. Several of these studies have found a greater reduction in risk with being physically active among women who were in the lower range of BMI.

Unfortunately, studies of obesity and breast cancer risk have rarely reported on the association of BMI stratified by physical activity. One exception is a study by Enger et al. that examined the interaction of BMI and physical activity for ER+/PR+ tumors; these researchers did not find statistically significant interaction but did observe the greatest reductions in risk among women with low BMI (defined as BMI < 23.7 kg/m^2 and higher levels of physical activity (17.6 + MET-hours/week) [37]. More work is needed among large studies with good measures of physical activity and BMI before conclusions can be reached on whether the effect of physical activity on breast cancer risk is different among lean as compared to overweight and obese women.

FUTURE RESEARCH DIRECTIONS

In the area of breast cancer incidence, research on the association of weight, BMI, and other measures of fat distribution and weight change during middle and older adult life has been extensive. New research on these measures in this time of life should focus on exploring underlying mechanisms by which these exposures may influence cancer risk. Although recent research has examined differences in association by exogenous estrogen exposure, few studies have examined whether risk associated with obesity and other measures varies by characteristics of the tumor, such as hormone receptor status [37]. As basic and clinical research identifies additional specific tumor markers that may influence disease progression, it will be important to design studies to examine the effect of BMI, weight gain, and measures of fat distribution on the relative proportion of tumors that express these markers.

In addition, the interactions among diet, physical activity, and weight and breast cancer risk have been minimally explored. Such studies require very large samples with good measures of all of these exposures to have the power to identify differential effects in population subgroups. Although adult weight gain from young adult to middle life has been a consistent risk factor for postmenopausal breast cancer, research is needed on the effect of changes in weight during different periods in time when the breast may be undergoing rapid change, such as during puberty and pregnancy (Figure 14.1). Only a limited number of studies have attempted to examine this issue and these have not had repeat measures of weight across all of these time periods or have had to rely on recall in weight from the distant past.

A recent study from the Framingham cohort [94] that examined weight change based on repeat measured weights, found an increased risk only with weight gain from age 25 through middle age,

	In utero/ birth	Childhood	Puberty	Young adult	Pregnancy	Middle age	Menopause	Older age
Extent of data	Limited	Limited	Limited	Moderate	None	Extensive	Extensive	Limited
Summary Relative Risks *Weight/BMI*	Inconsistent	Inconsistent	Inconsistent	0.6	No data	1.3	1.5	1.9

FIGURE 14.1 Summary of past and future research directions exploring the associations of body size and breast cancer risk across the life cycle.

but not for weight gain in the young adult period or in the later postmenopausal period. However, given the missing information about weight at younger ages, this study did not have the power to explore the effect of weight gain during puberty and pregnancy fully.

In order to examine the contribution of estrogen as the underlying mechanism by which obesity influences breast cancer risk, studies have examined the risk of obesity or weight gain in groups stratified by HRT or estrogen status of the tumor. However, few studies have examined whether the effect of insulin-related peptides vary by BMI. Research is beginning to be published on the role of metabolic syndrome (obesity, glucose intolerance, low-serum high-density lipoprotein cholesterol [HDL-C]) and breast cancer incidence [101]. Similarly, a limited number of studies have begun to explore the effect of high glycemic load or glycemic index and cancer risk for other cancers, such as colon and prostate cancer. Some evidence suggests that these dietary patterns are more likely to lead to abnormalities in glucose metabolism and insulin processing among obese as compared to normal weight individuals. Therefore, research should be designed to examine whether such differential effects occur for breast cancer outcomes in normal as compared to overweight women.

Research is beginning to explore whether measures postulated to relate to immune function, such as C-reactive protein, may be adversely affected in obesity and therefore be another mechanism by which obesity increases disease risk. In addition, the identification of biologically active cytokines produced by adipose tissue, such as leptin and adiponectin, is beginning to be examined for a possible role in breast cancer. For example, two small case-control studies have found that low serum adiponectin levels are associated with an increased risk of breast cancer, possibly through a nonestrogen-mediated mechanism [102,103]. At present, studies examining the role of cytokines and other inflammatory markers are very limited in breast cancer. However, such measures may be available in many large cohort and case-control studies and may be a promising area of exploration in the future.

Finally, most of the obesity-related research in breast cancer has been done based on general risk populations of white women. Future research is needed to examine how BMI, weight gain, and measures of regional adiposity influence risk for breast cancer among women from different racial and ethnic groups, as well as women at increased risk of cancer as assessed by family history or specific molecular markers of genetic susceptibility. One study has reported that, among women with inherited mutations in BRCA1 and BRCA2, women who were normal weight and physically active in adolescence had a delayed onset of breast cancer [104].

CONCLUSIONS AND POPULATION-ATTRIBUTABLE RISK

Extensive data from case-control and cohort studies provide convincing evidence of a modest 30% increased risk of postmenopausal breast cell cancer from overweight and obesity and a larger twofold increase in risk for adult weight gain. Estimates from a meta-analysis of cohort studies found gradual increases in risk of postmenopausal breast cancer to a BMI of 28, after which risk did not increase further. The relative risk for a BMI of 28 compared with a BMI of less than 21 was 1.26 [56]. However, risk estimates vary by age at diagnosis, history of HRT, and estrogen receptor status of the tumor with a much stronger risk observed among overweight and obese women who have never used HRT or who have estrogen-positive tumors.

Another meta-analysis found that this increased risk for postmenopausal breast cancer corresponded to a 12% increase for an overweight woman and a 25% increase for an obese woman [105]. A stronger association is seen for adult weight gain, with a doubling of risk among women who have never used HRT and who gained over 20 kg from age 18 [23]. A meta-analysis of cohort studies found an inverse association between BMI and premenopausal breast cancer, with a relative risk of 0.54 for women with a BMI higher than 31 compared to women with a BMI of less than 21 [56]. This estimate is consistent with the reduction in risk of 0.6 to 0.7 observed in many studies and does not appear to be present for BMIs less than 28. Data on the association of various measures of regional adiposity, such as waist or hip circumference, are limited and less consistent, with few finding associations among premenopausal women and some showing increases in risk among postmenopausal women with increased waist or hip circumferences.

Given the strength of the evidence from observational epidemiological studies on the role of obesity in postmenopausal breast cancer risk, a logical next question to be examined is the effect of weight loss in reducing risk. Few observational epidemiological studies have examined the effect of weight loss on disease risk because of the inability to distinguish intended from unintended weight loss related to coexisting disease. Because of this potential bias, reports of the association of weight loss with breast cancer outcomes from observational epidemiological studies must be interpreted with caution and few studies have examined this issue. In fact, most studies have included women with weight loss in the reference group when examining the association of changes in weight or BMI with breast cancer risk.

The limited number of studies that have examined the association of weight loss separately have not found statistically significant associations between weight loss and risk [23,65,67,69,72,90]. Only one study has examined the effect of intentional weight loss on breast cancer risk. In that study from the Iowa's Women's Health Study, intentional weight loss of 20 or more pounds was associated with a 21% reduction in risk of subsequent postmenopausal breast cancer (RR = 0.79 95% CI = 0.65 to 0.97) [106]. After adjustment for multiple other breast cancer risk factors, this reduced risk was essentially unchanged (RR = 0.82; 95% CI = 0.66 to 1.00). This study also found a reduction in risk among women who had lost at least 10 lb from their maximum weight (RR = 0.85; 95% CI = 0.73 to 0.98).

Research has begun to explore the effect of randomized controlled trials of weight loss and specific diet and physical activity changes on physiological factors that may influence breast cancer risk, such as estrogen, androgens, and insulin-related peptides. Evidence from these studies is summarized in Chapter 7 in this book. Conclusive evidence of the effect of weight loss on breast cancer risk will require randomized controlled trials of weight loss involving changes in diet and physical activity.

Only a few studies have attempted to estimate the population-attributable risk or what proportion of postmenopausal breast cancer can be attributed to overweight and obesity. In 2001, Bergstrom et al. estimated that about 9% of postmenopausal breast cancer could be attributed to overweight and obesity [105]. However, that estimate was based on rates of overweight and obesity in European countries throughout the 1980s and early 1990s. Current rates of overweight and obesity among women in the U.S. are much higher. For example, the rate of obesity among women in Europe in the Bergstrom study was 13%, but the rate of obesity among women in the U.S. today is about 33%. Therefore, a rough estimate of the population-attributable fraction of breast cancer due to overweight and obesity today in the U.S. may be closer to 15%. Given evidence of a continued increase in obesity in the U.S. and internationally, it is likely that obesity will become an increasingly important contributor to breast cancer risk worldwide.

REFERENCES

1. de Waard F, Baanders–van Halewijn EA. A prospective study in general practice on breast cancer in postmenopausal women. *Int J Cancer.* 1974; 14:153–160.
2. World Health Organization. Obesity: preventing and managing the global epidemic. Report of a WHO consultation, WHO technical reports series, no. 894. 894. 2000. Geneva, Switzerland, World Health Organization.
3. Ekbom A, Hsieh C-C, Lipworth L, Adami H-O, Trichopoulos D. Intrauterine environment and breast cancer risk in women: a population-based study. *J Natl.Cancer Inst.* 1997; 89:71–76.
4. Le Marchand L, Kolonel LN, Myers BC, Mi M-P. Birth characteristics of premenopausal women with breast cancer. *Br J Cancer.* 1988; 57:437–439.
5. Hilakivi–Clarke L, Clarke R, Lippman M. The influence of maternal diet on breast cancer risk among female offspring. *Nutrition.* 1999; 15:392–401.
6. Lawlor DA, Oaksah M, Gunnell D, Davey Smith G, Ebrahim S. Associations of adult measures of childhood growth with breast cancer: findings from the British Women's Heart and Health Study. *Br J Cancer.* 3 A.D.; 89:81–87.
7. Berstein LM. Newborn macrosomy and cancer. *Adv Cancer Res.* 1988; 50:231–278.
8. Ekbom A, Trichopoulos D, Adami H-O, Hsieh C-C, Lan S-J. Evidence of prenatal influences on breast cancer risk. *Lancet.* 1992; 340:1015–1018.
9. Innes K, Byers T, Schymura M. Birth characteristics and subsequent risk for breast cancer in very young women. *Am J Epidemiol.* 2000; 152:1121–1128.
10. Michels KB, Trichopoulos D, Robins JM et al. Birthweight as a risk factor for breast cancer. *Lancet.* 1996; 348:1542–1546.
11. Sanderson M, Williams MA, Malone KE et al. Perinatal factors and risk of breast cancer. *Epidemiology.* 1996; 7:34–37.
12. De Stavola BL, Hardy R, Kuh D, dos Santos Silva I, Wadsworth M, Swerdlow AJ. Birthweight, childhood growth and risk of breast cancer in a British cohort. *Br J Cancer.* 2000; 83:964–968.
13. Kaijser M, Lichtenstein P, Granath F, Erlandsson G, Cnattingius S, Ekbom A. *In utero* exposures and breast cancer: a study of opposite-sexed twins. *J Natl Cancer Inst.* 2001; 93:60–62.
14. Mellemkjaer L, Olsen ML., Sorensen HT, Thulstrup AM, Olsen J. Birth weight and risk of early-onset breast cancer (Denmark). *Cancer Causes Control.* 2003; 14:61–64.
15. Leong NM, Mignone LI, Newcomb PA et al. Early life risk factors in cancer: the relation of birth weight to adult obesity. *Int J Cancer.* 2003; 103:789–791.
16. Whitaker RC, Dietz WH. Role of the prenatal environment in the development of obesity. *J Pediatr.* 1998; 132:768–776.
17. Okasha M, McCarron P, Gunnell D, Smith GD. Exposures in childhood, adolescence and early adulthood and breast cancer risk: a systematic review of the literature. *Breast Cancer Res Treat.* 2003; 78:223–276.
18. Brinton LA, Swanson CA. Height and weight at various ages and risk of breast cancer. *Ann Epidemiol.* 1992; 2:597–609.
19. Choi NW, Howe GR, Miller AB, Matthews V, Morgan RW, Munan L. An epidemiologic study of breast cancer. *Am J Epidemiol.* 1978; 107:510–521.
20. Chu SY, Lee NC, Wingo PA, Senie RT, Greenberg RS, Peterson HB. The relationship between body mass and breast cancer among women enrolled in the Cancer and Steroid Hormone Study. *J Clin Epidemiol.* 1991; 44:1197–1206.
21. Folsom AR, Kaye SA, Prineas RJ, Potter JD, Gapstur SM, Wallace RB. Increased incidence of carcinoma of the breast associated with abdominal adiposity in postmenopausal women. *Am J Epidemiol.* 1990; 131:794–803.
22. Franceschi S, Favero A, La Vecchia C et al. Body size indices and breast cancer risk before and after menopause. *Int J Cancer.* 1996; 67:181–186.
23. Huang Z, Hankinson SE, Colditz GA et al. Dual effects of weight and weight gain on breast cancer risk. *JAMA.* 1997; 278:1407–1411.
24. Harris RE, Namboodiri KK, Wynder EL. Breast cancer risk: effects of estrogen replacement therapy and body mass. *J Natl Cancer Inst.* 1992; 84:1575–1582.

25. Hislop TG, Coldman AJ, Elwood JM, Grauer G, Kan L. Childhood and recent eating patterns and risk of breast cancer. *Cancer Detect Prev.* 1986; 9:47–58.
26. Le Marchand L, Kolonel LN, Earle ME, Mi MP. Body size at different periods of life and breast cancer. *Am J Epidemiol.* 1988; 128:137–152.
27. London SJ, Colditz GA, Stampfer MJ, Willett WC, Rosner BR, Speizer FE. Prospective study of relative weight, height, and risk of breast cancer. *JAMA.* 1989; 262:2853–2858.
28. Lund E, Adami HO, Bergstrom R, Meirik O. Anthropometric measures and breast cancer in young women. *Cancer Causes Control.* 1990; 1:169–172.
29. Paffenbarger RS, Kampert JB, Change HG. Characteristics that predict risk of breast cancer before and after the menopause. *Am J Epidemiol.* 1980; 112:258–268.
30. Sellers TA, Kushi LH, Potter JD, Kaye SA, Nelson CL, McGovern PG. Effect of family history, body-fat distribution, and reproductive factors on the risk of postmenopausal breast cancer. *N Engl J Med.* 1992; 326:1323–1329.
31. Willett WC, Browne ML, Bain C et al. Relative weight and risk of breast cancer among premenopausal women. *Am J Epidemiol.* 1985; 122:731–740.
32. Ursin G, Paganini–Hill A, Siemiatycki J, Thompson WD, Haile RW. Early adult body weight, body mass index, and premenopausal bilateral breast cancer: data from a case-control study. *Breast Cancer Res Treat.* 1995; 33:75–82.
33. Chie WC, Li CY, Huang CS, Chang KJ, Lin RS. Body size as a factor in different ages and breast cancer risk in Taiwan. *Anticancer Res.* 1998; 18:565–570.
34. Magnusson C, Baron J, Persson I et al. Body size in different periods of life and breast cancer risk in postmenopausal women. *Int J Cancer.* 1998; 76:29–34.
35. Coates RJ, Uhler RJ, Hall HI et al. Risk of breast cancer in young women in relation to body size and weight gain in adolescence and early adulthood. *Br J Cancer.* 1999; 81:167–174.
36. Peacock SL, White E, Daling JR, Voigt LF, Malone KE. Relation between obesity and breast cancer in young women. *Am J Epidemiol.* 1999; 149:339–346.
37. Enger SM, Ross RK, Paganini–Hill A, Carpenter CL, Bernstein L. Body size, physical activity, and breast cancer hormone receptor status: results from two case-control studies. *Cancer Epidemiol Biomarkers Prev.* 2000; 9:681–687.
38. HIrose K, Tajima K, Hamajima N et al. Association of family history and other risk factors with breast cancer risk among Japanese premenopausal and postmenopausal women. *Cancer Causes Control.* 2001; 12:349–358.
39. de Vasconcelos AB, Azevedo e Silva Mendonca, Sichieri R. Height, weight, weight change and risk of breast cancer in Rio de Janeiro, Brazil. *Sao Paulo Med J.* 2001; 119:62–66.
40. Wenten M, Gilliland FD, Baumgartner K, Samet JM. Associations of weight, weight change, and body mass with breast cancer risk in Hispanic and non-Hispanic white women. *Ann Epidemiol.* 2002; 12:435–434.
41. Morimoto LM, White E, Chen Z et al. Obesity, body size, and risk of postmenopausal breast cancer: the Women's Health Initiative (United States). *Cancer Causes Control.* 2002; 13:741–751.
42. Tretli S. Height and weight in relation to breast cancer morbidity and mortality: a prospective study of 570,000 women in Norway. *Int J Cancer.* 1989; 44:23–30.
43. Willett WC, Browne ML, Bain C et al. Relative weight and risk of breast cancer among premenopausal women. *Am J Epidemiol.* 1985; 122:731–740.
44. Swanson CA, Brinton LA, Taylor PR, Licitra LM, Zeigler RG, Schairer C. Body size and breast cancer risk assessed in women participating in the Breast Cancer Detection Demonstration Project. *Am J Epidemiol.* 1989; 130:1133–1141.
45. Bouchardy C, Le MG, Hill C. Risk factors for breast cancer according to age at diagnosis in a French case-control study. *J Clin Epidemiol.* 1990; 43:267–275.
46. Pathak DR, Whittemore AS. Combined effects of body size, parity and menstrual events on breast cancer incidence in seven countries. *Am J Epidemiol.* 1992; 135:153–167.
47. Vatten LJ, Kvinnsland S. Prospective study of height, body mass index and risk of breast cancer. *Acta Oncol.* 1992; 31:195–200.
48. Tornberg SA, Carstensen JM. Relationship between Quetelets index and cancer of breast and female genital tract in 47,000 women followed for 25 years. *Br J Cancer.* 1994; 69:358–361.

49. Swanson CA, Coates RJ, Schoenberg JB et al. Body size and breast cancer risk among women under age 45 years. *Am J Epidemiol.* 1996; 143:698–706.
50. Hall IJ, Newman B, Millikan RC, Moorman PG. Body size and breast cancer risk in black women and white women: the Carolina Breast Cancer Study. *Am J Epidemiol.* 2000; 151:754–764.
51. Friedenreich CM, Courneya KS, Bryant HE. Case-control study of anthropometric measures and breast cancer risk. *Int J Cancer.* 2002; 99:445–452.
52. Yoo K, Tajima K, Park S et al. Postmenopausal obesity as a breast cancer risk factor according to estrogen and progesterone receptor status (Japan). *Cancer Lett.* 2001; 167:57–63.
53. Hirose K, Tajima K, Hamajima N et al. Association of family history and other risk factors with breast cancer risk among Japanese premenopausal and postmenopausal women. *Cancer Causes Control.* 2001; 12:349–358.
54. Shu XO, Jin F, Dai Q et al. Association of body size and fat distribution with risk of breast cancer among Chinese women. *Int J Cancer.* 2001; 94:449–455.
55. Kolonel LN, Nomura AMY, Lee J, Hirohata T. Anthropometric indicators of breast cancer risk in postmenopausal women in Hawaii. *Nutr Cancer.* 1986; 8:247–256.
56. van den Brandt PA, Spiegelman D, Yaun SS et al. Pooled analysis of prospective cohort studies on height, weight, and breast cancer risk. *Am J Epidemiol.* 2000; 152:514–527.
57. Valaoras VD, MacMahon B, Trichopoulous D, Polychronpoulou A. Lactation and reproductive histories of breast cancer. *Int J Cancer.* 1969; 4:350–363.
58. Kalish LA. Relationships of body size with breast cancer. *J Clin Oncol.* 1984; 2:287–293.
59. Lubin F, Ruder AM, Wax Y, Modan B. Overweight and changes in weight throughout adult life life in breast cancer etiology. *Am J Epidemiol.* 1985; 122:579–588.
60. Tao SC, Yu MC, Ross RK, Xiu KW. Risk factors for breast cancer in Chinese women of Beijing. *Int J Cancer.* 1988; 42:495–8.
61. Negri E, La Vecchia C, Bruzzi P, Dardanoni G, Decarli A, Palli D. Risk factors for breast cancer: pooled results from three Italian case-control studies. *Am J Epidemiol.* 1988; 128:1207–1215.
62. Ingram D, Nottage E, Ng S, Sparrow L, Roberts A, Willcox D. Obesity and breast disease. The role of the female sex hormones. *Cancer.* 1989; 64:1049–1053.
63. Hseih C, Trichopoulos D, Katsouyanni K, Yuasa S. Age at menarche, age at menopause, height and obesity as risk factors for breast cancer: assciations and interactions in an international case-control study. *Int J Cancer.* 1990; 46:796–800.
64. Parazzini F, La Vecchia C, Negri E, Bruzzi P, Palli D, Boyle P. Anthropometric variables and risk of breast cancer. *Int J Cancer.* 1990; 45:397–402.
65. Radimer K, Siskind V, Bain C, Schofield F. Relation between anthropometric indicators and risk of breast cancer among Australian women. *Am J Epidemiol.* 1993; 138:77–89.
66. Yong LC, Brown CC, Schatzkin A, Schairer C. Prospective study of relative weight and risk of breast cancer: the Breast Cancer Detection Demonstration Project follow-up study, 1979 to 1987–1989. *Am J Epidemiol.* 1996; 143:985–995.
67. Ziegler RG, Hoover RN, Nomura AM et al. Relative weight, weight change, height, and breast cancer risk in Asian–American women. *J Natl Cancer Inst.* 1996; 88:650–660.
68. Galanis DJ, Kolonel LN, Lee J, Le Marchand L. Anthropometric predictors of breast cancer incidence and survival in a multi-ethnic cohort of female residents of Hawaii, United States. *Cancer Causes Control.* 1998; 9:217–224.
69. Trentham–Dietz A, Newcomb PA, Storer BE et al. Body size and risk of breast cancer. *Am J Epidemiol.* 1997; 145:1011–1019.
70. Li CI, Stanford JL, Daling JR. Anthropometric variables in relation to risk of breast cancer in middle-aged women. *Int J Epidemiol.* 2000; 29:208–213.
71. Lam PB, Vacek PM, Geller BM, Muss HB. The association of increased weight, body mass index, and tissue density with the risk of breast carcinoma in Vermont. *Cancer.* 2000; 89:369–375.
72. Trentham–Dietz A, Newcomb PA, Egan KM et al. Weight change and risk of postmenopausal breast cancer (United States). *Cancer Causes Control.* 2000; 11:533–542.
73. Sellers TA, Davis J, Cerhan JR et al. Interaction of waist/hip ratio and family history on the risk of hormone receptor-defined breast cancer in a prospective study of postmenopausal women. *Am J Epidemiol.* 2002; 155:225–233.

74. Lahmann PH, Lissner L, Gullberg B, Olsson H, Berglund G. A prospective study of adiposity and postmenopausal breast cancer risk: the Malmo Diet and Cancer Study. *Int J Cancer.* 2003; 103:246–252.
75. Feigelson HS JCTLTMCE. Weight gain, body mass index, hormone replacement therapy, and post-menopausal breast cancer in a large prospective study. *Cancer Epidemiol Biomarkers Prev.* 2004; 13:220–224.
76. Swerdlow AJ, De Stavola BL, Floderus B et al. Risk factors for breast cancer at young ages in twins: an international population-based study. *J Natl Cancer Inst.* 2002; 94:1238–1246.
77. Mannisto S, Pietinen P, Pyy M, Palmgren J, Eskelinen M, Uusitupa M. Body-size indicators and risk of breast cancer according to menopause and estrogen-receptor status. *Int J Cancer.* 1996; 68:8–13.
78. Ng EH, Gao F, Ji CY, Ho GH, Soo KC. Risk factors for breast carcinoma in Singaporean Chinese women: the role of central obesity. *Cancer.* 1997; 80:725–731.
79. Kaaks R, van Noord PA, Den T, I, Peeters PH, Riboli E, Grobbee DE. Breast-cancer incidence in relation to height, weight and body-fat distribution in the Dutch "DOM" cohort. *Int J Cancer.* 1998; 76:647–651.
80. Huang Z, Willett WC, Colditz GA et al. Waist circumference, waist:hip ratio, and risk of breast cancer in the Nurses' Health Study. *Am J Epidemiol.* 1999; 150:1316–1324.
81. Sonnenschein E, Toniolo P, Terry MB et al. Body fat distribution and obesity in pre- and postmenopausal breast cancer. *Int J Epidemiol.* 1999; 28:1026–1031.
82. Ballard–Barbash R, Schatzkin A, Carter CL, Kannel WB, Kreger BE, D'Agostino RB. Body fat distribution and breast cancer in the Framingham study. *J Natl Cancer Inst.* 1990; 82:286–290.
83. Schapira DV, Kumar NB, Lyman GH, Cox CE. Abdominal obesity and breast cancer risk. *Ann Intern Med.* 1990; 112:182–186.
84. Bruning PF, Bonfrer JMG, Van Moord PAH, Hart AAM, De Jong–Bakker M, Nooijen WJ. Insulin resistance and breast cancer risk. *Int J Cancer.* 1992; 52:511–516.
85. Bruning PF. Endogenous estrogen and breast cancer: a possible relationship between body fat distribution and estrogen availability. *J Steroid Biochem.* 1987; 27:487–492.
86. den Tonkelaar ID, Seidell J, Collette HJ, de Waard F. Obesity and subcutaneous fat patterning in relation to breast cancer in postmenopausal women participating in the diagnostic investigation of mammary cancer project. *Cancer.* 1992; 69:2663–2667.
87. Petrek JA, Peters M, Cirrincione C, Rhodes D, Bajorunas D. Is body fat topography a risk factor for breast cancer? *Ann Intern Med.* 1993; 118:356–362.
88. Sellers TA, Gapstur SM, Potter JD, Kushi LH, Bostick RM, Folsom AR. Association of body fat distribution and family histories of breast and ovarian cancer with risk of postmenopausal breast cancer. *Am J Epidemiol.* 1993; 138:799–803.
89. den Tonkelaar I, Seidell J, Collette HJ. Body fat distribution in relation to breast cancer in women participating in the DOM-project. *Breast Cancer Res Treat.* 1995; 34:55–61.
90. Ballard–Barbash R, Schatzkin A, Taylor PR, Kahle LL. Association of change in body mass with breast cancer. *Cancer Res.* 1990; 50:2152–2155.
91. Barnes–Josiah D, Potter JD, Sellers TA, Himes JH. Early body size and subsequent weight gain as predictors of breast cancer incidence (Iowa, United States). *Cancer Causes Control.* 1995; 6:112–118.
92. Jernstrom H, Barrett–Connor E. Obesity, weight change, fasting insulin, proinsulin, C-peptide, and insulin-like growth factor-1 levels in women with and without breast cancer: the Rancho Bernardo Study. *J Women's Health Gender-Based Med.* 1999; 8:1265–1272.
93. Shoff SM, Newcomb PA, Trentham–Dietz A et al. Early-life physical activity and postmenopausal breast cancer: effect of body size and weight change. *Cancer Epidemiol Biomarkers Prev.* 2000; 9:591–595.
94. Radimer K, Ballard–Barbash R, Miller JS et al. Weight change and the risk of late onset breast cancer in the original Framingham cohort. *Nutr Cancer.* 2004; 49:7–13.
95. Jones BA, Kasi SV, Curnen MG, Owens PH, Dubrow R. Severe obesity as an explanatory factor for the black/white difference in stage at diagnosis of breast cancer. *Am J Epidemiol.* 1997; 146:394–404.
96. Moorman P, Jones B, Millikan R, Hall I, Newman B. Race, anthropometric factors, and stage at diagnosis of breast cancer. *Am J Epidemiol.* 2001; 153:284–291.
97. Adebamowo CA, Ogundiran TO, Adenipekun AA et al. Obesity and height in urban Nigerian women with breast cancer. *Ann Epidemiol.* 2003; 13:455–461.

98. International Agency for Research on Cancer Working Group. IARC Working Group on the evaluation of cancer-preventive strategies. IARC handbooks of cancer prevention, vol. 6. *Weight Control and Physical Activity.* Lyon, France: IARC Press, 2002.
99. Lee IM. Physical activity and cancer prevention -- data from epidemiologic studies. *Med Sci Sports Exercise.* 2003; 35:1823–1827.
100. Friedenreich CM. Physical activity and breast cancer risk: the effect of menopausal status. *Exercise Sport Sci Rev.* 2004; 32:180–184.
101. Furberg AS, Veierod M, Wilsgaard T, Bernstein L, Thune I. Serum high-density lipoprotein cholesterol, metabolic profile and breast cancer risk. *J Natl Cancer Inst.* 2004; 96:1152–1160.
102. Mantzoros C, Petridou E, Dessypris N et al. Adiponectin and breast cancer risk. *J Clin Endocrinol Metab.* 2004; 89:1102–1107.
103. Miyoshi Y, Funahashi T, Kihara S et al. Association of serum adiponectin levels with breast cancer risk. *Clin Cancer Res.* 2003; 9:5699–5704.
104. King MC, Marks JH, Mandell JB. Breast and ovarian cancer risks due to inherited mutations in BRCA1 and BRCA2. *Science.* 2003; 302:643–645.
105. Bergstrom A, Pisani P, Tenet V, Wolk A, Adami HO. Overweight as an avoidable cause of cancer in Europe. *Int J Cancer.* 2001; 91:421–430.
106. Parker ED, Folsom AR. Intentional weight loss and incidence of obesity-related cancers: the Iowa Women's Health Study. *Int J Obesity.* 2003; 27:1447–1452.

15 Body Size, Obesity, and Colorectal Cancer

Anne McTiernan and Martha L. Slattery

CONTENTS

INTRODUCTION

Many aspects of the associations among body weight, obesity, and colorectal cancer have been examined. Colorectal cancer has been studied looking at the combined colon and rectal areas, as well as each site separately. Additionally, unlike many cancers, associations between body size and the precursor lesion, adenomous polyps, have been reported. Weight and height data using body mass index (BMI, kg/m^2), fat patterning using waist and hip circumference measurements, and weight change are indicators of body size that provide insight into the association and possible biological mechanisms underlying the association.

The literature is consistent in terms of reported associations between body size and colon and rectal cancers. Gender-specific associations have been observed almost universally, with stronger associations reported for men than for women [1]. Site-specific associations that have been reported suggest that obesity is associated mainly with colon cancer rather than rectal cancer, although studies that have examined proximal and distal colon cancers report stronger associations for distal rather than proximal tumors.

Most epidemiological studies examining the association with body weight and obesity have relied on self-reported height and weight. For case-control studies, the period of recalled height and weight varies from several years prior to diagnosis to the year prior to diagnosis; cohort studies usually use self-reported current height and weight, with varying individual time between reported data and cancer diagnosis. Height and weight measurements are converted to indicators of body mass, with BMI the most commonly used. Sometimes the World Health Organization (WHO) criteria for overweight (BMI > 25) and obesity (BMI ≥ 30) are used.

Unfortunately, most studies currently in the literature have not used WHO standards for determining obesity, thus making comparisons and interpretations across studies more difficult. Rather, most studies have categorized BMI based on distribution in the studied population. The upper range of BMI for many studies is close to the ≥30 set by WHO; however, sometimes the upper range is at 26, which would indicate overweight but not obesity by the WHO criteria. Limited data exist on waist or hip circumference measurements as indicators of fat pattern and its impact on colorectal cancer risk. Few studies have evaluated BMI and circumference measures simultaneously to determine the independent effects of each. Also, limited information is available on weight change or early life body size as possible risk factors for colon and rectal cancer.

COLON CANCER

Reported associations between body size and colon cancer have been fairly consistent across case-control and cohort studies. Studies of cases of 100 or more cases are shown in Table 15.1. Other studies with fewer cases provide similar estimates of association, although with less precision. Studies that have examined associations with obesity (a BMI of approximately ≥30) report slightly stronger associations than those that report associations for overweight or a BMI of over 25. For men, most studies report significantly increased risk, with relative risk estimates of around 2.0, although estimates range from 1.2 to 3.0. Most studies have adjusted for important confounding factors, including physical activity, dietary intake, and smoking; however, some report only age-adjusted estimates of association [1,2]. Most studies show evidence of a dose–response association.

Among women, associations are generally weaker than those observed for men and are often not statistically significant; point estimates are often around 1.4 and range from 0.7 to 2.7 [3–12]. Some variation in risk estimates among women may stem from ages of the women studied because stronger associations have been observed for pre- vs. postmenopausal women overall and postmenopausal women taking hormone replacement therapy are at higher risk if they are overweight or obese than if they are normal weight [9].

The association between body size and risk of colon cancer in African Americans is not well documented; only one study of 99 cases evaluated the association between BMI and colorectal cancer [12], with imprecise estimates of association. The cohort study by Chyou and colleagues [13] showed only a weak association between BMI and colorectal cancer risk among Asian men living in Hawaii. It is unknown whether this weaker association is from the lower levels of BMI observed in that population or whether the lack of association is the result of some other unknown factors. Data on associations between body size and colon cancer among other racial and ethnic groups are limited.

Some studies that have been adequately powered to look at associations for proximal and distal colon tumors show stronger associations for distal tumors than proximal tumors [4,6,11,14], although the study by Le Marchand et al. [3] showed stronger associations with proximal rather than distal tumors. The study by Terry [5] did not observe a significant association for proximal or distal tumors; however, the study population was restricted to women and, given the weaker associations usually detected for women, this is not inconsistent with the literature. In a study by Le Marchand et al. [15] the greatest risk associated with a large BMI was observed for sigmoid tumors, which most studies include as part of the distal colon. Although most studies report associations between body size and incident cancers, Murphy et al. [16] report associations for mortality similar to those reported for incidence.

The association between colorectal neoplasia and body fat distribution, as indicated by the waist-to-hip ratio, is shown in Table 15.1 as the set of relative risks or odds ratios with high vs. low or normal levels of waist-to-hip ratio [4,17,18]. Results from case-control as well as cohort studies suggest that a higher waist–hip ratio increases risk of colon cancer. The ranges and distributions of this ratio differ substantially across the various studies; however, as was observed with BMI, the waist-to-hip ratio also shows a pattern of a positive association with increased colon cancer risk. In the studies displaying a dose–response pattern, no specific threshold for this association was found except in the study of males by Giovannucci et al. [19].

A study conducted by MacInnis and colleagues [14] evaluated several indicators of body size and body composition in conjunction with colon cancer risk. In addition to the observation that

TABLE 15.1
Associations between Body Size and Colon Cancer

No. cases	Design	Obesity indicator: BMI	Obesity indicator: WHR	Weight change	Study (ref.)
M 205	CC	2.2 (1.2–4.1)			Graham (10)
F 223		1.8 (1.01–3.4)			
M 112	CC	2.1 (2.0–4.6)			West (70)
F 119		2.3 (1.1–4.9)			
M 388	CC	1.2 (0.5–2.9)			Kune (71)
F 327		0.7 (0.3–1.6)			
M and F: 452	CC	2.0 (1.3–3.1)			Gerhardsson de Verdier (21)
M 302	C	1.5 (1.1–2.2)			Lee (20)
F 212	C	1.4 (0.9–2.2)	1.3 (0.8–1.9)		Bostick (8)
F 289	C	1.2 (0.9–1.7)			Chyou (13)
F 779	CC	1.3 (1.0–1.7)		1.3 (1.0–1.6)	Dietz (11)
M 203	C	1.5 (0.9–2.5)	3.4 (1.5–7.7)		Giovannucci (19)
F 393	C	1.5 (1.02–2.1)	1.5 (0.9–2.5)		Martinez (6)
M 698	CC	2.2 (1.5–3.2)		1.6 (1.0–2.4)	Le Marchand (3)
F 494		1.2 (0.8–1.9)		0.8 (0.5–1.3)	
M 1095	CC	2.0 (1.5–2.6)	1.3 (0.98–1.7)		Caan (4)
F 888		1.5 (1.08–1.9)	1.7 (1.2–2.4)		
M 59	C	2.6 (1.1–6.1)			Singh (72)
F 83		1.1 (0.6–1.8)			
M 1124	CC	1.7 (1.3–2.3)	0.6 (0.4–0.8)		Russo (17)
F 819		0.9 (0.7–1.2)	1.7 (1.3–2.3)		
M 102	C	3.0 (1.0–8.7)	0.8 (0.2–3.5)		Ford (7)
F 117		2.7 (1.04–2.2)	0.9 (0.2–4.5)		
M 1792	C	1.8 (1.5–2.1)			Murphy (16)
F 1616		1.3 (1.1–1.5)			
F 291	C	1.2 (0.9–1.7)			Terry (24)
M 234	C	1.1 (0.7–1.7)			Nilsen (2)
F 277		1.1 (0.7–1.8)			
F 341	C		1.1 (0.8–1.6)		Parker (73)
M 153	C	1.7 (1.1–2.8)	2.1 (1.3–3.4)		MacInnis (14)

Notes: C = cohort; CC = case-control; BMI compares highest to lowest level; WHR = waist-to-hip ratio, compares highest to lowest level of risk; weight change as indicated by changes in weight over time.

BMI and waist-to-hip ratio increased risk of colon cancer, with the strongest associations for distal tumors, researchers looked at fat-free mass and fat mass, based on bioimpedance data, and observed increased risk for both. The associations with BMI and fat mass were attenuated when adjusted for other factors. However, the association with fat-free mass and waist–hip ratio remained after adjustment for other body composition measures. The authors proposed two independent effects of body composition on risk of colon cancer: one associated with nonadipose mass and the other with central adiposity.

Few studies have examined weight change and colon cancer risk. However, some studies have reported on BMI and obesity at different times in life. In general, no evidence suggests a stronger association between BMI earlier in life and colorectal neoplasia than one later in life. The cohort studies by Lee et al. [20] and Le Marchand et al. [15] show relative risks for BMI in the late second and the third decades of life similar to those for BMIs in later adulthood (all in the 1.4 to 1.6 range). Case-control studies suggest that elevated BMI in the later adult years and weight gain between early adult ages and later adult ages tends to increase risk for colon cancer [3,11].

RECTAL CANCER

Few studies have examined associations between body size and rectal cancer and those that have generally reported results for few cases. From existing data, it appears that body size is not associated with rectal cancer among men or women [11,15,17,21–24]. The study by Slattery et al. [23] is the largest study of rectal cancer reported to date. In that study of almost 1000 rectal cancer cases, no difference was found in risk of rectal cancer associated with being overweight (BMI of >25) or obese (BMI of >30). Other components of energy balance, energy intake and energy expenditure, were associated in a similar manner as was observed for colon cancer using the same study population and methods to collect data [25]. This implies that increased BMI and a positive energy balance may be less important risk factors for rectal cancer than for colon cancer. Studies that have combined colon and rectal tumors generally observe weaker associations than those that report associations for colon tumors only.

ADENOMAS

Studies of adenomas are important to provide evidence for the time (or times) in colorectal carcinogenesis when factors associated with body weight might be most important in colorectal cancer. Studies evaluating the association between body size and adenoma occurrence have examined associations by polyp size and type. Most studies have examined BMI with associations similar to those observed for colon cancer [26–29]. Some studies do not detect associations with adenomas and body size [30]. In a study that included cancer and adenomas, an increased risk with a large BMI was observed for large adenomas only, but not for colorectal tumors [31].

Most studies have observed a 1.5- to 2.5-fold increase in risk of adenomas among the group with the largest BMI. A large waist-to-hip ratio also has been associated with risk for adenomas, with stronger associations observed for larger adenomas [28,32]. The observation that BMI is more strongly associated with larger adenomas than with smaller ones suggests that obesity-related factors might be acting at a later stage in the development of cancer — perhaps by contributing to the promotion and progression of adenomas toward cancer. Alternatively, this pattern could be seen simply because there may be many other causes of small adenomas that do not progress; among people with small adenomas, those other causes serve to dilute-out the obesity association with risk.

INTERACTIONS

Evaluation of risk associated with body size in conjunction with other factors can provide insight into possible biological mechanisms. The factors most frequently evaluated with body size have included other components of energy balance, including physical activity and energy intake. Hormone replacement therapy, estrogen status, and use of nonsteroidal anti-inflammatory drugs (NSAIDs) also have been evaluated in conjunction with BMI [5,9]; Table 15.2 summarizes data from one large case-control study [9]. Given numbers of cases and controls available from that study, evaluation of interaction is possible. High levels of vigorous physical activity and low levels of energy intake have been shown to modify the colon cancer risk associated with obesity in several studies [3,20,25]. Studies further suggest that diet composition, specifically diets with a high glycemic index, may be important effect modifiers [33]. Hypothesis related to the assessment of these interactions stems from the energy balance equation that illustrates the relationship among energy intake, energy expenditure, and ability to maintain energy balance.

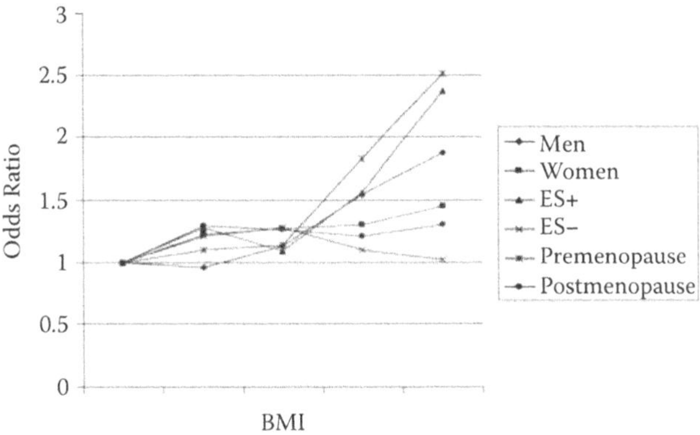

FIGURE 15.1 Association between BMI and colon cancer.

The hypothesis for assessing interactions between menopausal hormone use and estrogen developed from the observed gender-specific associations identified for BMI and colon cancer. Studies that have evaluated the interactions between obesity and estrogen or menopausal hormone use [5,9] have shown that being overweight or obese increases risk of colon cancer only among women who are estrogen positive (that is, premenopausal women or postmenopausal women using menopausal hormone therapy). As shown in Figure 15.1, among these women, risks associated with a large BMI are similar to associations observed in men, with risk estimates twice that of those for women who are lean. However, women who are estrogen negative (e.g., postmenopausal, not taking menopausal hormones) do not experience the same effect from being overweight or obese.

Further delineation between postmenopausal women who take and do not take menopausal hormones results in a risk for women not taking menopausal hormones that is not different from the referent; those who do take menopausal hormones have risk at the level of or slightly higher than that observed for men. In men it has been observed that, with advancing age, risk associated with being overweight or obese declines [9]. This could be the result of declining androgen levels that operate in a similar fashion to that of estrogen in regulating cancer risk associated with obesity because they have a similar influence as that of estrogen on insulin resistance [34]. The interaction

TABLE 15.2
Interaction between BMI and Other Exposures and Risk of Colon Cancer, Suggesting Mechanisms Involving Metabolic Pathways

		Low E/Low BMI	High E/Low BMI		Low E/High BMI		High E/High BMI	
Energy intake	M	1.0	2.1	(1.3–3.4)	1.9	(1.3–2.7)	3.0	(1.9–4.7)
	F	1.0	1.3	(0.8–2.2)	1.3	(0.7–2.2)	1.7	(0.9–3.2)
PAL (9.25)	M	1.0	1.7	(0.7–4.2)	1.9	(1.1–3.5)	3.6	(2.0–6.8)
	F	1.0	1.2	(0.7–1.9)	0.7	(0.4–1.2)	1.7	(1.1–2.7)
Estrogen Status		1.0	1.0	(0.4–2.5)	1.9	(0.9–4.2)	3.2	(1.5–7.0)
		1.0	1.1	(0.5–2.2)	0.6	(0.3–1.2)	1.3	(0.7–2.4)
NSAIDs		1.0	2.2	(1.5–3.2)	2.5	(1.7–3.6)	2.6	(1.8–3.8)

Notes: E = exposure; PAL = physical activity level. High exposure is defined as high energy intake, low energy expenditure, not using estrogen (HRT), not taking nonsteroidal anti-inflammatory medications. Thus, high E/low BMI reflects risk of exposure other than BMI, low E/high BMI reflects risk from high BMI (≥30); high E and high BMI is the relative risk from having the exposure and from having a high BMI.

between physical activity and BMI and estrogen and BMI suggests that BMI may influence colorectal risk through its influence on insulin.

Of interest also is the observed significant interaction between use of NSAIDs and BMI (Table 15.2). It is unclear whether this interaction indicates a mechanism involving inflammation or some other complex mechanism at play.

TUMOR MUTATIONS

Evaluation of the association between BMI and colon cancer looking at specific tumor mutations has provided insight into possible mechanisms of action and the role of body size in what may be specific disease pathways. Few studies have been reported to date, although those that have suggest that BMI may be involved in several pathways. One study reported that a large BMI was associated with Ki-*ras* mutations in codons 12 and 13 [35]. The BMI associations appeared to be more specific for Ki-*ras* mutations in women than in men. BMI appeared to be associated equally with tumors with and without p53 mutations [36]. Obesity was reported as associated only with tumors that were stable in women; however, in men, obesity was associated with stable as well as unstable tumors [37].

BIOLOGICAL MECHANISMS

It has been proposed that the influence of energy balance on risk of colon cancer may embrace endogenous hormone metabolism [38]. The mechanisms that relate obesity to risk of colon cancer most likely include a complex metabolic pathway involving estrogen, insulin, and inflammation.

Perhaps the mechanism that may have the greatest effect on the association between BMI and colon cancer involves the insulin pathway and the cross-talk between insulin and estrogen/androgen. Support for this association comes from data looking at BMI risk by exposure to estrogen and menopausal hormone use as previously described. This hypothesized mechanism is supported by the different in risk observed for men and women and the interaction with physical activity. High levels of BMI are associated with high levels of insulin; on the other hand, adipose tissue stores estrogen that may be turned on in a low-estrogen environment, such as that seen in postmenopausal women. However, if the findings by MacInnis et al. [14] are repeated in other studies, and the fat-free mass and central adiposity are more important than BMI, it is possible that the BMI-associated colon cancer risk is operating through high insulin levels. Because studies support a significant interaction between BMI and estrogen, it is possible that insulin and estrogen pathways are both operational.

Insulin-related genes may interact with BMI to alter risk of colorectal cancer. Insulin-like growth factor-1 (IGF-1), insulin-like growth factor-binding protein-3 (IGFBP-3), insulin receptor substrate-1 (IRS-1), and insulin receptor substrate-2 (IRS-2) have been proposed as involved in insulin-related pathways of cancer etiology. Polymorphisms of these genes have been identified, some of which have been shown to have effects on insulin resistance and/or diabetes. High serum IGF-1 levels have been associated with an increased risk of colorectal cancer, and variation in serum IGF-1 levels has been associated with a 19 CA repeat polymorphism 1 kb upstream of the transcription start site [39,40]. In men, serum IGF-1 concentrations were lower with the 19CA genotype than for other *IGF1* genotypes [41]. One could predict that this genotype might be associated with a decreased risk of colorectal cancer.

High levels of IGFBP-3 have been associated with a reduced risk of colorectal cancer [42,43]. An A/C polymorphism at nucleotide –202 is associated with different levels of IGFBP-3 in a dose–response fashion, i.e., AA > AC > CC [44,45]. A Gly972Arg (G972R) polymorphism in the *IRS-1* gene has been associated with insulin resistance and type-2 diabetes [46,47]. The G1057D *IRS-2* polymorphism has been associated with obesity and therefore a plausible link to insulin resistance and colorectal cancer [48]. Studies also have suggested that *IRS-2* is involved in insulin signaling and in the regulation of obesity [40]. One study evaluating the association between these genotypes and colon and rectal cancer risk observed a significant interaction between BMI and *IRS-2* and risk of rectal cancer and a borderline significant association with colon cancer (Slattery, under review). For colon cancer, those with the *DD* genotype had the greatest risk if they also had a BMI of 30 or more. Those with the *DD IRS-2* genotype were half as likely to develop rectal cancer at a BMI of <25 than those with the *GG* genotype.

Some studies suggest that the vitamin D receptor (VDR) also may be involved in insulin and insulin-like growth factor-mediated disease pathways. The VDR[4] is a nuclear receptor involved in the regulation of many physiological processes, including cell growth and differentiation and metabolic homeostasis [49–53]. Polymorphisms of the *VDR* gene most frequently studied include two restriction fragment length polymorphisms (RFLPs) in intron 8 (Bsm I and Apa I) and one in exon 9 (Taq I). These are in linkage disequilibrium with each other and with several 3′ untranslated region (3′ UTR) polymorphisms, including a poly A repeat [54].

At the start site of the gene, a polymorphism detected with a *Fok I* digest also has been studied and has been shown not to be in linkage disequilibrium with the other variants [54,55]. The polymorphism associated with lack of *Fok1* digestion (F) changes the start site from the first STG to one that is three codons downstream; thus the F genotype is associated with a protein three amino acids shorter than that associated with the f genotype. *VDR* polymorphisms have been examined in conjunction with colorectal adenomas and cancer and SS and BB variants have been shown to reduce adenoma/cancer risk [56–58].

The *ff* genotype of the Fok I polymorphism has been reported in one study to increase risk of colorectal cancer [59]. VDR genotypes, BMI, physical activity, and energy intake have been evaluated with energy balance and risk of colorectal cancer in one study (Slattery et al., in press). Data from a population-based case control study of colon (1174 cases and 1174 controls) and rectal (785 cases and 1000 controls) cancers was used to evaluate the associations. The *Bsm1*, polyA, and *Fok1 VDR* polymorphisms were evaluated. For colon cancer, those who were obese were at greater risk of colon cancer if they had the *SS* or *BB* (OR 3.50 95% CI 1.75 to 7.03; p interaction 0.03) or ff (OR 2.62 95% CI 1.15 to 5.99; p interaction 0.12) VDR genotypes. These findings are unexpected because the *SS*, *BB*, and *ff* alleles reduce risk of colon cancer overall.

Inflammation as a mechanisms related to obesity is being explored, although it is far from understood. Aspirin and other NSAIDs have been recognized as reducing risk of colorectal cancer for many years [60–65]. Although involvement in the COX-2 pathway has been thought to be the main biological mechanism underlying this association, it is possible that aspirin and NSAIDS may be involved in other biological mechanism. Cyclooxygenase-independent actions have been proposed, stimulated in part by the observations that NSAIDS inhibit tumor formation and growth in COX-deficient cell lines [59].

It has been proposed that aspirin and other NSAIDs reduce inflammation and that a reduction in inflammation decreases insulin resistance [47,66–68]. High doses of salicylates have been shown to reverse hyperglycemia, hyperinsulinemia, and dyslipidemia in obese rodents by sensitizing insulin signaling. In patients with type-2 diabetes, aspirin treatment has been shown to reduce fasting plasma glucose, total cholesterol, C-reactive protein, triglycerides, and insulin clearance; aspirin reduced hepatic glucose production and improved insulin-stimulated peripheral glucose uptake by 20% [59,65,69]. Aspirin/NSAID influence on insulin resistance appears to be independent of COX-2 inhibition; instead, it involves inhibition of NFKB and IKB and/or activation of PPARs. An interaction between aspirin and IRS-1 in antagonizing effects of tumor necrosis factor-α (TNF-α) has also been reported [47,66] TNF-α is a major cause of insulin resistance associated with obesity and inflammation.

As with all mechanisms reviewed, it is possible that obesity is in the causal pathway associated with mechanisms involving estrogen/androgen, insulin, and inflammation rather than the cause. However, studies that have examined BMI after adjusting for NSAIDs and aspirin continue to see direct associations between BMI and risk of colon cancer. To better understand the mechanisms involved in the obesity/body composition relationship with colon cancer, it is necessary to consider obesity and body composition alone. Research directed at understanding the components of energy balance and how they are mediated by factors such as estrogen and aspirin are needed.

SUMMARY

Failure to achieve energy balance is gaining momentum as an important consideration in the etiology of cancer. The concept of energy balance, or the ability to maintain body weight by balancing energy intake with energy expenditure, ties together important colon cancer risk factors. Elevated levels of body fat, as indicated by increased BMI during adult life and/or increased waist-to-hip ratio, are associated with increased risk for colon cancer and colon adenomas.

This association is seen for men and women, though it is higher for men. The reason for this difference by gender is not clear, although some data suggest that estrogen/androgen and aspirin/NSAIDs are involved in these differences. If obesity is simply an indicator of caloric imbalance then there should be no difference between the genders. On the other hand, obesity may have an offsetting beneficial effect among women. A factor such as the hyperestrogenemia associated with postmenopausal obesity could explain the gender differences — an estrogen benefit could be serving to blunt the obesity-related risk in women.

REFERENCES

1. International Agency for Research on Cancer. IARC Handbook of Cancer Prevention vol. 6, *Weight Control and Physical Activity.* Lyon, France: IARC Press, 2002.
2. Nilsen TI, Vatten LJ. Prospective study of colorectal cancer risk and physical activity, diabetes, blood glucose and BMI: exploring the hyperinsulinaemia hypothesis. *Br J Cancer* 2001; 84:417–422.
3. Le Marchand L, Wilkens LR, Kolonel LN, Hankin JH, Lyu LC. Associations of sedentary lifestyle, obesity, smoking, alcohol use, and diabetes with the risk of colorectal cancer. *Cancer Res* 1997; 57:4787–4794.
4. Caan BJ, Coates AO, Slattery ML, Potter JD, Quesenberry CP, Jr, Edwards SM. Body size and the risk of colon cancer in a large case-control study. *Int J Obesity Relat Metab Disord* 1998; 22:178–184.
5. Terry PD, Miller AB, Rohan TE. Obesity and colorectal cancer risk in women. *Gut* 2002; 51:191–194.
6. Martinez ME, Giovannucci E, Spiegelman D, Hunter DJ, Willett WC, Colditz GA. Leisure-time physical activity, body size, and colon cancer in women. Nurses' Health Study Research Group. *J Natl Cancer Inst* 1997; 89:948–955.
7. Ford ES. Body mass index and colon cancer in a national sample of adult U.S. men and women. *Am J Epidemiol* 1999; 150:390–398.
8. Bostick RM, Potter JD, Kushi LH, et al. Sugar, meat, and fat intake, and non-dietary risk factors for colon cancer incidence in Iowa women (United States). *Cancer Causes Control* 1994; 5:38–52.
9. Slattery ML, Ballard–Barbash R, Edwards S, Caan BJ, Potter JD. Body mass index and colon cancer: an evaluation of the modifying effects of estrogen (United States). *Cancer Causes Control* 2003; 14:75–84.
10. Graham S, Marshall J, Haughey B, et al. Dietary epidemiology of cancer of the colon in western New York. *Am J Epidemiol* 1988; 128:490–503.
11. Dietz AT, Newcomb PA, Marcus PM, Storer BE. The association of body size and large bowel cancer risk in Wisconsin (United States) women. *Cancer Causes Control* 1995; 6:30–36.
12. Dales LG, Friedman GD, Ury HK, Grossman S, Williams SR. A case-control study of relationships of diet and other traits to colorectal cancer in American blacks. *Am J Epidemiol* 1978; 109:132–144.
13. Chyou PH, Nomura AM, Stemmermann GN. A prospective study of colon and rectal cancer among Hawaii Japanese men. *Ann Epidemiol* 1996; 6:276–282.
14. MacInnis RJ, English DR, Hopper JL, Haydon AM, Gertig DM, Giles GG. Body size and composition and colon cancer risk in men. *Cancer Epidemiol Biomarkers Prev* 2004; 13:553–559.

15. Le Marchand L, Wilkens LR, Mi MP. Obesity in youth and middle age and risk of colorectal cancer in men. *Cancer Causes Control* 1992; 3:349–354.
16. Murphy TK, Calle EE, Rodriguez C, Kahn HS, Thun MJ. Body mass index and colon cancer mortality in a large prospective study. *Am J Epidemiol* 2000; 152:847–854.
17. Russo A, Franceschi S, La Vecchia C, et al. Body size and colorectal-cancer risk. *Int J Cancer* 1998; 78:161–165.
18. Martinez ME, Grodstein F, Giovannucci E, et al. A prospective study of reproductive factors, oral contraceptive use, and risk of colorectal cancer. *Cancer Epidemiol Biomarkers Prev* 1997; 6:1–5.
19. Giovannucci E, Ascherio A, Rimm EB, Colditz GA, Stampfer MJ, Willett WC. Physical activity, obesity, and risk for colon cancer and adenoma in men. *Ann Intern Med* 1995; 122:327–334.
20. Lee I-M, Paffenbarger RS, Jr. Quetelet's index and risk of colon cancer in college alumni. *J Natl Cancer Inst* 1992; 84:1326–1331.
21. de Verdier MG, Hagman U, Steineck G, Rieger Å, Norell SE. Diet, body mass and colorectal cancer: a case-referent study in Stockholm. *Int J Cancer* 1990; 45:832–838.
22. Graham S, Dayal H, Swanson M, Mittelman A, Wilkinson G. Diet in the epidemiology of cancer of the colon and rectum. *J Natl Cancer Inst* 1978; 61:709–714.
23. Slattery ML, Caan BJ, Benson J, Murtaugh M. Energy balance and rectal cancer: an evaluation of energy intake, energy expenditure, and body mass index. *Nutr Cancer* 2003; 46:166–171.
24. Terry P, Giovannucci E, Bergkvist L, Holmberg L, Wolk A. Body weight and colorectal cancer risk in a cohort of Swedish women: relation varies by age and cancer site. *Br J Cancer* 2001; 85:346–349.
25. Slattery ML, Potter J, Caan B, et al. Energy balance and colon cancer — beyond physical activity. *Cancer Res* 1997; 57:75–80.
26. Bird CL, Frankl HD, Lee ER, Haile RW. Obesity, weight gain, large weight changes, and adenomatous polyps of the left colon and rectum. *Am J Epidemiol* 1998; 147:670–680.
27. Davidow AL, Neugut AI, Jacobson JS, et al. Recurrent adenomatous polyps and body mass index. *Cancer Epidemiol Biomarkers Prev* 1996; 5:313–315.
28. Shinchi K, Kono S, Honjo S, et al. Obesity and adenomatous polyps of the sigmoid colon. *Jpn J Cancer Res* 1994; 85:479–484.
29. Giovannucci E, Colditz GA, Stampfer MJ, Willett WC. Physical activity, obesity, and risk of colorectal adenoma in women (United States). *Cancer Causes Control* 1996; 7:253–263.
30. Terry MB, Neugut AI, Bostick RM, et al. Risk factors for advanced colorectal adenomas: a pooled analysis. *Cancer Epidemiol Biomarkers Prev* 2002; 11:622–629.
31. Boutron–Ruault MC, Senesse P, Meance S, Belghiti C, Faivre J. Energy intake, body mass index, physical activity, and the colorectal adenoma-carcinoma sequence. *Nutr Cancer* 2001; 39:50–57.
32. Kono S, Handa K, Hayabuchi H, et al. Obesity, weight gain and risk of colon adenomas in Japanese men. *Jpn J Cancer Res* 1999; 90:805–811.
33. Slattery ML, Benson J, Berry TD, et al. Dietary sugar and colon cancer. *Cancer Epidemiol Biomarkers Prev* 1997; 6:677–685.
34. Polderman KH, Gooren LJG, Asscheman H, Bakker A, Heine RJ. Induction of insulin resistance by androgens and estrogens. *J Clin Endocrinol Metab* 1994; 79:265–271.
35. Slattery ML, Anderson K, Curtin K, et al. Lifestyle factors and Ki-*ras* mutations in colon cancer tumors. *Mutat Res* 2001; 483:73–81.
36. Slattery ML, Curtin K, Ma K, et al. Diet activity, and lifestyle associations with p53 mutations in colon tumors. *Cancer Epidemiol Biomarkers Prev* 2002; 11:541–548.
37. Slattery ML, Potter JD, Curtin K, et al. Estrogens reduce and withdrawal of estrogens increase risk of microsatellite instability-positive colon cancer. *Cancer Res* 2001; 61:126–130.
38. Kaaks R. Nutrition, energy balance and colon cancer risk: the role of insulin and insulin-like growth factor-I. *IARC Sci Publ* 2002; 156:289–293.
39. Kido Y, Nakae J, Hribal ML, Xuan S, Efstratiadis A, Accili D. Effects of mutations in the insulin-like growth factor signaling system on embryonic pancreas development and beta-cell compensation to insulin resistance. *J Biol Chem* 2002; 277:36740–36747.
40. White MF. Insulin signaling in health and disease. *Science* 2003; 302:1710–1711.
41. Jernstrom H, Chu W, Vesprini D, et al. Genetic factors related to racial variation in plasma levels of insulin-like growth factor-1: implications for premenopausal breast cancer risk. *Mol Genet Metab* 2001; 72:144–154.

42. Collard TJ, Guy M, Butt AJ, et al. Transcriptional upregulation of the insulin-like growth factor binding protein IGFBP-3 by sodium butyrate increases IGF-independent apoptosis in human colonic adenoma-derived epithelial cells. *Carcinogenesis* 2003; 24:393–3401.
43. Furstenberger G, Senn HJ. Insulin-like growth factors and cancer. *Lancet Oncol* 2002; 3:298–302.
44. Schernhammer ES, Hankinson SE, Hunter DJ, Blouin MJ, Pollak MN. Polymorphic variation at the –202 locus in IGFBP3: Influence on serum levels of insulin-like growth factors, interaction with plasma retinol and vitamin D and breast cancer risk. *Int J Cancer* 2003; 107:60–64.
45. Deal C, Ma J, Wilkin F, et al. Novel promoter polymorphism in insulin-like growth factor-binding protein-3: correlation with serum levels and interaction with known regulators. *J Clin Endocrinol Metab* 2001; 86:1274–1280.
46. Withers DJ. Insulin receptor substrate proteins and neuroendocrine function. *Biochem Soc Trans* 2001; 29:525–529.
47. Hotamisligil GS, Peraldi P, Budavari A, Ellis R, White MF, Spiegelman BM. IRS-1-mediated inhibition of insulin receptor tyrosine kinase activity in TNF-alpha- and obesity-induced insulin resistance. *Science* 1996; 271:665–668.
48. Lautier C, El Mkadem SA, Renard E, et al. Complex haplotypes of IRS2 gene are associated with severe obesity and reveal heterogeneity in the effect of Gly1057Asp mutation. *Hum Genet* 2003; 113:34–43.
49. Adachi R, Shulman AI, Yamamoto K, et al. Structural determinants for vitamin d receptor response to endocrine and xenobiotic signals. *Mol Endocrinol* 2004; 18:43–52.
50. Barger-Lux MJ, Heaney RP, Hayes J, DeLuca HF, Johnson ML, Gong G. Vitamin D receptor gene polymorphism, bone mass, body size, and vitamin D receptor density. *Calcif Tissue Int* 1995; 57:161–162.
51. Haussler MR, Haussler CA, Jurutka PW, et al. The vitamin D hormone and its nuclear receptor: molecular actions and disease states. *J Endocrinol* 1997; 154 Suppl:S57–73.
52. Hayes CE, Nashold FE, Spach KM, Pedersen LB. The immunological functions of the vitamin D endocrine system. *Cell Mol Biol* (Noisy-le-grand) 2003; 49:277–300.
53. Jurutka PW, Remus LS, Whitfield GK, et al. The polymorphic N terminus in human vitamin D receptor isoforms influences transcriptional activity by modulating interaction with transcription factor IIB. *Mol Endocrinol* 2000; 14:401–420.
54. Slattery ML, Yakumo K, Hoffman M, Neuhausen S. Variants of the VDR gene and risk of colon cancer (United States). *Cancer Causes Control* 2001; 12:359–364.
55. Whitfield GK, Remus LS, Jurutka PW, et al. Functionally relevant polymorphisms in the human nuclear vitamin D receptor gene. *Mol Cell Endocrinol* 2001; 177:145–159.
56. Peters U, McGlynn KA, Chatterjee N, et al. Vitamin D, calcium, and vitamin D receptor polymorphism in colorectal adenomas. *Cancer Epidemiol Biomarkers Prev* 2001; 10:1267–1274.
57. Kim HS, Newcomb PA, Ulrich CM, et al. Vitamin D receptor polymorphism and the risk of colorectal adenomas: evidence of interaction with dietary vitamin D and calcium. *Cancer Epidemiol Biomarkers Prev* 2001; 10:869–874.
58. Ingles SA, Wang J, Coetzee GA, Lee ER, Frankl HD, Haile RW. Vitamin D receptor polymorphisms and risk of colorectal adenomas (United States). *Cancer Causes Control* 2001; 12:607–614.
59. Yuan M, Konstantopoulos N, Lee J, et al. Reversal of obesity- and diet-induced insulin resistance with salicylates or targeted disruption of Ikkbeta. *Science* 2001; 293:1673–1677.
60. Marnett LJ. Aspirin and the potential role of prostaglandins in colon cancer. *Cancer Res* 1992; 52:5575–5589.
61. Baron JA, Greenberg ER. Could aspirin really prevent colon cancer [editorial]. *N Engl J Med* 1991; 325:1644–1646.
62. Ahnen DJ. Colon cancer prevention by NSAIDs: what is the mechanism of action? *Eur J Surg* Suppl 1998:111–114.
63. Thun MJ, Namboodiri MM, Heath CW, Jr. Aspirin use and reduced risk of fatal colon cancer. *N Engl J Med* 1991; 325:1593–1596.
64. Sandler RS. Aspirin and other nonsteroidal anti-inflammatory agents in the prevention of colorectal cancer. *Important Adv Oncol* 1996:123–137.
65. Hundal RS, Petersen KF, Mayerson AB, et al. Mechanism by which high-dose aspirin improves glucose metabolism in type 2 diabetes. *J Clin Invest* 2002; 109:1321–1326.

66. Gao Z, Zuberi A, Quon MJ, Dong Z, Ye J. Aspirin inhibits serine phosphorylation of insulin receptor substrate 1 in tumor necrosis factor-treated cells through targeting multiple serine kinases. *J Biol Chem* 2003; 278:24944–24950.
67. Xu H, Hotamisligil GS. Signaling pathways utilized by tumor necrosis factor receptor 1 in adipocytes to suppress differentiation. *FEBS Lett* 2001; 506:97–102.
68. Hotamisligil GS. The role of TNFalpha and TNF receptors in obesity and insulin resistance. *J Intern Med* 1999; 245:621–625.
69. Baron SH. Salicylates as hypoglycemic agents. *Diabetes Care* 1982; 5:64–71.
70. West DW, Slattery ML, Robison LM, et al. Dietary intake and colon cancer: sex- and anatomic site-specific associations. *Am J Epidemiol* 1989; 130:883–894.
71. Kune GA, Kune S, Watson LF. Body weight and physical activity as predictors of colorectal cancer risk. *Nutr Cancer* 1990; 13:9–17.
72. Singh PN, Fraser GE. Dietary risk factors for colon cancer in a low-risk population. *Am J Epidemiol* 1998; 148:761–774.
73. Parker ED, Folsom AR. Intentional weight loss and incidence of obesity-related cancers: the Iowa Women's Health Study. *Int J Obesity Relat Metab Disord* 2003; 27:1447–1452.

16 Endogenous Hormone Metabolism and Endometrial Cancer

Rudolf Kaaks and Annekatrin Lukanova

CONTENTS

INTRODUCTION

Endometrial cancer is very much a disease of affluence, with age-standardized incidence rates that are up to ten times higher in Western, industrialized countries than in rural Asia or Africa [1,2]. Studies on time trends, as well as on migrants from low- to high-risk areas, have clearly shown that nongenetic (lifestyle) factors are to be held responsible for the large international differences in incidence rates.

One of the key risk factors for endometrial cancer among pre- and postmenopausal women is excess body weight [3,4]. In many studies, endometrial cancer risk was found to rise approximately linearly with increasing body mass index (BMI), especially among postmenopausal women. Among premenopausal women, several studies have shown a threshold effect, with an increase in risk only among obese women with a BMI of about 30 kg/m^2 or higher [3]. Overall, excess body weight has been estimated to account for up to about half of endometrial cancer incidence in Western Europe and the U.S. [5].

The endometrial tissue consists of stroma, vascular endothelium, and glandular and surface epithelium. These various cell types respond to sex steroids and other hormones in the circulation and also secrete a variety of growth factors that act as paracrine and autocrine regulators of cellular proliferation, differentiation, and apoptosis. Inhibition of cellular differentiation and apoptosis, and stimulation of cell proliferation, enhance tumor development by favoring the accumulation and fixation of mutations in proto-oncogenes and tumor suppressor genes, by stimulating the clonal expansion of cells with mutations and by enhancing the growth of established tumors [6–9].

From a histological and molecular pathology perspective, the vast majority (>80%) of endometrial tumors (referred to as “type I”) are endometrioid carcinomas, which are generally associated with endometrial hyperplasia [10,11]. These carcinomas often show mutations in the *ras* proto-oncogene and in the *PTEN* tumor suppressor gene, but not in the *P53* tumor suppressor gene. Other (type-II) tumors are more often serous papillary, clear cell, or squamous carcinomas; these generally develop from atrophic endometrial tissue in older women [10,12,13] and often show *P53* mutations, but not *ras* or *PTEN* mutations. Most epidemiological studies did not distinguish between these two tumor types. Nevertheless, some evidence indicates that endocrine and nutritional lifestyle factors, including obesity, affect the risk of type-I but not type-II tumors [10,11].

Excess body weight is associated with a number of major changes in endocrine metabolism. Increasing evidence suggests that these endocrine changes — chronic hyperinsulinemia, decreased serum levels of sex hormone binding globulin (SHBG), and increased levels of total and bioavailable androgens and estrogens (see also Chapter 7) — may provide the metabolic link between excess body weight and endometrial cancer development. In the present chapter, the relationships among excess weight, endogenous sex hormones, and endometrial cancer risk are discussed.

THE UNOPPOSED ESTROGEN HYPOTHESIS

The predominant theory describing the relationship between endogenous steroid hormones and endometrial cancer risk is known as the *unopposed estrogen* theory [14]. This stipulates that endometrial cancer risk is increased in women who have high plasma bioavailable estrogens and/or low plasma progesterone so that mitogenic or proapoptotic effects of estrogens are insufficiently counterbalanced by progesterone.

A first observation upon which the unopposed estrogen theory was based is that endometrial proliferation rates are increased during the follicular phase of the menstrual cycle, when progesterone levels are low and estradiol levels are at normal premenopausal concentrations [14]. More recent studies showed that, to a large part, the proliferative action of estradiol on endometrial tissue is mediated by an increased local production (mostly by stromal tissue) of insulin-like growth factor-I (IGF-I) [15–20]. The antiproliferative action of progesterone, on the other hand, has been shown to be largely mediated by enhanced local synthesis of IGF-binding protein-1, which is the most abundant IGF-binding protein in endometrial tissue and inhibits IGF-I action [21–26].

A second major observation that led to the unopposed estrogen theory was that endometrial cancer risk is increased among women using exogenous estrogens, but no such increase occurs when the estrogens are combined with progestins. Studies in the 1970s showed an increase in endometrial cancer risk among users of sequential oral contraceptives containing a long-duration, relatively potent estrogen (ethinylestradiol) and a short-duration weak progestin (dimethisterone) [27]. By contrast, the use of combined oral contraceptives that contain progestins for at least 10 days per monthly cycle (in addition to estrogen) has been associated with no increase [27,28] or only a moderate increase [29] in endometrial cancer risk.

Among postmenopausal women, use of estrogen-only replacement therapy has been shown to increase endometrial cancer risk. No such increase has been found for women who used estrogen–progestin replacement therapy to which progestins were added sequentially for at least 10 days in a 1-month cycle (sequential estrogen plus progestin replacement therapy or continuously (combined estrogen plus progestin replacement therapy [27,30,31].

In addition to these observations, increasing evidence from epidemiological studies suggests that elevated postmenopausal levels of endogenous estrogens and reduced premenopausal levels of progesterone are risk factors for endometrial cancer (see following sections).

EXCESS WEIGHT, BIOAVAILABLE ESTROGENS, AND ENDOMETRIAL CANCER RISK

Relationships of endometrial cancer risk with blood levels of endogenous estrogens have been examined in a number of case-control studies and in two prospective cohort studies.

Among postmenopausal women, several case-control studies have shown decreased plasma levels of sex hormone-binding globulin (SHBG) [32,33], as well as increased total [32–39] and bioavailable [32,39] estrogens, in endometrial cancer patients compared to cancer-free control subjects. Similar observations were made in one prospective cohort study in New York [40] and in a subsequent extension of this study that combined a total of 124 cases and 236 controls from three prospective cohorts in New York, Northern Sweden, and Milan. In the extended study, endometrial cancer risk increased approximately sixfold for postmenopausal women in the top quintile of bioavailable estradiol (unbound to SHBG) compared to those in the bottom quintile [41].

Among premenopausal women, one large case-control study showed decreased total and bioavailable estradiol in endometrial cancer patients, although they also had lower levels of SHBG and higher levels of estrone [32]. Contrary to the observations made in postmenopausal women, the lack of direct association of premenopausal serum estradiol levels with endometrial cancer risk has been tentatively explained (with support of some other observations) by the possible existence of a nonlinear relationship of estrogen levels with endometrial cancer. According to the latter hypothesis, endometrial cancer risk would be directly related to serum estradiol levels only within the postmenopausal range of 5 to 20 pg/ml, whereas there would be no such relationship within the premenopausal range (above 50 pg/ml) [14].

Excess weight results in increased estrogen concentrations from peripheral conversion of androgens to estrogens in adipose tissue by aromatase enzyme [42–44]. After menopause, when ovarian production of estrogens stops, peripheral conversions in adipose tissue of Δ4-androstenedione to estrone and of estrone and testosterone into estradiol become the primary source of endogenous estradiol [42,45]. Thus, in postmenopausal women, degree of adiposity appears to be linearly related to plasma levels of estrone and estradiol, as well as to levels of bioavailable estradiol unbound to SHBG [38,42,46–58].

In premenopausal women, contrary to postmenopausal women, excess weight and chronic hyperinsulinemia have little effect on levels of total or bioavailable estradiol [59–62]. This is due to the relatively minor contribution of estrogen production by adipose tissue compared to the ovarian estrogen production, plus the fact that, in premenopausal women, total and bioavailable estrogen levels are also regulated through negative feedback of estradiol on the pituitary secretion of follicle-stimulating hormone.

EXCESS WEIGHT, OVARIAN HYPERANDROGENISM, AND ENDOMETRIAL CANCER RISK

Several case-control studies have shown that endometrial cancer risk is also increased in pre- and postmenopausal women with elevated plasma levels of Δ4-androstenedione [32,37,38] and testosterone [63,64]. Elevated circulating androgens have also been associated with hyperplasia of the endometrium, which generally precedes and accompanies the occurrence of type-I endometrial carcinomas [10,11,65,66]. In addition to these observations, there is clear evidence for an increase in endometrial cancer risk among women with polycystic ovary syndrome — a complex metabolic syndrome of ovarian hyperandrogenism characterized by elevated plasma levels of testosterone and Δ4-androstenedione and amenorrhea or oligomenorrhea (signs of anovulatory menstrual cycles) [67].

Due to chronic anovulation and thus the lack of ovarian corpus luteum formation, this syndrome is also related to a deficit of ovarian progesterone production and low plasma progesterone levels. Cases of polycystic ovary syndrome in women developing endometrial cancer have been frequently reported, especially in young patients below the age of 40 [68–76]. Furthermore, several case-control and cohort studies have shown an increased risk of endometrial cancer among women who have polycystic ovary syndrome or among infertile women who were clinically characterized by normal plasma estrogen levels but a deficiency of progesterone, with relative risk estimates between about 3.0 to 9.0 [77–80]. Prevalence estimates of clinical polycystic ovary syndrome in premenopausal women vary between 3 and 8%, ranking it among the most common female endocrine disorders [81–85]. On the basis of these prevalence figures and of estimated average fivefold increase in endometrial cancer risk among women with polycystic ovary syndrome, this syndrome can account for about 24% of endometrial cancer cases among young, premenopausal women.

Although endometrial tissue contains androgen receptors [86,87], androgens do not appear to have any direct stimulatory effect on endometrial cell proliferation; in fact, it is possible that they may even reduce proliferation rates [88–91]. The association of plasma androgen levels with endometrial cancer risk is thus more likely to be explained by an increase in estrogens, especially in postmenopausal women, for whom plasma androgen levels are a key determinant of the amounts of estrogens formed in the endometrium and adipose tissue. In premenopausal women, ovarian androgen excess most likely increases endometrial cancer risk through reductions in ovarian progesterone production.

Excess body weight generally has not been found to be strongly related to plasma levels of Δ4-andorstenedione and testosterone in postmenopausal women [46,92–94] or in normoandrogenic premenopausal women [95–100], although obesity-induced lowering of SHBG concentrations does result in increased levels of bioavailable T, unbound to SHBG [96,99,101–105]. In premenopausal women with ovarian hyperandrogenism polycystic ovary syndrome, however, excess weight and chronic hyperinsulinemia are related to increased absolute serum androgen concentrations (see next section).

CHRONIC HYPERINSULINEMIA AND ENDOMETRIAL CANCER RISK

One major metabolic consequence of excess body weight is insulin resistance, which in turn leads to chronically elevated fasting and nonfasting plasma insulin levels [106–108]. Several studies have shown that chronically elevated blood insulin concentrations can be a risk factor for endometrial cancer. Endometrial cancer risk is increased in pre- and postmenopausal women with non-insulin-dependent diabetes [109–113] — a condition generally associated with long periods of insulin resistance and hyperinsulinemia before as well as after its diagnosis.

Furthermore, the results from at least two epidemiological studies in postmenopausal women suggest an increased risk with hyperinsulinemia, even in nondiabetic subjects. One large case-control study showed endometrial cancer risk to be associated with serum levels of C-peptide, a marker of pancreatic insulin secretion [114]. A pooled, nested case-control study in cohorts in New York, Northern Sweden, and Milan (combining a total of 166 cases and 315 controls) showed a more than fivefold increase in endometrial cancer risk for women in the highest vs. the lowest quintile of plasma C-peptide [115]. This strong relationship persisted after adjustment for BMI.

Several mechanisms could explain the direct relationship of chronically elevated insulin with increased endometrial cancer risk. First, experiments *in vitro* have shown that insulin is a key regulator of IGFBP-1 gene expression and production in endometrial tissue [116–119]; thus, it seems likely that elevated insulin could increase IGF-I activity in endometrial tissue by downregulating endometrial IGFBP-1 levels [118,120]. Second, insulin is a key regulator of the hepatic synthesis and plasma levels of SHBG, downregulating SHBG levels, and is thus a direct determinant of bioavailable estradiol unbound to SHBG, especially among postmenopausal women [46,93,95,104,121–132]. Finally, studies *in vitro* have shown stimulatory effects of insulin on androgen synthesis by ovarian tissue [133–135]; in women with polycystic ovary syndrome (but not in normoandrogenic women), hyperinsulinemia has been shown to be a major cause of ovarian androgen excess [134].

Close to half the women with clinical diagnosis of polycystic ovary syndrome are severely overweight or obese. Insulin resistance and hyperinsulinemia are present in lean and obese women with polycystic ovary syndrome [100,136–139], but are more severe in the obese subgroup [100,137,139–141]. Furthermore, most studies with polycystic ovary syndrome patients have shown direct associations of obesity or plasma insulin with levels of total plasma testosterone and Δ4-androstenedione [97,136,142–147], and anovulatory cycles are also more frequent in the obese and more insulin-resistant polycystic ovary syndrome patients [148–151]. In many women with polycystic ovary syndrome, insulin-lowering drugs can be used successfully to reduce ovarian androgen excess and restore regular menstrual cycles [152]. These various observations suggest that hyperinsulinemia may be a direct cause of chronic anovulation and progesterone deficiency.

SUMMARY

Endometrial cancer is very much a disease of the economically developed world. Epidemiological studies have shown that the high incidence rates in high-risk countries are to be attributed to lifestyle factors. One major lifestyle factor associated with increased endometrial cancer risk is excess body weight, and this association is most likely due to adiposity-induced alterations in endogenous hormone metabolism.

Epidemiological studies have shown increased endometrial cancer risks among pre- and postmenopausal women who have elevated plasma androstenedione and testosterone, as well as among postmenopausal women who have increased levels of estrone and estradiol. Furthermore, evidence is strong that chronic hyperinsulinemia is also an important risk factor. These various relationships of endometrial cancer risk with endocrine metabolism can all be interpreted in the light of the "unopposed estrogen" hypothesis, which proposes that endometrial cancer may develop as a result of the mitogenic effects of estrogens when these are insufficiently counterbalanced by progesterone. In premenopausal women, excess weight may increase risk by inducing hyperinsulinemia, ovarian hyperandrogenism (polycystic ovary syndrome), chronic anovulation, and progesterone deficiency. Among postmenopausal women, excess weight most likely continues stimulating endometrial cancer development by increasing bioavailable estrogen levels through the aromatization of the androgens in adipose tissue and the reduction of serum levels of SHBG.

REFERENCES

1. Parkin DM, Whelan SL, Ferlay J, Raymond L, and Young J *Cancer Incidence in Five Continents.* Lyon, France: IARC Press. Eds. vol. VII, N143, 1–1240. 1997.
2. Pisani P, Parkin DM & Ferlay J 1993 Estimates of the worldwide mortality from eighteen major cancers in 1985. Implications for prevention and projections of future burden. *Int J Cancer* 55 891–903.
3. International Agency for Research on Cancer, IARC Handbook of Cancer Prevention, vol. 6, 2002 *Weight Control and Physical Activity.* Lyon, France: IARC Press, 2002.
4. Bergstrom A, Pisani P, Tenet V, Wolk A & Adami HO 2001 Overweight as an avoidable cause of cancer in Europe. *Int J Cancer* 91 421–430.
5. Calle EE & Kaaks R 2004 Overweight, obesity and cancer: epidemiological evidence and proposed mechanisms. *Natl Rev Cancer* 4 579–591.
6. Preston–Martin S, Pike MC, Ross RK, Jones PA & Henderson BE 1990 Increased cell division as a cause of human cancer. *Cancer Res* 50 7415–7421.
7. Ames BN, Shigenaga MK & Gold LS 1993 DNA lesions, inducible DNA repair, and cell division: three key factors in mutagenesis and carcinogenesis. *Environ Health Perspect* 101 Suppl 5 35–44.
8. Russo J, Tay LK & Russo IH 1982 Differentiation of the mammary gland and susceptibility to carcinogenesis. *Breast Cancer Res Treat* 2 5–73.
9. Scott RE & Maercklein PB 1985 An initiator of carcinogenesis selectively and stably inhibits stem cell differentiation: a concept that initiation of carcinogenesis involves multiple phases. *Proc Natl Acad Sci USA* 82 2995–2999.
10. Sherman ME 2000 Theories of endometrial carcinogenesis: a multidisciplinary approach. *Mod. Pathol* 13 295–308.
11. Emons G, Fleckenstein G, Hinney B, Huschmand A & Heyl W 2000 Hormonal interactions in endometrial cancer. *Endocr Relat Cancer* 7 227–242.

12. Bokhman JV 1983 Two pathogenetic types of endometrial carcinoma. *Gynecol Oncol* 15 10–17.
13. Deligdisch L & Cohen CJ 1985 Histologic correlates and virulence implications of endometrial carcinoma associated with adenomatous hyperplasia. *Cancer* 56 1452–1455.
14. Key TJ & Pike MC 1988 The dose–effect relationship between "unopposed" estrogens and endometrial mitotic rate: its central role in explaining and predicting endometrial cancer risk. *Br J Cancer* 57 205–212.
15. Giudice LC, Lamson G, Rosenfeld RG & Irwin JC 1991 Insulin-like growth factor-II (IGF-II) and IGF binding proteins in human endometrium. *Ann NY Acad Sci* 626 295–307.
16. Murphy LJ & Ghahary A 1990 Uterine insulin-like growth factor-1: regulation of expression and its role in estrogen-induced uterine proliferation. *Endocr Rev* 11 443–453.
17. Kleinman D, Karas M, Roberts-CT J, Leroith D, Phillip M, Segev Y, Levy J & Sharoni Y 1995 Modulation of insulin-like growth factor I (IGF-I) receptors and membrane-associated IGF-binding proteins in endometrial cancer cells by estradiol. *Endocrinology* 136 2531–2537.
18. Leone M, Costantini C, Gallo G, Voci A, Massajoli M, Messeni LM & de CL 1993 Role of growth factors in the human endometrium during aging. *Maturitas* 16 31–38.
19. Murphy LJ, Murphy LC & Friesen HG 1987 Estrogen induces insulin-like growth factor-I expression in the rat uterus. *Mol Endocrinol* 1 445–450.
20. Zhou J, Dsupin BA, Giudice LC & Bondy CA 1994 Insulin-like growth factor system gene expression in human endometrium during the menstrual cycle. *J Clin Endocrinol Metab* 79 1723–1734.
21. Suvanto–Luukkonen E, Sundstrom H, Penttinen J, Kauppila A & Rutanen EM 1995 Insulin-like growth factor-binding protein-1: a biochemical marker of endometrial response to progestin during hormone replacement therapy. *Maturitas* 22 255–262.
22. Rutanen EM, Nyman T, Lehtovirta P, Ammala M & Pekonen F 1994 Suppressed expression of insulin-like growth factor binding protein-1 mRNA in the endometrium: a molecular mechanism associating endometrial cancer with its risk factors. *Int J Cancer* 59 307–312.
23. Bell SC 1991 The insulin-like growth factor binding proteins — the endometrium and decidua. *Ann NY Acad Sci* 622 120–137.
24. Gao JG, Mazella J & Tseng L 1994 Activation of the human IGFBP-1 gene promoter by progestin and relaxin in primary culture of human endometrial stromal cells. *Mol. Cell Endocrinol* 104 39–46.
25. Liu HC, He ZY, Mele C, Damario M, Davis O & Rosenwaks Z 1997 Hormonal regulation of expression of messenger RNA encoding insulin-like growth factor binding proteins in human endometrial stromal cells cultured *in vitro*. *Mol Hum Reprod* 3 21–6.
26. Bell SC, Jackson JA, Ashmore J, Zhu HH & Tseng L 1991 Regulation of insulin-like growth factor-binding protein-1 synthesis and secretion by progestin and relaxin in long-term cultures of human endometrial stromal cells. *J Clin Endocrinol Metab* 72 1014–1024.
27. *IARC Monographs on the Evaluation of Carcinogenic Risks to Humans* 1999: Hormonal contraception and postmenopausal hormonal therapy. 72 IARC Press, Lyon, France.
28. Weiderpass E, Adami HO, Baron JA, Magnusson C, Lindgren A & Persson I 1999 Use of oral contraceptives and endometrial cancer risk (Sweden). *Cancer Causes Control* 10 277–284.
29. Persson I, Weiderpass E, Bergkvist L, Bergstrom R & Schairer C 1999 Risks of breast and endometrial cancer after estrogen and estrogen–progestin replacement. *Cancer Causes Control* 10 253–260.
30. Pike MC & Ross RK 2000 Progestins and menopause: epidemiological studies of risks of endometrial and breast cancer. *Steroids* 65 659–664.
31. Conover CA, Hartmann LC, Bradley S, Stalboerger P, Klee GG, Kalli KR & Jenkins RB 1998 Biological characterization of human epithelial ovarian carcinoma cells in primary culture: the insulin-like growth factor system. *Exp Cell Res* 238 439–449.
32. Potischman N, Hoover RN, Brinton LA, Siiteri P, Dorgan JF, Swanson CA, Berman ML, Mortel R, Twiggs LB, Barrett RJ, Wilbanks GD, Persky V & Lurain JR 1996 Case-control study of endogenous steroid hormones and endometrial cancer. *J Natl Cancer Inst* 88 1127–1135.
33. Pettersson B, Bergstrom R & Johansson ED 1986 Serum estrogens and androgens in women with endometrial carcinoma. *Gynecol Oncol* 25 223–233.
34. Benjamin F & Deutsch S 1976 Plasma levels of fractionated estrogens and pituitary hormones in endometrial carcinoma. *Am J Obstet Gynecol* 126 638–647.
35. Aleem FA, Moukhtar MA, Hung HC & Romney SL 1976 Plasma estrogen in patients with endometrial hyperplasia and carcinoma. *Cancer* 38 2101–4.

36. Oettinger M, Samberg I, Levitan Z, Eibschitz I & Sharf M 1984 Hormonal profile of endometrial cancer. *Gynecol Obstet Invest* 17 225–35.
37. Gimes G, Szarvas Z & Siklosi G 1986 Endocrine factors in the etiology of endometrial carcinoma. *Neoplasma* 33 393–397.
38. Austin H, Austin JM, Jr., Partridge EE, Hatch KD & Shingleton HM 1991 Endometrial cancer, obesity, and body fat distribution. *Cancer Res* 51 568–572.
39. Nyholm HC, Nielsen AL, Lyndrup J, Dreisler A, Hagen C & Haug E 1993 Plasma estrogens in postmenopausal women with endometrial cancer. *Br J Obstet Gynaecol* 100 1115–1119.
40. Zeleniuch–Jacquotte A, Akhmedkhanov A, Kato I, Koenig KL, Shore RE, Kim MY, Levitz M, Mittal KR, Raju U, Banerjee S & Toniolo P 2001 Postmenopausal endogenous oestrogens and risk of endometrial cancer: results of a prospective study. *Br J Cancer* 84 975–981.
41. Lukanova A, Lundin E, Micheli A, Arslan A, Ferrari P, Rinaldi S, Krogh V, Lenner P, Shore RE, Biessy C, Muti P, Riboli E, Koenig KL, Levitz M, Stattin P, Berrino F, Hallmans G, Kaaks R, Toniolo P & Zeleniuch–Jacquotte A 2004 Circulating levels of sex steroid hormones and risk of endometrial cancer in postmenopausal women. *Int J Cancer* 108 425–432.
42. Siiteri PK 1987 Adipose tissue as a source of hormones. *Am J Clin Nutr* 45 277–282.
43. Longcope C, Pratt JH, Schneider SH & Fineberg SE 1978 Aromatization of androgens by muscle and adipose tissue in vivo. *J Clin Endocrinol Metab* 46 146–152.
44. Perel E & Killinger DW 1979 The interconversion and aromatization of androgens by human adipose tissue. *J Steroid Biochem* 10 623–627.
45. Azziz R 1989 Reproductive endocrinologic alterations in female asymptomatic obesity. *Fertil Steril* 52 703–725.
46. Kaye SA, Folsom AR, Soler JT, Prineas RJ & Potter JD 1991 Associations of body mass and fat distribution with sex hormone concentrations in postmenopausal women. *Int J Epidemiol* 20 151–156.
47. Katsouyanni K, Boyle P & Trichopoulos D 1991 Diet and urine estrogens among postmenopausal women. *Oncology* 48 490–494.
48. Vermeulen A & Verdonck L 1978 Sex hormone concentrations in post-menopausal women. *Clin Endocrinol (Oxf)* 9 59–66.
49. MacDonald PC, Edman CD, Hemsell DL, Porter JC & Siiteri PK 1978 Effect of obesity on conversion of plasma androstenedione to estrone in postmenopausal women with and without endometrial cancer. *Am J Obstet Gynecol* 130 448–455.
50. Vermeulen A 1980 Sex hormone status of the postmenopausal woman. *Maturitas* 2 81–89.
51. Nisker JA, Hammond GL, Davidson BJ, Frumar AM, Takaki NK, Judd HL & Siiteri PK 1980 Serum sex hormone-binding globulin capacity and the percentage of free estradiol in postmenopausal women with and without endometrial carcinoma. A new biochemical basis for the association between obesity and endometrial carcinoma. *Am J Obstet Gynecol* 138 637–642.
52. Davidson BJ, Gambone JC, Lagasse LD, Castaldo TW, Hammond GL, Siiteri PK & Judd HL 1981 Free estradiol in postmenopausal women with and without endometrial cancer. *J Clin Endocrinol Metab* 52 404–408.
53. Kirschner MA, Schneider G, Ertel NH & Worton E 1982 Obesity, androgens, estrogens, and cancer risk. *Cancer Res* 42 3281s–3285s.
54. Klinga K, von Holst T & Runnebaum B 1983 Influence of severe obesity on peripheral hormone concentrations in pre- and postmenopausal women. *Eur J Obstet Gynecol Reprod Biol* 15 103–112.
55. Bruning PF, Bonfrer JM & Hart AA 1985 Nonprotein bound oestradiol, sex hormone binding globulin, breast cancer and breast cancer risk. *Br J Cancer* 51 479–84.
56. Enriori CL, Orsini W, del-Carmen CM, Etkin AE, Cardillo LR & Reforzo MJ 1986 Decrease of circulating level of SHBG in postmenopausal obese women as a risk factor in breast cancer: reversible effect of weight loss. *Gynecol Oncol* 23 77–86.
57. Toniolo PG, Levitz M, Zeleniuch–Jacquotte A, Banerjee S, Koenig KL, Shore RE, Strax P & Pasternack BS 1995 A prospective study of endogenous estrogens and breast cancer in postmenopausal women. *J Natl Cancer Inst* 87 190–197.
58. Zeleniuch–Jacquotte A, Bruning PF, Bonfrer JM, Koenig KL, Shore RE, Kim MY, Pasternack BS & Toniolo P 1997 Relation of serum levels of testosterone and dehydroepiandrosterone sulfate to risk of breast cancer in postmenopausal women. *Am J Epidemiol* 145 1030–1038.

59. Verkasalo PK, Thomas HV, Appleby PN, Davey GK & Key TJ 2001 Circulating levels of sex hormones and their relation to risk factors for breast cancer: a cross-sectional study in 1092 pre- and postmenopausal women (U.K.). *Cancer Causes Control* 12 47–59.
60. Dorgan JF, Reichman ME, Judd JT, Brown C, Longcope C, Schatzkin A, Albanes D, Campbell WS, Franz C & Kahle L. 1995 The relation of body size to plasma levels of estrogens and androgens in premenopausal women (Maryland, U.S.). *Cancer Causes Control* 6 3–8.
61. Thomas HV, Key TJ, Allen DS, Moore JW, Dowsett M, Fentiman IS & Wang DY 1997 Re: reversal of relation between body mass and endogenous estrogen concentrations with menopausal status [letter; comment]. *J Natl Cancer Inst* 89 396–398.
62. Nagata C, Kaneda N, Kabuto M & Shimizu H 1997 Factors associated with serum levels of estradiol and sex hormone-binding globulin among premenopausal Japanese women. *Environ Health Perspect* 105 994–997.
63. Mollerstrom G, Carlstrom K, Lagrelius A & Einhorn N 1993 Is there an altered steroid profile in patients with endometrial carcinoma? *Cancer* 72 173–181.
64. Nagamani M, Hannigan EV, Dillard EA, Jr. & Van Dinh T 1986 Ovarian steroid secretion in postmenopausal women with and without endometrial cancer. *J Clin Endocrinol Metab* 62 508–512.
65. Vitoratos N, Gregoriou O, Hassiakos D & Zourlas PA 1991 The role of androgens in the late-premenopausal woman with adenomatous hyperplasia of the endometrium. *Int J Gynaecol Obstet* 34 157–161.
66. Terada S, Suzuki N, Uchide K, Akasofu K & Nishida E 1993 Effects of testosterone on the development of endometrial tumors in female rats. *Gynecol Obstet Invest* 36 29–33.
67. Franks S 1995 Polycystic ovary syndrome. *N Engl J Med* 333 853–861.
68. Sommers SC, Hertig AT & Bengloff H 1949 Genesis of endometrial carcinoma. II. Cases 19 to 35 years old. *Cancer* 2 957–963.
69. Speert H 1949 Carcinoma of the endometrium in young women. *Surg Gynecol Obstet* 88 332–336.
70. DeVere RD & Dempster DR 1953 A case of the Stein–Leventhal syndrome associated with carcinoma of the endometrium. *J Obstet Gynaecol Br Emp* 60 865–867.
71. Jackson RL, Dockerty MB & Minn R 1957 The Stein–Leventhal Syndrome: Analysis of 43 cases with special reference to association with Endometrial Carcinoma. *Am J Obstet Gynecol* 73 161–173.
72. Castleman B & McNeely BU 1966 Case records of the Massachusetts General Hospital. Case 25–1966. *N Engl J Med* 274 1260–1267.
73. Wood GP & Boronow RC 1976 Endometrial adenocarcinoma and the polycystic ovary syndrome. *Am J Obstet Gynecol* 124 140–142.
74. Gallup DG & Stock RJ 1984 Adenocarcinoma of the endometrium in women 40 years of age or younger. *Obstet Gynecol* 64 417–420.
75. Farhi DC, Nosanchuk J & Silverberg SG 1986 Endometrial adenocarcinoma in women under 25 years of age. *Obstet Gynecol* 68 741–745.
76. Colafranceschi M, Taddei GL, Scarselli G, Branconi F, Tinacci G & Savino L 1989 Clinico-pathological profile of endometrial carcinoma in young women (under 40 years of age). *Eur J Gynaecol Oncol* 10 353–356.
77. Shu XO, Brinton LA, Zheng W, Gao YT, Fan J & Fraumeni JFJ 1991 A population-based case-control study of endometrial cancer in Shanghai, China. *Int J Cancer* 49 38–43.
78. Niwa K, Imai A, Hashimoto M, Yokoyama Y, Mori H, Matsuda Y & Tamaya T 2000 A case-control study of uterine endometrial cancer of pre- and postmenopausal women. *Oncol Rep* 7 89–93.
79. Coulam CB, Annegers JF & Kranz JS 1983 Chronic anovulation syndrome and associated neoplasia. *Obstet Gynecol* 61 403–407.
80. Modan B, Ron E, Lerner GL, Blumstein T, Menczer J, Rabinovici J, Oelsner G, Freedman L, Mashiach S & Lunenfeld B 1998 Cancer incidence in a cohort of infertile women. *Am J Epidemiol* 147 1038–1042.
81. Adams J, Polson DW & Franks S 1986 Prevalence of polycystic ovaries in women with anovulation and idiopathic hirsutism. *Br Med J Clin Res Ed* 293 355–359.
82. Polson DW, Adams J, Wadsworth J & Franks S 1988 Polycystic ovaries — a common finding in normal women. *Lancet* 1 870–872.
83. Conway GS, Honour JW & Jacobs HS 1989 Heterogeneity of the polycystic ovary syndrome: clinical, endocrine and ultrasound features in 556 patients. *Clin Endocrinol Oxf* 30 459–470.

84. Franks S 1989 Polycystic ovary syndrome: a changing perspective. *Clin Endocrinol Oxf* 31 87–120.
85. Asuncion M, Calvo RM, San Millan JL, Sancho J, Avila S & Escobar–Morreale HF 2000 A prospective study of the prevalence of the polycystic ovary syndrome in unselected Caucasian women from Spain. *J Clin Endocrinol Metab* 85 2434–2438.
86. Mertens HJ, Heineman MJ, Koudstaal J, Theunissen P & Evers JL 1996 Androgen receptor content in human endometrium. *Eur J Obstet Gynecol Reprod Biol* 70 11–13.
87. Horie K, Takakura K, Imai K, Liao S & Mori T 1992 Immunohistochemical localization of androgen receptor in the human endometrium, decidua, placenta and pathological conditions of the endometrium. *Hum Reprod* 7 1461–1466.
88. Hackenberg R, Beck S, Filmer A, Hushmand NA, Kunzmann R, Koch M, Slater EP & Schulz KD 1994 Androgen responsiveness of the new human endometrial cancer cell line MFE-296. *Int J Cancer* 57 117–122.
89. Legro RS, Kunselman AR, Miller SA & Satyaswaroop PG 2001 Role of androgens in the growth of endometrial carcinoma: an *in vivo* animal model. *Am J Obstet Gynecol* 184 303–308.
90. Tuckerman EM, Okon MA, Li T & Laird SM 2000 Do androgens have a direct effect on endometrial function? An *in vitro* study. *Fertil Steril* 74 771–779.
91. Neulen J, Wagner B, Runge M & Breckwoldt M 1987 Effect of progestins, androgens, estrogens and antiestrogens on 3H-thymidine uptake by human endometrial and endosalpinx cells *in vitro*. *Arch Gynecol* 240 225–232.
92. Newcomb PA, Klein R, Klein BE, Haffner S, Mares–Perlman J, Cruickshanks KJ & Marcus PM 1995 Association of dietary and life-style factors with sex hormones in postmenopausal women. *Epidemiology* 6 318–321.
93. Turcato E, Zamboni M, De Pergola G, Armellini F, Zivelonghi A, Bergamo–Andreis IA, Giorgino R & Bosello O 1997 Interrelationships between weight loss, body fat distribution and sex hormones in pre- and postmenopausal obese women. *J Intern Med* 241 363–372.
94. Cauley JA, Gutai JP, Kuller LH, LeDonne D & Powell JG 1989 The epidemiology of serum sex hormones in postmenopausal women. *Am J Epidemiol* 129 1120–1131.
95. Evans DJ, Hoffmann RG, Kalkhoff RK & Kissebah AH 1983 Relationship of androgenic activity to body fat topography, fat cell morphology, and metabolic aberrations in premenopausal women. *J Clin Endocrinol Metab* 57 304–310.
96. de Ridder CM, Bruning PF, Zonderland ML, Thijssen JH, Bonfrer JM, Blankenstein MA, Huisveld IA & Erich WB 1990 Body fat mass, body fat distribution, and plasma hormones in early puberty in females. *J Clin Endocrinol Metab* 70 888–893.
97. Holte J, Bergh T, Gennarelli G & Wide L 1994 The independent effects of polycystic ovary syndrome and obesity on serum concentrations of gonadotrophins and sex steroids in premenopausal women. *Clin Endocrinol Oxf* 41 473–481.
98. Zumoff B 1988 Hormonal abnormalities in obesity. *Acta Med Scand Suppl* 723 153–160.
99. Penttila TL, Koskinen P, Penttila TA, Anttila L & Irjala K 1999 Obesity regulates bioavailable testosterone levels in women with or without polycystic ovary syndrome. *Fertil Steril* 71 457–461.
100. Morales AJ, Laughlin GA, Butzow T, Maheshwari H, Baumann G & Yen SS 1996 Insulin, somatotropic, and luteinizing hormone axes in lean and obese women with polycystic ovary syndrome: common and distinct features. *J Clin Endocrinol Metab* 81 2854–2864.
101. Leenen R, van der KK, Seidell JC, Deurenberg P & Koppeschaar HP 1994 Visceral fat accumulation in relation to sex hormones in obese men and women undergoing weight loss therapy. *J Clin Endocrinol.Metab* 78 1515–1520.
102. Bernasconi D, Del Monte P, Meozzi M, Randazzo M, Marugo A, Badaracco B & Marugo M 1996 The impact of obesity on hormonal parameters in hirsute and nonhirsute women. *Metabolism* 45 72–75.
103. Ivandic A, Prpic–Krizevac I, Sucic M & Juric M 1998 Hyperinsulinemia and sex hormones in healthy premenopausal women: relative contribution of obesity, obesity type, and duration of obesity. *Metabolism* 47 13–19.
104. Seidell JC, Cigolini M, Charzewska J, Ellsinger BM, Di Biase G, Bjorntorp P, Hautvast JG, Contaldo F, Szostak V & Scuro LA 1990 Androgenicity in relation to body fat distribution and metabolism in 38-year-old women — the European Fat Distribution Study. *J Clin Epidemiol* 43 21–34.
105. Wajchenberg BL, Marcondes JA, Mathor MB, Achando SS, Germak OA & Kirschner MA 1989 Free testosterone levels during the menstrual cycle in obese versus normal women. *Fertil Steril* 51 535–537.

106. Abate N 1996 Insulin resistance and obesity. The role of fat distribution pattern. *Diabetes Care* 19 292–294.
107. Bjorntorp P 1992 Metabolic abnormalities in visceral obesity. *Ann Med* 24 3–5.
108. Unger R & Foster DW 1998 Diabetes mellitus. In *Williams Textbook of Endocrinology*, 8th ed., 1255–1333. JD Wilson & DW Foster, Eds. Philadelphia: W.B. Saunders Company.
109. O'Mara BA, Byers T & Schoenfeld E 1985 Diabetes mellitus and cancer risk: a multisite case-control study. *J Chronic.Dis* 38 435–441.
110. Adami HO, McLaughlin J, Ekbom A, Berne C, Silverman D, Hacker D & Persson I 1991 Cancer risk in patients with diabetes mellitus. *Cancer Causes Control* 2 307–314.
111. Franceschi S, La Vecchia C, Booth M, Tzonou A, Negri E, Parazzini F, Trichopoulos D & Beral V 1991 Pooled analysis of three European case-control studies of ovarian cancer: II. Age at menarche and at menopause. *Int J Cancer* 49 57–60.
112. Weiderpass E, Gridley G, Persson I, Nyren O, Ekbom A & Adami HO 1997 Risk of endometrial and breast cancer in patients with diabetes mellitus. *Int J Cancer* 71 360–363.
113. Shoff SM & Newcomb PA 1998 Diabetes, body size, and risk of endometrial cancer. *Am J Epidemiol* 148 234–240.
114. Troisi R, Potischman N, Hoover RN, Siiteri P & Brinton LA 1997 Insulin and endometrial cancer. *Am J Epidemiol* 146 476–482.
115. Lukanova A, Zeleniuch–Jacquotte A, Lundin E, Micheli A, Arslan AA, Rinaldi S, Muti P, Lenner P, Koenig KL, Biessy C, Krogh V, Riboli E, Shore RE, Stattin P, Berrino F, Hallmans G, Toniolo P & Kaaks R 2004 Prediagnostic levels of C-peptide, IGF-I, IGFBP -1, -2 and -3 and risk of endometrial cancer. *Int J Cancer* 108 262–268.
116. Lin J, Li R & Zhou J 2003 The influence of insulin on secretion of IGF-I and IGFBP-I in cultures of human endometrial stromal cells. *Chin Med J (Engl)* 116 301–304.
117. Lathi R, Hess A, Tulac S, Nayak N, Conti M & Giudice LC 2005 Dose-dependent insulin regulation of IGFBP-1 in human endometrial stromal cells is mediated by distinct signaling pathways. *J Clin Endocrinol Metab* 90 1599–1606.
118. Irwin JC, de las FL, Dsupin BA & Giudice LC 1993 Insulin-like growth factor regulation of human endometrial stromal cell function: coordinate effects on insulin-like growth factor binding protein-1, cell proliferation and prolactin secretion. *Regul Pept* 48 165–177.
119. Lee PD, Giudice LC, Conover CA & Powell DR 1997 Insulin-like growth factor binding protein-1: recent findings and new directions. *Proc Soc Exp Biol Med* 216 319–357.
120. Ayabe T, Tsutsumi O, Sakai H, Yoshikawa H, Yano T, Kurimoto F & Taketani Y 1997 Increased circulating levels of insulin-like growth factor-I and decreased circulating levels of insulin-like growth factor binding protein-1 in postmenopausal women with endometrial cancer. *Endocr J* 44 419–424.
121. Crave JC, Fimbel S, Lejeune H, Cugnardey N, Dechaud H & Pugeat M 1995 Effects of diet and metformin administration on sex hormone-binding globulin, androgens, and insulin in hirsute and obese women. *J Clin Endocrinol Metab* 80 2057–2062.
122. Pugeat M, Crave JC, Elmidani M, Nicolas MH, Garoscio CM, Lejeune H, Dechaud H & Tourniaire J 1991 Pathophysiology of sex hormone binding globulin (SHBG): relation to insulin. *J Steroid Biochem Mol Biol* 40 841–849.
123. Pasquali R, Vicennati V, Bertazzo D, Casimirri F, Pascal G, Tortelli O & Labate AM 1997 Determinants of sex hormone-binding globulin blood concentrations in premenopausal and postmenopausal women with different estrogen status. Virgilio Menopause Health Group. *Metabolism* 46 5–9.
124. Pasquali R, Casimirri F, Plate L & Capelli M 1990 Characterization of obese women with reduced sex hormone-binding globulin concentrations. *Horm Metab Res* 22 303–306.
125. Nestler JE, Powers LP, Matt DW, Steingold KA, Plymate SR, Rittmaster RS, Clore JN & Blackard WG 1991 A direct effect of hyperinsulinemia on serum sex hormone-binding globulin levels in obese women with the polycystic ovary syndrome. *J Clin Endocrinol Metab* 72 83–89.
126. Nestler JE 2000 Obesity, insulin, sex steroids and ovulation. *Int J Obes Relat Metab Disord* 24 Suppl 2 S71–S73.
127. Peiris AN, Sothmann MS, Aiman EJ & Kissebah AH 1989 The relationship of insulin to sex hormone-binding globulin: role of adiposity. *Fertil Steril* 52 69–72.

128. Kirschner MA, Samojlik E, Drejka M, Szmal E, Schneider G & Ertel N 1990 Androgen-estrogen metabolism in women with upper body versus lower body obesity. *J Clin Endocrinol Metab* 70 473–479.
129. Weaver JU, Holly JM, Kopelman PG, Noonan K, Giadom CG, White N, Virdee S & Wass JA 1990 Decreased sex hormone binding globulin (SHBG) and insulin-like growth factor binding protein (IGFBP-1) in extreme obesity. *Clin Endocrinol Oxf* 33 415–422.
130. Sharp PS, Kiddy DS, Reed MJ, Anyaoku V, Johnston DG & Franks S 1991 Correlation of plasma insulin and insulin-like growth factor-I with indices of androgen transport and metabolism in women with polycystic ovary syndrome. *Clin Endocrinol Oxf* 35 253–257.
131. Haffner SM, Dunn JF & Katz MS 1992 Relationship of sex hormone-binding globulin to lipid, lipoprotein, glucose, and insulin concentrations in postmenopausal women. *Metabolism* 41 278–284.
132. Preziosi P, Barrett CE, Papoz L, Roger M, Saint PM, Nahoul K & Simon D 1993 Interrelation between plasma sex hormone-binding globulin and plasma insulin in healthy adult women: the telecom study. *J Clin Endocrinol Metab* 76 283–287.
133. Kaaks R 1996 Nutrition, hormones, and breast cancer: is insulin the missing link? *Cancer Causes Control* 7 605–625.
134. Poretsky L, Cataldo NA, Rosenwaks Z & Giudice LC 1999 The insulin-related ovarian regulatory system in health and disease. *Endocr Rev* 20 535–582.
135. Cara JF 1994 Insulin-like growth factors, insulin-like growth factor binding proteins and ovarian androgen production. *Horm Res* 42 49–54.
136. Chang RJ, Nakamura RM, Judd HL & Kaplan SA 1983 Insulin resistance in nonobese patients with polycystic ovarian disease. *J Clin Endocrinol Metab* 57 356–359.
137. Dunaif A, Graf M, Mandeli J, Laumas V & Dobrjansky A 1987 Characterization of groups of hyperandrogenic women with acanthosis nigricans, impaired glucose tolerance, and/or hyperinsulinemia. *J Clin Endocrinol Metab* 65 499–507.
138. Dunaif A, Segal KR, Futterweit W & Dobrjansky A 1989 Profound peripheral insulin resistance, independent of obesity, in polycystic ovary syndrome. *Diabetes* 38 1165–1174.
139. Rittmaster RS, Deshwal N & Lehman L 1993 The role of adrenal hyperandrogenism, insulin resistance, and obesity in the pathogenesis of polycystic ovarian syndrome. *J Clin Endocrinol Metab* 76 1295–1300.
140. Grulet H, Hecart AC, Delemer B, Gross A, Sulmont V, Leutenegger M & Caron J 1993 Roles of LH and insulin resistance in lean and obese polycystic ovary syndrome. *Clin Endocrinol Oxf* 38 621–626.
141. Rajkhowa M, Bicknell J, Jones M & Clayton RN 1994 Insulin sensitivity in women with polycystic ovary syndrome: relationship to hyperandrogenemia. *Fertil Steril* 61 605–612.
142. Burghen GA, Givens JR & Kitabchi AE 1980 Correlation of hyperandrogenism with hyperinsulinism in polycystic ovarian disease. *J Clin Endocrinol Metab* 50 113–116.
143. Shoupe D, Kumar DD & Lobo RA 1983 Insulin resistance in polycystic ovary syndrome. *Am J Obstet Gynecol* 147 588–592.
144. Pasquali R, Casimirri F, Venturoli S, Paradisi R, Mattioli L, Capelli M, Melchionda N & Labo G 1983 Insulin resistance in patients with polycystic ovaries; its relationship to body weight and androgen levels. *Acta Endocrinol Copenhagen* 104 110–116.
145. Nagamani M, Van DT & Kelver ME 1986 Hyperinsulinemia in hyperthecosis of the ovaries. *Am J Obstet Gynecol* 154 384–389.
146. Wajchenberg BL, Giannella ND, Lerario AC, Marcondes JA & Ohnuma LY 1988 Role of obesity and hyperinsulinemia in the insulin resistance of obese subjects with the clinical triad of polycystic ovaries, hirsutism and *Acanthosis nigricans*. *Horm Res* 29 7–13.
147. Pasquali R, Casimirri F, Venturoli S, Antonio M, Morselli L, Reho S, Pezzoli A & Paradisi R 1994 Body fat distribution has weight-independent effects on clinical, hormonal, and metabolic features of women with polycystic ovary syndrome. *Metabolism* 43 706–713.
148. Kiddy DS, Sharp PS, White DM, Scanlon MF, Mason HD, Bray CS, Polson DW, Reed MJ & Franks S 1990 Differences in clinical and endocrine features between obese and nonobese subjects with polycystic ovary syndrome: an analysis of 263 consecutive cases. *Clin Endocrinol Oxf* 32 213–220.
149. Soler JT, Folsom AR, Kaye SA & Prineas RJ 1989 Associations of abdominal adiposity, fasting insulin, sex hormone binding globulin, and estrone with lipids and lipoproteins in post-menopausal women. *Atherosclerosis* 79 21–27.

150. Robinson S, Kiddy D, Gelding SV, Willis D, Niththyananthan R, Bush A, Johnston DG & Franks S 1993 The relationship of insulin insensitivity to menstrual pattern in women with hyperandrogenism and polycystic ovaries. *Clin Endocrinol Oxf* 39 351–355.
151. Barbieri RL, Smith S & Ryan KJ 1988 The role of hyperinsulinemia in the pathogenesis of ovarian hyperandrogenism. *Fertil Steril* 50 197–212.
152. Baillargeon JP, Iuorno MJ & Nestler JE 2003 Insulin sensitizers for polycystic ovary syndrome. *Clin Obstet Gynecol* 46 325–340.

17 Obesity and Pancreatic Cancer

Dominique S. Michaud and Edward Giovannucci

CONTENTS

INTRODUCTION

Pancreatic cancer is the fourth leading cause of cancer deaths in the U.S. [1] and the sixth leading cause of cancer death in Europe [2]. Most patients with pancreatic cancer are diagnosed late in the progression of the disease and have a life expectancy of several months. In Europe and in the U.S., the 1-year and 5-year survival rates for pancreatic cancer are less than 25 and 5%, respectively, and mortality rates are essentially identical to incidence rates [2,3]. Survival rates have only improved slightly over the past decade due to the lack of significant medical advancements in the early detection or treatment of pancreatic cancer. The majority of pancreatic cancers are exocrine adenocarcinomas of the pancreas. Islet tumors of the endocrine pancreas and other types of exocrine tumors (e.g., sarcomas) are very rare.

Pancreatic cancer is rare in the first three decades of life. After age 30, however, incidence rates increase exponentially and peak in the seventh and eighth decades [3]. Men consistently have higher incidence and mortality rates than women and, in the U.S., blacks have higher incidence and mortality rates than whites [3]. Pancreatic cancer rates are lower in developing countries than in developed countries [4]. Mortality rates in both sexes have increased over the past four decades in a number of countries where rates had been low in the mid-1950s, such as Japan, Spain, Italy, Bulgaria, Poland, and Yugoslavia [5]. In Japan, age-standardized mortality rates have jumped from 1.4 per 100,000 to 12.5 per 100,000 in men between 1950 and 1995 [6], demonstrating that environmental factors play an important role.

Tobacco smoking is the one of the few established risk factors for pancreatic cancer. Inherited susceptibility explains a small fraction (5 to 10%) of pancreatic cancers, but the genes responsible for familial pancreatic cancer have not yet been identified. Late onset diabetes, or type-2 diabetes, has been consistently associated with elevated risks of pancreatic cancer. In a meta-analysis of 20 studies with data on the duration of diabetes prior to pancreatic cancer, individuals with diabetic histories of 5 or more years had a twofold elevation in pancreatic cancer risk compared to those without a history of diabetes, or diabetes of less than 5 years duration (95% confidence interval 1.2 to 3.2) [7]. In several recent studies, including three cohort studies, relative risks for pancreatic cancer ranged between 1.3 and 1.7 for individuals with long-standing diabetes (10 or more years), compared to those with no diabetes [8–11]. The strength and consistency of these studies suggest that a diabetic state, which develops 10 or more years prior to cancer diagnosis, is likely to be related causally to the development of pancreatic tumors.

The association between type-2 diabetes and pancreatic cancer risk may be the result of years of elevated postload glucose concentration, hyperinsulinemia, and gradual impaired glucose tolerance. In a prospective study of nondiabetics in which blood was obtained an average of 25 years prior to pancreatic cancer diagnosis, postload glucose concentration was directly associated with pancreatic cancer risk in men and women [12]. In a similar prospective study with 10 years of follow-up, positive associations were observed between fasting serum glucose levels and pancreatic cancer mortality in men and women (trend test, p-value = 0.01) [13]. In that study, conducted in Korea, even modestly elevated fasting serum glucose levels were associated with higher pancreatic cancer mortality in women (RR = 1.45, 95% CI = 1.16 to 1.81, for fasting glucose levels between 90 and 109 compared to <90 mg/dL) [13] . These two studies, together with the well-established relation with late onset diabetes, suggest that body weight and insulin resistance may play an important role in the etiology of pancreatic cancer.

IN VITRO AND ANIMAL STUDIES

Human pancreatic tumors are believed to arise from ductal cells because tumors show ductal structure. However, it has been argued that tumors may arise from acinar cells [14], islets of Langerhans cells, or stem cells [15] and that they appear ductal in shape due to differentiation. In the hamster model (hamsters treated with the pancreatic carcinogen *N*-nitrosobis(2-oxopropyl)amine [BOP]), which in many aspects is identical to the human disease, most ductal-type cancers develop within islets [16]. The histogenesis of pancreatic cancer is not well understood and difficult to establish because tumors are not usually detected until late in the progression of the disease.

At least two different mechanisms could contribute to a positive association between obesity and pancreatic cancer. The first mechanism described here involves insulin and insulin resistance and may also explain the relation between type-2 diabetes and pancreatic cancer. The second mechanism involves gastrointestinal hormones.

In vitro studies show that insulin promotes growth of hamster, rat, and numerous human pancreatic cell lines [17–25]. Although insulin is known to stimulate cell proliferation, it does not appear to be directly responsible in promoting pancreatic cancer, given that administration of exogenous insulin has an inhibitory effect on tumor induction in the hamster pancreatic cancer model [26,27]. Studies suggest that islet cell turnover, associated with insulin resistance, may play an important role in pancreatic carcinogenesis. Stimulation of islet cell proliferation enhances pancreatic ductal carcinogenesis in hamsters [28], and the destruction of islet cells by streptozotocin or alloxan inhibits cancer induction [29–31].

In a recent study, hamster pancreatic cancer was inhibited by the drug metformin, which normalized insulin levels and the rate of islet cell turnover [32]. In a cohort study of patients with type-I diabetes (a disease in which islet cells are destroyed by the body), the number of pancreatic cancer cases observed was much lower than expected in those hospitalized with diabetes 15 or more years prior to cancer diagnosis (SIR = 0.1, 95% CI = 0.1 to 3.8) [33]. Although the number of cases is small and results are unstable, this finding supports the hypothesis that islet cell proliferation may play a role in pancreatic carcinogenesis.

The second mechanism that may explain the association between obesity and pancreatic cancer may be related to production of gastrointestinal hormones such as cholecystokinin or gastrin. Excess caloric intake, which can lead to weight gain, is likely to occur with frequent food consumption. With food intake, gastrointestinal hormones, such as gastrin and cholecystokinin, are elevated. Cholecystokinin, in turn, stimulates the secretion of enzymes from the exocrine pancreas. Cholecystokinin and gastrin promote growth of numerous pancreatic cancer cell lines [34–36]. In the rat model, endogenous hypergastrinaemia and hypercholecystokininemia induced carcinogenesis in acinar cells of the pancreas [37–39]. Hypergastrinaemia, however, did not enhance induced pancreatic carcinogenesis in the hamster model [40], and findings of hypercholecystokininemia in hamster models have been inconsistent [41–44].

LIMITATIONS OF STUDY DESIGNS IN EPIDEMIOLOGICAL STUDIES

Because of the rapidly fatal nature of pancreatic cancer, case-control studies on this cancer typically have low participation rates and rely heavily on next of kin (i.e., proxies) to obtain exposure data. In these circumstances, selection and recall biases are likely to occur. In an attempt to reduce error introduced when including proxy data, some case-control studies have chosen to keep only cases who responded directly to the questions asked. However, these case-control studies are more prone to survival bias because patients with the most aggressive cancers will be too ill or deceased by the time they are identified.

When studying body weight, case-control studies of pancreatic cancer may be more prone to recall bias because weight loss often occurs several years prior to pancreatic cancer diagnosis and is often a primary characteristic leading to the detection of this cancer. Similarly, use of proxies to obtain data on patients 2 years prior to interview may lead to weight misclassification because proxies are less likely to remember the patient's weight accurately. With proxy interviews, error in reporting weight may be random or biased if, for example, proxies consistently underestimate patients' weight. Recall bias due to weight loss and use of proxy interviews may explain why a number of case-control studies failed to observe associations between obesity and pancreatic cancer risk. In contrast, cohort studies are not prone to these types of errors because weight information is collected prior to disease and proxy interviews are not used.

Although the cohort study design is optimal to examine weight and pancreatic cancer, this type of study is often limited by power, given that pancreatic cancer incidence is ranked 11th out of all cancers (in the U.S., 2004) [1]. Consequently, men and women are often combined and numerous years of follow-up must be available to obtain reasonable sample sizes. Another potential limitation, which may apply to either type of study design but is perhaps more common in "healthy" cohorts, is weight range; some studies may not be suited to examine body weight if few participants classify as obese. In some cohort studies, the associations between weight and pancreatic cancer mortality have been reported, due to the lack of incidence data. However, mortality studies should lead to similar results, given the high fatality of pancreatic cancer.

CASE-CONTROL STUDIES

Results from case-control and cohort studies are summarized in Table 17.1. Four case-control studies observed no association between weight and pancreatic cancer risk [45–48]. All of these studies relied on proxy interviews to obtain body weight of cases. The largest was a collaborative case-control study that combined data from five studies in four different countries (Canada, Poland, The Netherlands, Australia) to obtain 802 pancreatic cancer cases [46]. No association with BMI was observed overall or in the five individual centers that contributed to the collaborative case-control study; detailed results from two of the five studies were published separately [45,47].

The four most recent case-control studies were conducted using only direct interviews and had over 300 cases of pancreatic cancer cases each (Table 17.1) [49–52]. Positive associations between body weight and pancreatic cancer risk were observed in men and women in all four studies. In two studies [49,51], "usual" adult weight was reported instead of current weight, which may have helped reduce bias associated with preclinical weight loss. In a U.S. study, a 50% increase in risk of pancreatic cancer was observed for men and women (individually) for the highest quartile of

TABLE 17.1
Case-Control and Cohorts Studies Examining the Association between Body Mass Index (BMI) and the Risk of Pancreatic Cancer

First author (year)	Country	Proxies[a]	Adjusted smoking/diabetes		Cases	Gender	RR (95% CI)	BMI category cutpoints (kg/m²)[b]
Case-control studies								
Bueno de Mesquita (1990)	Netherlands	48%	Y	N	90	M	0.88 (0.40–1.94)	>27.9 vs. ≤23.0
					74	F	1.13 (0.46–2.80)	>28.7 vs. ≤21.6
Ghadirian (1991)	Canada	75%	Y	N	179	M, F	0.88 (0.42–1.85)	>26.5 vs. ≤21
Howe (1991)[c]	Canada, Poland Netherlands, Australia	65%	Y	N	802	M, F	1.00 (0.73–1.36)	>27.9 vs. ≤21.9
Lyon (1993)	U.S.	100%	N	N	149 (M, F)	M	0.83 (0.43–1.58)	Top vs. bottom tertile
						F	1.05 (0.53–2.08)	Top vs. bottom tertile
Ji (1996)	China	No	Y	Y	255	M	1.46 (0.85–2.51)	>22.5 vs. ≤19.4 (usual)
					183	F	1.38 (0.91–2.08)	>23.2 vs. ≤19.4 (usual)
Silverman (1998)	U.S.	No	Y	Y	218	M	1.5 (1.0–2.3)	≥27.2 vs. <23.2 (usual)
					213	F	1.5 (0.9–2.5)	≥34.4 vs. <27.6[d] (usual)
Hanley (2001)	Canada	No	Y	N	173	M	1.90 (1.08–3.35)	≥28.3 vs. <23.7
					139	F	1.21 (0.70–2.06)	≥27.4 vs. <22.1
Pan (2004)	Canada	No	Y	N	355	M	1.43 (1.02–1.98)	≥30 vs. <25
					275	F	1.63 (1.14–2.34)	≥30 vs. <25
Cohort studies								
Friedman (1993)	U.S.		Y	Y	450	M, F	1.05 (1.00–1.10)	for 5 kg increment
Shibata (1994)	U.S.		Y	N	65	M, F	1.23 (0.66–2.28)	≥23.9 vs. <21.8 (M)
								≥23.2 vs. <20.4 (F)
Gapstur (2000)	U.S.		Y	Y	96	M	3.04 (1.52–6.08)	≥28.6 vs. <24.2
					43	F	0.73 (0.30–1.80)	≥26.2 vs. <21.0
Michaud (2001)	U.S.		Y	Y	140	M	1.76 (0.90–3.45)	≥30.0 vs. <23.0
					210	F	1.70 (1.09–2.64)	≥30.0 vs. <23.0

Stolzenberg-Solomon (2002)	Finland	Y	Y	172	M	0.91 (0.56–1.48)	>29.2 vs. ≤23.1
Isaksson (2002)	Sweden	Y	N	176	M, F	0.56 (0.2–1.52)	>30.0 vs. <18.5
Lee (2003)	U.S.	Y	Y	212	M, F[e]	0.99 (0.60–1.62)	≥27.5 vs. <22.5
Calle (2003)	U.S.	Y	N	1908	M	1.49 (0.99–2.22)	≥35.0 vs. <25.0
				1650	F	2.76 (1.74–4.36)	≥40.0 vs. <25.0
Patel (2005)	U.S.	Y	Y	137	M	2.38 (1.50–3.78)	>30.0 vs. <25.0
				105	F	1.73 (1.02–2.92)	>30.0 vs. <25.0
Obesity cohort studies[f]							
Moller (1994)	Denmark	N	N	34	M	1.8 (1.2–2.5)	Obese vs. nonobese
				67	F	1.7 (1.3–2.2)	Obese vs. nonobese
Wolk (2001)	Sweden	N	N	29	M	2.4 (1.6–3.4)	Obese vs. nonobese
				34	F	1.1 (0.8–1.5)	Obese vs. nonobese
Samanic (2004)	U.S.	N	N	5874	M (White)	1.20 (1.07–1.33)	Obese vs. nonobese
				1721	M (Black)	1.07 (0.86–1.34)	Obese vs. nonobese

[a]In case-control studies.

[b]BMI for case-control studies is based on weight 2 years prior to interview, unless specified otherwise (usual = usual adult weight); BMI for cohort studies is at cohort baseline.

[c]Collaborative study of five case-control studies; includes data from Ghadirian, P. et al., *Int J Cancer* 1991; 47:1–6 and Bueno de Mesquita, H.B. et al., *Int J Cancer* 1990; 46:435–444.

[d]BMI for women is kg/m$^{1.5}$.

[e]Only 5 cases are women.

[f]Obese is based on a medical diagnosis.

BMI, compared to the bottom quartile [49]. In this study, the association reported for the top BMI quartile and the linear test for trend were only statistically significant among men, possibly due to a smaller number of cases among women (n = 213). Positive associations of similar magnitude (relative risks ranging between 1.2 to 1.9) were observed for men and women in two Canadian studies using similar cutpoints for BMI (Table 17.1) [50,52]. The fourth study to show a positive association was conducted in an Asian population with relatively low BMI cutpoints for the highest category [51]. To date, this is the only study on weight and pancreatic cancer risk conducted in an Asian population. Studies suggest that Asian populations have a high percentage of body fat for a given BMI and also have higher diabetes or coronary heart disease risk than Europeans at the same BMI [53]. Therefore, it is conceivable that Asians may be at higher risk of pancreatic cancer with a smaller increase in BMI than Caucasians.

COHORT STUDIES

To date, nine cohort studies have examined the association between body weight and pancreatic cancer risk [12, 54–61]. In two of these studies, risks were calculated for pancreatic cancer mortality [59,60]. All but three [12,54,57] of the cohort studies relied on self-reported weight. The number of pancreatic cancer cases in these cohorts ranged between 65 and 3558 and cohort follow-up time ranged between 7 and 43 years. In the four largest cohorts, significantly elevated risks of pancreatic cancer were observed for obese individuals, compared to those with normal body weight [54,56,60,61].

The Cancer Prevention Study II (CPS-II) cohort, the largest study to examine weight and cancer death, included over 900,000 U.S. participants and detected 1908 male and 1650 female pancreatic cancer deaths over 16 years of follow-up [60]. At baseline, participants were asked to report their current weight and their weight 1 year earlier. Individuals who reported having lost more than 10 lb over the previous year were excluded from the analyses. The strongest relative risk of pancreatic cancer death was observed among women with BMI ≥ 40 kg/m^2 (considered "grade III overweight"), compared to women with BMI < 25 kg/m^2 (RR = 2.76, 95% CI = 1.74 to 4.36). Relative risks were also elevated among men with BMI ≥35 (RR = 1.49, 95% CI = 0.99 to 2.22) and women with BMI between 35 and 39.9 (RR = 1.41, 95% CI = 1.01 to 1.99), compared to men and women with normal BMI (<25; data were not given for men with BMI ≥ 40 because of low person-years in this group). Among men, the association between BMI and pancreatic cancer death was stronger when the analysis was restricted to those who had never smoked (RR = 2.61, 95% CI = 1.27 to 5.35, for BMI ≥ 35 compared to normal weight).

In a subset of the larger CPS-II cohort (Nutrition Cohort), 242 incident pancreatic cancer cases were detected over a 7-year follow-up period [61]. A similar association was observed in this study for obesity and risk of pancreatic cancer among men and women (RR = 2.08, 95% CI = 1.48 to 2.93, for BMI > 30 vs. BMI < 25). In addition, an independent association was observed for central weight gain, compared with peripheral weight gain, after adjusting for BMI (RR = 1.45, 95% CI = 1.02 to 2.07).

Obesity was also associated with elevated risk of incident pancreatic cancer in the Nurses' Health Study and the Health Professionals Follow-up Study cohorts [56]. Weight was reported at baseline in each cohort and a total of 350 incident pancreatic cancer cases were included in the analyses (both cohorts). Similar associations were observed for men and women with BMI ≥ 30, compared to BMI < 23 (see Table 17.1). Tests for trend were statistically significant in both cohorts.

Four cohorts reported no association between weight and pancreatic cancer risk [55,57–59]; in a fifth, an association was detected among men but not women [12]. A narrow weight range and limited statistical power may explain why some of these studies failed to detect an association between body weight and pancreatic cancer risk. In one of the studies, which consisted largely of elderly participants (65 to 85 years at baseline) living in a retirement community, few participants were overweight (top BMI cutpoint for men and for women was less than 24) [55]. Small case numbers (n = 65) were another limitation to this study. In the College Alumni Health Study, the top BMI category cutpoint was 27.5 and only 10% of participants fell into that category. In the Chicago Heart Association cohort study, in which no association was detected among women, the top BMI category cutpoint was 26.2 for women (compared to 28.6 for men) and only 43 cases were women.

In a study of male smokers, no association was detected for weight and pancreatic cancer risk, even with a wide range in BMI [57]. It is conceivable that the association between weight and pancreatic cancer risk does not apply to heavy smokers. As mentioned above, in the CPS-II cohort, men who had never smoked had a much stronger association between BMI and pancreatic cancer death [60].

Results from a Swedish Twin Registry cohort also reported no association with weight, even among obese individuals (BMI > 30) [58]. However, the same study found an increase in risk of pancreatic cancer among those who reported an adult weight gain of 12 kg or more compared to those who gained 2 to 5 kg (RR = 1.46, 95% CI = 0.87 to 2.45).

In a different Swedish cohort, body weight was not reported, but weight gain was [62]. This study consisted of 35,000 men and women who participated in a general health examination in Malmö, Sweden, between 1974 and 1992. Incidence and mortality of cancer were obtained through linkage with the Cause of Death Register and the National Cancer Register; 43 pancreatic cancer cases were detected during follow-up. The authors reported a relative risk of 2.4 (95% CI = 1.1 to 4.9) for a greater than 10 kg increase in body weight since age 30 years, compared to all others, after controlling for smoking.

OBESITY COHORT STUDIES

In three studies, pancreatic cancer rates of patients with a hospital diagnosis of obesity were compared to those of nonobese individuals from similar populations [63–65]. Two of these studies detected follow-up incident cancer cases by record linkage to nationwide Cancer and Death Registries (Sweden [64] and Denmark [63]). In the study conducted in Sweden, follow-up ranged between 1 and 29 years and the standardized incidence ratio (SIR) for pancreatic cancer was 2.4 (95% CI = 1.6 to 3.4) among men and 1.1 (95% CI = 0.8 to 1.5) among women [64]. The risk was higher among obese men and women who were less than 60 years old at the time of follow-up (SIR = 2.5, 95% CI = 1.5 to 4.0). In the study conducted in Denmark, follow-up ranged between 1 and 11 years and the standardized incidence ratio for pancreatic cancer was 1.8 (95% CI = 1.2 to 2.5) among men and 1.7 (95% CI = 1.3 to 2.2) among women [63]. In this cohort, the highest risk of pancreatic cancer was observed for men and women who were 60 to 69 years old at the time of the cancer diagnosis (SIR = 2.4).

The third obesity cohort study was conducted among male U.S. veterans [65]. Incident cases that occurred between 1 and 27 years of follow-up were included in the analysis; obesity was considered as a time-dependent variable. Among white men, the relative risk for pancreatic cancer given an obesity diagnosis was 1.20 (95% CI = 1.07 to 1.33) compared to nonobese men (5874 pancreatic cancer cases). The association between obesity and pancreatic cancer risk was not as strong among black men (RR = 1.07, 95% CI = 0.86 to 1.34; 1721 pancreatic cancer cases).

META-ANALYSIS

In a recent meta-analysis including 14 studies and 6391 pancreatic cancer cases, the summary estimated relative risk of pancreatic cancer using a random effects model was 1.19 for obese individuals (BMI ≥ 30) compared to those with a normal body weight (BMI ≤ 22; 95% CI = 1.10 to 1.29; or, RR = 1.02, 95% CI = 1.01 to 1.03 for a unit increase in BMI) [66]. The combined estimated relative risk was higher among studies that adjusted for smoking in the analyses (RR =

1.03, 95% CI = 1.02 to 1.03 for a unit increase in BMI), compared to those that did not adjust for smoking (RR = 1.00, 95% CI = 0.96 to 1.03). Similarly, estimated relative risks were higher among studies that did not use proxy data (RR = 1.03, 95% CI = 1.01 to 1.06 for a unit increase in BMI), compared to those that did (RR = 0.99, 95% CI = 0.97 to 1.02, for a unit increase in BMI).

SUMMARY

Besides tobacco smoking, type-2 diabetes is one of the strongest risk factors for pancreatic cancer. A causal association with type-2 diabetes is likely to exist because a number of studies observe elevated risks of pancreatic cancer with long-standing diabetes. The association between type-2 diabetes and pancreatic cancer risk may be due to elevated postload glucose concentration, hyperinsulinemia, and resulting insulin resistance, suggesting that body weight may also play a role in pancreatic carcinogenesis.

Earlier studies examining body weight and pancreatic cancer risk offered no indication that weight may be a risk factor of pancreatic cancer. Methodological issues in case-control studies, especially regarding the use of proxies, may explain the observed null results. More recent case-control studies using only direct interviews reported elevated risks of pancreatic cancer among men and women with elevated BMIs. A number of recent cohort studies observed similar associations. The largest cohort study (with smoking data), including 3558 pancreatic cancer cases, reported relative risks of mortality between 1.5 and 2.8 for obese men and women, compared to normal weight. The association in men was strongest among those who had never smoked.

Overall, animal and human studies suggest that a positive association between body weight and pancreatic cancer risk exists. The association may be strongest among men and women who are considered obese (i.e., BMI greater than 30). Future studies need to focus on the effects of physical activity.

REFERENCES

1. *Cancer Facts and Figures 2004*. Atlanta: American Cancer Society, Inc., 2004.
2. Bray, F, Sankila, R, Ferlay, J, and Parkin, DM. Estimates of cancer incidence and mortality in Europe in 1995. *Eur J Cancer* 2002; 38:99–166.
3. Ries, LAG, Eisner, MP, Kosary, CL, Hankey, BF, Miller, BA, Clegg, L, et al. (Eds.). *SEER Cancer Statistics Review, 1975–2000*. Bethesda, MD: National Cancer Institute, 2003.
4. Pisani, P, Parkin, DM, Bray, F, and Ferlay, J. Estimates of the worldwide mortality from 25 cancers in 1990. *Int J Cancer* 1999; 83:18–29.
5. Sahmoun, AE, D'Agostino, RA, Jr., Bell, RA, and Schwenke, DC. International variation in pancreatic cancer mortality for the period 1955–1998. *Eur J Epidemiol* 2003; 18:801–816.
6. Lin, Y, Tamakoshi, A, Wakai, K, Kawamura, T, Aoki, R, Kojima, M, et al. Descriptive epidemiology of pancreatic cancer in Japan. *J Epidemiol* 1998; 8:52–59.
7. Everhart, J, and Wright, D. Diabetes mellitus as a risk factor for pancreatic cancer. A meta-analysis. *JAMA* 1995; 273:1605–1609.
8. Silverman, DT. Risk factors for pancreatic cancer: a case-control study based on direct interviews. *Teratog Carcinog Mutagen* 2001; 21:7–25.
9. Calle, EE, Murphy, TK, Rodriguez, C, Thun, MJ, and Heath, CW, Jr. Diabetes mellitus and pancreatic cancer mortality in a prospective cohort of United States adults [see comments]. *Cancer Causes Control* 1998; 9:403–410.
10. Chow, WH, Gridley, G, Nyren, O, Linet, MS, Ekbom, A, Fraumeni, JF, Jr, et al. Risk of pancreatic cancer following diabetes mellitus: a nationwide cohort study in Sweden. *J Natl Cancer Inst* 1995; 87:930–931.
11. Wideroff, L, Gridley, G, Mellemkjaer, L, Chow, WH, Linet, M, Keehn, S, et al. Cancer incidence in a population-based cohort of patients hospitalized with diabetes mellitus in Denmark. *J Natl Cancer Inst* 1997; 89:1360–1365.

12. Gapstur, SM, Gann, PH, Lowe, W, Liu, K, Colangelo, L, and Dyer, A. Abnormal glucose metabolism and pancreatic cancer mortality. *JAMA* 2000; 283:2552–2558.
13. Jee, SH, Ohrr, H, Sull, JW, Yun, JE, Ji, M, and Samet, JM. Fasting serum glucose level and cancer risk in Korean men and women. *JAMA* 2005; 293:194–202.
14. Longnecker, DS, Shinozuka, H, and Dekker, A. Focal acinar cell dysplasia in human pancreas. *Cancer* 1980; 45:534–540.
15. Pour, PM, and Schmied, B. The link between exocrine pancreatic cancer and the endocrine pancreas. *Int J Pancreatol* 1999; 25:77–87.
16. Pour, PM. Experimental pancreatic cancer. *Am J Surg Pathol* 1989; 13 Suppl 1:96–103.
17. Fisher, WE, Muscarella, P, Boros, LG, and Schirmer, WJ. Variable effect of streptozotocin-diabetes on the growth of hamster pancreatic cancer (H2T) in the Syrian hamster and nude mouse. *Surgery* 1998; 123:315–320.
18. Fisher, WE, Boros, LG, and Schirmer, WJ. Insulin promotes pancreatic cancer: evidence for endocrine influence on exocrine pancreatic tumors. *J Surg Res* 1996; 63:310–313.
19. Takeda, Y, and Escribano, M. Effects of insulin and somatostatin on the growth and the colony formation of two human pancreatic cancer cell lines. *J Cancer Res Clin Oncol* 1991; 117:416–420.
20. Kornmann, M, Maruyama, H, Bergmann, U, Tangvoranuntakul, P, Beger, HG, White, MF, et al. Enhanced expression of the insulin receptor substrate-2 docking protein in human pancreatic cancer. *Cancer Res* 1998; 58:4250–4254.
21. Mossner, J, Logsdon, CD, Williams, JA, and Goldfine, ID. Insulin, via its own receptor, regulates growth and amylase synthesis in pancreatic acinar AR42J cells. *Diabetes* 1985; 34:891–897.
22. Ding, XZ, Fehsenfeld, DM, Murphy, LO, Permert, J, and Adrian, TE. Physiological concentrations of insulin augment pancreatic cancer cell proliferation and glucose utilization by activating MAP kinase, PI3 kinase and enhancing GLUT-1 expression. *Pancreas* 2000; 21:310–320.
23. Beauchamp, RD, Lyons, RM, Yang, EY, Coffey, RJ, Jr, and Moses, HL. Expression of and response to growth regulatory peptides by two human pancreatic carcinoma cell lines. *Pancreas* 1990; 5:369–380.
24. Wang, F, Larsson, J, Adrian, TE, Gasslander, T, and Permert, J. *In vitro* influences between pancreatic adenocarcinoma cells and pancreatic islets. *J Surg Res* 1998; 79:13–19.
25. Liehr, RM, Melnykovych, G, and Solomon, TE. Growth effects of regulatory peptides on human pancreatic cancer lines PANC-1 and MIA PaCa-2. *Gastroenterology* 1990; 98:1666–1674.
26. Pour, PM and Stepan, K. Modification of pancreatic carcinogenesis in the hamster model. VIII. Inhibitory effect of exogenous insulin. *J Natl Cancer Inst* 1984; 72:1205–1208.
27. Pour, PM, Kazakoff, K, and Carlson, K. Inhibition of streptozotocin-induced islet cell tumors and N-nitrosobis(2-oxopropyl)amine-induced pancreatic exocrine tumors in Syrian hamsters by exogenous insulin. *Cancer Res* 1990; 50:1634–1639.
28. Pour, PM and Kazakoff, K. Stimulation of islet cell proliferation enhances pancreatic ductal carcinogenesis in the hamster model. *Am J Pathol* 1996; 149:1017–1025.
29. Pour, PM, Donnelly, K, and Stepan, K. Modification of pancreatic carcinogenesis in the hamster model. 3. Inhibitory effect of alloxan. *Am J Pathol* 1983; 110:310–314.
30. Bell, RH, Jr., Sayers, HJ, Pour, PM, Ray, MB, and McCullough, PJ. Importance of diabetes in inhibition of pancreatic cancer by streptozotocin. *J Surg Res* 1989; 46:515–519.
31. Bell, RH, Jr., McCullough, PJ, and Pour, PM. Influence of diabetes on susceptibility to experimental pancreatic cancer. *Am J Surg* 1988; 155:159–164.
32. Schneider, MB, Matsuzaki, H, Haorah, J, Ulrich, A, Standop, J, Ding, XZ, et al. Prevention of pancreatic cancer induction in hamsters by metformin. *Gastroenterology* 2001; 120:1263–1270.
33. Zendehdel, K, Nyren, O, Ostenson, CG, Adami, HO, Ekbom, A, and Ye, W. Cancer incidence in patients with type 1 diabetes mellitus: a population-based cohort study in Sweden. *J Natl Cancer Inst* 2003; 95:1797–1800.
34. Smith, JP, Fantaskey, AP, Liu, G, and Zagon, IS. Identification of gastrin as a growth peptide in human pancreatic cancer. *Am J Physiol* 1995; 268:R135–141.
35. Smith, JP, Shih, A, Wu, Y, McLaughlin, PJ, and Zagon, IS. Gastrin regulates growth of human pancreatic cancer in a tonic and autocrine fashion. *Am J Physiol* 1996; 270:R1078–1084.
36. Smith, JP, Kramer, ST, and Solomon, TE. CCK stimulates growth of six human pancreatic cancer cell lines in serum-free medium. *Regul Pept* 1991; 32:341–349.

37. Stewart, ID, Flaks, B, Watanapa, P, Davies, PW, and Williamson, RC. Pancreatobiliary diversion enhances experimental pancreatic carcinogenesis. *Br J Cancer* 1991; 63:63–66.
38. Chu, M, Franzen, L, Sullivan, S, Rehfeld, JF, Ihse, I, and Borch, K. Effects of pancreaticobiliary diversion and gastric fundectomy on azaserine-induced pancreatic carcinogenesis in the rat. *Pancreas* 1993; 8:330–337.
39. Chu, M, Franzen, L, Sullivan, S, Wingren, S, Rehfeld, JF, and Borch, K. Pancreatic hypertrophy with acinar cell nodules after longterm fundectomy in the rat. *Gut* 1993; 34:988–993.
40. Chu, M, Kullman, E, Rehfeld, JF, and Borch, K. Effect of chronic endogenous hypergastrinaemia on pancreatic growth and carcinogenesis in the hamster. *Gut* 1997; 40:536–540.
41. Chu, M, Rehfeld, JF, and Borch, K. Chronic endogenous hypercholecystokininemia promotes pancreatic carcinogenesis in the hamster. *Carcinogenesis* 1997; 18:315–320.
42. Pour, PM, Lawson, T, Helgeson, S, Donnelly, T, and Stepan, K. Effect of cholecystokinin on pancreatic carcinogenesis in the hamster model. *Carcinogenesis* 1988; 9:597–601.
43. Meijers, M, van Garderen–Hoetmer, A, Lamers, CB, Rovati, LC, Jansen, JB, and Woutersen, RA. Role of cholecystokinin in the development of BOP-induced pancreatic lesions in hamsters. *Carcinogenesis* 1990; 11:2223–2226.
44. Takahashi, M, Imaida, K, Furukawa, F, and Hayashi, Y. Inhibitory effects of soybean trypsin inhibitor during initiation and promotion phases of N-nitrosobis(2-oxopropyl)amine-induced hamster pancreatic carcinogenesis. *Prog Clin Biol Res* 1991; 369:145–154.
45. Bueno de Mesquita, HB, Moerman, CJ, Runia, S, and Maisonneuve, P. Are energy and energy-providing nutrients related to exocrine carcinoma of the pancreas? *Int J Cancer* 1990; 46:435–444.
46. Howe, GR, Ghadirian, P, Bueno de Mesquita, HB, Zatonski, WA, Baghurst, PA, Miller, AB, et al. A collaborative case-control study of nutrient intake and pancreatic cancer within the search programme. *Int J Cancer* 1992; 51:365–372.
47. Ghadirian, P, Simard, A, Baillargeon, J, Maisonneuve, P, and Boyle, P. Nutritional factors and pancreatic cancer in the francophone community in Montreal, Canada. *Int J Cancer* 1991; 47:1–6.
48. Lyon, JL, Slattery, ML, Mahoney, AW, and Robison, LM. Dietary intake as a risk factor for cancer of the exocrine pancreas. *Cancer Epidemiol Biomarkers Prev* 1993; 2:513–518.
49. Silverman, DT, Swanson, CA, Gridley, G, Wacholder, S, Greenberg, RS, Brown, LM, et al. Dietary and nutritional factors and pancreatic cancer: a case-control study based on direct interviews. *J Natl Cancer Inst* 1998; 90:1710–1719.
50. Hanley, AJ, Johnson, KC, Villeneuve, PJ, and Mao, Y. Physical activity, anthropometric factors and risk of pancreatic cancer: results from the Canadian enhanced cancer surveillance system. *Int J Cancer* 2001; 94:140–147.
51. Ji, BT, Hatch, MC, Chow, WH, McLaughlin, JK, Dai, Q, Howe, GR, et al. Anthropometric and reproductive factors and the risk of pancreatic cancer: a case-control study in Shanghai, China. *Int J Cancer* 1996; 66:432–437.
52. Pan, SY, Johnson, KC, Ugnat, AM, Wen, SW, and Mao, Y. Association of obesity and cancer risk in Canada. *Am J Epidemiol* 2004; 159:259–268.
53. WHO, EC. Appropriate body-mass index for Asian populations and its implications for policy and intervention strategies. *Lancet* 2004; 363:157–163.
54. Friedman, GD and van den Eeden, SK. Risk factors for pancreatic cancer: an exploratory study. *Int J Epidemiol* 1993; 22:30–37.
55. Shibata, A, Mack, TM, Paganini–Hill, A, Ross, RK, and Henderson, BE. A prospective study of pancreatic cancer in the elderly [see comments]. *Int J Cancer* 1994; 58:46–49.
56. Michaud, DS, Giovannucci, E, Willett, WC, Colditz, GA, Stampfer, MJ, and Fuchs, CS. Physical activity, obesity, height and the risk of pancreatic cancer. *JAMA* 2001; 286:921–929.
57. Stolzenberg–Solomon, RZ, Pietinen, P, Taylor, PR, Virtamo, J, and Albanes, D. A prospective study of medical conditions, anthropometry, physical activity, and pancreatic cancer in male smokers (Finland). *Cancer Causes Control* 2002; 13:417–426.
58. Isaksson, B, Jonsson, F, Pedersen, NL, Larsson, J, Feychting, M, and Permert, J. Lifestyle factors and pancreatic cancer risk: a cohort study from the Swedish Twin Registry. *Int J Cancer* 2002; 98:480–482.
59. Lee, IM, Sesso, HD, Oguma, Y, and Paffenbarger, RS, Jr. Physical activity, body weight, and pancreatic cancer mortality. *Br J Cancer* 2003; 88:679–683.

60. Calle, EE, Rodriguez, C, Walker–Thurmond, K, and Thun, MJ. Overweight, obesity, and mortality from cancer in a prospectively studied cohort of U.S. adults. *N Engl J Med* 2003; 348:1625–1638.
61. Patel, AV, Rodriguez, C, Bernstein, L, Chao, A, Thun, MJ, and Calle, EE. Obesity, recreational physical activity, and risk of pancreatic cancer in a large U.S. Cohort. *Cancer Epidemiol Biomarkers Prev* 2005; 14:459–466.
62. Ogren, M, Hedberg, M, Berglund, G, Borgstrom, A, and Janzon, L. Risk of pancreatic carcinoma in smokers enhanced by weight gain. Results from 10-year follow-up of the Malmo Preventive Project Cohort Study. *Int J Pancreatol* 1996; 20:95–101.
63. Moller, H, Mellemgaard, A, Lindvig, K, Olsen, JH, and Moller, H. Obesity and cancer risk: a Danish record-linkage study. *Eur J Cancer* 1994; 30A:344–350.
64. Wolk, A, Gridley, G, Svensson, M, Nyren, O, McLaughlin, JK, Fraumeni, JF, et al. A prospective study of obesity and cancer risk (Sweden). *Cancer Causes Control* 2001; 12:13–21.
65. Samanic, C, Gridley, G, Chow, WH, Lubin, J, Hoover, RN, and Fraumeni, JF, Jr. Obesity and cancer risk among white and black United States veterans. *Cancer Causes Control* 2004; 15:35–43.
66. Berrington de Gonzalez, A, Sweetland, S, and Spencer, E. A meta-analysis of obesity and the risk of pancreatic cancer. *Br J Cancer* 2003; 89:519–523.

18 Obesity and Overweight in Relation to Adenocarcinoma of the Esophagus

Cathrine Hoyo and Marilie D. Gammon

CONTENTS

INTRODUCTION

Esophageal cancer is the eighth most common cause of cancer-related morbidity and the sixth most common cause of cancer-related death. Squamous cell carcinoma is still the predominant histological subtype worldwide, although incidence of this subtype is stable or decreasing [1,2]. Among men, African Americans are at a nearly sixfold increased risk of squamous cell carcinoma of the esophagus compared to white men; however, risk among white men is four times higher for adenocarcinomas compared to that of African Americans. Among women, the risk of squamous cell carcinoma is lower than that of men, but is similar by race [3].

Incidence of adenocarcinomas of the esophagus and in the closely linked gastric cardia has increased rapidly for at least 30 years. In the United States, Devesa [4] reported a crossover of the esophageal histological subtypes in the mid-1990s; adenocarcinomas became the predominant subtype, rather than squamous cell carcinoma, making it the fastest increasing cancer to date. These patterns are evident among men and women, although rates are much lower among women [3].

Reasons for the rapid increase in the incidence of esophageal adenocarcinoma reported in most industrialized countries are not clear, but parallel an equally rapid increase in the prevalence of obesity and overweight status. Based on a representative sample of adult Americans, the estimated prevalence of obesity, defined as a body mass index (BMI; weight in kilograms divided by height in meters squared) of 30 kg/m^2 or more, increased from 12% in 1991 to 18% in 1998 [5]. By 2001, this prevalence had increased to 21% [6], representing a 75% increase in a 10-year period. In the U.S., approximately 60% of the adult population is currently overweight (25 kg/m^2) or obese [7]. Among obese individuals, the steepest increases have been reported among those with BMI of >40 kg/m^2, for whom prevalence has increased by a factor of four in the last 10 years [8]. Because of under-reporting of weight increases with the respondent's actual weight, a prevalence estimate of 60%, which is based on self-reports, is likely an underestimate.

Obesity is associated with all-cause mortality [9] and with increased risk of cardiovascular diseases [10], diabetes, cancers of the colon, rectum, liver, gall bladder, pancreas, breast, corpus uterus, cervix, ovary, and kidney, and non-Hodgkin's lymphoma [11]. As reviewed in this chapter, obesity has also been recently associated with adenocarcinomas of the esophagus and gastric cardia; these associations are independent of known risk factors, including cigarette smoking and alcohol consumption.

Up to 90% of squamous cell carcinoma of the esophagus can be attributed to the synergistic effect of alcohol and tobacco use [12], and the precipitous decrease in the incidence of this histological subtype in the U.S. has been attributed to decreases in tobacco use. The strength of the association between alcohol and adenocarcinomas of the esophagus or gastric cardia is weaker [13]. Recent evidence suggests that the risk of such adenocarcinomas is also inversely associated with gastrointestinal infection with *Helicobacter pylori* (*H. pylori*) [14]. However, strong evidence also implicates overweight and obesity in the etiology of these adenocarcinomas [15–18]. Cases of adenocarcinomas of the esophagus and gastric cardia are more likely than controls to have a history of gastroesophageal reflux disease, hiatal hernia, or Barrett's metaplasia [17–19]. These conditions, which are considered precursors to esophageal adenocarcinoma [20], are also common among overweight and obese individuals.

The mechanisms by which obesity could increase risk of esophageal adenocarcinoma are unclear; mechanical as well as biochemical hypotheses have been proposed. Central obesity may predispose individuals to adenocarcinoma of the esophagus by initiating a cascade of events, beginning with hiatal hernia and gastroesophageal reflux disease, which predominantly affects the gastroesophageal junction [15,21]. Constant irritation of squamous cells in the lower third of the esophagus is thought to invoke a compensatory response that gives rise to Barrett's metaplasia, in which squamous cells are gradually replaced by columnar cells.Although a small proportion of patients with Barrett's metaplasia eventually develop esophageal adenocarcinoma, the condition is considered a precursor for this adenocarcinoma. In this model, digestive enzymes, including gastric and bile acids, may irritate and cause inflammation on the esophagus, leading to hyperproliferation of columnar cells less vulnerable to refluxate, constituting the first "hit." This may eventually lead to low-grade and then premalignant, high-grade dysplastic changes in the esophagus, which in turn may lead to esophageal adenocarcinoma. This hypothesis is consistent with the multistep process of carcinogenesis [22]. Some epidemiological evidence implicates obesity in the etiology of Barrett's metaplasia and gastroesophageal reflux disease, as reviewed next.

METHODS

A comprehensive literature search was conducted to identify epidemiological studies that examined obesity or overweight status in relation to: (1) esophageal adenocarcinoma; (2) the closely related tumor, gastric cardia adenocarcinoma; (3) the precursor lesion, Barrett's esophagus; and (4) gastroesophageal reflux disease. A computerized search of English language publications was performed up to June 2004 using MEDLINE online database (National Library of Medicine, Bethesda, MD) as well as manual searches of abstract lists for recent cancer or epidemiology conferences and the reference lists of all relevant articles. Most articles evaluated the risk of adenocarcinoma of the esophagus separately from those of the gastric cardia; however, some early studies combined the two anatomical subtypes together in a single outcome group because of the belief that the two share a common etiology. Whether this latter assumption is correct remains unresolved.

The standard clinical and epidemiological assessment of obesity, weight for height or BMI, was used in many of the studies identified for this review. The World Health Organization defines a BMI of 25 kg/m^2 or greater as overweight and a BMI of 30 kg/m^2 as obese [23]. Circumferences of the hip and waist have traditionally been used to estimate fat distribution in epidemiological studies. Centralized obesity, as assessed by the waist circumference or waist-to-hip ratio, has been shown to be associated strongly with adult weight gain [24]. Although the validity of each of these measures remains an active topic of investigation, the test and retest reliability of BMI with total body fat and waist-to-hip ratio with central obesity and visceral adipose tissue accumulation are high [24]. Central obesity, which represents an aberrant fat accumulation, may be as important as BMI and may be a more potent adiposity phenotype and a better predictor of chronic disease.

RESULTS

Esophageal Adenocarcinoma

Table 18.1 summarizes results from 13 case-control studies and one cohort study that investigated the association between esophageal adenocarcinoma risk and obesity [15–18,25–33]. The investigations were conducted between 1986 and 2001 in a variety of Western countries, including the U.S., Sweden, Norway, Italy, Great Britain, and Germany. Most studies estimated obesity using BMI, which was calculated based on the study participants' recall of usual adult weight, defined as weight ranging from 1 to 20 years prior to the study interview. Weight at specific ages, such as 20 or 40 years of age, was also based on recall. Height, measured or self-reported at interview following disease onset, together with recalled weight, was commonly used to compute BMI.

Using BMI 1 year prior to the interview as a proxy for usual BMI, all [15–18,26,27,30–33] but three studies [25,28,29] reported a dose-dependent increase in the risk of esophageal adenocarcinoma in relation to obesity. The estimates of the magnitude of the association ranged from an odds ratio (OR) of 2.5 to 3.1, when individuals in the lowest quartile of usual or current BMI were compared to those in the highest quartiles. Although fourfold increases in risk were also reported among German men [33], these findings were based on a small number of cases. The two- to threefold increase in risk varied little across populations, despite different cut-points, suggesting perhaps that the relative fat deposits, and not absolute cut-point values of BMI, are important.

The timing of obesity relative to the onset of esophageal adenocarcinoma also appeared to influence risk. When the association between esophageal adenocarcinoma and BMI at specific ages, such as BMI at age 20 [17], was evaluated, the magnitude of the association between obesity and esophageal adenocarcinoma was even stronger. In a Swedish case-control study, Lagergren [17] reported a 16-fold increase in risk of adenocarcinoma of the esophagus among individuals with a BMI greater than 30 kg/m^2 some 20 years before the interview, when compared to those with a BMI less than 22 kg/m^2. The significance of these findings is unclear because others [16] have reported that the magnitude of the association between esophageal adenocarcinoma and obesity at age 20 or at age 40 years was similar; however, the association was slightly stronger among subjects who reported obesity at age 20 than among those who were obese at age 40. One interpretation of these findings is that the duration of obesity during adulthood, rather than obesity in the period surrounding diagnosis, may be the important factor in the etiology of esophageal adenocarcinoma.

Few studies evaluated duration of obesity directly, and instead relied on participants to recall weight at different ages to estimate duration. A very strong association between duration of obesity and risk of esophageal adenocarcinoma was found among British women [31], although the highest quartile included those with a BMI of <23 kg/m^2. Confirming these results, Chak [32] reported a dose-dependent increase in risk with increasing duration of obesity. However, in these studies [31,32], the number of cases involved was small and estimates were imprecise.

Although most studies combined men and women in the final analyses, studies that provided results stratified by sex suggest that obesity may have a less detrimental effect among women than among men, although these findings are not consistent. In a cohort study, Tretli [18] reported a more than twofold increase in risk of esophageal adenocarcinoma among men in the fourth BMI quartile and no evidence of such an association in women. In the British study that included only women, however, BMI at age 20 was associated with a more than sixfold increase in esophageal

TABLE 18.1
Summary of Results from Studies of Obesity and Esophageal Adenocarcinoma

Location	Design/sample size	Obesity estimation	Results: OR (95% CI) by quantile of obesity estimate	Study ref. and year
U.S.	Hospital case control; 122 gastric and esophageal male cases; 4544 controls	BMI 5 years prior to diagnosis	Combined gastric and esophageal adenocarcinomas BMI >28 = ref; BMI 25–27.9 OR = 0.7 (0.4–1.1); BMI 22–24.9 OR = 0.7 (0.4–1.2); BMI < 22 OR = 1.2 (0.6–2.4)	25 (1993)
U.S.	Case control; 162 gastric cardia and esophagus cases; 685 controls; whites only	BMI; <23.1 kg/m^2 as referents	BMI 23.1-25 = OR =1.1 (0.6–2.1); BMI 25.1–26.6 = OR 1.2 (0.6–2.3); BMI >26.6 = OR 3.1 (1.8–5.3)	26 (1995)
U.S.	Case control; 298 cases; 133 cases (28 blacks)	BMI 1 year before diagnosis	1–10%le — OR = 1.6 (0.7–3.6) 10–49%le — ref 50–89%le — OR = 1.2 (0.7–2.1) 90%le+ — OR = 2.5 (1.2–5.0)	27 (1995)
U.S.	Case control; 28 adenocarcinoma; 67 gastric cardia; 132 controls	BMI, weight, height	OR = 0.93 (0.8–1.0) Association with height	28 (1996)
U.S.	Case control; 292 cases; 685 controls	Weight, BMI, weight change	Men: Q1 = ref; Q2 OR = 1.5 (0.8–2.5); Q3 OR = 2.0 (1.2–3.5); Q4 OR = 3.0 (1.7–5.0) Women: Q1 = ref; Q2 OR = 0.8 (0.2–3.4); Q3 OR = 2.1 (0.6–7.4); Q4 = 2.6 (0.8–8.5)	15 (1998)
Sweden	Case control; 189 cases; 820 controls (whites only)	BMI @ age 20 BMI 20 years before interview	At age 20 yrs: Q1 = ref; Q2 OR = 0.9 (0.5–1.6); Q3 OR = 1.6(0.9–2.8); Q4 OR = 2.7 (1.6–4.6) 20 yrs before interview: Q1 = ref; Q2 OR = 2.2 (1.0–4.7) ;Q3 OR = 3.8 (1.9–7.7); Q4 OR = 7.6 (3.8–15.2)	17 (1999)
Norway	Cohort, 119 (94 men, 25 women, whites only)	BMI in men BMI in women	Q1 = ref; Q2 OR = 1.74 (0.9–3.4); Q3 OR = 1.32 (0.6–2.8); Q4 OR = 1.1 (0.6–2.4); Q5 OR = 2.40 (1.3–4.4)	18 (1999)

U.S.	222 esophagus 1356 controls	BMI current, at age 40 and age 20 in quartiles	BMI at age 20: Q1 = ref; Q2 OR = 1.23 (0.8–1.9); Q3 OR = 1.34 (0.9–2.1); Q4 OR = 1.77 (1.1–2.7); BMI at age 40 years Q1 = ref; Q2 OR = 1.13 (0.7–1.7); Q3 OR = 1.76 (1.1–2.9); Q4 OR = 2.78 (1.7–4.4)	16 (2001)
Italy	262 cases; 262 controls; hospital based	BMI, weight	BMI cases 25.7 kg/m^2 vs. controls 25.4 kg/m^2	29 (2000)
U.S.	Case control; 124 cases; 449 controls	Usual BMI	BMI in cases = 26.4 kg/m^2 vs. controls = 25.0 kg/m^2 OR = 1.1 (1.04–1.18)	30 (2002)
U.K.	Case control; 74 cases; 74 controls	BMI at age 20	Q1 = ref; Q2 OR = 0.86 (0.17–4.32); Q3 OR = 4.9 (0.9–28.0) Q4 OR = –6.04 (1.28–28.5	31 (2000)
U.S.	58 adenocarcinoma, and Barrett's cases; 106 controls	BMI	Current OR = 0.63; p-value = 0.23 1 year ago OR = 1.03; p-value = 0.9 5 years ago OR = 1.25; p-value = 0.6 10 years ago OR = 2.31;p-value = 0.02 20 yrs ago OR = 3.16; p-value = 0.004	32 (2002)
Germany	Case control; 47 cases; 50 controls (men only)	BMI	25 kg/m^2 = ref; 25.1–27.5 OR = 4.52 (1.29–15.93); >27.5 kg/m^2 OR = 14.72 (4.18–51.93)	33 (2002)

Note: BMI = body mass index (wt/ht^2); OR = odds ratio; Q = quantile; ref = reference group.

adenocarcinoma risk, although the number of study cases was small [31]. Differences between men and women suggest that, rather than total body fat, central adiposity, which is more common in men, may be the important factor involved in the etiology of esophageal adenocarcinoma.

The few studies unable to document an association with obesity were hospital based [29], or combined adenocarcinomas of the gastric cardia with those of the esophagus to form a single outcome group [25,26]. Because obesity is associated with many chronic conditions, the prevalence of obesity among hospital-based controls may be higher than that in the general population. Thus, case-control studies that utilize hospital-based controls in an investigation of obesity would be expected to underestimate an association. In addition, due to the anatomical proximity of esophageal and gastric cardia adenocarcinomas, the earlier studies presented findings from analyses that combined these as a single disease endpoint [25,26]. Collapsing the two tumors into a single outcome may increase statistical power; however, the etiology of esophageal adenocarcinoma may be distinct from those of the gastric cardia. Thus, if the relation with obesity varies by anatomical subtype, findings from studies combining the two could be misleading. It is therefore not surprising that, of the three studies that combined anatomical sites or used hospital-based controls, only one [26] found statistically significant differences in obesity between cases and controls.

Gastric Cardia Adenocarcinoma

Table 18.2 summarizes results from the six case-control studies that evaluated the association between obesity and the risk of gastric cardia adenocarcinoma [15–17,21,27,28]. These studies were conducted in China, Sweden, and the U.S. Five of the six studies [15–17,21,27] found a weak to moderate, dose-dependent increase in risk of gastric cardia adenocarcinoma with increasing obesity. In four studies [15–17,27], these associations were weaker than those reported for the association between BMI and esophageal adenocarcinoma.

TABLE 18.2
Summary of Results from Studies of Obesity and Gastric Cardia Adenocarcinoma

Location	Design/sample size	Obesity estimation	Results: OR (95% CI) by quantile of obesity estimate	Study ref. and year
China	Case control; 1124 cases; 1451 controls	Usual, maximum, and minimum BMI quartiles; referents < 19.38 kg/m^2; highest 22.1	Usual weight in all men; Q1 = ref Q2 — 1.3 (0.8–2.3) Q3 — 2.1 (1.2–3.8) Q4 — 3.5 (1.9–6.1) In men <60 years; Q1 = ref Q2 — 3.3 (1.0–10.6) Q3 — 2.8 (0.8–9.3) Q4 — 6.5 (2.1–20.6) No increased risk in women	21 (1997)
U.S.	Case control; 261 cases and 685 controls	Usual BMI, weight, weight change/adult	BMI quartiles; women: Q1 = ref; Q2 OR = 0.9 (0.2–3.2); Q3 OR = 2.2 (0.7–7.1); Q4 OR = 1.3 (0.4–4.2). Men: Q1 = ref; Q2 OR = 0.9 (0.6–1.6); Q3 OR = 1.3 (0.8–2.2); Q4 OR = 1.1–2.9	15 (1998)
Sweden	Case control; 262 cases; 820 controls	BMI at age 20, 20 years before interview	20 years < interview 1.3; 2.2 (1.4–3.40); 4.3 (2.1–8.7) At age 20: 0.9; 1.3; 2.0 (1.3–2.9)	17 (1999)
U.S.	Case control; 165 cases; 724 controls	BMI 1 year before interview	1–10%le — 0.8 (0.4–1.8) 11–49%le — ref 50–89%le — 1.3 (0.8–2.1) >89%le — 1.6 (0.8–3.0)	27 (1995)
U.S.	Case control; 277 cases, 1356 controls, only 3 AA EA, and 10 GC; 7 and 17 for Asians	BMI current, at age 20, and at 40 years in quartiles	BMI at age 40 years: Q1 = ref; Q2 OR = 1.49 (1.0–2.1); Q3 OR = 1.45 (0.9–2.3); Q4 OR = 2.08 (1.4–3.2): BMI at age 20: Q1 = ref; Q2 OR = 1.13 (0.8–1.7); Q3 OR = 1.36 (0.9–2.0); Q4 OR + 1.71 (1.2–2.6)	16 (2001)
U.S.	Case control; 132 controls, 67 gastroesophageal, gastric cardia	BMI Height	BMI — no association Height — OR = 2.8 in top quartile	28 (1996)

Note: BMI = body mass index (wt/ht^2); OR = odds ratio; Q = quantile; ref = reference group.

These epidemiological studies usually included assessment of BMI at interview, or relied on an estimate of usual adult BMI, which was commonly based on self-reported weight in the year prior to the interview. In some studies, participants were also asked to recall their weight at age 20 or 40 years or 20 years prior to the interview; thus, estimates of adult weight change could also be calculated.

In studies that evaluated duration, the risk of gastric cardia adenocarcinoma increased with time since the participant was first obese. The magnitude of the association for an increased BMI 1 year prior to the interview was weak to moderate, whereas the magnitude in relation to increased BMI some 20 to 50 years prior to disease onset was moderate to strong [16,17]. Compared to individuals in the lowest quartile of BMI 1 year prior to the interview [16], those in the highest category of BMI were at 60% increased risk of gastric cardia adenocarcinoma. BMI at age 40 years [16] or 20 years prior to the interview [17] was associated with two- to threefold increase in risk. Recalled usual BMI was associated with up to a fourfold increase in risk of gastric cardia adenocarcinoma in men, suggesting that prolonged periods of central obesity in adulthood may be etiologically linked to these tumors. As would be expected if the association was causal, duration of obesity during the course of adulthood appears important.

Most, but not all, studies found that the risk of gastric cardia adenocarcinoma associated with obesity varied by sex. In a generally lean Chinese population-based case-control study, Ji and colleagues [21] reported up to sixfold increased risk of gastric cardia cancers associated with increasing BMI, but the association was stronger among men than women. As with esophageal adenocarcinoma, weight change during adulthood was not associated with increased risk of gastric cardia adenocarcinoma [15].

Although theses studies show a positive association between obesity and gastric cardia adenocarcinoma, particularly among men, a limitation among them is that body fat was more commonly assessed using BMI rather than the more pertinent waist circumference or waist-to-hip ratio. Central obesity is more common in men and is more relevant to the postulated hypothesis of intra-abdominal pressure. However, estimates of central obesity are particularly difficult to obtain accurately and reliably in a case-control study. Future studies may benefit from inquiring retrospectively about waist and hip circumference using proxy measures such as clothing size, similar to breast cancer studies that include assessment of brassiere size. Although precise estimates could not be obtained from such an inquiry, the relative measure and duration could be evaluated.

Barrett's Metaplasia

Table 18.3 summarizes the results from four studies evaluating the association between obesity and Barrett's esophagus that were conducted in the U.S. and the U.K. [34–37]. In these studies, obesity was estimated using BMI, weight, weight change, and waist-to-hip ratio. In a British cross-sectional study of Barrett's esophagus patients, Caygill [34] reported a strong association with high BMI among patients younger than 50 years, but this association was not apparent among patients 50 years and older. These findings were corroborated in a study based on 51 Barrett's esophagus patients that was conducted by Moe [35]. The authors [35] found that diet and nutritional status were associated with elevated cell proliferative fractions in patients. Among these patients, 45% of cases had a high BMI (>27.6 kg/m^2) and elevated waist-to-hip ratio was significantly associated with the mean and maximum %S phase cells. Weight change was also associated with the mean and maximum percentage of cells in the G2 phase.

In contrast, Gerson [36] reported no association between adult weight change and Barrett's in a study of 110 individuals aged 50 years or more who were undergoing sigmoidoscopy. Finally, in a much larger follow-up study of over 400 Barrett's esophagus patients, Vaughan [37] found a consistent association with higher waist-to-hip ratio that was stronger among men than women. Vaughan [37] also reported a strong association between waist-to-hip ratio and other high-risk

TABLE 18.3
Summary of Results from Studies of Obesity and Barrett's Esophagus

Location	Design/sample size	Obesity estimation	Results: OR (95% CI) by quantile of obesity estimate	Study ref. and year
U.S.	350 patients with Barrett's metaplasia; case only	BMI, waist-to-hip ratio, weight change from age 25 years	%S phase for WHR r = 0.33; BMI *r* = 0.03; weight change *r* = 0.01	35 (2000)
U.S.	110 Barrett's esophagus patients age 50 to 80 years; cross sectional	Weight	No association Obese = 17% Nonobese = 16%	36 (2002)
U.K.	102 Barrett's esophagus patients (69 men and 33 women)	BMI	No association; BMI > 30 vs. ≤ 30; % Barrett's esophagus BMI > 30 in 50+-year-olds = 16%; BMI > 30 in < 50-year-olds = 39%	34 (2002)
U.S.	429 patients Barrett's metaplasia	WHR, BMI; distribution of adipose tissue more important than overall BMI	WHR and not BMI associated with high-grade dysplasia, OR = 1.5 (0.6–3.7); increased aneuploidy, OR = 4.3 (1.2–15.6); and loss of heterozygosity on *17*p; OR = 3.9 (1.3–11.4) No association with BMI	37 (2002)

Note: BMI = body mass index (wt/ht^2); OR = odds ratio; r = correlation coefficient; WHR = waist-hip ratio.

markers of Barrett's esophagus, including higher grade esophageal dysplasia, increased aneuploidy, and loss of heterozygosity in tumor suppressors *9p* and *17p*.

Taken together, these findings suggest that obesity increases the risk of esophageal and gastric cardia adecarcinoma by acting early and influencing risk of Barrett's esophagus. Although this cascade of events may be initiated by intra-abdominal pressure, it might also occur through alteration of growth factors, hormones, or metabolic factors that regulate cell growth [20]. Abdominal obesity is associated with hyperinsulinemia, leptin, and free fatty acids [20]. Insulin also affects the levels of circulating insulin-like growth factors (IGFs) and their binding protein. Association studies relating these factors to Barrett's esophagus are currently underway [37].

Obesity's effects may act early in the pathogenesis of esophageal adenocarcinoma, possibly by increasing risk of hiatal hernia and subsequent gastroesophageal reflux disease [38,39]. Obesity has also been associated with cell cycle abnormalities assessed using content flow cytometry to estimate the proportion of proliferating cells, fraction of cells in each phase of the cell cycle (G0, G1, S, and G2). Also, the presence of aneuploid cell populations is more common among patients with Barrett's esophagus compared to otherwise healthy individuals [37]. Recent studies [37,40] have reported an association between genetic and cell cycle abnormalities, including aneploidy (OR = 4.3) and loss of heterozygosity on *9p* and *17p* (OR = 3.9), in relation to increased central obesity as measured by waist-to-hip ratio. In one of these studies [37], women had on average a larger BMI (mean = 28.9); however, their waist-to-hip ratio was lower (0.87 vs. 0.97). This may explain in part the preponderance of esophageal and gastric cardia adenocarcinomas among men. These findings also suggest that, in the presence of Barrett's esophagus, fat distribution may be more important than BMI.

Gastroesophageal Reflux Disease (GERD)

Table 18.4 summarizes observational and experimental studies evaluating the relationship between obesity and gastroesophageal reflux symptoms. These studies were conducted in Italy, the U.K., Norway, The Netherlands, Sweden, and the U.S. Eight of the ten studies, of which some were randomized clinical trials, reported a moderate to strong dose-dependent increase in risk of gastroesophageal reflux disease among overweight and obese individuals. When compared to those who were in the lowest category of BMI [41–44], individuals at the highest category of BMI had an increased risk of gastroesophageal reflux disease, heartburn, or hiatal hernia.

In a large U.K. population-based cross-sectional study of over 27,000 individuals, a larger BMI was associated with nearly threefold increase in risk of gastroesophageal reflux disease symptoms, including heartburn and regurgitation, that was independent of confounding factors such as dyspeptic symptoms [41]. In a cross-sectional study of 1524 otherwise healthy individuals, Locke [45] also reported a strong association between gastroesophageal reflux disease and BMI. NHANES 1 follow-up data of nearly 20 years showed that hospitalization for gastroesophageal reflux disease was related to BMI [44]. Most importantly, a British study [46] found that, among obese patients who lost an average of 4 kg, gastroesophageal reflux disease symptoms were reduced significantly. These latter findings have since been confirmed in another investigation in which a higher frequency of lower esophageal sphincter dysfunction and gastroesophageal reflux disease was found among patients who remained obese, compared to those who lost weight during the 8-month study period [43].

The association between obesity and gastroesophageal reflux disease has not been found in all studies, however, including several large population-based studies and randomized clinical trials [29,47,48]. Among a Swedish population [47], no significant changes in gastroesophageal reflux disease symptoms were noted after an average weight loss of more than 9 kg.

A limitation in the interpretation of these findings is that none of the studies evaluated the role of central obesity as measured by waist circumference or waist-to-hip ratio. The timing of the relevant exposure period varies across studies, with some assessing obesity at diagnosis and others assessing obesity at varying adult ages. Furthermore, the randomized clinical trials [43,46,47] evaluated the effect of obesity on gastroesophageal reflux disease predominantly among the morbidly obese, making generalizability difficult. Despite these shortcomings, on the whole, these studies suggest that obesity increases the risk of gastroesophageal reflux disease.

DISCUSSION

The available epidemiological evidence suggests a positive association between obesity and the risk of esophageal and gastric cardia adenocarcinomas, as well as with the precursors, including Barrett's metaplasia and gastroesophageal reflux disease. As would be expected if the association were causal, this association increases with severity and duration of obesity. It also appears to be more common among men than women, suggesting that central obesity may be the important factor.

The mechanism underlying the association between obesity and adenocarcinomas of the esophagus and gastric cardia is unknown; however, several competing hypotheses have been proposed. One is that obesity exacerbates gastroesophageal reflux disease through increased intra-abdominal pressure [50] and the subsequent development of hiatal hernia [51]. More characteristic of Western populations, mechanical pressure from central obesity is exacerbated by tight belts [52] and is hypothesized to give rise to the encroachment of columnar metaplasia, a compensatory response to the corrosive effects of digestive enzymes, including gastric and bile acids. The encroachment

TABLE 18.4
Summary of Results from Studies of Obesity and Gastroesophageal Reflux Disease

Location	Design/sample size	Obesity estimation	Results: OR (95% CI) by quantile of obesity estimate	Study ref. and year
Italy	238 cases, 262 controls	BMI, weight	BMI, weight of GERD group similar to controls	29 (2000)
U.K.	Cross-sectional, n = 10,537	BMI 25–29.9 and 30+ kg/m² compared to normal and underweight	<25 kg/m² = ref; 25–<30 kg/m²; OR = 1.82 (1.33–2.5) OR 30+ kg/m² OR = 2.91 (2.0–4.1)	41 (2003)
Norway	Cross-sectional, 3113 GERD symptoms	BMI	Dose dependent increase in risk of GERD with increased obesity — men: <25 kg/m² = ref; 25–30 kg/m² OR = 2.2 (2.0–2.6); 30–35 OR = 3 3.1 (2.6–3.6); >35kg/m OR = 2 3.3 (2.4–4.7) In women, <25 = ref; 25–30 OR = 2.0 (1.7–2.4); 30–35 OR = 3.9 (3.3–4.7); >35 OR = 6.3 (4.9–8.0)	42 (2003)
Netherlands	Randomized placebo, controlled trial of obese; 42 untreated patients	BMI, WHR, waist	52% had evidence of GERD; weight loss and visceral fat loss were associated with reduction in symptoms and normal pH	43 (2002)
Sweden	Out of 820 interviewees, 135 reflux cases	BMI at age 20, and 20 years before interview	No association	48 (2000)
U.S.	Case control; 189 cases, 1024 controls; 151 hiatal hernia cases	BMI < 20; 20 to 25; 26–30; and >30 kg/m²	<20 kg/m² = ref; 20–25 kg/m² OR = 1.1 (0.7–1.6); 25–30 kg/m² OR = 1.8 (1.4–2.3); >30 kg/m² OR = 2.1 (1.5–2.6)	49 (2000)
U.S.	Cohort of 12,347 followed for 18 years	BMI	GERD hospitalizations associated with overweight or obese status; < 22 kg/m² = ref; 22–<25 OR = 1.17 (0.87–1.56); 25–28.2 OR = 1.45 (1.10–1.91); >28.2 OR = 1.93 (1.49–2.52)	44 (1999)

U.K.	Cross-sectional; 34 patients	Current BMI	Strong association; <24 kg/m² = ref; 24–27 kg/m² OR = 1.4 (0.9–2.3); 27–30 kg/m² OR = 2.0 (1.2–3.3); >30 kg/m² OR = 2.8 (1.7–4.5)	45 (1999)
U.K.	Randomized clinical trials	Current BMI	Moderate association with loss of each 4 kg in weight	46 (1999)
Sweden	Randomized clinical trials	Current BMI	No association	47 (1999)

Note: BMI = body mass index (wt/ht²); OR = odds ratio; GERD = gastroesophageal reflux disease; WHR = waist-hip ratio.

of columnar epithelium (Barrett's esophagus) is a recognized precursor for esophageal and gastric cardia adenocarcinomas. This model is compatible with the multistep process of carcinogenesis, in which central obesity and then gastroesophageal disease are the initial steps that may be followed by the development of low-grade and then high-grade dysplastic changes in the gastrointestinal tract. This hypothesis is also compatible with disease preponderance among men. However, it does not explain the lower incidence among African American men who have a larger body size [7].

Overweight status and obesity are a result of energy balance stores that are too large compared to energy output. Obesity results from high energy intake or low expenditure, or both, and reflects an interplay between heritable genetic factors involved in growth, and environmental factors that may alter endocrine function, including secretion of insulin, sex steroid, and growth hormone [53]. Approximately 25% of obesity can be attributed to genetic factors [54], although the precise loci involved are unknown. The most atherogenic fat deposit of the human body is thought to be in the abdominal cavity, around the viscera, particularly the fat deposits with small blood vessels draining into the portal vein that carries blood back to the liver [24]. This hypothesis is supported by findings that men, who tend to have a large waist circumference, are at greater risk of esophageal and gastric cardia adenocarcinomas compared to women, in whom excess fat is predominantly deposited on thighs and buttocks.

First proposed by Mercer [55], the prolonged esophageal transit time observed for solid foods is longer, on average, in obese persons compared to lean individuals. This could theoretically increase contact time for carcinogens present in food. Mercer [56] reported observing a significantly longer esophageal transit time among obese individuals compared to lean patients, even though both patient groups had been diagnosed with gastroesophageal reflux disease. However, the authors did not provide usual food types consumed or their composition to enable speculation on possible carcinogens that may have been involved. Some evidence suggests a slower transit time for foods with a high fat content compared to those without it, so disease risk may be associated with dietary fat rather than transit time. Testing this hypothesis has not received much attention because differences in the duration of exposure to any given carcinogen is probably marginal during swallowing.

Another hypothesis posited is that of increased cell proliferation [57] and inhibition of apoptosis. Elevated IGF circulating levels may enhance cell proliferation, resulting in a larger than normal number of cell divisions and increased opportunities for genetic accidents [58]. Also, because insulin-like growth factors inhibit apoptosis, the probability of survival of cells with the "single hit" is increased, thus increasing the pool of cells available for subsequent "hits" and consequent transformation. Elevated circulating levels of insulin-like growth factors may also influence the probability of progression to clinically apparent or aggressive disease.

Obese individuals are characterized by insulin resistance, compensatory hyperinsulinemia, and increased production of insulin-like growth factors [59]. A recent study on the oversecretion of IGF-I and IGF-II in gastric cancer cells [60] reported that the major binding protein, IGFBP-3, was secreted only in approximately half of the cells. Inoculation of cells with IGF-I and IGF-II resulted in proliferation. Elevated levels of IGF-I have been associated with increased risk of cancers of the breast in younger women [61–64], prostate [65–70], and colon [71–73]. Elevated levels of IGFBP-3, relative to IGF-I, have also been associated with decreased risk of breast and prostate cancer.

In addition, IGF-II has been implicated in the paracrine growth of non-small-cell lung cancer cells *in vitro* [74]. Dose-dependent, two- to threefold increases in risk have also been reported with colorectal cancer among individuals with elevated IGF-II levels [71,75], although the relationships failed to achieve statistical significance. Intra-abdominal fat stores may act as the first "hit" by altering metabolism of insulin, increasing generalized proliferative response as a result of elevated insulin or IGF levels. IGFs may also inhibit apoptosis so that the theoretical probability of survival of cells with a single hit is increased, thus increasing the pool of cells available for subsequent hits and consequent transformation. However, the prevalence of hyperinsulinemia or elevated IGF levels is unknown and, although the contribution of hyperinsulinemia to esophageal and gastric cardia adenocarcinomas has been speculated about widely, this remains unknown.

Excess body fat may also increase risk of esophageal adenocarcinoma by modifying the effect of a yet unidentified environmental carcinogen. If such an agent were sequestered in fat tissue, body fat could be associated with increased risk of esophageal adenocarcinoma. Based on this hypothesis, differences in risk among various subpopulations could therefore reflect differences in the intensity and duration of obesity. This hypothesis remains intriguing, despite the lack of data to support it, because of its potential to explain racial differences in disease risk. For example, although obesity is a plausible underlying cause of adenocarcinomas of the esophagus and gastric cardia, it is still unclear why incidence differs markedly between African Americans and whites living in the U.S., given that recent national data suggest that African American men have a higher BMI than white men do [7]. Of note, however is that abdominal visceral adiposity rather than overall size by BMI may explain, in part, racial differences in risk of these adenocarcinomas. Recent evidence suggests that, at a given BMI, white males and females have a higher waist circumference than African Americans and, presumably, visceral fat [76].

DNA damage caused by a mixture of environmental exposures may require the base excision or strand break repair. In epidemiological and animal studies, oxidative stress and lipid peroxidation are associated with increased obesity, and weight loss among the morbidly obese decreases oxidative stress and increases antioxidant activity [77]. Base excision repair targets DNA damage associated with oxidative stress, although it may also repair strand breaks and nonbulky adducts induced by exogenous agents such as ionizing radiation and tobacco smoke [78]. Carcinogen-induced DNA damage and cellular damage induced by inflammation during hyperkeritization may play a role in the carcinogenesis of the esophagus and gastric cardia. The precise mechanism involved in obesity and oxidative stress is complex; however, the insulin resistance common in obesity is associated with oxidative stress in humans [79,80].

DNA repair capacity is variable in human populations and a part of that variation is believed to be genetic. A reduction in efficiency of any one pathway may increase risk of replicating damaged or transformed cells. DNA repair capacity has been evaluated by comparing polymorphisms in base excision and nucleotide excision repair pathways in relation to risk of cancers of the breast [81,82], prostate [83,84], lung [85,86], skin [87], and head and neck [88]. *In vitro* studies of other adenocarcinomas, including pancreatic and prostate tissue, have shown that DNA adducts form after exposure to environmental toxins [89,90] and intake of diets with antioxidative properties has been shown to decrease prostate cancer risk through inactivation of reactive oxygen species [91]. In support of this hypothesis, Brown [26] reported an inverse association between increased fiber intake and adenocarcinomas of the esophagus and gastric cardia. To date, no studies have evaluated whether DNA repair capacity may play an important role in the development of esophageal and gastric cardia adenocarcinomas.

A suboptimal ability to mount a cellular immune response has been implicated in the development of several adenocarcinomas and has also been associated with obesity [92]. Several animal studies have also linked obesity with impaired immune response [93,94]. Cytokines and other proinflammatory mediators have been implicated in inflammatory Barrett's metaplasia [95]. Cytokines, chemokines, and their receptors have various biological functions, including the inflammatory response, immune cell trafficking, angiogenesis, and metastasis. Proinflammatory chemokines and their receptors are expressed in esophageal and gastric cancer cells and infiltrating immune cells within esophageal tumors. Proinflammatory gene polymorphisms in combination with proinflammatory conditions exacerbated by obesity-related gastroesophageal reflux, accompanied by sloughing of basal cells, hyperkeratinization and hyperproliferation, may influence the development of esophageal and gastric cardia adenocarcinoma.

Humoral immunity in tissue found in the gastrointestinal tract is characterized by the production of immunoglobulin A (IgA) and the CC chemokines CCR2, CCR4, and CCR9 are expressed by esophageal and intestinal epithelial cells [96]. Solid tumor and leukemic cells expressing chemokine receptors have been shown to metastasize to chemokine-secreting organs [96,97]. Chemokines may indirectly affect tumor development by attracting immunocompetent cells with pro- or antitumoral activities. Chemokine receptors mediate the migration of lymphocytes through the binding of ligands, and the expression is differentially regulated in lymphocyte subsets.

Cytokines such as interferon (IFN)-alpha and gamma are also known potent immune modulators that can inhibit or enhance immune cell activity within the tightly regulated microenvironment of inflammation, depending upon the concentration of the cytokine and the activation stage of the cell. Among B-cell chronic lymphocytic leukemia patients, increases in several cytokines and chemokines, including IFN-alpha-2b, CC chemokines CXR3, CCR7, and CXR4, were shown to increase with increasing disease severity [98]. Animals deficient in CCR4 and CCR9 have also shown a reduced IgA immune response [99]. CCR9 has been identified as the chemokine receptor regulating lymphocyte trafficking during T-cell development and in mucosal immunity [100].

SUMMARY AND FUTURE DIRECTIONS

The incidence of esophageal and gastric cardia adenocarcinomas has been increasing rapidly in the last 30 years, and the etiology of these adenocarcinomas is not fully understood. The temporal, gender, and geographic variation for adenocarcinomas of gastric cardia and esophagus, together with suggestions of familial aggregation of these adenocarcinomas, suggests the importance of environmental factors whose intensity of exposure has increased in the last 30 to 40 years. Obesity has been associated with esophageal and gastric cardia risk as well as its precursors, including Barrett's esophagus and gastroesophageal reflux disease. If causally related, obesity may act early in carcinogenesis through increased intra-abdominal pressure, followed by gastroesophageal reflux disease, the deregulation of the cell cycle, Barrett's esophagus, and the dysplasia, and eventually leading to adenocarcinoma.

The lower incidence among women, despite a similar prevalence of obesity in specific subpopulations, and the high prevalence of adenocarcinomas in geographic regions where the prevalence of obesity is moderate suggest that central obesity, more frequently occurring in men, may be the important factor in the etiology of adenocarcinomas of the esophagus and gastric cardia. However, correlates of central obesity, such as waist-to-hip ratio and weight gain, have not been consistently linked to risk of these tumors. Whether this is due to the challenges associated with accurately assessing these latter measures in epidemiological research, particularly using a case-control design, needs to be clarified. Furthermore, if obesity is causally related to gastric cardia and esophageal adenocarcinomas, the lower risk of cancer among African Americans, who generally have a higher prevalence of obesity, needs to be reconciled. Molecular epidemiological studies of esophageal cancer may help to elucidate these issues.

Assessment of obesity in epidemiological research is subject to misclassification, and may vary by gender, in that women may under-report and men may over-report body size. Consistent with this possibility, such misclassification would result in an overestimation of the risk associated with obesity among men and an underestimation of risk among women. Although long-term cohort studies would be ideal, determining the role of obesity in the development of adenocarcinomas of the esophagus and gastric cardia can be achieved by carefully designed, population-based, case-control studies. Disentangling the effects of obesity from other competing factors will require studies to capture retrospectively fat distribution parameters and changes in these parameters over time during adulthood.

REFERENCES

1. Parkin DM. Bray F. Ferlay J. Pisani P. Estimating the world cancer burden: Globocan 2000. *Int J Cancer*, 2001; 94(2):153–156.
2. Parkin DM. Bray FI. Devesa SS. Cancer burden in the year 2000. The global picture. *Eur J Cancer*, 2001; 37 Suppl 8:S4–66.
3. Vizcaino AP. Moreno V. Lambert R. Parkin DM. Time trends incidence of both major histologic types of esophageal carcinomas in selected countries, 1973–1995. *Int J Cancer*, 2002; 99:860–868.
4. Devesa SS. Blot WJ. Fraumeni JF. Jr. Changing patterns in the incidence of esophageal and gastric carcinoma in the U.S. 1998; *Cancer*, 1998; 83(10):2049–2053.
5. Mokdad AH. Serdula MK. Dietz WH. Bowman BA. Marks JS. Koplan JP. The spread of obesity epidemic in the U.S. 1991–1998. *JAMA*, 1999; 282:1519–1522.
6. Mokdad AH. Ford ES. Bowman BA. Dietz WH. Vinicor F. Bales VS. Marks JS. Prevalence of obesity, diabetes and obesity-related health risk factors. *JAMA*, 2003; 289:76–79.
7. National Center for Health Statistics. http://www.fedstats.gov/key_stats/NCHSkey.html.
8. Sturm R. Increases in clinically severe obesity in the U.S., 1986–2000. *Arch Intern Med*, 2003; 16:2146–2148.
9. Bray GA. Commentary on classics in obesity. Life insurance and overweight. *Obesity Res*, 1995; 3:97–99.
10. De Michele M. Panico S. Iannuzzi A. Celentano E. Ciardullo AV. Galasso R. Sacchetti L. Zarrilli F. Bond MG. Rubba P. Association of obesity and central fat distribution with carotid artery wall thickening in middle-aged women. *Stroke*, 2002; 33(12):2923–2928.
11. Calle EE. Rodriguez C. Walker–Thurmond K. Thun MJ. Overweight, obesity, and mortality from cancer in a prospectively studied cohort of U.S. adults. *N Engl J Med*, 2003; 348(17):1625–1638.
12. Munoz N. Day NE. Esophageal cancer. In: Fraumeni JF. Jr. Ed. *Cancer Epidemiology and Prevention*. New York. Oxford University Press, 1996; 681–706.
13. Gammon MD. Schoenberg JB. Ahsan H. Risch HA. Vaughan TL. Chow WH. Rotterdam H. et al. Tobacco, alcohol, and socioeconomic status and adenocarcinomas of the esophagus and gastric cardia. *J Natl Cancer Inst*, 1997; 89(17):1277–1284.
14. Chow WH. Blaser MJ. Blot WJ. Gammon MD. Vaughan TL. Risch HA. Perez–Perez GI. Schoenberg JB. Stanford JL. Rotterdam H. West AB. Fraumeni JF. Jr. An inverse relation between cagA+ strains of *Helicobacter pylori* infection and risk of esophageal and gastric cardia adenocarcinoma. *Cancer Res*, 1998; 58:588–90.
15. Chow WH. Blot WJ. Vaughan TL. Risch HA. Gammon MD. Stanford JL. et al. Body mass index and risk of adenocarcinoma of the esophagus and gastric cardia. *J Natl Cancer Inst*, 1998; 90:150–155.
16. Wu AH. Wan P. Bernstein L. A multiethnic population-based study of smoking, alcohol and body size and risk of adenocarcinomas of the stomach and esophagus (U.S.). *Cancer Causes Control*, 2001; 12:721–732.
17. Lagergren J. Bergstrom R. Nyren O. Association between body mass and adenocarcinoma of the esophagus and gastric cardia. *Ann Intern Med*, 1999; 130:883–890.
18. Tretli S. Robsahm TE. Height, weight and cancer of the esophagus and stomach: a follow-up study in Norway. *Eur J Cancer Prev*, 1999; 8:115–122.
19. Farrow DC. Vaughan TL. Sweeney C. Gammon MD. Chow WH. Risch HA. Stanford JL. Hansten PD. Mayne ST. Schoenberg JB. Rotterdam H. Ahsan H. West AB. Dubrow R. Fraumeni JF. Jr. Blot WJ. Gastroesophageal reflux disease, use of H2 receptor antagonists, and risk of esophageal and gastric cancer. *Cancer Causes Control*, 2000; 11(3):231–238.

20. Vaughan TL. Esophagus. In: Franco EL. Rohan TE. Eds. *Cancer Precursors — Epidemiology, Detection, and Prevention*, 2002. Springer–Verlag. New York; p. 96–116.
21. Ji BT. Chow WH. Yang G. McLaughlin JK. Gao RN. Zheng W. Shu XO. et al. Body mass index and risk of cancers of the gastric cardia and distal stomach in Shanghai, China. *Cancer Epidemiol Biomarkers Prev*, 1997; 6:481-485.
22. Knudson AG. Jr. Mutation and cancer: statistical study of retinoblastoma. *Proc Nat Acad Sci USA*, 1971; 68:820–823.
23. Kuczmarski RJ. Flegal KM. Criteria for definition of overweight in transition: background and recommendations for the U.S. *Am J Clin Nutr*, 2000; 72:1074–1081.
24. Bray GA. Bouchard C. James WPT. Definition and proposed current classification of obesity. In: Bray GA. Bouchard C. James WPT. Eds. *Handbook of Obesity*. New York: Marcel Dekker, 1998; 31–40.
25. Kabat GC. Ng SK. Wynder EL. Tobacco, alcohol intake, and diet in relation to adenocarcinoma of the esophagus and gastric cardia. *Cancer Causes Control*, 1993; 4:123–132.
26. Brown LM. Silverman DT. Pottern LM. Schoenberg JB. Greenberg RS. Swanson GM. et al. Adenocarcinoma of the esophagus and esophagogastric junction in white men in the U.S.: alcohol, tobacco, and socioeconomic factors. *Cancer Causes Control*, 1994; 5:333–340.
27. Vaughan TL. Davis S. Kristal A. Thomas DB. Obesity, alcohol, and tobacco as risk factors for cancers of the esophagus and gastric cardia: adenocarcinoma vs. squamous cell carcinoma. *Cancer Epidemiol Biomarkers Prev*, 1995; 4:85–92.
28. Zhang ZF. Kurtz RC. Sun M. Karpeh M. Jr. Yu GP et al. Adenocarcinomas of the esophagus and gastric cardia: medical conditions, tobacco, alcohol, and socioeconomic factors. *Cancer Epidemiol Biomarkers Prev*, 1996; 5:761–768.
29. Incarbone R. Bonavina L. Szachnowicz S. Saino G. Peracchia A. *Dis Esophagus*, 2000; 13:275–278.
30. Chen H. Ward MH. Graubard BI. Heineman EF. Markin RM. Potischman NA. et al. Dietary patterns and adenocarcinoma of the esophagus and distal stomach. *Am J Clin Nutr*, 2002; 75:137–144.
31. Cheng KK. Sharp L. McKinney PA. Logan RFA. Chilvers CED. Cook–Mozaffari P. et al. A case-control study of oesophageal adenocarcinoma in women: a preventable disease. *Br J Cancer*, 2000; 83:127–132.
32. Chak A. Lee T. Kinnard MF. Brock W. Faulx A. Willis J. Cooper GS. Sivak MV. Goddard KAB. Familial aggregation of Barrett's esophagus, esophageal adenocarcinoma and esophagogastric junction adenocarcinoma in Caucasian adults. *Gut*, 2002; 51:323–328.
33. Bollschweiler E. Wolfgarten E. Nowroth T. Rosendahl U. Monig SP. Holscher AH. Vitamin intake and risk of esophageal cancer in Germany. *J Cancer Res Clin Oncol*, 2002; 128:575–580.
34. Caygill CPJ, Johnston DA, Lopez M, Johnsto BJ, Watson A, Reed PI, Hill M. Lifestyle factors and Barrett's esophagus. *Am J Gatsroenerol*, 2002; 97:1328–1331.
35. Moe GL. Kristal AR. Levine DS. Vaughan TL. Reid BJ. Waist-to-hip ratio and dietary and serum selenium are associated with DNA content flow cytometry in Barrett's esophagus. *Nutr Cancer*, 2000; 36:7–13.
36. Gerson LB. Shetler K. Triadafilopoulos G. Prevalence of Barrett's esophagus in asymptomatic individuals. *Gastroentorology*, 2002; 123:636–639.
37. Vaughan TL. Kristal AR. Blount PL. Levine DS. Galipeau PC. Prevo LJ. Sanchez CA. Rabinovitch PS. Reid BJ. Nonsteroidal anti-inflammatory drug use, body mass index, and anthropometry in relation to genetic and flow cytometric abnormalities in Barrett's esophagus. *Cancer Epidemiol Biomarkers Prev*, 2002; 11:745–752.
38. Farrow DC. Vaughan TL. Sweeney C. Gammon MD. Chow WH. Risch HA. Stanford JL. Hansten PD. Mayne ST. Schoenberg JB. Rotterdam H. Ahsan H. West AB. Dubrow R. Fraumeni JF. Jr. Blot WJ. Gastroesophageal reflux disease, use of H2 receptor antagonists, and risk of esophageal and gastric cancer. Cancer Causes Control, 2000; 11:231–238.
39. Avidan B. Sonnenberg A. Schnell TG. Chejfec G. Metz A. Sontag SJ. Hiatal hernia size, Barrett's length, and severity of acid reflux are all risk factors for esophageal adenocarcinoma. Am J Gastroenterol, 2002; 97(8):1930–1936.
40. Bjorntorp P. Hormonal control of regional fat distribution. Hum reprod. 1997; 12 Suppl 1:21–25.
41. Murray L. Johnston B. Lane A. Harvey I. Donovan J. Nair P. Harvey R. Relationship between body mass and gastroesophageal reflux symptoms: the Bristol Helicobacter Project. Int J Epidemiol, 2003; 32:645–650.

42. Nilsson M. Johnston R. Ye W. Hveem K. Lagergren J. Obesity and estrogen as risk factors for gastroesophageal reflux symptoms. *JAMA*, 2003; 290:66–72.
43. Mathus–Vliegen EM. Tygat GN. Gastroesophageal reflux in obese subjects: influence of overweight, weight, weight loss and chronic gastric balloon distension. *Scand J Gastroenterol*, 2002; 37:1246–1252.
44. Ruhl CE. Everhat JE. Overweight, but not high fat intake, incraeses risk of gastroesophageal reflux disease hospitalization: the NHANES I Epidemiologic Follow-Up Study. First National Health and Nutrition Examination Survey. *Ann Epidemiol*, 1999; 9:424–435.
45. Locke GR. III. Talley NJ. Fett SL. Zinsmeister AR. Melton LJ. III. Risk factors associated with symptoms of gastroesophageal reflux. *Am J Med*, 1999; 106:642–649.
46. Fraser–Moddie CA, Norton B. Gornall C. Magnago S. Weale AR. Holmes GK. Weight loss has an independent beneficial effect on symptoms of gastro-oesophageal reflux in patients who are overweight. *Scand J Gatsroenterol*, 1999; 34:337–340.
47. Kjellin A. Ramel S. Rossner S. Thor K. Gastroesophageal reflux in obese patients is not reduced by weight reduction. *Scand J Gastroenterol*, 1996; 31:1047–1051.
48. Lagergren J. Bergstrom R. Nyren O. No relation between body mass index and gastroesophageal reflux symptoms in a Swedish population based study. *Gut*, 2000; 47:26–29.
49. Wilson LJ. Ma W. Hirschowitz BI. Association of obesity with hiatal hernia and esophagitis. *Am J Gastroenterol*, 1999; 94:2840–2844.
50. Mayne ST. Navarro SA. Diet, obesity and reflux in the etiology of adenocarcinomas of the esophagus and gastric cardia in humans. *J Nutr*, 2002; 132(11 Suppl):3467S–3470S
51. Bowers SP. Mattar SG. Smith CD. Waring JP. Hunter JG. Clinical and histologic follow-up after antireflux surgery for Barrett's esophagus. *J Gastrointestinal Surg*, 2002; 6:532–8.
52. La Veccia C. Negri E. Lagiou P. Trichopolos D. Oesophageal adenocarcinoma: a paradigm of mechanical carcinogenesis. *Int J Cancer*, 2002; 102:269–270.
53. Kopelman PG. Finer N. Reply: is obesity a disease? *Int J Obesity Relat Metab Disorders*, 2001; 25:1405–1406.
54. Bouchard C. Bray GA. Hubbard VS. Basic and clinical aspects of regional fat distribution. *Am J Clin Nutr*, 1990; 52:946–950.
55. Mercer CD. Wren SF. DaCosta LR. Beck IT. Lower esophageal sphincter pressure and gastroesophageal pressure gradients in excessively obese patients. *J Med*, 1987;18(3–4):135–146.
56. Mercer CD. Rue C. Hanelin L. Hill LD. Effect of obesity on esophageal transit. *Am J Surg*, 1985; 149:177–181.
57. Preston–Martin S. Pike MC. Ross RK. Jones PA. Henderson BE. Increased cell division as a cause of human cancer. *Cancer Res*, 1990; 50:7415–7421.
58. Pollak M. Insulin-like growth factors and prostate cancer. *Epidemiologic Rev*, 2001; 23:59–66.
59. Yu H. Mistry J. Nicar MJ. Khosravi MJ. Diamandis A. van Doorn J. Juul A. Insulin-like growth factors (IGF-I, free IGF-I and IGF-II) and insulin-like growth factor binding proteins (IGFBP-2, IGFBP-3, IGFBP-6, and ALS) in blood circulation. *J Clin Lab Anal*, 1999; 13:166–172.
60. Yi HK. Hwang PH. Yang DH. Kang CW. Lee DY. Expression of the insulin-like growth factors (IGFs) and the IGF-binding proteins (IGFBPs) in human gastric cancer cells. *Eur J Cancer*, 2001; 37:2257–2263.
61. Hankinson SE. Willett WC. Colditz GA. Hunter DJ. Michaud DS. Deroo B. Rosner B. Speizer FE. Pollak M. Circulating concentrations of insulin-like growth factor-I and risk of breast cancer. *Lancet*, 1998; 351(9113):1393–1396.
62. Bruning PF. Van Doorn J. Bonfrer JM. Van Noord PA. Korse CM. Linders TC. Hart AA. Insulin-like growth-factor-binding protein 3 is decreased in early-stage operable premenopausal breast cancer. *Int J Cancer*, 1995; 62(3):266–270.
63. Toniolo P. Bruning PF. Akhmedkhanov A. Bonfrer JM. Koenig KL. Lukanova A. Shore RE. Zeleniuch–Jacquotte A. Serum insulin-like growth factor-I and breast cancer. *Int J Cancer*, 2000; 88:828–832.
64. Bohlke K. Cramer DW. Trichopoulos D. Mantzoros CS. Insulin-like growth factor-I in relation to premenopausal ductal carcinoma *in situ* of the breast. *Epidemiology*, 1998; 9(5):570–573.
65. Chan JM. Stampfer MJ. Giovannucci E. Gann PH. Ma J. Wilkinson P. Hennekens CH. Pollak M. Plasma insulin-like growth factor-I and prostate cancer risk: a prospective study. *Science*, 1998; 279:563–566.

66. Stattin P. Stenman UH. Riboli E. Hallmans G. Kaaks R. Ratios of IGF-I, IGF binding protein-3, and prostate-specific antigen in prostate cancer detection. *J Clin Endocrinol Metab*, 2001; 86:5745–5748.
67. Mantzoros CS. Tzonou A. Signorello LB. Stampfer M. Trichopoulos D. Adami HO. Insulin-like growth factor 1 in relation to prostate cancer and benign prostatic hyperplasia. *Br J Cancer*, 1997; 76:1115–1118.
68. Harman SM. Metter EJ. Blackman MR. Landis PK. Carter HB. Baltimore Longitudinal Study on Aging. Serum levels of insulin-like growth factor I (IGF-I), IGF-II, IGF-binding protein-3, and prostate-specific antigen as predictors of clinical prostate cancer. *J Clin Endocrinol Metab*, 2000; 85:4258–4265.
69. Wolk A. Mantzoros CS. Andersson SO. Bergstrom R. Signorello LB. Lagiou P. Adami HO. Trichopoulos D. Insulin-like growth factor 1 and prostate cancer risk: a population-based, case-control study. *J Natl Cancer Inst*, 1998; 90:911–915.
70. Djavan B. Susani M. Bursa B. Basharkhah A. Simak R. Marberger M. Predictability and significance of multifocal prostate cancer in the radical prostatectomy specimen. *Tech Urol*, 1999; 5:139–142.
71. Ma J. Pollak MN. Giovannucci E. Chan JM. Tao Y. Hennekens CH. Stampfer MJ. Prospective study of colorectal cancer risk in men and plasma levels of insulin-like growth factor (IGF)-I and IGF-binding protein-3 [see comment]. *J Natl Cancer Inst*, 1999; 91:620–625.
72. Giovannucci E. Pollak MN. Platz EA. Willett WC. Stampfer MJ. Majeed N. Colditz GA. Speizer FE. Hankinson SE. A prospective study of plasma insulin-like growth factor-1 and binding protein-3 and risk of colorectal neoplasia in women. *Cancer Epidemiol Biomarkers Prev*, 2000; 9:345–349.
73. Kaaks R. Toniolo P. Akhmedkhanov A. Lukanova A. Biessy C. Dechaud H. Rinaldi S. Zeleniuch–Jacquotte A. Shore RE. Riboli E. Serum C-peptide, insulin-like growth factor (IGF)-I, IGF-binding proteins, and colorectal cancer risk in women. *J Natl Cancer Inst*, 2000; 92:1592–1600.
74. Reeve JG. Morgan J. Schwander J. Bleehen NM. Role for membrane and secreted insulin-like growth factor-binding protein-2 in the regulation of insulin-like growth factor action in lung tumors. *Cancer Res*, 1993; 53:4680–4685.
75. Manousos O. Souglakos J. Bosetti C. Tzonou A. Chatzidakis V. Trichopoulos D. Adami HO. Mantzoros C. IGF-I and IGF-II in relation to colorectal cancer. *Int J Cancer*, 1999; 83:15–17.
76. Okosun IS. Anochie LK. Chandra KM. Racial/ethnic differences in prehypertension in American adults: Population and relative attributable risk of abdominal adiposity. J Hum Hypertension, 2004;18:849-855.
77. Dandona P. Mohanty P. Ghanim H. Aljada A. Browne R. Hamouda W. Prabhala A. Afzal A. Garg R. The suppressive effect of dietary restriction and weight loss in the obese on the generation of reactive oxygen species by leukocytes, lipid peroxidation, and protein carbonylation. *J Clin Endocrinol Metab*, 2001; 86:355–362.
78. Wiencke JK. DNA adduct burden and tobacco carcinogenesis. *Oncogene*, 2002; 21(48):7376–7391.
79. Urakawa H. Katsuki A. Sumida Y. Gabazza EC. Murashima S. Morioka K. Maruyama N. Kitagawa N.Tanaka T. Hori Y. Nakatani K. Yano Y. Adachi Y. Oxidative stress is associated with adiposity and insulin resistance in men. *J Clin Endocrinol Metab*, 2003; 88(10):4673–4676.
80. Dandona P. Aljada A. Bandyopadhyay A. Inflammation: the link between insulin resistance, obesity and diabetes. *Trends Immunol*, 2004; 25(1):4–7.
81. Tang D. Cho S. Rundle A. Chen S. Phillips D. Zhou J. Hsu Y. Schnabel F. Estabrook A. Perera FP. Polymorphisms in the DNA repair enzyme XPD are associated with increased levels of PAH–DNA adducts in a case-control study of breast cancer. *Breast Cancer Res Treatment*, 2002; 75:159–166.
82. Duell EJ. Millikan RC. Pittman GS. Winkel S. Lunn RM. Tse CK. Eaton A. Mohrenweiser HW. Newman B. Bell DA. Polymorphisms in the DNA repair gene XRCC1 and breast cancer. *Cancer Epidemiol Biomarkers Prev*, 2001; 10(3):217–222.
83. van Gils CH. Bostick RM. Stern MC. Taylor JA. Differences in base excision repair capacity may modulate the effect of dietary antioxidant intake on prostate cancer risk: an example of polymorphisms in the XRCC1 gene. *Cancer Epidemiol Biomarkers Prev*, 2002; 11:1279–1284.
84. Rybicki BA. Conti DV. Moreira A. Cicek M. Casey G. Witte JS. DNA repair gene XRCC1 and XPD polymorphisms and risk of prostate cancer. *Cancer Epidemiol Biomarkers Prev*, 2004; 13:23–29.
85. Chen S. Tang D. Xue K. Xu L. Ma G. Hsu Y. Cho SS. DNA repair gene XRCC1 and XPD polymorphisms and risk of lung cancer in a Chinese population. *Carcinogenesis*, 2000; 23(8):1321–1325.

86. David–Beabes GL. Lunn RM. London SJ. No association between the XPD (Lys751G1n) polymorphismor the XRCC3 (Thr241Met) polymorphism and lung cancer risk. *Cancer Epidemiol Biomarkers Prev*, 2001; 10(8):911–912.
87. Winsey SL. Haldar NA. Marsh HP. Bunce M. Marshall SE. Harris AL. Wojnarowska F. Welsh KI. A variant within the DNA repair gene XRCC3 is associated with the development of melanoma skin cancer. *Cancer Res*, 2000; 60(20):5612–5616.
88. Sturgis EM. Castillo EJ. Li L. Zheng R. Eicher SA. Clayman GL. Strom SS. Spitz MR. Wei Q. Polymorphisms of DNA repair gene XRCC1 in squamous cell carcinoma of the head and neck. *Carcinogenesis*, 1999; 20:2125–129.
89. Wang M. Abbruzzese JL. Friess H. Hittelman WN. Evans DB. Abbruzzese MC. Chiao P. Li D. DNA adducts in human pancreatic tissues and their potential role in carcinogenesis. *Cancer Res*, 1998; 58(1):38–41.
90. DeWeese TL. Hruszkewycz AM. Marnett LJ. Oxidative stress in chemoprevention trials. *Urology*, 2001; 57(4 Suppl 1):137–140.
91. Fleshner NE. Kucuk O. Antioxidant dietary supplements: rationale and current status as chemopreventive agents for prostate cancer. *Urology*, 2001; 57(4 Suppl 1):90–94.
92. Nieman DC. Nehlsen–Cannarella SI. Henson DA. Butterworth DE. Fagoaga OR. Warren BJ. Rainwater MK. Immune response to obesity and moderate weight loss. *Int J Obesity Relat Metabolic Disorders: J Int Assoc Study Obesity*, 1996; 20(4):353–360.
93. Plotkin BJ. Paulson D. Chelich A. Jurak D. Cole J. Kasimos J. Burdick JR. Casteel N. Immune responsiveness in a rat model for type II diabetes (Zucker rat, fa/fa): susceptibility to *Candida albicans* infection and leucocyte function. *J Med Microbioly*, 1996; 44:277–283.
94. Moriguchi S. Kato M. Sakai K. Yamamoto S. Shimizu E. Exercise training restores decreased cellular immune functions in obese Zucker rats. *J Appl Physiol*, 1998; 84:311–317.
95. Oka M. Attwood SE. Kaul B. Smyrk TC. DeMeester TR. Immunosuppression in patients with Barrett's esophagus. *Surgery*, 1992; 112(1):11–17.
96. Letsch A. Keilholz U. Schadendorf D. Assfalg G. Asemissen AM. Thiel E. Scheibenbogen C. Functional CCR9 expression is associated with small intestinal metastasis. *J Invest Dermatol*, 2004;122:685–690.
97. Murakami T. Cardones AR. Hwang ST. Chemokine receptors and melanoma metastasis. *J Dermatol Sci*, 2004; 36:71–78.
98. Ghobrial IM. Bone ND. Stenson MJ. Novak A. Hedin KE. Kay NE. Ansell SM. Expression of the chemokine receptors CXCR4 and CCR7 and disease progression in B-cell chronic lymphocytic leukemia/small lymphocytic lymphoma. *Mayo Clinic Proc*, 2004; 79:318–325.
99. Van Damme J, Struyf S, Opdenakker G. Chemokine-protease interaction in cancer. *Semin Cancer Biol*, 2004; 14:201–208.
100. Zabel Zella D. Barabitskaja O. Casareto L. Romerio F. Secchiero P. Reitz MS., Jr. Gallo RC. Weichold FF. Recombinant INF-alpha 2b increases the expression of apoptosis CD95 and chemokine receptors CCR1 and CCR3 in momocytoid cells. *J Immunol*, 1999; 163:3169–3175.

Section V

Mechanisms Associating Obesity with Cancer Incidence

19 Obesity and Sex Hormones

Rudolf Kaaks and Anne McTiernan

CONTENTS

INTRODUCTION

Overweight and obesity increase risk for the development of several types of cancer, including postmenopausal breast, colon, endometrium, kidney, lower esophagus, pancreas, and, perhaps, ovary and thyroid cancers [1]. Once individuals develop cancer, depending on the site, they may be at increased risk of recurrence and poorer survival if they are overweight or obese. Several potential mechanisms might explain the link between increased adiposity and increased cancer risk, including hormonal, inflammatory, and immune system effects. This chapter reviews the scientific literature on the association between excess adiposity and sex hormone concentrations in women and men.

ADIPOSE TISSUE

Adipose tissue constitutes an active endocrine and metabolic organ that can have far-reaching effects on the physiology of other tissues [2]. In response to endocrine and metabolic signals from other organs, adipose tissue responds by increases or decreases in the release of free fatty acids — an energy-providing fuel for skeletal muscle and other tissues. It plays an active role in the regulation of energy balance and lipid metabolism through the release of several peptide hormones, including leptin, adiponectin, resistin, and tumor necrosis factor alpha (TNFα). Increased adipose tissue release of free fatty acids, resistin, and TNFα, as well as reduced release of adiponectin, in turn give rise to insulin resistance — a metabolic state characterized by reduced metabolic response of tissues (muscle, liver, adipose) to insulin — and to compensatory hyperinsulinemia [3,4].

In addition to its role in regulating energy balance, lipid metabolism, and insulin sensitivity, adipose tissue expresses various steroid hormone metabolizing enzymes and, especially in postmenopausal women and men, is an important source of circulating estrogens (Table 19.1).

TABLE 19.1
Associations of Obesity with Selected Hormones and Binding Globulins

Hormone or binding globulin	Obesity vs. normal weight
Insulin	↑
Insulin-like growth factor-I (IGF-I)	Nonlinear, peak around BMI 24–27 kg/m^2
Free IGF-I	↑
IGF binding protein-1	↓
IGF binding protein-3	↑ or NE
Sex hormone-binding globulin	↓
Total testosterone	↓ (M), NE (F); ↑ (PCOS)
Free testosterone	↓ (M), ↑ (F)
Total estradiol	↑ (M, postmenopausal F) NE (premenopausal F)
Free estradiol	↑ (M, postmenopausal F) NE (premenopausal F)

Notes: ↑ = increased levels; ↓ = decreased levels; NE = no observed effect; M = males; F = females; PCOS = premenopausal women with polycystic ovary syndrome.

SEX HORMONES AND CANCER

Epidemiological studies have provided substantial evidence that adiposity-induced alterations in circulating levels of sex steroids could in large part explain the associations observed between anthropometric indices of excess weight and risks of cancers of the breast (postmenopasual women only) and endometrium pre- and postmenopasual women) [1]. For these two tissue types, a large body of experimental and clinical evidence also indicates the central role of estrogens, androgens, and progesterone in regulating cellular differentiation, proliferation, and apoptosis induction [5–7].

A recent combined analysis of nested case-control data from nine cohort studies, with data from 663 breast cancer cases and 1765 women without breast cancer, showed that postmenopausal women with elevated estrogen or androgen levels have increased risk for developing breast cancer [8]. Women with blood hormone concentrations in the top quintile for estradiol, free estradiol, testosterone, androstenedione, dehydroepiandrosterone (DHEA), and dehydroepiandrosterone sulfate (DHEAS) were approximately twice as likely to develop breast cancer compared with women with serum hormones in the bottom quintile, and the trends were highly statistically significant. Furthermore, risk was inversely related to blood levels of sex hormone-binding globulin (SHBG) [8,9].

Further analyses of these nine pooled cohort studies indicated that the association of body mass index (BMI, kg/m^2) with breast cancer risk could be attributed almost entirely to increasing blood levels of total or bioavailable estradiol with increasing BMI [10]. Taken together, these studies indicate that much, if not all, of the BMI–breast cancer relationship can be explained by the adiposity-related increase in endogenous estrogen levels.

Further evidence that increased estrogen levels may underlie the association between BMI and breast cancer comes from studies of menopausal hormone therapy. BMI is more strongly related to risk of breast cancer among postmenopausal women who have never used menopausal hormone therapy, compared to women who did use these hormones [11–15]. A likely interpretation of this is that only among women whose levels of estrogens are low (i.e., after menopause, and among nonusers of menopausal hormone therapy) does increased adiposity lead to a rise in breast cancer risk, but not among women whose circulating estrogens are already high due to menopausal hormone therapy use. Finally, mortality is higher among heavier women with breast cancer than among leaner women, and some studies indicate that the association of elevated BMI with poorer prognosis is more pronounced among women with estrogen receptor (ER)-positive tumors [17–19].

With regard to endometrial cancer, a number of case-control studies [20] and prospective studies [21,22] have shown increased cancer risks among pre- and postmenopausal women who have comparatively low plasma levels of SHBG and high levels of the androgens Δ4-androstenedione and testosterone. In one prospective study, risk was also found to be directly related to postmenopausal serum levels of estrone and total and bioavailable estradiol [20,21] with estimated relative risks up to about 5.0 for women in the upper quartiles or quintiles of estradiol levels [21]. In premenopausal women, endometrial cancer risk is also elevated among women with polycystic ovary syndrome [20], which often develops together with, and in large extent as a consequence of, chronic hyperinsulinemia and is generally related to progesterone deficiency.

These various relationships all fit a coherent physiologic model in line with the "unopposed estrogen" theory and endometrial cancer [20,23,24]. This widely accepted theory is based on a diverse body of evidence, including the association between endometrial cancer and the use of unopposed estrogen therapy. It stipulates that endometrial cancer development is enhanced by the mitogenic effects of estrogens when these are insufficiently counterbalanced by progesterone.

Among men, prostate cancer development is also thought to be related to endogenous hormone metabolism, such as by androgen production [25–28]. However, excess weight does not appear to be a key risk factor for prostate cancer, with the possible exception of advanced disease. Indeed, one hypothesis is that obese men, who have high estrogen and low testosterone levels compared with lighter weight men, may have lower risk of prostate cancer due to these hormonal imbalances [29]. Furthermore, risk for prostate cancer is not consistently associated with increase in circulating total or bioavailable testosterone, or other androgens [26–28]. One prospective cohort study suggests that men with high estradiol levels and men with low testosterone levels may be at reduced risk for prostate cancer [28].

ESTROGENS

Adiposity and Estrogens in Women

Estrogens can promote growth of several hormone-dependent tumors, particularly breast and endometrium; conversely, antiestrogens or withdrawal of endogenous estrogens are effective adjuvant treatments for breast cancer [30,31]. Postmenopausal women produce estrogens in fat and other tissue through the aromatization of androgens to estrogens [32,33]. The enzyme aromatase is abundantly present in adipose tissue, especially subcutaneous fat. Estrogens are tumor promoters *in vitro* and *in vivo*, and women with high circulating levels of estrogens are at increased risk of developing breast cancer [8].

After menopause, the ovarian production of estrogen and progesterone ceases, but the production of various androgens continues. Most women continue to have detectable concentrations of circulating estrogen after menopause, however; the most prevalent is estrone [32]. After menopause, estrone is produced predominantly through the peripheral conversion, mostly in adipose tissue of adrenal androstenedione [33]. Estradiol, the most metabolically active of the estrogens, is produced in postmenopausal women through the reduction of estrone and the aromatization of ovarian and adrenal testosterone. In postmenopausal women, about 55% of circulating estradiol is bound to SHBG, whereas only a small fraction (2 to 3%) circulates in the "free" (unbound) state; most of the remainder is bound to albumin (45%) [34]. The free and albumin-bound fractions can diffuse from the circulation toward target tissues, and is termed "bioavailable" estradiol. Testosterone is produced in postmenopausal women in the ovaries and adrenals; women who have had bilateral oophorectomies have lower concentrations of testosterone compared with women with intact ovaries [35].

Several cross-sectional epidemiological studies have found that postmenopausal women who are overweight or obese have elevated concentrations of estrogens compared with lighter weight women. Researchers in the Oxford component of the European Prospective Investigation into Cancer and Nutrition (EPIC) study investigated the relationship between plasma concentrations of estradiol and SHBG and breast cancer risk factors in 456 healthy postmenopausal women [36]. Increased adiposity was directly associated with increased estradiol and decreased SHBG concentrations (both p trend < 0.001). Women whose BMI was more than 27.5 kg/m^2 had a mean estradiol concentration that was almost two times greater than that of women whose BMI was less than 20 kg/m^2. The greatest increase in estradiol concentration was observed between those with BMI greater than 27.5 kg/m^2 compared with those with BMI lower than this level. SHBG concentrations were also negatively associated with increasing tertile of waist-to-hip ratio (p trend < 0.001).

In a study of 420 postmenopausal women without cancer in the Shanghai Breast Cancer Study, BMI, weight, waist circumference, and hip circumference were positively associated with concentrations of estrone and estradiol and significantly negatively associated with SHBG concentrations, although not all of the associations were statistically significant [37]. A cross-sectional analysis of 443 postmenopausal women in New York, Sweden, and Italy found that increased adiposity was significantly positively associated with estrone, estradiol, and free estradiol [38]. SHBG was significantly negatively associated with BMI. In a subsample of 217 participants in the Nurses Health Study, BMI was positively associated with plasma concentrations of estrogens, with multivariate-adjusted correlations ranging from 0.37 for estrone and estrone sulfate to 0.63 for bioavailable estradiol, with all p ≤ 0.01 [39].

In a cross-sectional study of 144 healthy postmenopausal Chinese women, estrone and estradiol levels increased with high BMI; the respective levels were 41% (two-sided P = 0.02) and 17% higher (P = 0.34) among women in the highest BMI category (BMI 24) compared with those in the lowest category (BMI < 20) [40]. In a study of 663 postmenopausal women with and without impaired fasting glucose, impaired glucose tolerance, or type-2 diabetes from the Rancho Bernardo Study, those with a BMI ≥ 27 had higher serum estradiol (27.6 vs. 21.2 pmol/l) and bioavailable estradiol (16.3 vs. 11.1 pmol/l, p ≤ 0.001) compared with leaner men [41]. Women with a waist-to-hip ratio of 0.85 or greater had statistically significantly higher levels of estradiol (24.2 vs. 22.5 pmol/l, p ≤ 0.05) and bioavailable estradiol (13.6 vs. 12.1 pmol/l, p ≤ 0.05). Several other cross-sectional studies have also found a positive association between increased adiposity and increased levels of estrogen and decreased levels of SHBG in healthy postmenopausal women [42–49].

Adiposity has also been found to be similarly related to sex hormone blood concentrations in breast cancer patients [50,51]. In a population-based cohort of 505 postmenopausal women with Stage 0-3a breast cancer (the Health, Eating, Activity, Lifestyle [HEAL] Study), adiposity was positively and statistically significantly associated with circulating levels of estrone, estradiol, and free estradiol (Figure 19.1 through Figure 19.3) [50]. Women were identified to this study through the SEER cancer registries of Western Washington and New Mexico and were primarily non-Hispanic and Hispanic whites. Between 4 and 12 months after diagnosis, anthropometric measures and blood draws were obtained on all women and dual energy x-ray absorptiometry (DEXA) scans were obtained on 415 women. Obese women (BMI ≥ 30) had 35% higher concentrations of estrone and 130% higher concentrations of estradiol, compared with lighter women (BMI < 22.0) (p trend, 0.005 and 0.002, respectively). Similar associations were observed for DEXA-derived body fat mass and percent body fat, and waist circumference. Concentrations of free estradiol were doubled to tripled in overweight and obese women compared with lighter weight women (p trend = 0.0001).

Further evidence of an association between adipose tissue stores and circulating estrogen concentrations comes from intervention studies resulting in fat loss. Wu et al. conducted a meta-analysis of low-fat dietary intervention studies, of which four were in postmenopausal women [52]. None of the data in these publications included randomized controls. Three of the four studies found significant reductions in estradiol level after 3 weeks to 5 months of intervention. All of these three interventions also produced weight loss, ranging from 1.4 to 3.4 kg [53–55]. In the one

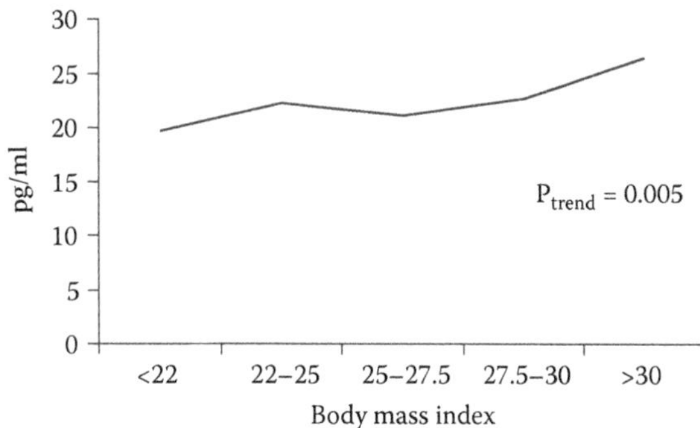

FIGURE 19.1 Estrone concentrations by BMI in postmenopausal breast cancer survivors.

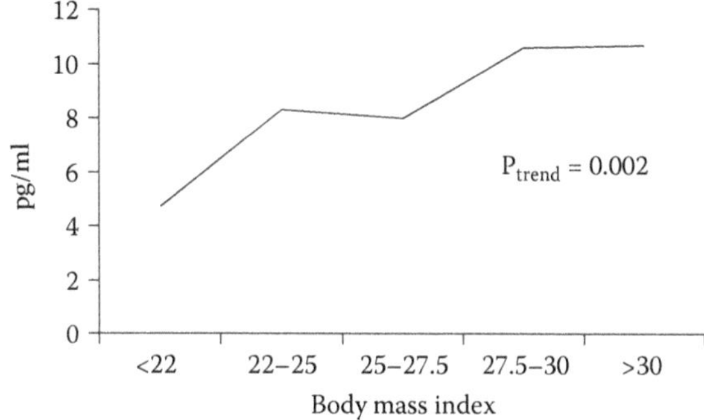

FIGURE 19.2 Estradiol concentrations by BMI in postmenopausal breast cancer survivors.

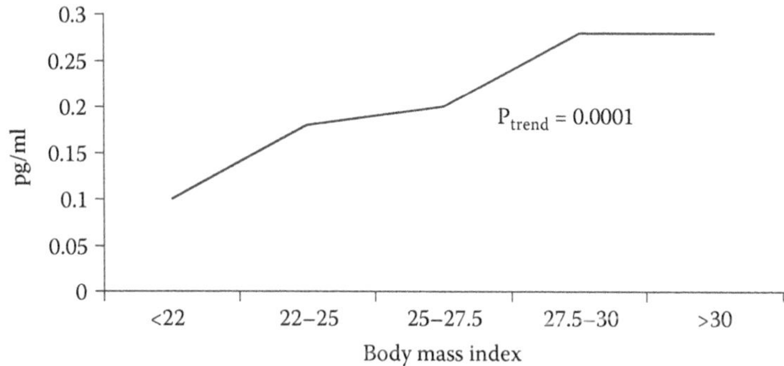

FIGURE 19.3 Free estradiol concentrations by BMI in postmenopausal breast cancer survivors.

study that did not produce weight loss, estradiol levels increased after 2 months [56]. Therefore, a reasonable question remains of whether the change in estradiol was due to the dietary fat change or to the loss of adipose tissue.

Exercise-induced fat loss also results in reductions in circulating estrogens. In the Physical Activity for Total Health Study (a randomized controlled clinical trial in 173 postmenopausal, sedentary, overweight/obese women), a 1-year moderate-intensity aerobic exercise program (45 minutes/day, 5 days/week) produced statistically significant reductions in estrogens. The effect was limited to women who lost body fat: women whose percentage of body fat (DEXA) decreased by >2% had statistically significant (comparing exercisers vs. controls) decreases at 12 months of 11.9, 13.7, and 16.7% for serum estrone, estradiol, and free estradiol, respectively [57].

Adiposity and Estrogens in Men

In men, estradiol is produced primarily through tissue aromatization of testosterone, and estrone is produce through tissue aromatization of adrenal androstenedione [58]. In overweight and obese men, as in overweight and obese postmenopausal women, increased aromatase activity results in higher circulating levels of estrogens. In a study of 775 men with and without impaired fasting glucose, impaired glucose tolerance, or type-2 diabetes from the Rancho Bernardo Study, those with a BMI ≥ 27 had slightly higher serum estradiol (75.8 vs. 74.4 pmol/l) and bioavailable estradiol (49.8 vs. 46.4 pmol/l, $p \leq 0.001$) compared with leaner men [41]. Other large cross-sectional studies have also shown direct correlations of BMI with serum levels of estrone and estradiol in men [59–61].

Mechanisms of Adiposity Effect on Sex Steroid Synthesis and Bioavailability

Adiposity influences the synthesis and bioavailability of endogenous sex steroids (estrogens, androgens, progesterone) (Table 19.1) through at least three mechanisms. First, adipose tissue expresses a variety of sex steroid metabolizing enzymes for the formation of estrogens from androgenic precursors secreted by the gonads or adrenal glands. In postmenopausal women and in men, adipose tissue is a major site of estrogen synthesis and BMI is directly related to circulating levels of estrone and estradiol as described earlier (Table 19.1) [62–64].

Second, through an increase in circulating insulin, adiposity reduces the hepatic synthesis and blood concentrations of SHBG, a plasmatic binding protein with high specific affinity for testosterone and estradiol [65]. In men and women, adiposity-related decreases in SHBG levels generally increase the fraction of bioavailable estradiol unbound to SHBG. In women only, decreases in SHBG generally also lead to increased levels of bioavailable testosterone [24,62,65,66]. In men, by contrast, decreases in SHBG generally entail reductions in total testicular testosterone production and no increase in bioavailable testosterone [62,66,67].

Finally, elevated insulin has been shown to enhance androgen synthesis in ovarian cell and tissue *in vitro* [68] and chronic hyperinsulinemia has been strongly implicated in the development of syndromes of excess ovarian androgen production (polycystic ovary syndrome). The polycystic ovary syndrome is characterized by ovarian hyperandrogenism, chronic anovulation, and progesterone deficiency [68–70]; it is a relatively frequent syndrome, with an estimated prevalence of around 4 to 6% of premenopausal women. In women with polycystic ovary syndrome, fasting serum insulin levels are directly correlated with serum androgen concentrations, but in normoandrogenic women, such correlation has not generally been observed [24]. Nevertheless, because of reductions in serum SHBG, insulin levels do generally correlate positively with levels of bioavailable testosterone, unbound to SHBG, in women with or without polycystic ovary syndrome.

ANDROGENS

Adiposity and Androgens in Women

Overweight, obese, and sedentary postmenopausal women have elevated concentrations of circulating total and free androgens, which may be due to increased amounts of 17β-hydroxysteroid dehydrogenase in subcutaneous and intra-abdominal fat. A combined analysis of nested case-control studies within nine cohort studies, which included data from 663 breast cancer cases and 1765 women without breast cancer, found that postmenopausal women with serum hormone concentrations in the top quintile for testosterone, androstenedione, DHEA, and DHEAS were approximately twice as likely to develop breast cancer compared with women with serum hormones in the bottom quintile [8]. In the same analysis, a doubling of androgen concentration resulted in a 20 to 40% increase in risk for breast cancer.

When estradiol and testosterone were included in the same model, the effect of doubling of testosterone on breast cancer risk was greater than that of estradiol (RR 1.32 and 1.18, respectively), and similar results were observed for androstenedione when combined in a model with estradiol. These androgens may increase cell proliferation by being converted to estradiol and estrone in the circulation or target tissue. In addition, androgens may affect breast cancer risk by directly stimulating the growth and division of breast cells.

In the cross-sectional analysis of 443 postmenopausal women in New York, Sweden, and Italy described earlier, increased adiposity was positively associated with bioavailable testosterone (p trend = 0.009), free testosterone, (p trend < 0.001), androstenedione (p trend = 0.01), and DHEAS (p trend = 0.13) [38]. In the study of 420 postmenopausal women without cancer in the Shanghai Breast Cancer Study, BMI, weight, waist circumference, and hip circumference were positively associated with concentrations of testosterone, although the associations were not statistically significant. The greatest effect of adiposity on testosterone level appeared to be in the women whose BMI was greater than 25.8 vs. lighter weight women. In that same study, concentrations of DHEAS rose slightly but nonstatistically significantly with increasing measures of adiposity [37].

In the Health, Eating, Activity, Lifestyle (HEAL) cohort of breast cancer patients, overweight and obese women had statistically significantly elevated levels of total testosterone, free testosterone, and DHEAS (Figure 19.4 and Figure 19.5) [59]. Levels of DHEAS and free testosterone were higher in women in the top quartiles for body fat mass compared with the leanest women.

In the Physical Activity for Total Health Study described earlier, a 1-year moderate-intensity aerobic exercise program (45 minutes/day, 5 days/week) produced statistically significant reductions in androgens with fat loss. Among women who lost >2% body fat, testosterone and free testosterone concentrations fell by 10.1 and 12.2% between baseline and 12 months in exercisers compared

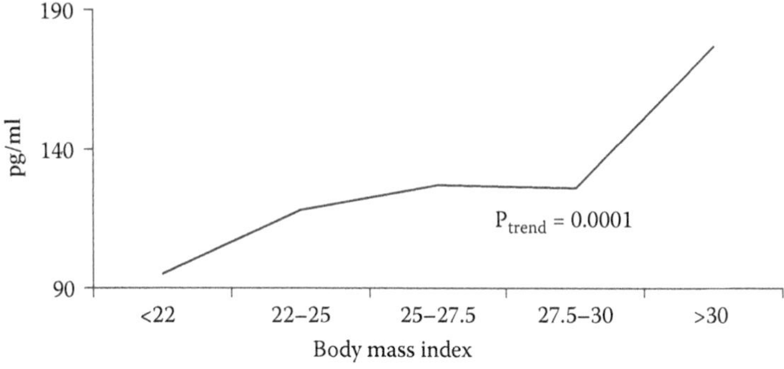

FIGURE 19.4 Testosterone concentrations by BMI in postmenopausal breast cancer survivors.

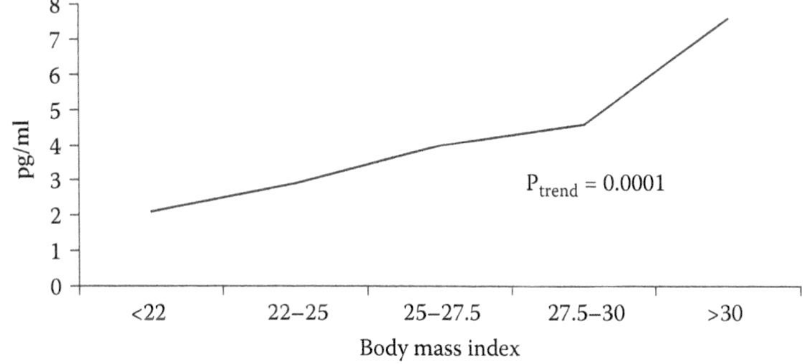

FIGURE 19.5 Free testosterone concentrations by BMI in postmenopausal breast cancer survivors.

with a decrease of 1.6 and 8.0% in controls ($P = 0.02$ and 0.03 compared with exercisers, respectively). Concentrations of testosterone and free testosterone among exercisers who lost between 0.5 and 2% body fat declined by 4.7 and 10.4%. In controls who lost this amount of body fat, concentrations of testosterone and free testosterone declined by only 2.8 and 4.3% ($P = 0.03$ and 0.01 compared with exercisers, respectively) [71].

Adiposity and Androgens in Men

In a subsample of 1548 men, aged 25 to 84 years, participating in the Tromso study, testosterone and SHBG were measured, free testosterone was calculated, and all were correlated with BMI and waist circumference [72]. Both adiposity measures were statistically significantly negatively associated with concentrations of testosterone, free testosterone, and SHBG, although the associations with free testosterone were weak. The lowest concentrations of testosterone and free testosterone were seen in men whose waist circumference was in the highest tertile and whose BMI was in the lowest tertile, e.g., those with the most disproportionate amount of abdominal adiposity.

Among 178 men sampled from the San Antonio Heart Study, free testosterone, but not total testosterone, was inversely associated with central adiposity [73]. In a sample of 511 men in the Rancho Bernardo Study, total testosterone was inversely associated with subsequent central obesity (measured after 12 years) [74].

In another report from the Rancho Bernardo Study in 775 men with and without prediabetes or diabetes, those with BMI ≥ 27 had lower testosterone (9.7 vs. 11.4 nmol/l, $p \leq 0.001$) and bioavailable testosterone (3.16 vs. 3.26 nmol/l, $p \leq 0.05$). Waist-to-hip ratio showed similar, but attenuated, associations [41]. In a population-based random sample of 1241 middle-aged U.S. men, androstenedione, total plasma testosterone, albumin-bound testosterone, dihydrotestosterone, and SHBG decreased with increasing quintile of BMI [75]. In a cross-sectional study of 250 nonobese men and 50 obese men, BMI was negatively associated with testosterone and DHEAS [76]. In a population-based series of 1127 older African–American, white, Chinese–American, and Japanese–American men without cancer, age-adjusted concentrations of testosterone (total, free, and bioavailable), dihydrotestosterone, the ratio of dihydrotestosterone to total testosterone, and SHBG decreased with increasing levels of adiposity [77].

Small weight loss intervention studies in obese men, who tend to be hypoandrogenemic, have reported that significant weight loss through diet or bariatric surgery results in increases in testosterone, free testosterone, and other androgens, and normalization of SHBG [78].

SUMMARY

Adipose tissue is a significant source of estrogens for women, especially after menopause. These elevations are significant enough to increase risk for several hormone-related cancers, particularly postmenopausal breast and endometrial cancers. These associations are seen in healthy women as well as in women with breast cancer. Overweight and obese women also have elevated circulating androgen concentrations. Preliminary evidence suggests that these elevated hormones can be reversed through weight loss, through diet or exercise, although the exact dietary and exercise patterns most likely to limit excess hormone production are not known. In men, excess adiposity increases circulating estrogens and lowers testosterone, which may be protective against prostate cancer occurrence.

REFERENCES

1. International Agency for Research on Cancer. IARC *Handbooks of Cancer Prevention*, Vol. 6, *Weight Control and Physical Activity*, Lyon, IARC Press, 2002.
2. Rajala, M. and Scherer, P. Minireview: the adipocyte — at the crossroads of energy homeostasis, inflammation, and atherosclerosis. *Endocrinology* 144, 3765, 2003.
3. Reaven, G.M. Banting lecture 1988. Role of insulin resistance in human disease. *Diabetes* 37, 1595, 1988.
4. Wajchenberg, B.L. Subcutaneous and visceral adipose tissue: their relation to the metabolic syndrome. *Endocr Rev* 21, 697, 2000.
5. Dickson, R.B. and Stancel, G.M. Estrogen receptor-mediated processes in normal and cancer cells. *J Natl Cancer Inst Monogr*, 27, 135–145, 2000.
6. Flototto, T. et al. Hormones and hormone antagonists: mechanisms of action in carcinogenesis of endometrial and breast cancer. *Horm Metab Res* 33, 451, 2001.
7. Key, T. and Pike, M. The dose–effect relationship between "unopposed" estrogens and endometrial mitotic rate: its central role in explaining and predicting endometrial cancer. *Br J Cancer* 57, 205, 1988.
8. Endogenous Hormones and Breast Cancer Collaborative Group. Endogenous sex hormones and breast cancer in postmenopausal women: reanalysis of nine prospective studies. *J Natl Cancer Inst* 94, 606, 2002.
9. Zeleniuch–Jacquotte, A. et al. Postmenopausal levels of estrogen, androgen, and SHBG and breast cancer: long-term results of a prospective study. *Br J Cancer* 90, 153, 2004.
10. Key, T.J. et al. Body mass index, serum sex hormones, and breast cancer risk in postmenopausal women. *J Natl Cancer Inst* 95, 1218, 2003.
11. Collaborative Group on Hormonal Factors in Breast Cancer. Breast cancer and hormone replacement therapy: collaborative reanalysis of data from 51 epidemiological studies of 52,705 women with breast cancer and 108,411 women without breast cancer. *Lancet* 350, 1047, 1997.
12. Schairer, C. et al. Menopausal estrogen and estrogen–progestin replacement therapy and breast cancer risk. *JAMA* 283, 485, 2000.
13. Huang, Z. et al. Dual effects of weight and weight gain on breast cancer risk. *JAMA* 278, 1407, 1997.
14. Feigelson, H. et al. Weight gain, body mass index, hormone replacement therapy, and postmenopausal breast cancer in a large prospective study. *Cancer Epidemiol Biomarkers Prev* 13, 220, 2004.
15. Morimoto, L. et al. Obesity, body size, and risk of postmenopausal breast cancer: the Women's Health Initiative. *Cancer Causes Control.* 13, 741, 2002.
16. MacInnis, R.J. et al. Body size and composition and risk of postmenopausal breast cancer. *Cancer Epidemiol Biomarkers Prev* 13, 2117, 2004.
17. Coates, R. et al. Race, nutritional status, and survival from breast cancer. *J Natl Cancer Inst* 82, 1684, 1990.
18. Tretli, S., Haldorsen, T. and Ottestad, L. The effect of premorbid height and weight on the survival of breast cancer patients. *Br J Cancer* 62, 299, 1990.
19. Maehle, B.O. and Tretli, S. Premorbid body mass index in breast cancer: reversed effect on survival in hormone receptor negative patients. *Breast Cancer Res Treat* 41, 123, 1996.
20. Reeves, M. et al. Body mass and breast cancer, relationship between method of detection and stage of disease. *Cancer* 77, 301, 1996.
21. Lukanova, A. et al. Circulating levels of sex steroid hormones and risk of endometrial cancer in postmenopausal women. *Int J Cancer* 108, 425, 2004.
22. Zeleniuch–Jacquotte, A. et al. Postmenopausal endogenous estrogens and risk of endometrial cancer: results of a prospective study. *Br J Cancer* 84, 975, 2001.
23. Key, T. and Pike, M. The dose–effect relationship between "unopposed" estrogens and endometrial mitotic rate: its central role in explaining and predicting endometrial cancer. *Br J Cancer* 57, 205, 1988.
24. Kaaks, R., Lukanova, A., and Kurzer, M.S. Obesity, endogenous hormones, and endometrial cancer risk: a synthetic review. *Cancer Epidemiol Biomarkers Prev* 11, 1531, 2002.
25. Kaaks, R., Lukanova, A. and Sommersberg, B. Plasma androgens, IGF-1, body size, and prostate cancer risk: a synthetic review. *Prostate Cancer Prostatic Dis* 3, 157, 2000.
26. Hsing, A.W., Reichardt, J.K. and Stanczyk, F.Z. Hormones and prostate cancer: current perspectives and future directions. *Prostate* 52, 213, 2002.

27. Bosland, M.C. The role of steroid hormones in prostate carcinogenesis. *J Natl Cancer Inst Monogr*, 39, 2000.
28. Gann, P.H. et al. Prospective study of sex hormone levels and risk of prostate cancer. *J. Natl Cancer Inst* 88, 1118, 1996.
29. Porter, M.P. and Stanford, J.L. Obesity and the risk of prostate cancer. *Prostate* 62, 316, 2004.
30. Howell, A., on behalf of the ATAC Trialists' Group A. The ATAC ("Arimidex," Tamoxifen, alone or in combination) trial in postmenopausal women with early breast cancer — updated efficacy results based on a median follow-up of 5 years. *Breast Cancer Res Treat* 88, 1S, 2004.
31. Chlebowski, R.T. et al. American Society of Clinical Oncology technology assessment of pharmacologic interventions for breast cancer risk reduction including tamoxifen, raloxifene, and aromatase inhibition. *J Clin Oncol* 20, 3328, 2002.
32. Meldrum, D. et al. Changes in circulating steroids with aging in postmenopausal women. *Obstet Gynecol* 57, 624, 1981.
33. Siiteri, P.K. Adipose tissue as a source of hormones. *Am J Clin Nutr* 45, 277, 1987.
34. Siiteri, P.K. et al. The serum transport of steroid hormones. *Recent Program Horm Res* 38, 457, 1982.
35. Judd, H.L. et al. Origin of serum estradiol in postmenopausal women. *Obstet Gynecol* 59, 680, 1982.
36. Verkasalo, P.K. et al. Circulating levels of sex hormones and their relation to risk factors for breast cancer: a cross-sectional study in 1092 pre- and postmenopausal women (United Kingdom). *Cancer Causes Control* 12, 47, 2001.
37. Boyapati, S.M. et al. Correlation of blood sex steroid hormones with body size, body fat distribution, and other known risk factors for breast cancer in postmenopausal Chinese women. *Cancer Causes Control* 15, 305, 2004.
38. Lukanova, A. et al. Body mass index, circulating levels of sex-steroid hormones, IGF-I and IGF-binding protein-3: a cross-sectional study in healthy women. *Eur J Endocrinol.* 150, 161, 2004.
39. Hankinson, S.E. et al. Alcohol, height, and adiposity in relation to estrogen and prolactin levels in postmenopausal women. *J Natl Cancer Inst.* 87, 1297, 1995.
40. Wu, A.H. et al. Soy intake and other lifestyle determinants of serum estrogen levels among postmenopausal Chinese women in Singapore. *Cancer Epidemiol Biomarkers Prev* 11, 844, 2002.
41. Goodman–Gruen, D. and Barrett–Connor, E. Sex differences in the association of endogenous sex hormone levels and glucose tolerance status in older men and women. *Diabetes Care* 23, 912, 2000.
42. Madigan, M.P. et al. Serum hormone levels in relation to reproductive and lifestyle factors in postmenopausal women (United States). *Cancer Causes Control.* 9, 199, 1998.
43. Cauley, J.A. et al. The epidemiology of serum sex hormones in postmenopausal women. *Am J Epidemiol* 129, 1120, 1989.
44. Kaye, S.A. et al. Associations of body mass and fat distribution with sex hormone concentrations in postmenopausal women. *Int J Epidemiol* 20, 151, 1991.
45. Newcomb, P.A. et al. Association of dietary and life-style factors with sex hormones in postmenopausal women. *Epidemiology* 6, 318, 1995.
46. Potischman, N. et al. Reversal of relation between body mass and endogenous estrogen concentrations with menopausal status. *J Natl Cancer Inst* 88, 756, 1996.
47. Kirschner, M.A. et al. Androgen–estrogen metabolism in women with upper body vs. lower body metabolism. *J Clin Endocrinol Metab* 70, 473, 1990.
48. Haffner, S.M., Katz, M.S., and Dunn, J.F. Increased upper body and overall adiposity is associated with decreased sex hormone binding globulin in postmenopausal women. *Int J Obesity* 15, 417, 1991.
49. Pasqueli, R. et al. Determinants of sex hormone binding globulin concentrations in premenopausal and postmenopausal women with different estrogen status. *Metabolism* 46, 5, 1997
50. McTiernan, A. et al. Adiposity and sex hormones in postmenopausal breast cancer survivors. *J Clin Oncol* 21, 1961, 2003,
51. Shapira, D.V., Kumar, N.B., Lyman, G.H. Obesity, body fat distribution, and sex hormones in breast cancer patients. *Cancer* 67, 2215, 1991.
52. Wu, A.H., Pike, M.C., and Stram, D.O. Meta-analysis: dietary fat intake, serum estrogen levels, and the risk of breast cancer. *J Natl Cancer Inst* 91, 529, 1999.
53. Crighton, I.L. et al. The effect of a low-fat diet on hormone levels in healthy pre- and postmenopausal women: relevance for breast cancer. *Eur J Cancer* 28A, 2024, 1992.

54. Prentice, R. et al. Dietary fat reduction and plasma estradiol concentration in healthy postmenopausal women. The Women's Health Trial Study Group. *J Natl Cancer Inst* 82, 129, 1990.
55. Heber, D., Ashley, J.M., Leaf, D.A., Barnard, R.J. Reduction of serum estradiol in postmenopausal women given free access to low-fat high-carbohydrate diet. *Nutrition* 7, 137, 1991.
56. Ingram, D.M. et al. Effect of low-fat diet on female sex hormone levels. *J Natl Cancer Inst* 79, 1225, 1987.
57. McTiernan, A. et al. Effect of exercise on serum estrogens in postmenopausal women: a 12-month randomized clinical trial. *Cancer Res.* 64, 2923, 2004.
58. Vermeulen, A. et al. Estradiol in elderly men. *Aging Male* 5, 98, 2002.
59. Shono, N. et al. The relationships of testosterone, estradiol, dehydroepiandrosterone-sulfate and sex hormone-binding globulin to lipid and glucose metabolism in healthy men. *J Atherosclerosis Thrombosis* 3, 45, 1996.
60. Haffner, S.M. et al. Obesity, body fat distribution and sex hormones in men. *Int J Obes Relat Metab Disord.* 17, 643, 1993.
61. Ferrini, R.L. and Barrett–Connor, E. Sex hormones and age: a cross-sectional study of testosterone and estradiol and their bioavailable fractions in community-dwelling men. *Am J Epidemiol* 147, 750, 1998.
62. Tchernof, A. and Despres, J.P. Sex steroid hormones, sex hormone-binding globulin, and obesity in men and women. *Horm Metab Res* 32, 526, 2000.
63. Key, T.J. et al. Body mass index, serum sex hormones, and breast cancer risk in postmenopausal women. *J Natl Cancer Inst* 95, 1218, 2003.
64. Key, T.J. et al. Energy balance and cancer: the role of sex hormones. *Proc Nutr Soc* 60, 81, 2001.
65. Pugeat, M. et al. Pathophysiology of sex hormone binding globulin (SHBG): relation to insulin. *J Steroid Biochem Mol Biol* 40, 841, 1991.
66. Kokkoris, P. and Pi–Sunyer, F.X. Obesity and endocrine disease. *Endocrinol Metab Clin North Am* 32, 895, 2003.
67. Kaaks, R., Lukanova, A., and Sommersberg, B. Plasma androgens, IGF-1, body size, and prostate cancer risk: a synthetic review. *Prostate Cancer Prostatic Dis* 3, 157, 2000.
68. Ehrmann, D.A., Barnes, R.B., and Rosenfield, R.L. Polycystic ovary syndrome as a form of functional ovarian hyperandrogenism due to dysregulation of androgen secretion. *Endocr Rev* 16, 322, 1995.
69. Dunaif, A. Insulin resistance and the polycystic ovary syndrome: mechanism and implications for pathogenesis. *Endocr Rev* 18, 774, 1997.
70. Robinson, S. et al. The relationship of insulin insensitivity to menstrual pattern in women with hyperandrogenism and polycystic ovaries. *Clin Endocrinol (Oxf)* 39, 351, 1993.
71. McTiernan, A. et al. Effect of exercise on serum androgens in postmenopausal women: a 12-month randomized clinical trial. *Cancer Epidemiol Biomarkers Prev* 13, 1099, 2004.
72. Svartberg, J. et al. Waist circumference and testosterone levels in community dwelling men. The Tromso study. *Eur J Epidemiol* 19,657, 2004.
73. Haffner, S.M. et al. Obesity, body fat distribution and sex hormones in men. *Int J Obes Relat Metab Disord* 17, 643, 1993.
74. Khaw, K.T. and Barrett–Connor, E. Lower endogenous androgens predict central adiposity in men. *Ann Epidemiol* 2, 675, 1992.
75. Field, A.E. et al. The relation of smoking, age, relative weight, and dietary intake to serum adrenal steroids, sex hormones, and sex hormone-binding globulin in middle-aged men. *J Clin Endocrinol Metab* 79, 1310, 1994.
76. Vermeulen, A., Kaufman, J.M., and Giagulli, V.A. Influence of some biological indexes on sex hormone-binding globulin and androgen levels in aging or obese males. *J Clin Endocrinol Metab* 81, 1821, 1996.
77. Wu, A.H. et al. Serum androgens and sex hormone-binding globulins in relation to lifestyle factors in older African–American, white, and Asian men in the United States and Canada. *Cancer Epidemiol Biomarkers Prev* 4, 735, 1995.
78. Pasquali, R. et al. Weight loss and sex steroid metabolism in massively obese man. *J Endocrinol Invest* 11, 205, 1988.

79. Pasquali, R. et al. Achievement of near-normal body weight as the prerequisite to normalize sex hormone-binding globulin concentrations in massively obese men. *Int J Obesity Relat Metab Disord* 21, 1, 1997.
80. Hankinson, S.E. et al. Plasma prolactin levels and subsequent risk of breast cancer in postmenopausal women. *J Natl Cancer Inst* 91, 629, 1999.
81. Manjer, J. et al. Postmenopausal breast cancer risk in relation to sex steroid hormones, prolactin and SHBG (Sweden). *Cancer Causes Control.* 14, 599, 2003.

20 Obesity and Insulin Resistance

George Blackburn and Belinda Waltman

CONTENTS

An estimated 10 to 40% of cancer cases are attributed to obesity. Excess adipose tissue, a central feature of obesity, increases the release of free fatty acids and certain cytokines, which leads to hyperinsulinemia and insulin resistance. Elevated concentrations of insulin result in elevated concentrations of biologically active insulin-like growth factor-1 and, through their respective receptors, both of these factors may contribute to tumorigenesis by inhibiting apoptosis and promoting cell proliferation. Fortunately, a few pivotal studies indicate that lifestyle intervention can delay or prevent the onset of tumor growth and metastasis. Reduced caloric intake, adherence to a prudent dietary pattern, and increased physical activity are particularly effective strategies to reverse insulin resistance. Data suggest that implementing these lifestyle intervention strategies may help reduce the risk of chronic disease, including cancer.

INTRODUCTION

Obesity is one of the most daunting health challenges of the 21st century.[1] An estimated 64% of American adults are overweight or obese.[2] Between 1986 and 2000, the prevalence of severe obesity (body mass index (BMI) ≥ 40 kg/m^2) quadrupled from 1 in 200 Americans to 1 in 50. Adults with a BMI ≥ 50 kg/m^2 (superobese) increased by a factor of 5, from 1 in 2000 to 1 in 400.[3,4] Children and adolescents suffered a similar fate. In the last 30 years, the prevalence of overweight children has nearly tripled.[5] At present, approximately 9 million children over 6 years of age are considered obese.[6] Each year, the U.S. spends an estimated $117 billion in direct and indirect costs on health problems associated with excess weight.[7] The health risks of overweight or obesity are second only to tobacco use as the leading cause of preventable death in the U.S.[8] Increasing numbers of people recognize that nutrition plays a critical role in maintaining good health and that overweight or obesity is associated with diabetes, heart disease, and stroke.

Awareness is growing that excess weight may also increase cancer risk. In fact, an estimated 10 to 40% of cancer cases are attributed to obesity.[9] Obesity has been linked to a number of different cancers[9–13]; the most compelling evidence of an increased risk is seen in studies of esophageal,[14–17] kidney,[18–21] endometrial,[22–25] colon,[26–31] and certain breast cancers.[32–35] Obesity may also be associated with pancreatic,[36–38] ovarian,[39–41] and gallbladder[42–44] cancers. The relative risks of these obesity-associated cancers are summarized in Table 20.1, based on the International Agency for Research on Cancer's (IARC) *Handbook of Cancer Prevention; Weight Control and Physical Activity*, as published in the Institute of Medicine's recent report on *Cancer Prevention and Early Detection*.[9,45] The association between obesity and prostate cancer is not conclusive, but a few large studies support a statistically significant increased risk of prostate cancer in obese men.[46–49]

FOOD INTAKE AND PHYSICAL INACTIVITY: WEIGHT GAIN, OBESITY, AND THE METABOLIC SYNDROME

Obesity is a complex disorder characterized by the accumulation of excess adipose tissue.[50] In Western countries, much of the problem stems from eating "too much of a bad thing." Fueling this unfortunate habit is the current trend toward increased portion sizes and the widespread availability of inexpensive convenience or "fast" foods, which are often high in fat and calories. Studies suggest that Americans get 30% of their daily calories from junk food[51] (now also called "foods of minimal nutritional value".[52]

Lack of adequate exercise is the other central problem. Of American adults, 28% lead sedentary lifestyles[53]; this is intricately linked to obesity.[54] Only one-quarter of Americans meet the current recommendations for physical activity, which call for 30 to 60 minutes of moderate activity a day.[55,56] Improper nutrition, inadequate physical activity, and the resulting increase in body weight are also the root causes of metabolic syndrome, a major health risk factor that precedes cardiovascular disease, diabetes, and certain cancers.[57–59] Having at least three of the following five risk factors qualifies an individual for metabolic syndrome (see Table 20.2)[60]:

TABLE 20.1
Increase in Risk of Incident Cancer Associated with Obesity

Relative risk (RR) level of evidence	Moderate (RR 1.35–1.99)	Large (RR 2.0+)
Convincing[a]	Colon	Breast Endometrial Kidney Esophageal
Possible[b]	Prostate (mortality)	

[a]Convincing: evidence that is consistently supported by a large number of well-designed studies and laboratory evidence, with biologically plausible mechanisms and a demonstrated dose–response relationship.
[b]Possible: evidence is supported by epidemiological findings and/or laboratory evidence, but in a limited fashion.
Source: Reprinted with permission from Institute of Medicine. National Cancer Policy Board, Curry SJ, Byers T, Hewitt M, Eds. *Fulfilling the Potential of Cancer Prevention and Early Detection*. Institute of Medicine, National Academies Press. Courtesy of National Academies Press, Washington, D.C.

TABLE 20.2
Clinical Identification of the Metabolic Syndrome

Risk factor	Defining level
Abdominal obesity[a] (waist circumference)[b]	>102 cm (40 in.) in men; >88 cm (35 in.) in women
Triglycerides	≥150 mg/dL
HDL-cholesterol	<40 mg/dL in men, <50 mg/dL in women
Blood pressure	≥130/85 mm Hg
Fasting glucose	≥110 mg/dL

[a]Overweight and obesity are associated with insulin resistance and the metabolic syndrome. However, the presence of abdominal obesity is more highly correlated with the metabolic risk factors than is an elevated body mass index (BMI). Therefore, the simple measure of waist circumference is recommended to identify the body weight component of the metabolic syndrome.

[b]Some male patients can develop multiple metabolic risk factors when the waist circumference is only marginally increased, e.g., 94 to 102 cm (37 to 40 in.). Such patients may have strong genetic contribution to insulin resistance and they should benefit from changes in life habits, similarly to men with categorical increases in waist circumference.

Source: *JAMA*. May 16, 2001, 285:2486–2497.

- Abdominal obesity, determined by waist circumference
- Dyslipidemia, classified by
  - Elevated triglyceride levels
  - Low high-density lipoprotein cholesterol levels
- Elevated blood pressure
- High fasting glucose levels indicative of insulin resistance

Metabolic syndrome is often used interchangeably with insulin resistance syndrome, a broader term characterized by insulin resistance and other symptoms or risk factors. Whereas the metabolic syndrome is used as a diagnostic tool to indicate subsequent diseases like cardiovascular disease, insulin resistance syndrome is a physiological condition that increases the chances of developing associated health problems.[61] Insulin resistance caused by excess weight, particularly abdominal or visceral fat, may explain the increased cancer risk among overweight and obese individuals.

INSULIN RESISTANCE PATHOPHYSIOLOGY

Insulin is a peptide hormone secreted by beta cells of the pancreas in response to elevated levels of glucose in the blood. Insulin and the structurally homologous insulin-like growth factors (IGFs) reside as a family of growth hormones.[62,63] Insulin controls the movement of glucose into muscle cells and suppresses the liver's production of glucose. It also regulates the breakdown of fat cells in adipose tissue. Therefore, skeletal muscle, the liver, and adipose tissue are the main organs affected by insulin resistance.

Adipocytes

There is good evidence that overweight and obesity can lead to insulin resistance.[64,65] Weight gain leads to an increase in adipose tissue and adipocytes.[66] Adipose tissue serves as a storage depot for energy in the form of triglycerides. The size and metabolic activity of adipocytes vary depending on their location in the body. Compared to subcutaneous adipocytes, abdominal (visceral) adipocytes are characterized by enlarged cells that are less sensitive to insulin-mediated antilypolysis, are more sensitive to catecholamine-induced lipolysis, and display increased metabolic activity via this elevated lypolytic activity and the increased release of free fatty acids.[67] Because visceral adipocytes uniquely contribute to the pathophysiology of insulin resistance, many physicians prefer to use abdominal circumference rather than BMI to assess the severity of potential health risks associated with overweight and obesity.

Fatty Acids

Excess adipose tissue results in the increased concentration of serum free fatty acids, partly due to an impaired inhibition of lipolysis in adipose tissue.[68] During normal lipolysis, adipose tissue hormone-sensitive lipase, activated by glucagon or epinephrine, hydrolyzes triclycerides into glycerol and free fatty acids, increasing the release of free fatty acids into the blood. Insulin exerts the opposite effect of glucagon by inactivating hormone sensitive lipase, inhibiting the mobilization of fat from adipose tissue. Once released into the blood, free fatty acids must be (1) oxidized (primarily in muscle tissue and the liver) for energy use; or (2) re-esterified to triglycerides in the liver. Failure of these metabolic pathways will result in elevated serum free fatty acids. This is particularly true for individuals with a genetically based impaired lipoprotein lipase, a condition associated with obesity and insulin resistance.[69–72] Elevated serum concentrations of free fatty acids inhibit insulin-stimulated glucose uptake and glycogen synthesis, leading to hyperinsulinemia and insulin resistance.[73,74]

Cytokines

Adipose tissue also harbors a warehouse of cytokines, or signaling hormones, that are key to energy regulation,[75] including tumor necrosis factor alpha (TNFα), resistin, and adiponectin.[66] Excess adipose tissue causes an increase in the release of TNFα[76] and resistin[77,78] and a decrease in the release of adiponectin.[79,80] These cytokines, particularly TNFα, stimulate the upregulation of preadipocytes to adipocytes. Increased levels of TNFα, derived from increasing numbers of fat cells, particularly in visceral tissue, also increase the release of free fatty acids. This, in turn, increases lipolysis, creating a vicious cycle of more fat cells and more free fatty acids.[81] Through these mechanisms, elevated serum levels of free fatty acids, TNFα, and other cytokines impair insulin sensitivity. These elevated serum concentrations of insulin and TNFα also target receptors on cells that promote cell proliferation and decrease apoptosis, leading to tumor development.

INSULIN RESISTANCE AND CANCER: PROPOSED MECHANISMS

Because insulin resistance decreases the organs' sensitivity to the actions of insulin, the body compensates by secreting more insulin. Elevated serum concentrations of insulin lead to a state of hyperinsulinemia. Chronic hyperinsulinemia is associated with certain colon,[82] breast,[83,84] pancreatic,[85] and endometrial[86] cancers. Increased blood levels of insulin cause a reduction in insulin-like growth-factor-binding proteins, resulting in an increase of the metabolically active protein, IGF-1, a molecule that regulates cell proliferation in response to energy from diet and body reserves.[11]

Insulin's tumorigenic effects may be direct, through signaling via the insulin receptor, or indirect, via insulin's influence on IGF-1 and insulin-like growth factor-I receptor (IGF1R), and the steroid hormones.[87] Research on certain cancers demonstrates that IGF-1 appears to mediate insulin's ability to promote cell division.[88,89] Together, these growth factors promote cell proliferation and inhibit programmed cell death.[90,91] Through these mechanisms, overweight and obesity lead to insulin resistance, which may promote cancer (Figure 20.1).

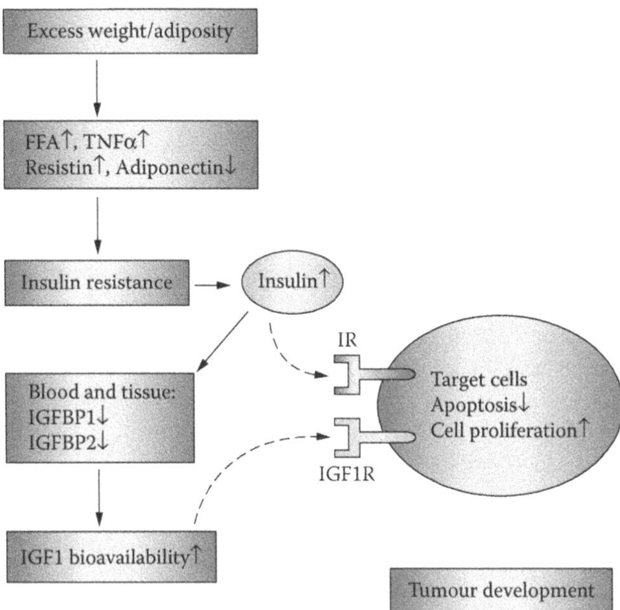

FIGURE 20.1 Effects of obesity on growth-factor production. In obesity, increased release from adipose tissue of free fatty acids (FFA), tumor necrosis factor α (TNFα), and resistin, and reduced release of adiponectin lead to the development of insulin resistance and compensatory, chronic hyperinsulinemia. Increased insulin levels, in turn, lead to reduced liver synthesis and blood levels of insulin-like growth factor-binding protein 1 (IGFBP1) and probably also reduced IGFBP1 synthesis locally in other tissues. Increased fasting levels of insulin in the plasma are generally also associated with reduced levels of IGFBP2 in the blood. This results in increased levels of bioavailable IGF1. Insulin and IGF1 signal through the insulin receptors (IRs) and IGF1 receptor (IGF1R), respectively, to promote cellular proliferation and inhibit apoptosis in many tissue types. These effects might contribute to tumorigenesis. (From Calle, E.E. and Kaaks, R., *Natl Rev Cancer*, 4, 579, 2004. With permission from Nature Publishing Group.)

Breast Cancer and Insulin Resistance

Breast cancer, the most common invasive cancer diagnosed among American women, is the second leading cause of cancer deaths in women. Several studies suggest a strong association between breast cancer and insulin resistance; however, more studies are needed to validate a causal relationship.[92] Through its negative effect on proper cell functioning, hyperinsulinemia appears to play a role in the etiology of breast cancer. Most breast cancer cells overexpress the insulin receptor[93,94] and the IGF-1 receptor,[95] that contribute to the pathophysiology of breast cancer.[94,96,97] Insulin and IGF-1 regulate cell proliferation via a tyrosine kinase growth factor cascade in breast cancer,[88] which may explain evidence of insulin's tumorigenic effects.[88,94,96]

Obesity and Breast Cancer

Obesity is responsible for an estimated 10 to 25% of all breast cancers.[9,98] More than 100 studies have examined the associations between breast cancer risk and weight or BMI, including those looking at weight gain at different ages and location of weight gain (i.e., visceral vs. subcutaneous fat). Taken together, the findings suggest that women who are overweight or obese have a 30 to 50% increased risk for postmenopausal breast cancer compared with leaner women.[33,99,100] Furthermore, lifetime weight gain in excess of 9.7 BMI points (as seen in the Women's Health Initiative) or 20 kg (as demonstrated in the Nurses Health Study) was associated with doubling of the risk of breast cancer.

Obesity, particularly abdominal obesity, plays a role in the biology of breast cancer by increasing circulating concentrations of androgens, as well as insulin, IGF-I, and other growth factors. Obesity is also associated with steroid hormonal profiles thought to favor breast cancer growth,[101] including higher concentrations of female hormones in postmenopausal women who are estrogen receptor positive and increased risk of breast cancer in women over age 50.

Weight also influences breast cancer survival. Women who are overweight, obese, or gain weight after diagnosis have poorer survival from breast cancer compared with women who maintain an appropriate BMI.[101,102] Race is another important factor. Obesity and obesity-related disorders, including breast cancer, are more prevalent in African American women[103,104] than in their white counterparts, a disparity even more pronounced among middle-aged women (55 vs. 28%, respectively).[105] African American women develop breast cancer an average of 10 years earlier than white women. They also present at a higher stage, with an increased number of positive nodes and more estrogen receptor/progesterone receptor-negative tumors.[106] African American women appear to be at greatest risk for weight gain in their second and third decades of life.

Metabolic syndrome, in which excess weight is a central feature, is common among minority women. The prevalence among African American women is approximately 57% higher than in African American men. Hispanic women have a prevalence about 26% higher than that of their male counterparts (Figure 20.2).[107] Finally, African American women have poorer outcomes from breast cancer than their white counterparts. These racial disparities in survival may stem from hormonal and genetic differences in African American women that affect their response to breast cancer therapy.[106]

Tall women and those who experienced rapid growth during adolescence (independent of final height) may also be at increased risk of developing breast cancer.[108] In this respect, height and rate of growth in early life potentially may be added to obesity and race as risk factors for developing breast cancer. Because Americans have become taller and fatter over the last four decades[109] and both factors may contribute to breast cancer incidence, increasing numbers of the U.S. population are at risk. Fortunately, a few pivotal studies indicate that lifestyle intervention can delay or prevent the onset of tumor growth and metastasis.

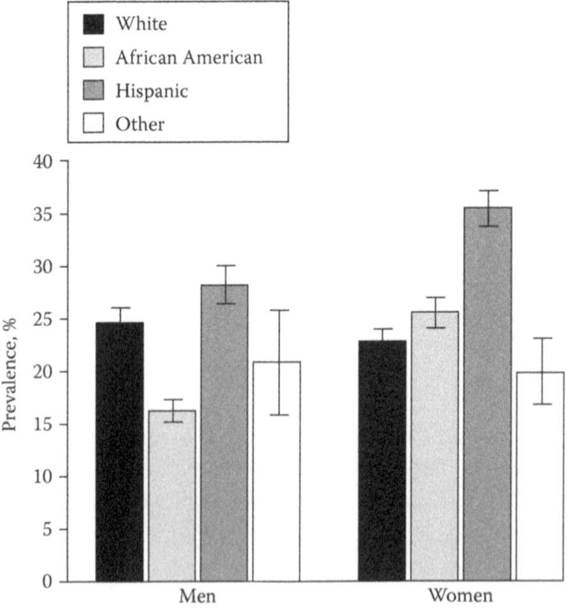

FIGURE 20.2 Age-adjusted prevalence of the metabolic syndrome among U.S. adults by sex and race or ethnicity. (From Ford, E.S. et al., *JAMA*, 287, 358, ©2002, American Medical Association. All rights reserved.)

THE WOMEN'S INTERVENTION NUTRITION STUDY (WINS)

The evidence linking breast cancer and dietary fat, particularly saturated and unsaturated fatty acids, was strong enough to warrant intervention through WINS and other studies such as the Women's Health Initiative (WHI) and the Women's Healthy Eating Lifestyle Study (WHEL). Launched in 1987, WINS is a National Cancer Institute–funded trial investigating the effect of a low-fat diet on the recurrence of breast cancer in postmenopausal women with stage I and II disease. Participants were randomized to a diet in which 15% of caloric intake is from fat or to a nonintervention group (control diet) in which approximately 30% of caloric intake is from fat.[110] All had previously received currently recommended treatment with tamoxifen or chemotherapy. The study required accrual of 2500 participants at 30 participating cancer centers. Recent data from the WINS trial suggest that lifestyle intervention resulting in dietary fat intake reduction may improve the relapse-free survival of postmenopausal breast cancer patients.

In a recent substudy of the WINS trial, 200 subjects were randomly selected from the low-fat diet arm of WINS to reduce their fat intake even further to examine the successful dietary strategies made by these women. Foods were divided into main groups and subgroups based on the USDA Food Guide Pyramid. The most substantial dietary changes made by the women in the strictly adherent low-fat group included a statistically significant decrease in the number of servings of high-fat foods from the following subgroups: sweet breads, snack foods, cheese, red meats, nuts and seeds, and eggs.[112] The strictly adherent group appears to have achieved this reduction in fat intake by shifting the number of overall servings consumed from each food group and significantly decreasing servings from the fats/oils/sweets and the bread food groups[112] (Table 20.3). Consumption of "other fruits" including apples, pears, and bananas increased. Women in the study were able to maintain sufficient nutrient intake while reducing dietary fat.

TABLE 20.3
Number of Servings from the Food Guide Pyramid at Baseline and 12 Months by WINS[a] Study Group

	Baseline (mean ± SD[b])		12 Months (mean ± SD)	
Food group	SA[c] (*n* = 50)	NSA[d] (*n* = 113)	SA (*n* = 50)	NSA (*n* = 113)
Bread	5.7 ± 2.2[f]	5.7 ± 2.3	4.8 ± 2.1[ef]	5.5 ± 1.9[e]
Vegetables	3.4 ± 1.3	3.5 ± 1.9	3.4 ± 1.5	3.2 ± 1.6
Fruits	2.3 ± 1.4	2.5 ± 1.6	2.7 ± 1.4	2.1 ± 1.6
Dairy	1.8 ± 1.1	1.6 ± 1.0	2.0 ± 1.6	1.7 ± 1.5
Meat	2.0 ± 0.9	2.1 ± 1.3	1.7 ± 1.0	1.9 ± 0.8
Fats, oils, sweets	4.8 ± 3.6[f]	5.4 ± 3.1[g]	3.0 ± 2.4[ef]	4.2 ± 3.0[e]

[a]WINS = Women's Intervention Nutrition Study.
[b]SD = standard deviation.
[c]SA = strictly adherent group (*n* = 50).
[d]NSA = not strictly adherent group (*n* = 113).
[e]Means are significantly different between groups within a time period.
[f]Means are significantly different for SA group across time.
[g]Means are significantly different for NSA group across time.

Source: Reprinted from Winters, B.L. et al., *J. Am. Diet Assoc.*, 104, 551–559, 2004, with permission from the American Dietetic Association.

THE WOMEN'S HEALTH INITIATIVE (WHI)

The WHI is a 15-year exploration of how to prevent coronary heart disease, breast and colon cancer, and fractures from osteoporosis. Sponsored by the National Institutes of Health, the WHI is one of the largest studies of its kind ever undertaken in the U.S. It involves more than 40 centers nationwide and over 162,000 American women aged 50 to 79. Enrollment began in 1993 and ended in 1998. First results of the Dietary Modification Trial are expected in 2006.[113]

The WHI Dietary Modification Trial is less a test of the dietary fat hypothesis than it is of the impact of a low-fat dietary pattern[114] high in fruits, vegetables, and grains on disease prevention. The trial involves approximately 49,000 women followed for 8 to 12 years, who followed their usual eating pattern or a diet low in fat but high in fruits, vegetables, and grains. The modified diet reduces daily fat intake to 20% of total calories, boosts fruits and vegetables to five or more daily servings, and increases grains to six or more daily servings. Structured telephone counseling, supported by print materials and monthly cooking classes, provides the principal instrument for maintaining the intervention.

To examine the associations among physical activity, diet, and insulin more closely, researchers studied a subsample from the WHI participants — 2996 postmenopausal women with no prior cancer history. Dietary intake was determined with a food frequency questionnaire and physical activity by questionnaire with fasting insulin regressed on physical activity and caloric intake. Figure 20.3 shows the differences in insulin levels in each quintile of physical activity and caloric intake, with approximately 120 values in each subgroup. Controlling for body weight, increased physical activity and reduced caloric intake independently ($p < 0.001$) predicted lower insulin concentrations. These results suggest that it is possible to manipulate and lower insulin levels through common weight loss strategies.

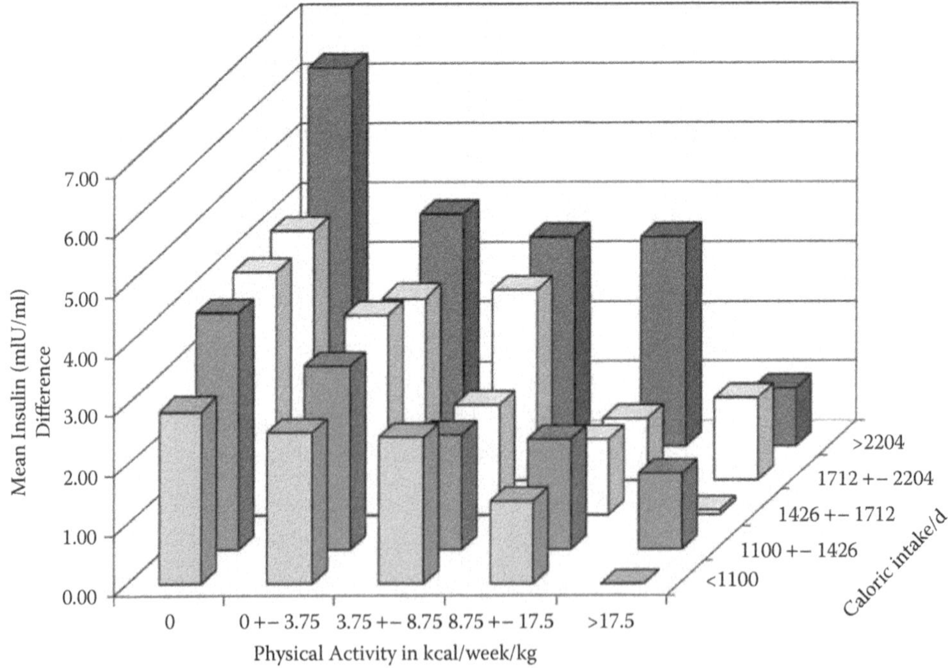

FIGURE 20.3 Differences in fasting insulin levels as mean values by quintiles of physical activity (kilocalories per week per kilogram) and caloric intake (kilocalories per day). All categories are compared with the lowest caloric intake and highest physical activity quintile. (From Chlebowski, R.T. et al., *J Clin Oncol.*, 2004; 22(22), 4507–4513, 2004. Reprinted with permission from the American Society of Clinical Oncology.)

FOOD INTAKE MEASUREMENT TOOLS

An editorial in the *Journal of the National Cancer Institute*[115] highlights the potential inaccuracy of the food frequency questionnaire (FFQ) as an exposure assessment tool in studies associating dietary intake with chronic disease risk. The authors illustrate that nutritional epidemiology involves complex multivariate models, and the measurement error of the instrument could be greatly amplified in this multivariate analysis, confounding associations between dietary intake and disease incidence. This may explain why a protective association between fruit and vegetable intake and cancer incidence was not evident in one study.[116] A similar effect was observed in the European Prospective Investigation of Cancer and Nutrition (EPIC) Study, when researchers discovered that an association between saturated fat intake and breast cancer risk was being obscured by the measurement error of the FFQ.[117]

The WINS trial methodology employs a dietary reporting system of serial, unannounced, 24-hour dietary recalls over the telephone. Through careful background research and analysis, this measurement tool was found to be more accurate and reliable than the FFQ.[111,118] Dietary intake was assessed by the mean of three recalls (one weekend and two weekdays) using the multiple-pass 24-hour recall system previously shown to be useful in this population.[119] Women in the low fat diet arm experienced a 24% reduction in recurrence risk over 5 years compared with controls.[111]

THE PRUDENT DIETARY PATTERN AS INTERVENTION STRATEGY FOR OBESE, INSULIN-RESISTANT INDIVIDUALS

Compliance with "prudent" dietary patterns based on current national guidelines is associated with decreased risk of chronic diseases[120–122] and is a crucial step in the prevention of cancer, cardiovascular disease, diabetes, and stroke.[123] The 2005 Dietary Guidelines for Americans[124] feature Institute of Medicine reference intakes for macronutrients[125] and nine, easy-to-understand key messages for good health. The thrust of the 2005 Dietary Guidelines for Americans is away from the Western diet, which is higher in saturated fats, red meat, and refined flours, and toward a diet rich in fruits, vegetables, whole grains, and lean meats. The latter is classified as a prudent dietary pattern.[126,127]

In terms of reducing the risk of cancer, the strategy of adhering to a prudent dietary pattern is supported by a study that examined subjects from the Iowa Women's Health Study, suggesting that better compliance with the Dietary Guidelines for Americans is linked to a lower risk of cancer.[128] Compliance with the "cluster of nutrition-related behaviors" recommended by the Dietary Guidelines was associated with a 15% overall reduction in cancer incidence among postmenopausal women in the top quintile of degree of adherence to the guidelines. Those who followed the physical activity, weight control, and diet recommendations cut their risk of cancer by 15%. In so doing, they underscored the power of lifestyle modification to protect middle-aged or older women against cancer.

A wealth of research indicates that diets reduced in calories, low in saturated fats, and high in fruits, vegetables, and whole grains offer a safe, effective way to maintain a healthy body weight.[123] Reduced caloric intake, adherence to a prudent dietary pattern, and increased physical activity are particularly effective weight loss strategies for the obese, insulin-resistant individual.[123] Weight loss will result in lower insulin[129] and IGF-I[130] levels, the reversal of insulin resistance,[131,132] and, thus, a reduction of the risk of cancer.[119,120,133,134]

SUMMARY

In obesity, increased release of free fatty acids, TNFα, and resistin and reduced release of adiponectin from adipose tissue lead to the development of insulin resistance and compensatory, chronic hyperinsulinemia. Increased insulin concentrations result in increased concentrations of bioavailable IGF-1, which signal through respective receptors to promote cellular proliferation and inhibit apoptosis in a way that might contribute to tumorigenesis.[11] Because many cancers do not respond to cancer therapy, it is important to recognize that the risk of developing obesity-associated diseases can be diminished or avoided through lifestyle interventions. Among the crucial factors are

- Maintaining a daily energy balance in which calories consumed do not exceed calories burned
- Following a prudent dietary pattern high in fruits, vegetables, and whole-grain fiber, and low in saturated fats, refined carbohydrates, and junk food
- Performing sufficient physical activity

The crux of this healthy living message can be boiled down to "CQE": cut calories, choose quality foods, and exercise daily.[135] Leading a healthy lifestyle is a challenge in the current environment, but it may be the most important and effective means to achieve cancer control.

ACKNOWLEDGMENTS

The authors would like to thank Julie Corliss for assistance with medical editing. Chapter preparation was supported in part by the Center for Healthy Living at Harvard Medical School, the Women's Intervention Nutrition Study (WINS) R01-CA45504, and the Boston Obesity Nutrition Research Center (BONRC) P30DK46200.

REFERENCES

1. Strategic plan for NIH obesity research. A report of the NIH Obesity Research Task Force: U.S. Department of Health and Human Services. National Institutes of Health, NIH Publication No. 04-5493, 2004.
2. Flegal KM, Carroll MD, Ogden CL, Johnson CL. Prevalence and trends in obesity among US adults, 1999–2000. *JAMA*, 288, 1723, 2002.
3. Sturm R. Increases in clinically severe obesity in the United States, 1986–2000. *Arch Intern Med*, 163, 2146, 2003.
4. Hedley AA, Ogden CL, Johnson CL, Carroll MD, Curtin LR, Flegal KM. Prevalence of overweight and obesity among US children, adolescents, and adults, 1999–2002. *JAMA*, 291, 2847, 2004.
5. Inge TH, Garcia V, Daniels S, Langford L, Kirk S, Roehrig H, Amin R, Zeller M, Higa K. A multidisciplinary approach to the adolescent bariatric surgical patient. *J Pediatr Surg*, 39, 442, 2004.
6. Committee on Prevention of Obesity in Children and Youth. Food and Nutrition Board. Board on Health Promotion and Disease Prevention. Institute of Medicine of the National Academies. In: Koplan JP, Liverman CT, Kraak VI, Eds. *Preventing Childhood Obesity. Health in the Balance*. Washington, D.C., Institute of Medicine, The National Academies Press, 2004.
7. Statistics related to overweight and obesity. NIDDK Weight Control Information Network. U.S. Department of Health and Human Services, National Institutes of Health. Available at: http://www.niddk.nih.gov/health/nutrit/pubs/statobes.htm. Accessed December 12, 2004.\
8. Flegal KM, Graubard BI, Williamson DF, Gail MH, Excess deaths associated with underweight, overweight, and obesity. *JAMA*, 293, 1861, 2005.
9. Vainio H, Bianchini F. Weight control and physical activity. *IARC Handbook of Cancer Prevention*, Vol. 6. Lyon, France, International Agency for Research on Cancer, 2002.
10. Calle EE, Rodriguez C, Walker–Thurmond K, Thun MJ. Overweight, obesity, and mortality from cancer in a prospectively studied cohort of U.S. adults. *N Engl J Med*, 348, 1625, 2003.
11. Calle EE, Kaaks R. Overweight, obesity and cancer: epidemiological evidence and proposed mechanisms. *Nat Rev Cancer*, 4, 579, 2004.
12. Bray GA. Medical consequences of obesity. *J Clin Endocrinol Metab*, 89, 2583, 2004.

13. National Cancer Institute. Obesity and cancer. U.S. National Institutes of Health. Available at: http://www.cancer.gov/newscenter/obesity1. Accessed November 2, 2004.
14. Brown LM, Swanson CA, Gridley G, Swanson GM, Schoenberg JB, Greenberg RS, Silverman DT, Pottern LM, Hayes RB, Schwartz AG, et al. Adenocarcinoma of the esophagus: role of obesity and diet. *J Natl Cancer Inst*, 87, 104, 1995.
15. Chow WH, Blot WJ, Vaughan TL, Risch HA, Gammon MD, Stanford JL, Dubrow R, Schoenberg JB, Mayne ST, Farrow DC, Ahsan H, West AB, Rotterdam H, Niwa S, Fraumeni JF Jr. Body mass index and risk of adenocarcinomas of the esophagus and gastric cardia. *J Natl Cancer Inst*, 90, 150, 1998.
16. Li SD, Mobarhan S. Association between body mass index and adenocarcinoma of the esophagus and gastric cardia. *Nutr Rev*, 58, 54, 2000.
17. Lagergren J, Bergström R, Nyrén O. Association between body mass and adenocarcinoma of the esophagus and gastric cardia. *Ann Intern Med*, 130, 883, 1999.
18. Chow WH, McLaughlin JK, Mandel JS, Wacholder S, Niwa S, Fraumeni JF Jr. Obesity and risk of renal cell cancer. *Cancer Epidemiol Biomarkers Prev*, 5, 17, 1996.
19. Yuan JM, Castelao JE, Gago-Domingues M, Ross RK, Yu MC. Hypertension, obesity and their medications in relation to renal cell carcinoma. *Brit J Cancer*, 77, 1508, 1998.
20. Lindblad P, Wolk A, Bergstrom R, Persson I, Adami HO. The role of obesity and weight fluctuations in the etiology of renal cell cancer: a population-based case-control study. *Cancer Epidemiol Biomarkers Prev*, 3, 631, 1994.
21. Mellemgaard A, Lindblad P, Schlenhofer B, Bergstrom R, Mandel JS, McCredie M, McLaughlin JK, Niwa S, Odaka N, Pommer W, et al. International renal-cell cancer study. III. Role of weight, height, physical activity, and use of amphetamines. *Int J Cancer*, 60, 350, 1995.
22. Goodman MT, Hankin JH, Wilkens LR, Lyu LC, McDuffie K, Liu LQ, Kolonel LN. Diet, body size, physical activity, and the risk of endometrial cancer. *Cancer Res*, 57, 5077, 1997.
23. Salazar–Martínez E, Lazcano–Ponce EC, Lira–Lira GG, Escudero–De los Rios P, Salmeron–Castro J, Larrea F, Hernandez–Avila M. Case-control study of diabetes, obesity, physical activity and risk of endometrial cancer among Mexican women. *Cancer Causes Control*, 11, 707, 2000.
24. Shoff SM, Newcomb PA. Diabetes, body size, and risk of endometrial cancer. *Am J Epidemiol*, 148, 234, 1998.
25. Weiderpass E, Persson I, Adami HO, Magnusson C, Lindgren A, Baron JA. Body size in different periods of life, diabetes mellitus, hypertension, and risk of postmenopausal endometrial cancer (Sweden). *Cancer Causes Control*, 11, 185, 2000.
26. Ford ES. Body mass index and colon cancer in a national sample of adult U.S. men and women. *Am J Epidemiol*, 150, 390, 1999.
27. Caan BJ, Coates AO, Slattery ML, Potter JD, Quesenberry Jr CP, Edwards SM. Body size and the risk of colon cancer in a large case-control study. *Int J Obesity Relat Metab Disord*, 22, 178, 1998.
28. Kono S, Handa K, Kayabuchi H, Kiyohara C, Inoue H, Marugame T, Shinomiya S, Hamada H, Onuma K, Koga H. Obesity, weight gain and risk of colon adenomas in Japanese men. *Jpn J Cancer Res*, 90, 805, 1999.
29. Shike M. Body weight and colon cancer. *Am J Clin Nutr*, 63, 442S, 1996.
30. Giacosa A, Franceschi S, La Vecchia C, Favero A, Andreatta R. Energy intake, overweight, physical exercise and colorectal cancer risk. *Eur J Cancer Prev*, 8, S53, 1999.
31. Murphy TK, Calle EE, Rodriguez C, Kahn HS, Thun MJ. Body mass index and colon cancer mortality in a large prospective study. *Am J Epidemiol*, 152, 847, 2000.
32. van den Brandt PA, Spiegelman D, Yuan SS, et al. Pooled analysis of prospective cohort studies on height, weight, and breast cancer risk. *Am J Epidemiol*, 152, 514, 2000.
33. Trentham–Dietz A, Newcomb PA, Storer BE, Longnecker MP, Baron J, Greenberg ER, Willett WC. Body size and risk of breast cancer. *Am J Epidemiol*, 145, 1011, 1997.
34. Friedenreich CM. Review of anthropometric factors and breast cancer risk. *Eur J Cancer Prev*, 10, 15, 2001.
35. Yoo KY, Tajima K, Park S, Kang D, Kim S, Hirose K, Takeuchi T, Miura S. Postmenopausal obesity as a breast cancer risk factor according to estrogen and progesterone receptor status (Japan). *Cancer Lett*, 167, 57, 2001.

36. Silverman DT, Swanson CA, Gridley G, Wacholder S, Greenberg RS, Brown LM, Hayes RB, Swanson GM, Schoenberg JB, Pottern LM, Schwartz AG, Fraumeni JF Jr, Hoover RN. Dietary and nutritional factors and pancreatic cancer: a case-control study based on direct interviews. *J Natl Cancer Inst*, 90, 1710, 1998.
37. Hanley AJ, Johnson KC, Villeneuve PJ, Mao Y. Physical activity, anthropometric factors and risk of pancreatic cancer: results from the Canadian enhanced cancer surveillance system. *Int J Cancer*, 94, 140, 2001.
38. Michaud DS, Giovannucci E, Willett WC, Colditz GA, Stampfer MJ, Fuchs CS. Physical activity, obesity, height, and the risk of pancreatic cancer. *JAMA*, 286, 921, 2001.
39. Mink PJ, Folsom AR, Sellers TA, Kushi LH. Physical activity, waist-to-hip ratio, and other risk factors for ovarian cancer: a follow-up study of older women. *Epidemiology*, 7, 38, 1996.
40. Fairfield KM, Willett WC, Rosner BA, Manson JE, Speizer FE, Hankinson SE. Obesity, weight gain, and ovarian cancer. *Obstet Gynecol*, 100, 288, 2002.
41. Lubin F, Chetrit A, Freedman LS, Alfandary E, Fishler Y, Nitzan H, Zultan A, Modan B. Body mass index at age 18 years and during adult life and ovarian cancer risk. *Am J Epidemiol*, 157, 113, 2003.
42. Moerman CJ, Bueno-de-Mesquita HB. The epidemiology of gallbladder cancer: lifestyle-related risk factors and limited surgical possibilities for prevention. *Hepato-Gastroenterology*, 46, 1533, 1999.
43. Zatonski WA, Lowenfels AB, Boyle P, Maisonneuve P, Bueno de Mesquita HB, Ghadirian P, Jain M, Przewozniak K, Baghurst P, Moerman CJ, Simard A, Howe GR, McMichael AJ, Hsieh CC, Walker AM. Epidemiologic aspects of gallbladder cancer: a case-control study of the SEARCH Program of the International Agency for Research on Cancer. *J Natl Cancer Inst*, 89, 1132, 1997.
44. Wolk A, Gridley G, Svensson M, Nyren O, McLaughlin JK, Fraumeni JF, Adam HO. A prospective study of obesity and cancer risk (Sweden). *Cancer Causes Control*, 12, 13, 2001.
45. Institute of Medicine. National Cancer Policy Board, Curry SJ, Byers T, Hewitt M, Eds. *Fulfilling the Potential of Cancer Prevention and Early Detection*. Institute of Medicine, National Academies Press. Available at: http://www.nap.edu/books/0309091713/html/. Accessed December 15, 2004.
46. Engeland A, Tretli S, Bjorge T. Height, body mass index, and prostate cancer: a follow-up of 950,000 Norwegian men. *Br J Cancer*, 89, 1237, 2003.
47. Samanic C, Gridley G, Chow WH, Lubin J, Hoover RN, Fraumeni JF Jr. Obesity and cancer risk among white and black United States veterans. *Cancer Causes Control*, 15, 35, 2004.
48. Pan SY, Johnson KC, Ugnat AM, Wen SW, Mao Y. Association of obesity and cancer risk in Canada. *Am J Epidemiol*, 159, 259, 2004.
49. Presti JC Jr. Obesity and prostate cancer. *Curr Opin Urol*, 15, 13, 2005.
50. Korner J, Aronne LJ. The emerging science of body weight regulation and its impact on obesity treatment. *J Clin Invest*, 111, 565, 2003.
51. Block G. Foods contributing to energy intake in the US: data from NHANES III and NHANES 1999–2000. *J Food Composition Anal*, 17, 439, 2004.
52. Goldberg RA, Hogan H. Restricting foods of minimal nutritional value in Texas public schools. Harvard Business School, Case Study 9-904-420, Aug 2, 2004.
53. National Center for Chronic Disease Prevention and Health Promotion. Behavioral Risk Factor Surveillance System. Available at: http://www.cdc.gov/brfss/. Accessed December 12, 2004.
54. Manson JE, Skerrett PJ, Greenland P, VanItallie TB. The escalating pandemics of obesity and sedentary lifestyle. A call to action for clinicians. *Arch Intern Med*, 164, 249, 2004.
55. National Heart, Lung, and Blood Institute (NHLBI), National Institutes of Health. *The Practical Guide to the Identification, Evaluation, and Treatment of Overweight and Obesity in Adults*, 2000.
56. Physical activity trends — United States 1990–1998. *Morb Mortal Wkly Rep*, 50, 166, 2001.
57. Laukkanen JA, Laaksonen DE, Niskanen L, Pukkala E, Hakkarainen A, Salonen JT. Metabolic syndrome and the risk of prostate cancer in Finnish Men: a population-based study. *Cancer Epidemiol Biomarkers Prev*, 13, 1646, 2004.
58. Reaven GM. Insulin resistance, compensatory hyperinsulinemia, and coronary heart disease: syndrome X revisited. In: Jefferson LS, Cherrington AD, Eds. *Handbook of Physiology*, Section 7, The Endocrine System, Vol. U, *The Endocrine Pancreas and Regulation of Metabolism*. Oxford, England: University Press, 1169, 2001.
59. Hammarsten J, Hogstedt B. Clinical, haemodynamic, anthropometric, metabolic and insulin profile of men with high-stage and high-grade clinical prostate cancer. *Blood Press*, 13, 47, 2004.

60. Executive Summary of the Third Report of the National Cholesterol Education Program (NCEP) Expert Panel on Detection, Evaluation, and Treatment of High Blood Cholesterol in Adults (Adult Treatment Panel III). *JAMA*, 285, 2486, 2001.
61. Reaven GM. The metabolic syndrome or the insulin resistance syndrome? Different names, different concepts, and different goals. *Endocrinol Metab Clin North Am*, 33, 283, 2004.
62. Menon RK, Sperling MA. Insulin as a growth factor. *Endocrinol Metab Clin North Am*, 25, 633, 1996.
63. Le Roith D. Insulin-like growth factors. *N Engl J Med*, 336, 633, 1997.
64. Reaven GM. Banting lecture 1988: role of insulin resistance in human disease. *Diabetes*, 37, 1595, 1988.
65. Reaven GM. Pathophysiology of insulin resistance in human disease. *Physiol Rev*, 75, 473, 1995.
66. Rajala MW, Scherer PE. Minireview: the adipocyte — at the crossroads of energy homeostasis, inflammation, and atherosclerosis. *Endocrinology*, 144, 3765, 2003.
67. Wajchenberg BL. Subcutaneous and visceral adipose tissue: their relation to the metabolic syndrome. *Endocr Rev*, 21, 697, 2000.
68. Mook S, Halkes CC, Bilecen S, Cabezas MC. *In vivo* regulation of plasma free fatty acids in insulin resistance. *Metabolism*, 53, 1197, 2004.
69. Berman DM, Nicklas BJ, Ryan AS, Rogus EM, Dennis KE, Goldberg AP. Regulation of lipolysis and lipoprotein lipase after weight loss in obese, postmenopausal women. *Obesity Res*, 12, 32, 2004.
70. Eckel RH. Lipoprotein lipase: a multifunctional enzyme relevant to common metabolic diseases. *N Engl J Med*, 320, 1060, 1989.
71. Large V, Arner P. Regulation of lipolysis in humans: pathophysiological modulation in obesity, diabetes, and hyperlipidaemia. *Diabetes Metab Rev*, 24, 409, 1998.
72. Kern PA. High adipose tissue lipoprotein lipase activity plays a causal role in the etiology of obesity. In: Angel A, Anderson H, Bouchard C, Lau D, Leiter L, Mendelson R, Eds. *Progress in Obesity Research: Proceedings of the Seventh International Congress on Obesity*. Toronto, Canada, August 20–25, 1994. John Libbey & Company, London, Vol 7, 89, 1996.
73. Boden G, Chen X, Ruiz J, White JV, Rossetti L. Mechanisms of fatty acid-induced inhibition of glucose uptake. *J Clin Invest*, 93, 2438, 1994.
74. Roden M, Price TB, Perseghin G, Petersen KF, Rothman DL, Cline GW, Shulman GI. Mechanism of free fatty acid-induced insulin resistance in humans. *J Clin Invest*, 97, 2859, 1996.
75. Gale SM, Castracane VD, Mantzoros CS. Energy homeostasis, obesity and eating disorders: recent advances in endocrinology. *J Nutr*, 134, 295, 2004.
76. Hotamisligil GS, Arner P, Caro JF, Atkinson RL, Spiegelman BM. Increased adipose tissue expression of tumor necrosis factor-alpha in human obesity and insulin resistance. *J Clin Invest*, 95, 2409, 1995.
77. Steppan CM, Bailey ST, Bhat S, Brown EJ, Banerjee RR, Wright CM, Patel HR, Ahima RS, Lazar MA. The hormone resistin links obesity to diabetes. *Nature*, 409, 307, 2001.
78. McTernan PG, McTernan CL, Chetty R, Jenner K, Fisher FM, Lauer MN, Crocker J, Barnett AH, Kumar S. Increased resistin gene and protein expression in human abdominal adipose tissue. *J Clin Endocrinol Metab*, 87, 2407, 2002.
79. Tsao TS, Lodish HF, Fruebis J. ACRP30, a new hormone controlling fat and glucose metabolism. *Eur J Pharmacol*, 440, 213, 2002.
80. Arita Y, Kihara S, Ouchi N, Takahashi M, Maeda K, Miyagawa J, Hotta K, Shimomura I, Nakamura T, Miyaoka K, Kuriyama H, Nishida M, Yamashita S, Okubo K, Matsubara K, Muraguchi M, Ohmoto Y, Funahashi T, Matsuzawa Y. Paradoxical decrease of an adipose-specific protein, adiponectin, in obesity. *Biochem Biophys Res Commun*, 257, 79, 1999.
81. Green A, Rumberger JM, Stuart CA, Ruhoff MS. Stimulation of lipolysis by tumor necrosis factor-alpha in 3T3-L1 adipocytes is glucose dependent: implications for long-term regulation of lipolysis. *Diabetes*, 53, 74, 2004.
82. Giovannucci E. Insulin and colon cancer. *Cancer Causes Control*, 6, 164, 1995.
83. Kaaks R. Nutrition, hormones, and breast cancer: is insulin the missing link? *Cancer Causes Control*, 7, 605, 1996.
84. Stoll BA. Western nutrition and the insulin resistance syndrome: a link to breast cancer. *Eur J Clin Nutr*, 53, 83, 1999.

85. Weiderpass E, Partanen T, Kaaks R, Vainio H, Porta M, Kauppinen T, Ojajarvi A, Boffetta P, Malats N. Occurrence, trends and environment etiology of pancreatic cancer. *Scand J Work Environ Health*, 24, 165, 1998.
86. Kaaks R, Lukanova A, Kurzer MS. Obesity, endogenous hormones, and endometrial cancer risk: a synthetic review. *Cancer Epidemiol Biomarkers Prev*, 11, 1531, 2002.
87. Moschos SJ, Mantzoros CS. The role of the IGF system in cancer: from basic to clinical studies and clinical applications. *Oncology*, 63, 317, 2002.
88. Zhang X, Yee D. Tyrosine kinase signaling in breast cancer: insulin-like growth factors and their receptors in breast cancer. *Breast Cancer Res Treat*, 2, 170, 2002.
89. Yu H, Rohan TE. Role of the insulin-like growth factor family in cancer development and progression. *J Natl Cancer Inst*, 92, 1472, 2000.
90. Gooch JL, Van Den Berg CL, Yee D. Insulin-like growth factor (IGF)-I rescues breast cancer cells from chemotherapy-induced cell death — proliferative and anti-apoptotic effects. *Breast Cancer Res Treat*, 56, 1, 1999.
91. Ibrahim YH, Yee D. Insulin-like growth factor-I and cancer risk. *Growth Horm IGF Res*, 14, 261, 2004.
92. Goodwin PJ, Ennis M, Pritchard KI, Trudeau ME, Koo J, Madarnas Y, Hartwick W, Hoffman B, Hood N. Fasting insulin and outcome in early-stage breast cancer: results of a prospective cohort study. *J Clin Oncol*, 20, 42, 2002.
93. Papa V, Pezzino V, Constantino A, Belfiore A, Giuffrida D, Frittitta L, Vannelli GB, Brand R, Goldfine ID, Vigneri R. Elevated insulin receptor content in human breast cancer. *J Clin Invest*, 86, 1503, 1990.
94. Papa V, Belfiore A. Insulin receptors in breast cancer: biological and clinical role. *J Endocrinol Invest*, 19, 324, 1996.
95. Papa V, Gliozzo B, Clark GM, McGuire WL, Moore D, Fujita–Yamaguchi Y, Vigneri R, Goldfine ID, Pezzino V. Insulin-like growth factor-I receptors are overexpressed and predict a low risk in human breast cancer. *Cancer Res*, 53, 3736, 1993.
96. Cullen KJ, Yee D, Sly WS, Perdue J, Hampton B, Lippman ME, Rosen N. Insulin-like growth factor receptor expression and function in human breast cancer. *Cancer Res*, 50, 48, 1990.
97. Milazzo G, Giorgino F, Damante G, Sung C, Stampfer MR, Vigneri R, Goldfine ID, Belfiore A. Insulin receptor expression and function in human breast cancer cell lines. *Cancer Res*, 52, 3924, 1992.
98. Brown JK, Byers T, Doyle C, Coumeya KS, Demark–Wahnefried W, Kushi LH, McTieman A, Rock CL, Aziz N, Bloch AS, Eldridge B, Hamilton K, Katzin C, Koonce A, Main J, Mobley C, Morra ME, Pierce MS, Sawyer KA. Nutrition and physical activity during and after cancer treatment: an American Cancer Society guide for informed choices. *Calif Cancer J Clin*, 53, 268, 2003.
99. Hunter DJ, Willett WC. Diet, body size, and breast cancer. *Epidemiol Rev*, 15, 110, 1993.
100. Ballard–Barbash R, Swanson CA. Body weight: estimation of risk for breast and endometrial cancers. *Am J Clin Nutr*, 63, 437S, 1996.
101. McTiernan A, Rajan KB, Tworoger SS, Irwin M, Bernstein L, Baumgartner R, Gilliland F, Stanczyk FZ, Yasui Y, Ballard–Barbash R. Adiposity and sex hormones in postmenopausal breast cancer survivors. *J Clin Oncol*, 21, 1961, 2003.
102. Goodwin PJ, Boyd NF. Body size and breast cancer prognosis: a critical review of the evidence. *Breast Cancer Res Treat*, 16, 205, 1990.
103. Kumanyika SK. The impact of obesity on hypertension management in African Americans. *J Health Care Poor Underserved*, 8, 352, 1997.
104. Heck KE, Wagener DK, Schatzkin A, Devesa SS, Breen N. Socioeconomic status and breast cancer mortality, 1989 through 1993: an analysis of education data from death certificates. *Am J Public Health*, 87, 1218, 1997.
105. National Center for Health Statistics. Public Health Service. *Health Promotion and Disease Prevention: United States, 1985. Vital and Health Statistics*. Hyattsville, U.S. Government Printing Office, 1985.
106. Aziz H, Hussain F, Sohn C, Mediavillo R, Saitta A, Hussain A, Brandys M, Homel P, Rotman M. Early onset of breast carcinoma in African American women with poor prognostic factors. *Am J Clin Oncol*, 22, 436, 1999.
107. Ford ES, Giles WH, Dietz WH. Prevalence of the metabolic syndrome among U.S. adults: findings from the Third National Health and Nutrition Examination Survey. *JAMA*, 287, 356, 2002.
108. Michels KB, Willett WC. Breast cancer — early life matters. *N Engl J Med*, 351, 1679, 2004.

109. Ogden CL, Fryar CD, Carroll MD, Flegal KM. Mean body weight, height, and body mass index, United States 1960–2002. Advance data from vital and health statistics, no. 347. Hyattsville, Maryland, National Center for Health Statistics, 2004.
110. Chlebowski RT, Blackburn GL, Buzzard IM, Rose DP, Martino S, Khandekar JD, York RM, Jeffery RW, Elashoff RM, Wynder EL. Adherence to a dietary fat intake reduction program in postmenopausal women receiving therapy for early stage breast cancer. *J Clin Oncol*, 11, 2072, 1993.
111. Chlebowski RT, Blackburn GL, Elashoff RE, Thomson C, Goodman MT, Shapiro A, Giuliano AE, Karanja N, Hoy MK, Nixon DW. Dietary fat reduction in postmenopausal women with primary breast cancer: phase III women's intervention nutrition study (WINS). *Proc. Amer Soc Clin Oncol,* 24(10), 2005.
112. Winters BL, Mitchell DC, Smiciklas-Wright H, Grosvenor MB, Liu W, Blackburn GL. Dietary patterns in women treated for breast cancer who successfully reduce fat intake: the Women's Intervention Nutrition Study (WINS). *J Am Diet Assoc*, 104, 551, 2004.
113. American Cancer Society. Facts about the Women's Health Initiative, National Institutes of Health. National Heart, Lung, and Blood Institute, 2001.
114. Hunter DJ, Spiegelman D, Willett WC. Dietary fat and breast cancer. *J Natl Cancer Inst*, 90, 1303, 1998.
115. Schatzkin A, Kipnis V. Could exposure assessment problems give us wrong answers to nutrition and cancer questions? *J Natl Cancer Inst*, 96, 1564, 2004.
116. Hung HC, Joshipura KJ, Jiang R, Hu FB, Hunter D, Smith-Warner SA, Colditz GA, Rosner B, Spiegelman D, Willett WC. Fruit and vegetable intake and risk of major chronic disease. *J Natl Cancer Inst*, 96, 1577, 2004.
117. Bingham SA, Luben R, Welch A, Wareham N, Khaw KT, Day N. Are imprecise methods obscuring a relation between fat and breast cancer? *Lancet*, 362, 182, 2003.
118. Buzzard IM, Faucett CL, Jeffery RW McBane L, McGovern P, Baxter JS, Shapiro AC, Blackburn GL, Chlebowski RT, Elashoff RM, Wynder EL. Monitoring dietary change in low-fat diet intervention study: advantages of using 24-hour recalls vs. food records. *J Am Diet Assoc*, 96, 574, 1996.
119. Copeland T, Grosvenor M, Mitchell DC, Smiciklas–Wright H, Marsoobian V, Blackburn G, Winters B. Designing a quality assurance system for dietary data in a multicenter clinical trial: Women's Intervention Nutrition Study. *J Am Diet Assoc*, 100, 1186, 2000.
120. Byers T, Nestle M, McTiernan A, Doyle C, Currie–Williams A, Gansler T, Thun M. American Cancer Society guidelines on nutrition and physical activity for cancer prevention: Reducing the risk of cancer with healthy food choices and physical activity. *Calif Cancer J Clin*, 52, 92, 2002.
121. Krauss RM, Eckel RH, Howard B, Appel LJ, Daniels SR, Deckelbaum RJ, Erdman JW Jr, Kris–Etherton P, Goldberg IJ, Kotchen TA, Lichtenstein AH, Mitch WE, Mullis R, Robinson K, Wylie–Rosett J, St Jeor S, Suttie J, Tribble DL, Bazzarre TL. AHA Dietary Guidelines: revision 2000: a statement for healthcare professionals from the Nutrition Committee of the American Heart Association. *Stroke*, 31, 2751, 2000.
122. McCullough ML, Giovannucci EL. Diet and cancer prevention. *Oncogene*, 23, 6349, 2004.
123. Eyre H, Kahn R, Robertson RM, Clark NG, Doyle C, Hong Y, Gansler T, Glynn T, Smith RA, Taubert K, Thun MJ. Preventing cancer, cardiovascular disease, and diabetes: a common agenda for the American Cancer Society, the American Diabetes Association, and the American Heart Association. *Stroke*, 35, 1999, 2004.
124. U.S. Department of Health and Human Services and the U.S. Department of Agriculture. Dietary Guidelines for Americans 2005. Available at: http://www.healthierus.gov/dietaryguidelines/. Accessed January 31, 2005.
125. Institute of Medicine. Food and Nutrition Board. *Dietary Reference Intakes for Energy, Carbohydrate, Fiber, Fat, Fatty Acids, Cholesterol, Protein, and Amino Acids (Macronutrients).* The National Academies of Sciences. Available at: http://books.nap.edu/catalog/10490.html. Accessed December 14, 2004.
126. Hu FB. Dietary pattern analysis: a new direction in nutritional epidemiology. *Curr Opin Lipidol*, 13, 3, 2002.
127. Fung TT, Rimm EB, Spiegelman D, Rifai N, Tofler GH, Willett WC, Hu FB. Association between dietary patterns and plasma biomarkers of obesity and cardiovascular disease risk. *Am J Clin Nutr*, 73, 61, 2001.

128. Harnack L, Nicodemus K, Jacobs DRJ, Folsom AR. An evaluation of the Dietary Guidelines for Americans in relation to cancer occurrence. *Am J Clin Nutr*, 6, 889, 2002.
129. Chlebowski RT, Pettinger M, Stefanick ML, Howard BV, Mossavar–Rahmani Y, McTiernan A. Insulin, physical activity, and caloric intake in postmenopausal women: breast cancer implications. *J Clin Oncol*, 22, 4507, 2004.
130. Nemet D, Connolly PH, Pontello–Pescatello AM, Rose–Gottron C, Larson JK, Galassetti P, Cooper DM. Negative energy balance plays a major role in the IGF-I response to exercise training. *J Appl Physiol*, 96, 276, 2004.
131. Monzillo LU, Hamdy O, Horton ES, Ledbury S, Mullooly C, Jarema C, Porter S, Ovalle K, Moussa A, Mantzoros CS. Effect of lifestyle modification on adipokine levels in obese subjects with insulin resistance. *Obesity Res*, 11, 1048, 2003.
132. Esposito K, Pontillo A, Di Palo C, Giugliano G, Masella M, Marfella R, Giugliano D. Effect of weight loss and lifestyle changes on vascular inflammatory markers in obese women: a randomized trial. *JAMA*, 289, 1799, 2003.
133. Chlebowski RT, Aiello E, McTiernan A. Weight loss in breast cancer patient management. *J Clin Oncol*, 20, 1128, 2002.
134. Bianchini F, Kaaks R, Vainio H. Weight control and physical activity in cancer prevention. *Obesity Rev*, 3, 5, 2002.
135. Blackburn GL, Waltman BA. Expanding the limits of treatment — new strategic initiatives. *J Am Diet Assoc*. 105, 5131–5135, 2005.

21 Obesity, Cytokines, and Other Inflammatory Markers

Elisa L. Priest and Timothy S. Church

CONTENTS

BACKGROUND

With the advent of inexpensive assays for an ever expanding number of immune system proteins, the field of immunology has grown exponentially over the last few decades. The growth of this field has also been promoted by research implicating immune factors in a variety of chronic diseases. For example, the acute phase reactant C-reactive protein (CRP) has been identified as a strong risk factor for the development of future heart attacks and strokes, the cytokine interleukin-6 (IL-6) has been linked to diabetes, and other cytokines are implicated in clinical depression and the development of certain cancers (Figure 21.1).[1] It is unclear at this point which cytokines and other immune measures are potential targets for therapeutic intervention and which are markers of physiological disturbances. Regardless, research is likely to continue to focus on these factors on a variety of fronts for the foreseeable future.

ACUTE AND CHRONIC INFLAMMATION

The human body's protection system can be divided into two broad categories: innate (nonspecific) and acquired (specific). The acquired immune system is capable of recognizing and eliminating specific foreign microorganisms and molecules. Nonspecific immune events result in inflammation and occur in response to an injury or infection; they comprise local (heat, swelling) and systemic changes. These systemic events, called the acute phase response, are responsible for the release of an array of proteins from the liver called acute phase proteins.[2] Classically, the inflammatory response was considered an acute phenomenon designed to limit tissue damage or infection. However, researchers are now focusing on chronic inflammation and inflammatory molecules as playing significant roles in a variety of acute and chronic diseases.

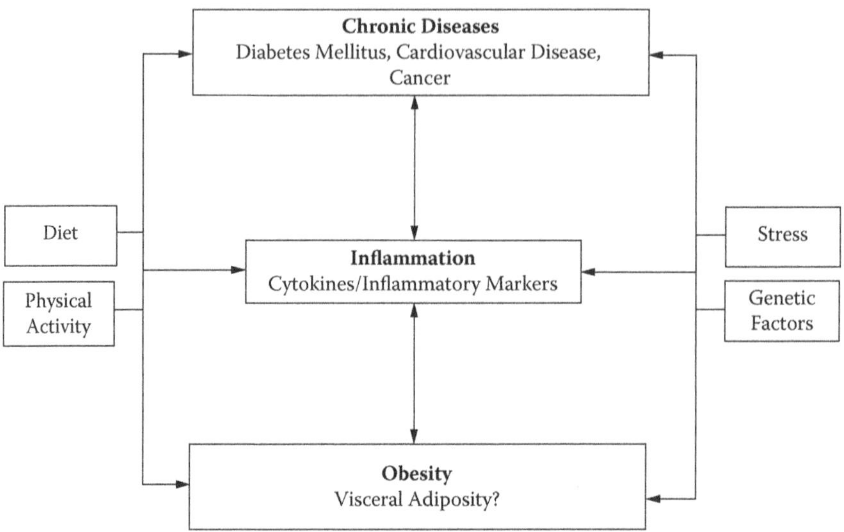

FIGURE 21.1 The relation of inflammation and chronic disease with other factors.

Cytokines

Innate and specific immune responses involve a multitude of cells. The primary channel of communication between these cells in both types of responses is through a group of secreted low-molecular-weight proteins called cytokines. Previously, cytokines were thought to be involved only with immune functions, but it is now believed that some cytokines interact with the immune and endocrine systems and are constitutively expressed. In general, cytokines bind to receptors on target cells and trigger signaling cascades that alter gene expression in the cells. They have high affinity for their receptors that allows a very small concentration of cytokines to have a significant biological effect.[3]

The role of cytokines and other inflammatory markers in the immune response and in the endocrine system is difficult to study for many reasons. Cytokines are pleiotropic in nature. One cytokine, for example IL-6, can have multiple effects on multiple cells. Next, cytokine action is often redundant, with two or more cytokines signaling similar cascades. Cytokines often act synergistically; two or more cytokines can have a greater effect than either can alone. Finally, cytokine signaling depends on the presence and availability of cytokine receptors on the cells. Cytokine receptors are highly specific and are found in cell membranes, where they trigger a signal cascade, and also in the bloodstream, where they serve to down-regulate an immune response by binding up floating cytokines.[3]

Hundreds of cytokines and other inflammatory markers are known and an exhaustive review of each one is beyond the scope of this chapter. Thus, this chapter is limited to well-studied inflammatory markers thought to play a role in obesity and its related comorbidities. A list of commonly studied inflammatory markers, cytokines, and hormones, as well as the type of study in which they were examined, is provided in Table 21.1.

Common Markers of Inflammation

Three of the most commonly studied inflammatory makers in relation to obesity and physical activity are CRP, IL-6, and TNF-α. CRP is produced in the liver and mediates activation of monocytes and macrophages, activates the complement system, blunts endothelial vasoreactivity, and increases the expression of adhesion molecules and monocyte chemoattractants in human endothelial cells.[4–12] Elevated CRP concentration has been shown to be an independent and strong

TABLE 21.1
Common Inflammatory Markers, Cytokines, and Hormones Studied in Obesity Research by Study Design

	Cross-sectional	Case-control	Clinical trial
Cytokines			
IL-6	X	X	X
IL-6sR	X		X
IL-18	X		
TNF-α	X	X	X
sTNFR1	X	X	X
sTNFR2	X	X	X
Complement components			
CRP	X	X	X
Complement C3	X		
Factor B	X		
Other immune components			
sICAM-1	X	X	X
sVCAM-1	X	X	X
PAI-1	X		
E-selectin		X	
P-selectin		X	X
Factor VIII		X	
MIF			X
VonWillebrand factor		X	
Hormones			
Adiponectin	X	X	X
Cortisol			X
Ghrelin		X	X
Insulin	X		
Leptin	X	X	X
Resistin		X	X

Notes: Interleukin 6 (IL-6); interleukin 6 soluble receptor (IL-6sR); tumor necrosis factor alpha (TNF-α); soluble tumor necrosis factor receptors 1 and 2 (sTNFR1, sTNFR2); C-reactive protein (CRP); soluble intercellular adhesion molecule-1 (sICAM-1); soluble vascular cell adhesion molecule-1 (sVCAM-1); plasminogen activator inhibitor-1 (PAI-1); macrophage migration inhibitory factor (MIF).

risk factor for CVD events and mortality, and it is gaining traction as a marker that should be considered when assessing CVD risk.[1,13–15] CRP release from the liver is largely regulated by IL-6, the most abundant cytokine in the plasma.

IL-6 is a pleiotropic cytokine influencing antigen-specific immune responses and inflammatory reactions. It is one of the major physiological mediators of acute phase reactions. IL-6 is secreted by a number of different cells, including circulating white blood cells, and by adipose tissue — specifically, visceral adipose tissue, which has a greater capacity for IL-6 production than peripheral adipose tissue does.[16,17] Stimulation by sympathetic input is also known to increase circulating IL-6 levels, and B-adrenergic stimulation has been found to increase IL-6 release from adipose tissue.[18,19] IL-6 is also involved in the cortisol-stress response (hypothalamus–pituitary axis), and glucose metabolism.

TNF-α is a potent proinflammatory cytokine and historically has been thought to be produced primarily by monocytes and macrophages. However, hypertrophied adipocytes have been shown to produce significant amounts of TNF-α.[20–22] TNF-α is a strong stimulator of IL-6 release, which feeds back to inhibit TNF-α production. It has been hypothesized that IL-6 production from adipose tissue is a consequence of TNF-α levels.[22]

Adipose Tissue as an Endocrine Organ

White adipose tissue was once considered to be a storage unit that responded primarily to hormones signaling fatty acid uptake and release. However, it is now known that adipocytes responsd to numerous cellular signals and actively secrete many proteins, called adipokines. Despite the similarity in name, adipokines should not be confused with cytokines. Adipokines may be cytokines, enzymes, hormones, or other inflammatory parameters. They play an integral role in physiological and metabolic processes, including[23]:

- Appetite and energy balance
- Immunity (IL-6, IL-8, TNF-α, transforming growth factor B [TGF-B])
- Insulin sensitivity and glucose homeostasis (adiponectin, resistin)
- Vascular haemostasis (plasminogen activator inhibitor-1 [PAI-1])
- Angiogenesis (vascular endothelial growth factor [VEGF])
- Blood pressure
- Lipid metabolism

Researchers are just beginning to unravel the roles that adipokines play in the evolving science of obesity. Every new discovery brings more questions than answers. For example, all locations of secretion, sites of action, binding receptors, and interactions with other proteins remain largely unknown for even the most studied inflammatory markers and adipokines. This chapter is a starting point for the study of inflammatory markers and obesity in a rapidly advancing field.

RESEARCH ON OBESITY AND INFLAMMATION

Cross-Sectional and Observational Studies

A selection of studies that examined the cross-sectional association between markers of inflammation or cytokines and obesity was reviewed.[24–52] Among the most commonly studied markers are CRP and IL-6. In a number of recent studies, CRP has been reported to be associated positively with BMI.[28,30,31,36,38,39,45,46,50,51] In a study of 2205 women and 1940 men from the 1999–2000 National Health and Nutrition Examination Survey (NHANES), significant and independent associations existed between CRP concentrations and both waist circumference and BMI.[31] In a sample of 61 obese postmenopausal women, Tchernof et al. found plasma CRP levels were positively associated with body weight, BMI, fat-free mass, total fat mass, and the intra-abdominal adipose tissue area.[45]

Similarly, CRP has been reported to be associated with measures of central adiposity such as waist-to-hip ratio, waist circumference, and visceral adiposity.[24,36,43,50,53] Saijo et al. studied 119 Japanese men and women and found CRP to be associated with visceral adiposity (waist circumference, waist-to-hip ratio, and visceral adipose tissue accumulation) even after adjustment for age, gender, and smoking.[43] Forouhi et al. compared South Asian and European men and women. In South Asians, waist girth and visceral fat area were highly associated with CRP. In contrast, in Europeans, BMI and percentage body fat were more significantly associated with CRP.[53]

In a study of postmenopausal women from the Healthy Women Study, measures of central adiposity (waist-to-hip ratio, waist girth, visceral fat) and overall adiposity (BMI, subcutaneous fat, weight, percent body fat) were all associated with CRP levels. Interestingly, CRP levels increased linearly across quartiles of visceral adipose tissue, BMI, and waist-to-hip ratio.[24]

Other measures of inflammation, such as IL-6 and TNF-α, have also been examined cross-sectionally for association with body composition. In general, the results are similar to those of CRP. IL-6 correlated with measures of obesity in several cross-sectional studies.[38,39,44,47,50,52] In a population of 107 healthy men and women, Yudkin et al. found that concentrations of IL-6, CRP, and TNF-α were strongly related to measures of total and central obesity.[50] Similarly, TNF-α is associated with obesity in a number of studies.[35,38,50,52]

Few cohort studies have specifically investigated the development of obesity and changes in inflammatory markers. One study by Duncan et al. studied weight gain and white blood cell count, fibrinogen, factor VIII, and von Willebrand factors in the 13,017 men and women aged 45 to 64 in the Atherosclerosis Risk in Communities (ARIC) cohort. Adjusted odds of a large weight gain for those in the highest quartile of fibrinogen were 1.65 (95% confidence interval [1.38 to 1.97]) when compared with the lowest quartile. Similar results were found for those in the highest quartile of white blood cell count, factor VIII, and von Willebrand factor.[54]

Intervention Studies

Intervention studies of inflammatory variables and obesity have primarily involved small weight loss trials in obese females (Table 21.2). The most common markers of inflammation studied were CRP, IL-6, and TNF-α. However, other relevant immune parameters and hormones such as leptin, insulin, and resistin have also been examined. Trials have used a variety of weight loss interventions, including exercise, diet, and behavioral modifications, as well as surgical procedures such as liposuction and bariatric surgery. Length of follow-up has varied greatly, from 3 weeks[55] to 24 months.[56] The majority of the trials were nonrandomized trials without control groups.

When a negative caloric balance is achieved and weight is lost, regardless of type of weight loss intervention, CRP and IL-6 have consistently been shown to decrease[35,39,45,56–66] and TNF-α has decreased[33,39,66–68] or remained unchanged.[57,60,61,63,65,69] Hormones such as leptin and insulin consistently decreased with weight loss.[35,57,58,64–66] One of the largest trials of weight loss consisted of 316 sedentary, older (>60) men and women with a follow-up time of 18 months; participants were randomized to a control group or weight loss intervention group. In this study, participants in the diet-induced weight loss group had significant reductions in CRP, IL-6, and soluble TNFR-1 compared to those who had no weight loss treatment.[61]

In a novel study by Klein et al. published in the *New England Journal of Medicine*, numerous plasma markers of cardiovascular disease risk were assessed in 15 obese females before and after undergoing abdominal liposuction.[69] They found no change in CRP, IL-6, TNF-α, adiponectin, or insulin levels despite an overall reduction in weight and subcutaneous adipose tissue. Interestingly, subjects with normal glucose tolerance had a larger reduction in subcutaneous abdominal adipose tissue compared with those with abnormal glucose tolerance (44 vs. 28%). The volume of abdominal visceral adipose tissue and thigh adipose tissue did not change in either of the groups. This study showed that weight loss through a reduction in subcutaneous adipose tissue is not sufficient to reduce elevated inflammatory parameters in obese women. In addition, it reinforces the current view that visceral adipose tissue is more active than subcutaneous adipose tissue in the secretion of metabolic and inflammatory parameters.

THE INTERACTION OF FITNESS AND FATNESS

Excess body fat is the result of caloric imbalance and is typically the consequence of too much energy intake and not enough caloric expenditure. An intriguing question that follows from this assumption is whether the relation between inflammation and body fat is due to the excess body fat or the behaviors that lead to it. In other words, is the heightened state of inflammation observed

TABLE 21.2
Summary of Weight Loss Trials and Inflammatory Markers

Population characteristics					Intervention type				Change in Inflammatory parameters					
N	% Female	BMI	Age	Follow-up	Exercise	Diet	Behavioral	Surgery	CRP	IL6	TNF-α	Adiponectin	Other	Author
14	100	39.5 ± 1.1	45 ± 4	3 weeks		X			↓	↓	↔		Leptin ↓	Bastard, 2000
20	100	40.4	43	12 weeks	X	X			↓				Leptin ↓	Davi, 2002
38	100	35.7 ± 5.6	25–54	12–24 months	X	X	X				↓			Dandona 1998
83	100	33.8 ± 0.4	48 ± 0.9	12 weeks		X			↓					Heilbronn, 2001
15	100	37.5	47 ± 3	10–12 weeks				Liposuction	↔	↔	↔	↔	Insulin ↔	Klein, 2004
37	89	49 ± 7	41 ± 7	14 months	X	X		X	↓	↓	↔		Insulin ↓	Kopp, 2003
11	58.9	41 ± 2	38.9 ± 9.8	>3 months		X	X				↓			Kern, 1995
20	100	41.6 ± 5.4	40.5 ± 9.1	12 months				X	↓	↔	↔			Laimer, 2002
67	100	37.6 ± 2.1	36.5 ± 4.6	12 months	X	X	X		↓	↓	↓		IL18 ↓	Marfella, 2004
316	62	34.4	>60	18 months	X	X	X		↓	↓	↔		sTNFR1 ↓ sTNFR2 ↔ IL-6sR ↓	Nicklas, 2004
25	100	35.2 ± 4.0	57.2 ± 5.5	13 months		X			↓					Tchernof, 2002
12	50	35.9 ± 0.9	49 (median)	8–14 weeks		X							Cortisol ↔	Tomlinson, 2004
27	81.5	46.7 ± 5.8	38.2 ± 7.5	3–24 months				X	↓				MIF ↑ sTNFR1 ↓ sTNFR2 ↓ PAI-1 ↓ AGP ↓	van Dielen, 2004
26	88.5	46.2	39 ± 10	4 months				X	↓	↔	↔		TNFR1 ↔ TNFR2 ↔	Vazquez, 2005
34	86	49.6 ± 5.9	42. ± 9.2 years	6 months				X		↓		↑	Leptin ↓ Resistin↔ sTNFR1↓ sTNFR2 ↔ ghrelin ↑	Vendrell, 2004
80	70	47.1 ± 0.9	38.3 ± 0.7	4–6 weeks		X	X		↓		↔	↔	Leptin ↓ Insulin ↓	Xydakis, 2004
27	85	36.3 ± 5.7	48.2 ± 11.7	3 months	X	X	X				↓		sTNFR1 ↑ sTNFR2 ↑	Zahorska–Markiewicz, 2000
56	100	37.2 ± 2.2	25ñ44	12 months	X	X	X	X		↓	↓		ICAM1 ↓ VCAM1 ↓ P-selectin ↓ Insulin ↓	Ziccardi, 2002

with excess body weight due to the presence of excess body fat or due to the poor nutrition, excess caloric intake, and physical inactivity responsible for overweight and obesity?

A number of cross-sectional studies have looked at this issue and it is clear that regular exercise explains a large part of the obesity–inflammation connection.[70–77] Many studies have found an inverse relation between regular physical activity (or cardiorespiratory fitness) and markers of systemic inflammation in men and women. However, although the observed fitness–inflammation association is usually only moderately attenuated, if at all, by adjustment for body habitus in men, in women this adjustment often eliminates the fitness–inflammation association. Gender differences in the physical activity–fatness–inflammation relation deserve further research. Current research suggests that systemic inflammation appears to be driven largely by physical activity habits in men (Figure 21.2), but body weight may be the primary driver in women. The source of the gender difference, if indeed one exists, is subject to speculation. However, potential starting points for investigation include location of fat mass (intramuscular, visceral, liver, etc.), effect of hormones (in particular, sex hormones), and stress.

Though not a randomized trial, Milani et al. reported that participation in a 3-month cardiac rehabilitation program reduced CRP in individuals with cardiovascular disease ($n = 235$) compared to no change in a control group ($n = 42$) of individuals with cardiovascular disease who elected not to participate in cardiac rehabilitation. In the group that attended cardiac rehabilitation, the reduction in CRP was similar in individuals who took statin medications and those who did not, and the reduction in CRP in those that lost weight was similar to that in those who did not (Figure 21.3).[70] Currently, no randomized, blinded, controlled clinical trials exist in the literature that are specifically designed to examine the ability of physical activity to reduce inflammation. With the growing importance of inflammatory markers such as CRP as clinical predictors of morbidity, there is a need for well-designed trials that examine the role of exercise in reducing inflammation in men and women from different ethnicities in a variety of populations.

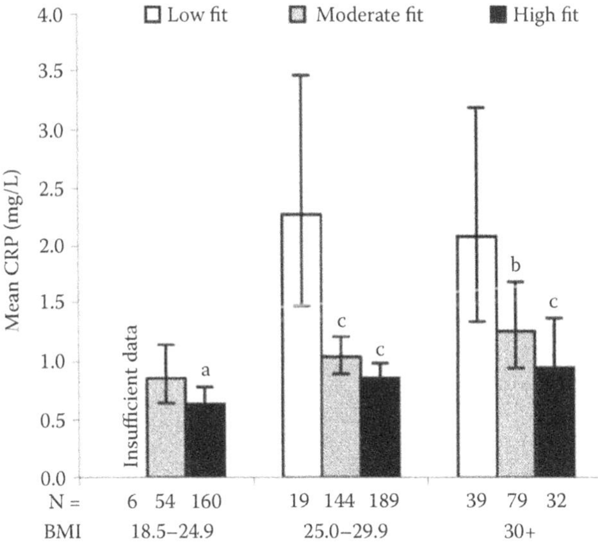

FIGURE 21.2 Adjusted geometric mean CRP values for categories of fitness and fatness. Data adjusted for age, BMI, vitamin use, statin medication use, aspirin use, presence of inflammatory disease, CVD, diabetes, and smoking. The number of individuals in the low fit–normal weight category was insufficient ($n = 6$) to generate a meaningful analysis. Error bars represent 95% confidence intervals. (a) $P < 0.05$ compared to moderate fit; (b) $p = 0.01$ compared to low fit; (c) $p \leq 0.001$ compared to low fit. (From Church, T. et al., *Arteriosclerosis, Thrombosis Vasc Biol* 2002; 22:1896–1876. With permission.)

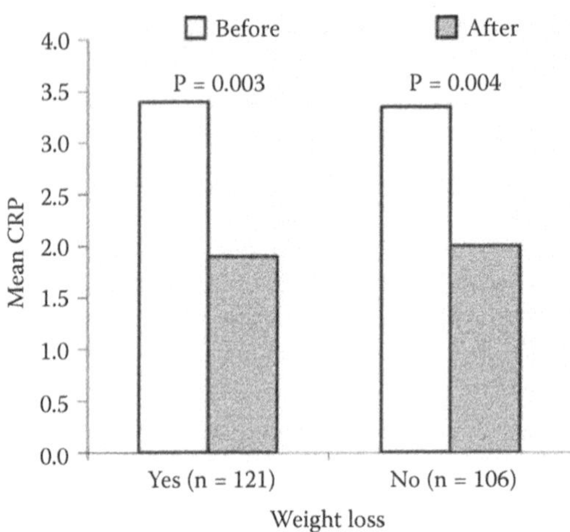

FIGURE 21.3 Change in mean C-reactive protein for individuals with CVD who completed a comprehensive cardiac rehabilitation program grouped by weight loss during the program. There were no substantial differences in changes in C-reactive protein between the group that reduced weight and the group that did not. (From Milani, R.V. et al., *J Am Coll Cardiol* 2004; 23:1056–1061. With permission.)

SUMMARY

Modern technology has made the measurement of markers of inflammation and cytokines cheap and widely accessible. Many chronic disease conditions are associated with an elevated state of inflammation and, for some conditions, inflammation may be part of the causal pathway. Extensive cross-sectional data demonstrate a strong association between markers of inflammation and measures of body fatness. Furthermore, weight loss intervention studies demonstrate reductions in plasma markers of inflammation with reductions in weight. However, the relative contributions to the development of an elevated state of inflammation of the behaviors responsible for overweight and obesity, such as poor diet and physical inactivity, remain poorly understood. Interventional studies are needed to examine the role of diet, physical activity, and weight loss in reducing inflammation in both genders across a variety of study populations.

REFERENCES

1. Ridker PM. Clinical application of C-reactive protein for cardiovascular disease detection and prevention. *Circulation*. 2003; 107:363–369.
2. Kuby J. Overview of the immune system, in Allen D, Ed: *Immunology*. New York: W.H. Freeman and Company; 1997:3–24.
3. Kuby J. Cytokines, in Allen D, Ed: *Immunology*. New York: W.H. Freeman and Company; 1997:312–334.
4. Lagrand WK, Visser CA, Hermens WT, et al. C-reactive protein as a cardiovascular risk factor: More than an epiphenomenon? *Circulation*. 1999; 100:96–102.
5. Munford RS. Statins and the acute-phase response. *N Engl J Med*. 2001; 344:2016–2018.
6. Yeh ET, Anderson HV, Pasceri V, et al. C-reactive protein: linking inflammation to cardiovascular complications. *Circulation*. 2001; 104:974–975.
7. Pasceri V, Cheng JS, Willerson JT, et al. Modulation of C-reactive protein-mediated monocyte chemoattractant protein-1 induction in human endothelial cells by anti-atherosclerosis drugs. *Circulation*. 2001; 103:2531–2534.
8. Pasceri V, Willerson JT, Yeh ET. Direct proinflammatory effect of C-reactive protein on human endothelial cells. *Circulation*. 2000; 102:2165–2168.

9. Cleland SJ, Sattar N, Petrie JR, et al. Endothelial dysfunction as a possible link between C-reactive protein levels and cardiovascular disease. *Clin Sci* (Lond). 2000; 98:531–535.
10. Fichtlscherer S, Zeiher AM. Endothelial dysfunction in acute coronary syndromes: association with elevated C-reactive protein levels. *Ann Med.* 2000; 32:515–518.
11. Fichtlscherer S, Rosenberger G, Walter DH, et al. Elevated C-reactive protein levels and impaired endothelial vasoreactivity in patients with coronary artery disease. *Circulation.* 2000; 102:1000–1006.
12. Hingorani AD, Cross J, Kharbanda RK, et al. Acute systemic inflammation impairs endothelium-dependent dilatation in humans. *Circulation.* 2000; 102:994–999.
13. Ridker PM, Hennekens CH, Buring JE, et al. C-reactive protein and other markers of inflammation in the prediction of cardiovascular disease in women. *N Engl J Med.* 2000; 342:836–843.
14. Ridker PM, Rifai N, Clearfield M, et al. Measurement of C-reactive protein for the targeting of statin therapy in the primary prevention of acute coronary events. *N Engl J Med.* 2001; 344:1959–1965.
15. Ridker PM. High-sensitivity C-reactive protein: potential adjunct for global risk assessment in the primary prevention of cardiovascular disease. *Circulation.* 2001; 103:1813–1818.
16. Fried SK, Bunkin DA, Greenberg AS. Omental and subcutaneous adipose tissues of obese subjects release interleukin-6: Depot difference and regulation by glucocorticoid. *J Clin Endocrinol Metab.* 1998; 83:847–850.
17. Tsigos C, Kyrou I, Chala E, et al. Circulating tumor necrosis factor alpha concentrations are higher in abdominal versus peripheral obesity. *Metabolism.* 1999; 48:1332–1335.
18. Halle M, Berg A, Northoff H, et al. Importance of TNF-alpha and leptin in obesity and insulin resistance: a hypothesis on the impact of physical exercise. *Exercise Immunol Rev.* 1998; 4:77–94.
19. Mohamed–Ali V, Bulmer K, Clarke D, et al. β-Adrenergic regulation of proinflammatory cytokines in humans. *Int J Obesity Relat Metab Disord.* 2000; 24 Suppl 2:S154–S155
20. Spiegelman BM, Choy L, Hotamisligil GS, et al. Regulation of adipocyte gene expression in differentiation and syndromes of obesity/diabetes. *J Biol Chem.* 1993; 268:6823–6826.
21. Hotamisligil GS, Budavari A, Murray D, et al. Reduced tyrosine kinase activity of the insulin receptor in obesity–diabetes: Central role of tumor necrosis factor-alpha. *J Clin Invest.* 1994; 94:1543–1549.
22. McCarty MF. Interleukin-6 as a central mediator of cardiovascular risk associated with chronic inflammation, smoking, diabetes, and visceral obesity: Down-regulation with essential fatty acids, ethanol and pentoxifylline. *Med Hypotheses.* 1999; 52:465–477.
23. Trayhurn P, Wood IS. Adipokines: inflammation and the pleiotropic role of white adipose tissue. *Br J Nutr.* 2004; 92:347–355.
24. Barinas–Mitchell E, Cushman M, Meilahn EN, et al. Serum levels of C-reactive protein are associated with obesity, weight gain, and hormone replacement therapy in healthy postmenopausal women. *Am J Epidemiol.* 2001; 153:1094–1101.
25. Bastard JP, Jardel C, Delattre J, et al. Evidence for a link between adipose tissue interleukin-6 content and serum C-reactive protein concentrations in obese subjects. *Circulation.* 1999; 99:2221–2222.
26. Chambers JC, Eda S, Bassett P, et al. C-reactive protein, insulin resistance, central obesity, and coronary heart disease risk in Indian Asians from the United Kingdom compared with European whites. *Circulation.* 2001; 104:145–150.
27. Cote M, Mauriege P, Bergeron J, et al. Adiponectinemia in visceral obesity: impact on glucose tolerance and plasma lipoprotein–lipid levels in men. *J Clin Endocrinol Metab.* 2005; 90:1434–1439.
28. Danesh J, Wheeler JG, Hirschfield GM, et al. C-reactive protein and other circulating markers of inflammation in the prediction of coronary heart disease. *N Engl J Med.* 2004; 350:1387–1397.
29. Engeli S, Feldpausch M, Gorzelniak K, et al. Association between adiponectin and mediators of inflammation in obese women. *Diabetes.* 2003; 52:942–947.
30. Ford ES. Body mass index, diabetes, and C-reactive protein among U.S. adults. *Diabetes Care.* 1999; 22:1971–1977.
31. Ford ES, Giles WH, Mokdad AH, et al. Distribution and correlates of C-reactive protein concentrations among adult U.S. women. *Clin Chem.* 2004; 50:574–581.
32. Hak AE, Pols HA, Stehouwer CD, et al. Markers of inflammation and cellular adhesion molecules in relation to insulin resistance in nondiabetic elderly: the Rotterdam study. *J Clin Endocrinol Metab.* 2001; 86:4398–4405.

33. Kern PA, Saghizadeh M, Ong JM, et al. The expression of tumor necrosis factor in human adipose tissue. Regulation by obesity, weight loss, and relationship to lipoprotein lipase. *J Clin Invest.* 1995; 95:2111–2119.
34. Kern PA, Ranganathan S, Li C, et al. Adipose tissue tumor necrosis factor and interleukin-6 expression in human obesity and insulin resistance. *Am J Physiol Endocrinol Metab.* 2001; 280:E745–E751
35. Kopp HP, Kopp CW, Festa A, et al. Impact of weight loss on inflammatory proteins and their association with the insulin resistance syndrome in morbidly obese patients. *Arteriosclerosis Thrombosis Vasc Biol.* 2003; 23:1042–1047.
36. Kriketos AD, Greenfield JR, Peake PW, et al. Inflammation, insulin resistance, and adiposity: a study of first-degree relatives of type 2 diabetic subjects. *Diabetes Care.* 2004; 27:2033–2040.
37. Lemieux I, Pascot A, Prud'homme D, et al. Elevated C-reactive protein: another component of the atherothrombotic profile of abdominal obesity. *Arteriosclerosis Thrombosis Vasc Biol.* 2001; 21:961–967.
38. Maachi M, Pieroni L, Bruckert E, et al. Systemic low-grade inflammation is related to both circulating and adipose tissue TNFalpha, leptin and IL-6 levels in obese women. *Int J Obesity Relat Metab Disord.* 2004; 28:993–997.
39. Marfella R, Esposito K, Siniscalchi M, et al. Effect of weight loss on cardiac synchronization and proinflammatory cytokines in premenopausal obese women. *Diabetes Care.* 2004; 27:47–52.
40. Mohamed–Ali V, Goodrick S, Rawesh A, et al. Subcutaneous adipose tissue releases interleukin-6, but not tumor necrosis factor-alpha, *in vivo. J Clin Endocrinol Metab.* 1997; 82:4196–4200.
41. Ouchi N, Kihara S, Funahashi T, et al. Reciprocal association of C-reactive protein with adiponectin in blood stream and adipose tissue. *Circulation.* 2003; 107:671–674.
42. Pradhan AD, Cook NR, Buring JE, et al. C-reactive protein is independently associated with fasting insulin in nondiabetic women. *Arteriosclerosis Thrombosos Vasc Biol.* 2003; 23:650–655.
43. Saijo Y, Kiyota N, Kawasaki Y, et al. Relationship between C-reactive protein and visceral adipose tissue in healthy Japanese subjects. *Diabetes Obesity Metab.* 2004; 6:249–258.
44. Straub RH, Hense HW, Andus T, et al. Hormone replacement therapy and interrelation between serum interleukin-6 and body mass index in postmenopausal women: a population-based study. *J Clin Endocrinol Metab.* 2000; 85:1340–1344.
45. Tchernof A, Nolan A, Sites CK, et al. Weight loss reduces C-reactive protein levels in obese postmenopausal women. *Circulation.* 2002; 105:564–569.
46. Visser M, Bouter LM, McQuillan GM, et al. Elevated C-reactive protein levels in overweight and obese adults. *JAMA.* 1999; 282:2131–2135.
47. Vozarova B, Weyer C, Hanson K, et al. Circulating interleukin-6 in relation to adiposity, insulin action, and insulin secretion. *Obesity Res.* 2001; 9:414–417.
48. You T, Ryan AS, Nicklas BJ. The metabolic syndrome in obese postmenopausal women: relationship to body composition, visceral fat, and inflammation. *J Clin Endocrinol Metab.* 2004; 89:5517–5522.
49. You T, Yang R, Lyles MF, et al. Abdominal adipose tissue cytokine gene expression: relationship to obesity and metabolic risk factors. *Am J Physiol Endocrinol Metab.* 2005; 288:E741–747.
50. Yudkin JS, Stehouwer CD, Emeis JJ, et al. C-reactive protein in healthy subjects: associations with obesity, insulin resistance, and endothelial dysfunction: a potential role for cytokines originating from adipose tissue? *Arteriosclerosis Thrombosis Vasc Biol.* 1999; 19:972–978.
51. Festa A, D'Agostino R, Jr., Howard G, et al. Chronic subclinical inflammation as part of the insulin resistance syndrome: the Insulin Resistance Atherosclerosis Study (IRAS). *Circulation.* 2000; 102:42–47.
52. Visser M, Pahor M, Taaffe DR, et al. Relationship of interleukin-6 and tumor necrosis factor-alpha with muscle mass and muscle strength in elderly men and women: the Health ABC Study. *J Gerontol A Biol Sci Med Sci.* 2002; 57:M326–M332.
53. Forouhi NG, Sattar N, McKeigue PM. Relation of C-reactive protein to body fat distribution and features of the metabolic syndrome in Europeans and South Asians. *Int J Obesity Relat Metab Disord.* 2001; 25:1327–1331.
54. Duncan BB, Schmidt MI, Chambless LE, et al. Fibrinogen, other putative markers of inflammation, and weight gain in middle-aged adults — the ARIC study. Atherosclerosis risk in communities. *Obesity Res.* 2000; 8:279–286.
55. Bastard JP, Jardel C, Bruckert E, et al. Variations in plasma soluble tumour necrosis factor receptors after diet-induced weight loss in obesity. *Diabetes Obesity Metab.* 2000; 2:323–325.

56. van Dielen FM, Buurman WA, Hadfoune M, et al. Macrophage inhibitory factor, plasminogen activator inhibitor-1, other acute phase proteins, and inflammatory mediators normalize as a result of weight loss in morbidly obese subjects treated with gastric restrictive surgery. *J Clin Endocrinol Metab.* 2004; 89:4062–4068.
57. Bastard JP, Jardel C, Bruckert E, et al. Elevated levels of interleukin 6 are reduced in serum and subcutaneous adipose tissue of obese women after weight loss. *J Clin Endocrinol Metab.* 2000; 85:3338–3342.
58. Davi G, Guagnano MT, Ciabattoni G, et al. Platelet activation in obese women: role of inflammation and oxidant stress. *JAMA.* 2002; 288:2008–2014.
59. Heilbronn LK, Noakes M, Clifton PM. Energy restriction and weight loss on very-low-fat diets reduce C-reactive protein concentrations in obese, healthy women. *Arteriosclerosis Thrombosis Vasc Biol.* 2001; 21:968–970.
60. Laimer M, Ebenbichler CF, Kaser S, et al. Markers of chronic inflammation and obesity: a prospective study on the reversibility of this association in middle-aged women undergoing weight loss by surgical intervention. *Int J Obesity Relat Metab Disord.* 2002; 26:659–662.
61. Nicklas BJ, Ambrosius W, Messier SP, et al. Diet-induced weight loss, exercise, and chronic inflammation in older, obese adults: a randomized controlled clinical trial. *Am J Clin Nutr.* 2004; 79:544–551.
62. Tomlinson JW, Moore JS, Clark PM, et al. Weight loss increases 11beta-hydroxysteroid dehydrogenase type 1 expression in human adipose tissue. *J Clin Endocrinol Metab.* 2004; 89:2711–2716.
63. Vazquez LA, Pazos F, Berrazueta JR, et al. Effects of changes in body weight and insulin resistance on inflammation and endothelial function in morbid obesity after bariatric surgery. *J Clin Endocrinol Metab.* 2004;
64. Vendrell J, Broch M, Vilarrasa N, et al. Resistin, adiponectin, ghrelin, leptin, and proinflammatory cytokines: relationships in obesity. *Obesity Res.* 2004; 12:962–971.
65. Xydakis AM, Case CC, Jones PH, et al. Adiponectin, inflammation, and the expression of the metabolic syndrome in obese individuals: the impact of rapid weight loss through caloric restriction. *J Clin Endocrinol Metab.* 2004; 89:2697–2703.
66. Ziccardi P, Nappo F, Giugliano G, et al. Reduction of inflammatory cytokine concentrations and improvement of endothelial functions in obese women after weight loss over one year. *Circulation.* 2002; 105:804–809.
67. Dandona P, Weinstock R, Thusu K, et al. Tumor necrosis factor-alpha in sera of obese patients: fall with weight loss. *J Clin Endocrinol Metab.* 1998; 83:2907–2910.
68. Zahorska–Markiewicz B, Janowska J, Olszanecka–Glinianowicz M, et al. Serum concentrations of TNF-alpha and soluble TNF-alpha receptors in obesity. *Int J Obesity Relat Metab Disord.* 2000; 24:1392–1395.
69. Klein S, Fontana L, Young VL, et al. Absence of an effect of liposuction on insulin action and risk factors for coronary heart disease. *N Engl J Med.* 2004; 350:2549–2557.
70. Milani RV, Lavie CJ, Mehra MR. Reduction in C-reactive protein through cardiac rehabilitation and exercise training. *J Am Coll Cardiol.* 2004; 43:1056–1061.
71. Pischon T, Hankinson SE, Hotamisligil GS, et al. Leisure-time physical activity and reduced plasma levels of obesity-related inflammatory markers. *Obesity Res.* 2003; 11:1055–1064.
72. Aronson D, Sella R, Sheikh–Ahmad M, et al. The association between cardiorespiratory fitness and C-reactive protein in subjects with the metabolic syndrome. *J Am Coll Cardiol.* 2004; 44:2003–2007.
73. Wannamethee SG, Lowe GD, Whincup PH, et al. Physical activity and hemostatic and inflammatory variables in elderly men. *Circulation.* 2002; 105:1785–1790.
74. LaMonte MJ, Durstine JL, Yanowitz FG, et al. Cardiorespiratory fitness and C-reactive protein among a tri-ethnic sample of women. *Circulation.* 2002; 106:403–406.
75. Ford ES. Does exercise reduce inflammation? Physical activity and C-reactive protein among U.S. adults. *Epidemiology.* 2002; 13:561–568.
76. Tomaszewski M, Charchar FJ, Przybycin M, et al. Strikingly low circulating CRP concentrations in ultramarathon runners independent of markers of adiposity: how low can you go? *Arteriosclerosis Thrombosis Vasc Biol.* 2003; 23:1640–1644.
77. Church TS, Barlow CE, Earnest CP, et al. Associations between cardiorespiratory fitness and C–reactive protein in men. *Arteriosclerosis Thrombosis Vascul Biol.* 2002; 22:1869–1876.

22 Mechanisms Associating Obesity with Cancer Incidence: Animal Models

Henry J. Thompson, Weiqin Jiang, and Zongjian Zhu

CONTENTS

INTRODUCTION

The prevalence of obesity is increasing at an unprecedented rate [1,2], and the occurrence of this disorder in humans is reported to be associated with an increased risk for a number of chronic diseases, including several types of cancer [3]. The goal of this review is to identify mechanisms that may account for the observed relationship between obesity and the occurrence of cancer. The obese state may affect the clinical characteristics of a carcinoma and/or on cancer treatment outcomes [3]; however, the extrapolation of such effects to understanding how obesity modulates the disease process resulting in cancer may obscure critical relationships and/or generate false leads about candidate mechanisms. Therefore, no consideration will be given to how obesity may affect the characteristics of detected cancers, cancer therapy, or cancer prognosis.

Obesitogenesis is a complex disorder resulting from the chronic misregulation of energy balance that results in obesity. Carcinogenesis also is a multifaceted disease process operationally divided into initiation, promotion, and progression; one particular stage of this disease is cancer. Obesitogenesis and carcinogenesis develop over a period of years. Given their complexity and time frame for occurrence, it is not surprising that the investigation of the relationship between obesity and cancer incidence in human populations is laden with difficulties and that the elucidation of causal mechanisms from such studies is even more problematic.

Animal models for obesitogenesis and carcinogenesis are well established; thus, a significant opportunity exists for experiments using these models to inform clinical understanding about potential cause and effect relationships between these diseases because key variables difficult to control in human populations can be manipulated using animal models. As will be discussed in subsequent sections, available preclinical evidence fails to support a direct relationship between obesity per se, i.e., body fatness and the occurrence of cancer. This observation illustrates the potential for preclinical studies to inform, challenge, and reshape current understanding about two very complex disorders. This chapter will be narrowly focused in order to advance a mechanistic hypothesis about the linkage between obesity and the occurrence of cancer.

OBESITY AND CANCER INCIDENCE

Obesity is an operationally defined stage in obesitogenesis characterized by the excessive accumulation of body fat [4]. Accumulation of energy in the body is due to an excess intake of energy relative to the amount of energy expended, a condition referred to as positive energy balance. In the adult, a lifestyle characterized by chronic positive energy balance leads to the development of overweight and obesity.

In a number of animal studies, models for obesity have been combined with carcinogenesis models to study the effects of obesity on the development of cancer [5–12]. In those experiments, animals ate excessive amounts of diet, usually as the result of a genetic defect that is a component of the obesity model. Over time, sufficient carcass energy was accumulated and the animals were considered obese. At time points after the obese state was attained, cancer endpoints were measured. The majority of studies in which a cancer endpoint was assessed concluded that a higher incidence of cancer occurred in obese animals.

However, in a subset of these studies, an effort was made to determine whether body fatness was the determinant of increased cancer rates; a direct relationship between body fatness and the occurrence of cancer was not found [8–12]. Consistent with these preclinical data, an expert panel on the role of weight control and physical activity in cancer prevention concluded that adult weight gain in excess of 5 kg, not obesity per se, is associated with an increased risk for cancer [3]. This implies that positive energy balance resulting in weight gain rather than obesity per se is a determinant of risk.

POSITIVE ENERGY BALANCE AND CANCER

Although there is a natural tendency to focus on the relationship between obesity per se and the development of cancer, the designation of the obese state is arbitrary — i.e., an operational definition — and indicates only that a particular magnitude of excess energy accumulation, frequently measured as body weight relative to height, has been attained in a disease process that, in most cases, has been ongoing for many years. Given the lack of evidence that obesity per se is linked mechanistically to the occurrence of cancer, an alternative explanation is that positive energy balance is a causal factor that permits the development of cancer.

The effects of different magnitudes of positive energy balance that result in different rates of energy accumulation in the body on the carcinogenic process have been investigated in animal models. However, those experiments, known as studies of caloric restriction, are generally not thought of in this light. Rather, given this nomenclature, the understandable perception is that studies of caloric restriction provide a model for starvation, famine, and/or profound undernutrition. Scientific literature contains examples of experiments in which it can legitimately be argued that this was the case; however, in a body of preclinical data on caloric restriction, experiments have been carefully designed so that the magnitude of positive energy balance is altered by regulating the amount of energy ingested while providing animals the same amounts of all other dietary components [13]. Moreover, in some experiments, this approach has been refined by introducing the concept of meal feeding all animals in an experiment [14]. For the purposes of this discussion, studies in which the only variable was the intake of calories and in which animals were meal fed are referred to as studies of dietary energy restriction; those experiments will be the basis for the remainder of this discussion of mechanisms.

Because mechanistic studies of dietary energy restriction have been primarily conducted in animal models for breast cancer, this chapter is based on studies of experimentally induced breast cancer. Nonetheless, the mechanisms discussed are likely to be applicable to cancer at organ sites other than the breast because the underlying mechanism responsible for the energy balance–cancer linkage appears unlikely to be driven by effects on the metabolism of sex steroid hormones [15–17]. Rather, available data indicate that such effects are secondary and may serve to amplify the primary effects of different states of energy balance on chemical mediators that modulate cancer risk, depending on the responsiveness to these hormones of the target tissue of interest.

It has been reported [13,14] that female rats fed 60 to 90% of the number of calories consumed by their counterparts allowed to eat *ad libitum* for the same number of meals and same duration of time each day do not lose weight. Rather, they are in positive energy balance and grow at a constant, although slower rate, depending on the number of calories consumed per day. Animals in these different states are maintained on different levels of positive energy balance. For this discussion, animals that consume 40% fewer calories than animals fed *ad libitum* are referred to as having a low positive energy balance. They provide a model to identify and study mechanisms that may be operative in individuals that limit weight gain resulting in the accumulation of body fat by monitoring their caloric intake and balancing it with energy expenditure.

On the other hand, animals allowed to eat *ad libitum* experience a high positive energy balance and provide a model to identify and study mechanisms relevant to the effects of increased energy availability on the carcinogenic process. As summarized in Figure 22.1, candidate mechanisms being reported to account for the effects of different positive energy balance on carcinogenesis are presented in subsequent sections with the goal of identifying how positive energy balance affects the process of tissue size homeostasis, the failure of which is a prerequisite for the development of cancer.

CELLULAR PROCESSES AND CARCINOGENESIS

Carcinogenesis is characterized by a failure in the regulation of tissue size homeostasis in which a clone of transformed cells achieves growth advantage due to an increased rate of cell proliferation and/or a decreased rate of cell death in comparison to neighboring populations of cells [18,19]. The development of a carcinoma can be considered a failure of tissue size regulation attributed to the formation, selection, expansion, and progression of clones of transformed cells [18]. In addition, it appears that a co-requisite event in the progression of premalignant clones of cells to those diagnosed as malignant is the induction of vascularization [19]. Evidence is now presented that excessive caloric intake (high positive energy balance) creates a permissive environment in which normal controls to cellular proliferation are abrogated, the checks on cell number accumulation by apoptosis are diminished, and restraints on the vascular system to increase blood supply are relaxed.

CELL PROLIFERATION

Rates of cell proliferation are generally low in populations of mammary epithelial cells at low risk for the development of cancer, but during premalignant and malignant stages of this disease process, cell proliferation is markedly increased [20]. In animals maintained on low positive energy balance,

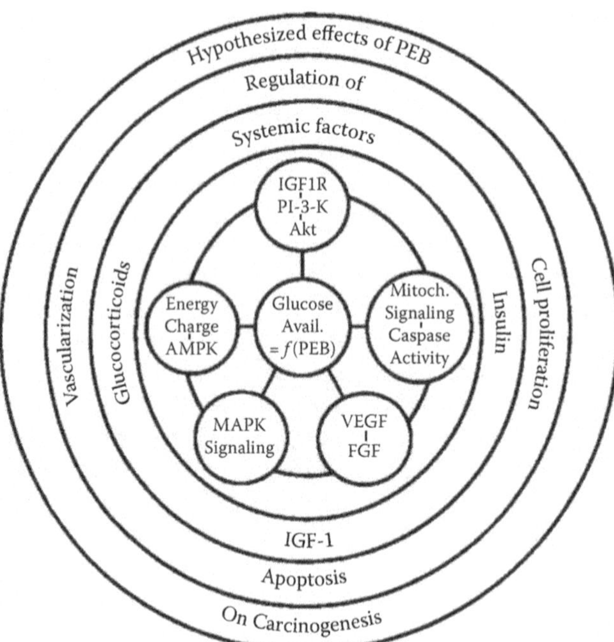

FIGURE 22.1 An overview of candidate mechanisms that may be involved in accounting for the effects of obesity on the development of cancer: the cellular processes, systemic factors, and intracellular signaling pathways that may be involved are shown. PEB = positive energy balance; IGF-1 = insulin-like growth factor-1.

rates of cell proliferation remain low despite the fact that cells harbor the genetic defects requisite for the development of cancer. On the other hand, high positive energy balance is associated with increased rates of cell proliferation [20,21]. Emerging evidence indicates that low positive energy balance slows progression of cells through the cycle cell by retarding passage at the G1/S checkpoint [22]. Mammary carcinomas that emerge in low positive energy balance-treated rats are only 15% the size of age-matched carcinomas that occur in animals receiving high positive energy balance.

When these carcinomas were used to mirror the effects of low positive energy balance on the carcinogenic process, levels of phosphorylated Rb and E2F-1 were observed to be significantly reduced by low positive energy balance [23]. Reductions in CDK2 and CDK4 kinase activity in low positive energy balance carcinomas were likely to account for the observed effects on Rb and E2F-1. Both Cip1/p21 and Kip1/p27, and levels of these proteins complexed with CDK2 were significantly elevated in low positive energy balance carcinomas, and levels of cyclin E were reduced. On the other hand, regulation of CDK4 kinase activity by low positive energy balance was likely due to a reduction in cyclin D1 protein as well as increased binding of P16 and P19 to CDK4. The majority of changes induced were reported to be reversed when animals were changed to high positive energy balance.

Thus, it appears that high positive energy balance is permissive to increases in levels of cyclin D and E, to lower levels of proteins in the Kip/Cip and p16 families of CKIs; these effects work in concert to promote higher levels of activity of the cyclin D-CDK4 and cyclin E-CDK2 complexes. Such changes result in the phosphorylation of the Rb protein and the release of E2F and related transcription factors — all of which support the sustained increase in cell proliferation considered a prerequisite for the development of cancer. These observations are consistent with the hypothesis that high positive energy balance, which if unchecked will lead to overweight and obesity, increases cancer risk by perpetuating an environment permissive to the deregulation of the cell cycle that is characteristic of carcinogenesis.

APOPTOSIS

Apoptosis is a critical process in the regulation of tissue size and defects in this cell death pathway are a prerequisite for the clinical manifestation of cancer [19]. Available data indicate that low positive energy balance favors the maintenance of constraints on the expansion of cell populations through the upregulation of cellular machinery that facilitates the activation of caspases and the suppression of caspase inhibitors. Low positive energy balance has been reported to induce apoptosis in premalignant and malignant mammary gland pathologies [20], and the pathway by which cell death was induced has been investigated [24] using the experimental approach reported in Zhu et al. [25]. Using caspase activity assays, it was shown that the activities of caspases 9 and 3 were elevated approximately twofold in carcinomas from low positive energy balance rats compared to carcinomas from animals receiving high positive energy balance; caspase 8 activity was similar in carcinomas from both groups.

This finding implies that low positive energy balance induces the mitochondrial pathway of apoptosis activation and is consistent with the finding that levels of Bcl-2 and Bcl-XL protein were significantly lower and levels of Bax and Apaf-1 were elevated in carcinomas from low positive energy balance- vs. high positive energy balance-treated animals. Expression levels of transcripts for IAP1, IAP2, X-linked IAP, and survivin — proteins that can block the activity of activated caspases — were also found to be significantly lower in mammary carcinomas from low positive energy balance vs. high positive energy balance animals. Thus, high positive energy balance favors a growth environment that permits the expansion of nontransformed and transformed cell populations within a tissue. Given that high positive energy balance is permissive to suppression of apoptotic pathways and the relaxation of cell cycle restraints observed in transformed cell populations, it is not surprising that the magnitude of positive energy balance has been reported to be proportional to the magnitude of the carcinogenic response [14].

VASCULARIZATION

Spatial limitations on the diffusion of nutrients and metabolic wastes between the vascular system and the cells that it supplies impose restraints on the growth of nontransformed and transformed cell populations [19]. Vascular supply to a tissue and its component cells can be induced via the expansion in size of existing blood vessels and/or the formation of new vessels. It has been reported [26] that premalignant mammary pathologies and mammary adenocarcinomas from low positive energy balance- vs. high positive energy balance-maintained animals were assessed for pathology-associated differences in vascularity. The density of blood vessels associated with premalignant mammary pathologies, as well as the density of blood vessels in immediate proximity to mammary carcinomas, was lower in animals maintained on low positive energy balance vs. high positive energy balance, although positive energy balance had no effect on intratumoral vascular density.

However, it remains unclear whether these differences in vascular density were due to differences in concentrations of growth factors required for maintenance or growth of blood vessels or to the inability of endothelial cells to respond to growth factors when low positive energy balance is maintained. Efforts to identify effects of positive energy balance on the expression of an array of genes involved in vascularization were inconclusive, although the evidence suggested involvement of signaling pathways of which VEGF is a component [26]. Based on the effects of positive energy balance on vascular density, it can be inferred that low positive energy balance imposes limitations on the supply of nutrients to and elimination of wastes from developing pathologies; these limitations could exert direct effects on cell proliferation and apoptosis in transformed epithelial cell populations undergoing clonal selection and expansion. High positive energy balance appears to relax restraints to vascularization, thereby maintaining an environment conducive to the expansion of cell populations. This effect is consistent with a positive association between energy balance and the risk for cancer.

The work presented in preceding sections is consistent with the view that high positive energy balance promotes the development of the cancer phenotype by fostering conditions favorable to the clonal expansion of transformed cell populations. It does this by inducing cells to leave the G_0 (quiescent) phase of the cell cycle. For cells that enter the cell cycle, high positive energy balance favors cell cycle progression due to its effects on the phosphorylation of Rb and the release of E2F1 from its binding to Rb. Increased phosphorylation of Rb is a consequence of the effects of high positive energy balance on the activity of CDK-4 and CDK-2 per the mechanisms described earlier.

In addition, high positive energy balance promotes the maintenance of the cellular antiapoptotic machinery by inducing changes in the metabolism of the Bcl-2 and IAP families of proteins. It is speculated that the effects of high positive energy balance on cell proliferation and apoptosis affect not only the expansion of transformed clones of cells, but also the ability of endothelial cells to respond to growth factors that induce vascular expansion. The coordinated regulation of proliferation, apoptosis, and vascularization is responsible for the promotional activity of high positive energy balance.

UNDERLYING MECHANISMS

That the activity of three cellular processes is coordinately regulated suggests that a common molecular mechanism is at work; the hypothesis advanced is that these effects are a direct consequence of the effects of positive energy balance on glucose homeostasis (Figure 22.2). In response to low positive energy balance, glucose availability is reduced, circulating levels of insulin and Insulin-like growth factor-1 (IGF-1) are reduced and of glucocorticoids are increased. One outcome of these changes is the limitation within a tissue of intracellular growth and survival factors. If this general hypothesis is valid, then it is important to determine whether the effects on carcinogenesis are due to changes in systemic factors involved in glucose homeostasis or to direct effects of glucose availability on cellular metabolism. Evidence addressing each possibility is reviewed in subsequent sections.

SYSTEMICALLY DRIVEN MECHANISMS

Insulin and Insulin-Like Growth Factors (IGFs)

Studies in rodents have shown that high positive energy balance accelerates DMBA- and MNU-induced mammary tumorigenesis in proportion to the magnitude of positive energy balance. In those studies, high positive energy balance was associated with higher plasma insulin levels again in proportion to the magnitude of positive energy balance maintained [27,28]. The relevance of these observations is based in part on reports that the development of DMBA-induced mammary tumors was inhibited by alloxan-induced diabetes and that alloxan- or streptozotocin-induced diabetes in rats caused a regression of 60 to 90% of DMBA-induced mammary tumors [29–32]. Tumor growth was restored and tumor latency reduced upon administration of insulin to diabetic rats.

The effects of different positive energy balances that modulate mammary carcinoma development on IGF metabolism have also been investigated. In a number of model systems, low positive energy balance is associated with a decrease in circulating levels of IGF-1. For example, Ruggeri and coworkers [27] reported that positive energy balances that inhibited DMBA-induced mammary tumorigenesis were associated with reduced circulating levels of insulin and IGF-1, but not IGF-II. A causal role of IGF-1 in mediating the protective effects of low positive energy balance was hypothesized; in that paradigm, the effects of positive energy balance were hypothesized to be mediated via a change in the availability of IGF-1, which in turn modulated tissue size homeostasis by decreasing cell proliferation and increasing the rate of apoptosis [33].

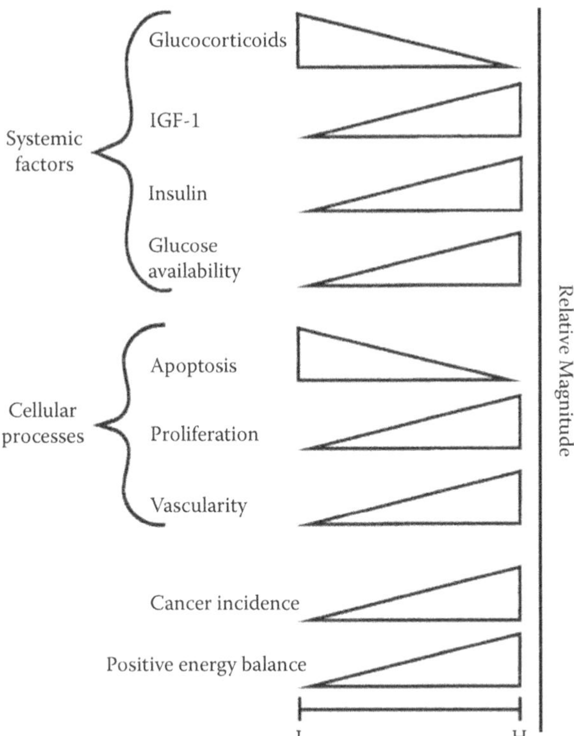

FIGURE 22.2 Magnitude of positive energy balance (low, L, to high, H) is positively associated with cancer incidence in the majority of organ sites investigated using animal models. Associations between positive energy balance and cellular processes and systemic factors that have been reported to influence the carcinogenic process are illustrated.

Zhu and coworkers have recently reported that protection against cancer is lost and plasma IGF-1 levels are restored to control values when animals are switched from low positive energy balance to high positive energy balance — also supporting a causal role of IGF-1 in accounting for the effects of positive energy balance on the carcinogenic response. However, in recent work, those investigators found that infusion of recombinant human IGF-1 to low positive energy balance-treated animals failed to mimic the effects on the carcinogenic response of switching animals from low positive energy balance to high positive energy balance. Collectively, these data imply a permissive but not obligatory role of insulin and its related growth factors in accounting for the effects of positive energy balance on the carcinogenic response.

Adrenal Cortical Steroids

A role for the adrenal gland in accounting for the effects of low positive energy balance in preventing tumor development has been proposed [34]. As Zhu et al. reported [14], in comparison to high positive energy balance, low positive energy balance has been shown to increase urinary excretion of immunoreactive adrenal cortical steroids and levels of urinary corticosteroids were reported to be associated inversely with mammary carcinoma multiplicity. These observations were followed by a series of reports by the same laboratory [22,35,36]. Briefly, it was shown that, *in vivo* [22,35] and *in vitro* [36], provision of supplemental corticosterone has effects on cell proliferation but not apoptosis similar to those observed in response to low positive energy balance. In particular, corticosterone induced higher levels of the CKI p27 and lower levels of cyclin D1 — effects that would be expected to occur when cell cycle progression is arrested at the G1/S transition.

However, two recently published observations from this laboratory raise questions about the degree to which increased adrenal cortical steroid activity alone accounts for the protective effects of low positive energy balance against mammary carcinogenesis [37,38]:

- In an animal study in which dietary corticosterone was fed to rats at a concentration that increased plasma corticosterone to levels comparable to those observed in animals that were low positive energy balance, mammary carcinogenesis was inhibited; however, the degree of inhibition was markedly less than that observed in response to low positive energy balance.
- Unlike observations reported in Pashko and Schwartz [39], adrenalectomy failed to negate the inhibitory activity of low positive energy balance against mammary carcinogenesis.

INTRACELLULAR MECHANISMS

Over seven decades ago, classical biochemical studies showed that tumors have altered metabolic profiles and display high rates of glucose uptake and glycolysis [40]. Although these metabolic changes are not the fundamental defects that cause cancer, they may confer a common advantage that allows colonies of transformed cells to expand, survive, and progress to cancer. Consistent with those early biochemical studies, PET tumor imaging using the fluorinated analogue of 2-deoxyglucose on a large number of tumor types has provided substantial documentation of the increased uptake of glucose by malignant cells [41–43]. This implies that a relationship exists between glucose utilization and the development of cancer [44].

Evidence from recent molecular studies has revealed that several of the multiple genetic alterations that cause tumor development directly affect glycolysis, the cellular response to hypoxia, and the ability of tumor cells to recruit new blood vessels [44]. Oncogene activation and/or changes in tumor suppressor gene function result in alterations in glucose metabolism at an early stage during carcinogenesis. It is likely that these effects are due to the development of oxygen gradients that result in reduced oxygen availability in developing clones of cells and that these changes result in the stabilization of constitutively produced HIF-1α. In turn, stabilization of HIF-1α leads to increased transcription of genes involved in glycolysis, glucose transport, and angiogenesis. Induction of enzymes involved in glycolysis results in a progressive dependence on glucose in those emerging clones because of the production of ATP via aerobic glycolysis rather than oxidative phosphorylation; to support the increased requirement for glucose, expression of genes involved in glucose transport is also increased.

If transformed cells have an increased requirement for glucose but low positive energy balance reduces glucose availability, it is possible that low positive energy balance would decrease cellular energy charge (the ratio of AMP to ATP) in emerging populations of transformed cells with a consequent activation of AMPK. Available evidence, although limited, indicates that activation of AMPK not only conserves the use of glucose, but also regulates, at least in part, cell cycle transit, cell death, and vascularization via effects on the phosphorylation of regulatory proteins. Candidate targets of AMPK include p53, Akt/PKB, and Raf. As noted earlier, low positive energy balance retards cell cycle progression at the G1/S transition, induces apoptosis via the mitochondrial activation pathway, and has differential effects on blood vessel formation and growth.

FINAL COMMENTS

As indicated at the outset of this chapter, this review and analysis was intended to be narrowly focused. Accordingly, no consideration has been given to the effects of positive energy balance on cellular oxidation or inflammation, two processes that may contribute significantly to the development of cancer. Suffice it to say that these processes should not be neglected in efforts to determine how obesitogenesis modulates the carcinogenic process.

SUMMARY

Just as cancer research has tended to focus on the end stage of the disease (cancer) rather than on the disease process (carcinogenesis), weight control research has tended to focus on the end stages of obesitogenesis rather than on consequences of different levels of positive energy balance that, over time, result in obesity. The investigation of weight control on the development of cancer requires an understanding of the effects of positive energy balance on the carcinogenic process; suitable preclinical models exist in which to conduct the needed research. Work summarized in this chapter indicates that positive energy balance affects the carcinogenic process by modulating cell proliferation, apoptosis, and tissue vascularity. It remains to be determined why these cellular processes are modulated by positive energy balance, but the role of glucose homeostasis in mediating the effects of positive energy balance clearly merits investigation.

ACKNOWLEDGMENTS

The excellent technical assistance of John McGinley in the preparation of this manuscript is greatly appreciated. This work was supported by PHS grants CA52626 and CA100693 from the National Cancer Institute.

REFERENCES

1. Mokdad AH, Bowman BA, Ford ES, Vinicor F, Marks JS, Koplan JP. The continuing epidemics of obesity and diabetes in the United States. *JAMA*, 2001; 286:1195–1200.
2. Statistics Related to Overweight and Obesity. NIH Publication No. 03-4158, http://www.niddk.nih.gov/health/nutrit/pubs/statobes.htm. 2003.
3. IARC. *Weight Control and Physical Activity.* Lyon: IARC Press, 2002.
4. *Clinical Guidelines on the Identification, Evaluation, and Treatment of Overweight and Obesity in Adults.* NIH Publication No. 98-4083. 1998.
5. Waxler SH. The relationship of obesity to liver tumors in mice. *Stanford Med Bull*, 1960; 18:1–4.
6. Seilkop SK. The effect of body weight on tumor incidence and carcinogenicity testing in B6C3F1 mice and F344 rats. *Fundam Appl Toxicol*, 1995; 24:247–259.
7. Wolff GL, Kodell RL, Cameron AM, Medina D. Accelerated appearance of chemically induced mammary carcinomas in obese yellow (Avy/A) (BALB/c X VY) F1 hybrid mice. *J Toxicol Environ Health*, 1982; 10:131–142.
8. Klurfeld DM, Lloyd LM, Welch CB, Davis MJ, Tulp OL, Kritchevsky D. Reduction of enhanced mammary carcinogenesis in LA/N-cp (corpulent) rats by energy restriction. *Proc Soc Exp Biol Med*, 1991; 196:381–384.
9. Lee WM, Lu S, Medline A, Archer MC. Susceptibility of lean and obese Zucker rats to tumorigenesis induced by N-methyl-N-nitrosourea. *Cancer Lett*, 2001; 162:155–160.
10. Cleary MP, Phillips FC, Getzin SC, Jacobson TL, Jacobson MK, Christensen TA, Juneja SC, Grande JP, Maihle NJ. Genetically obese MMTV-TGF-alpha/Lep(ob)Lep(ob) female mice do not develop mammary tumors. *Breast Cancer Res Treat*, 2003; 77:205–215.
11. Cleary MP, Juneja SC, Phillips FC, Hu X, Grande JP, Maihle NJ. Leptin receptor-deficient MMTV-TGF-alpha/Lepr(db)Lepr(db) female mice do not develop oncogene-induced mammary tumors. *Exp Biol Med* (Maywood), 2004; 229:182–193.
12. Freedman LS, Clifford C, Messina M. Analysis of dietary fat, calories, body weight, and the development of mammary tumors in rats and mice: a review. *Cancer Res*, 1990; 50:5710–5719.

13. Thompson HJ, Zhu Z, Jiang W. Protection against cancer by energy restriction: all experimental approaches are not equal. *J Nutr*, 2002; 132:1047–1049.
14. Zhu Z, Haegele AD, Thompson HJ. Effect of caloric restriction on pre-malignant and malignant stages of mammary carcinogenesis. *Carcinogenesis*, 1997; 18:1007–1012.
15. Sylvester PW, Aylsworth CF, Meites J. Relationship of hormones to inhibition of mammary tumor development by underfeeding during the "critical period" after carcinogen administration. *Cancer Res*, 1981; 41:1384–1388.
16. Sarkar NH, Fernandes G, Telang NT, Kourides IA, Good RA. Low-calorie diet prevents the development of mammary tumors in C3H mice and reduces circulating prolactin level, murine mammary tumor virus expression, and proliferation of mammary alveolar cells. *Proc Natl Acad Sci USA*, 1982; 79:7758–7762.
17. Sinha DK, Gebhard RL, Pazik JE. Inhibition of mammary carcinogenesis in rats by dietary restriction. *Cancer Lett*, 1988; 40:133–141.
18. Thompson HJ, Strange R, Schedin PJ. Apoptosis in the genesis and prevention of cancer. *Cancer Epidemiol Biomarkers Prev*, 1992; 1:597–602.
19. Hanahan D, Weinberg RA. The hallmarks of cancer. *Cell*, 2000; 100:57–70.
20. Zhu Z, Jiang W, Thompson HJ. Effect of energy restriction on tissue size regulation during chemically induced mammary carcinogenesis. *Carcinogenesis*, 1999; 20:1721–1726.
21. Lok E, Scott FW, Mongeau R, Nera EA, Malcolm S, Clayson DB. Calorie restriction and cellular proliferation in various tissues of the female Swiss Webster mouse. *Cancer Lett*, 1990; 51:67–73.
22. Zhu Z, Jiang W, Thompson HJ. Effect of energy restriction on the expression of cyclin D1 and p27 during premalignant and malignant stages of chemically induced mammary carcinogenesis. *Mol Carcinog*, 1999; 24:241–245.
23. Jiang W, Zhu Z, Thompson HJ. Effect of energy restriction on cell cycle machinery in 1-methyl-1-nitrosourea-induced mammary carcinomas in rats. *Cancer Res*, 2003; 63:1228–1234.
24. Thompson HJ, Zhu Z, Jiang W. Identification of the apoptosis activation cascade induced in mammary carcinomas by energy restriction. *Cancer Res*, 2004; 64:1541–1545.
25. Zhu Z, Jiang W, Thompson HJ. An experimental paradigm for studying the cellular and molecular mechanisms of cancer inhibition by energy restriction. *Mol Carcinog*, 2002; 35:51–56.
26. Thompson HJ, McGinley JN, Spoelstra NS, Jiang W, Zhu Z, Wolfe P. Effect of dietary energy restriction on vascular density during mammary carcinogenesis. *Cancer Res*, 2004; 64:5643–5650.
27. Ruggeri BA, Klurfeld DM, Kritchevsky D, Furlanetto RW. Caloric restriction and 7,12-dimethylbenz(a)anthracene-induced mammary tumor growth in rats: alterations in circulating insulin, insulin-like growth factors I and II, and epidermal growth factor. *Cancer Res*, 1989; 49:4130–4134.
28. Klurfeld DM, Welch CB, Davis MJ, Kritchevsky D. Determination of degree of energy restriction necessary to reduce DMBA-induced mammary tumorigenesis in rats during the promotion phase. *J Nutr*, 1989; 119:286–291.
29. Heuson JC, Legros N. Influence of insulin deprivation on growth of the 7,12-dimethylbenz(a)anthracene-induced mammary carcinoma in rats subjected to alloxan diabetes and food restriction. *Cancer Res*, 1972; 32:226–232.
30. Cohen ND, Hilf R. Influence of insulin on growth and metabolism of 7,12-dimethylbenz(α)anthracene-induced mammary tumors. *Cancer Res*, 1974; 34:3245–3252.
31. Hilf R, Hissin PJ, Shafie SM. Regulatory interrelationships for insulin and estrogen action in mammary tumors. *Cancer Res*, 1978; 38:4076–4085.
32. Gibson SL, Hilf R. Regulation of estrogen-binding capacity by insulin in 7,12-dimethylbenz(α)anthracene-induced mammary tumors in rats. *Cancer Res*, 1980; 40:2343–2348.
33. Kari FW, Dunn SE, French JE, Barrett JC. Roles for insulin-like growth factor-1 in mediating the anticarcinogenic effects of caloric restriction. *J Nutr Health Aging*, 1999; 3:92–101.
34. Boutwell RK, Brush MK, Rusch HP. The stimulating effect of dietary fat on carcinogenesis. *Cancer Res*, 1949; 9:741–746.
35. Zhu Z, Jiang W, Thompson HJ. Effect of corticosterone administration on mammary gland development and p27 expression and their relationship to the effects of energy restriction on mammary carcinogenesis. *Carcinogenesis*, 1998; 19:2101–2106.
36. Jiang W, Zhu Z, Bhatia N, Agarwal R, Thompson HJ. Mechanisms of energy restriction: effects of corticosterone on cell growth, cell cycle machinery, and apoptosis. *Cancer Res*, 2002; 62:5280–5287.

37. Jiang W, Zhu Z, McGinley JN, Thompson HJ. Adrenalectomy does not block the inhibition of mammary carcinogenesis by dietary energy restriction in rats. *J Nutr*, 2004; 134:1152–1156.
38. Zhu Z, Jiang W, Thompson HJ. Mechanisms by which energy restriction inhibits rat mammary carcinogenesis: in vivo effects of corticosterone on cell cycle machinery in mammary carcinomas. *Carcinogenesis*, 2003; 24:1225–1231.
39. Pashko LL, Schwartz AG. Reversal of food restriction-induced inhibition of mouse skin tumor promotion by adrenalectomy. *Carcinogenesis*, 1992; 13:1925–1928.
40. Walberg O. *The Metabolism of Tumors*. Constable, London 1930.
41. Weber WA, Schwaiger M, Avril N. Quantitative assessment of tumor metabolism using FDG-PET imaging. *Nucl Med Biol*, 2000; 27:683–687.
42. Wahl RL, Henry CA, Either SP. Serum glucose: effects on tumor and normal tissue accumulation of 2-[F-18]-fluoro-2-deoxy-D-glucose. *Radiology*, 1992; 183:643–647.
43. Wahl RL. Current status of PET in breast cancer imaging, staging, and therapy. *Semin Roentgenol*, 2001; 36:250–260.
44. Dang CV, Semenza GL. Oncogenic alterations of metabolism. *Trends Biochem Sci*, 1999; 24:68–72.

23 Genetics, Obesity, and Cancer

Shelley Tworoger and Monica McGrath

CONTENTS

INTRODUCTION

Obesity is a common, yet complex and multifactorial disease whose development is modulated by contributions from genetic and environmental influences. This chapter discusses the genetic components of obesity — a complex area with more than 430 genes, polymorphisms, and chromosomal regions identified as linked to or associated with obesity in humans [1]. Given the breadth of the available knowledge, we focus on the genetic aspects of obesity that are most likely to be related to cancer and its prevention. First, the genetic contributions to obesity, based on data from twin and family studies, and how genetics and the environment may interact in the development of obesity are discussed. Then, current approaches and their challenges to detect genetic mutations involved in obesity are reviewed and select genes of interest, particularly with respect to cancer, are highlighted. Finally, the importance of genetic variability in the success of lifestyle interventions to reduce obesity and cancer risk is discussed. In the interest of space, review papers rather than original articles are cited whenever possible.

GENETIC CONTRIBUTIONS TO OBESITY

HERITABILITY OF OBESITY

Although obesity is controlled in part by environmental and behavioral exposures, strong evidence indicates that genetic factors account for a substantial portion of the variation in human adiposity. Several study designs, including twin, adoption, and family studies, have been used to determine the correlation of obesity measures between different family members and the heritability of obesity, which is the variation in a certain trait e.g., body mass index (BMI) that is attributable to genetic factors. For example, a twin study compares how similar the obesity measure is between identical vs. fraternal twin pairs.

A detailed review of these study designs, including their advantages and disadvantages, can be found in Maes et al. [2]. These researchers determined pooled correlation estimates for various family member pairs across multiple studies of different designs that included more than 25,000 twin pairs and 50,000 biological and adoptive family members. The correlation for BMI (Figure 23.1) was smallest among genetically unrelated pairs (e.g., spouses), followed by partially genetically related pairs (e.g., siblings); it was highest among monozygotic (identical) twins [2]. This is consistent with a role of genetic factors in human obesity. Heritability of BMI also supports the role of genetics, although estimates differ by study design. The highest estimates are from twin studies (~70%), the lowest from adoption studies (~30%), and midrange estimates are from other family study designs (~40%) [2–4]. Several analyses combining multiple study designs with large sample sizes suggest that the heritability for BMI is between 40 and 65% [2,5].

Weight gain over time also appears to have a genetic component; among male twins, the heritability of adult weight gain over 40 years was 55 to 87% [6] and, among female twins, the heritability of change in BMI over 10 years was 57 to 86% [7]. Several studies have suggested that the heritability of BMI and waist-to-hip ratio is higher among women vs. men [8,9], but is similar for African–Americans and Caucasians [10]. Twin studies suggest that the heritability of BMI is higher in children and adolescents (~90%) vs. adults (~60 to 70%) and that, among adults, herita-

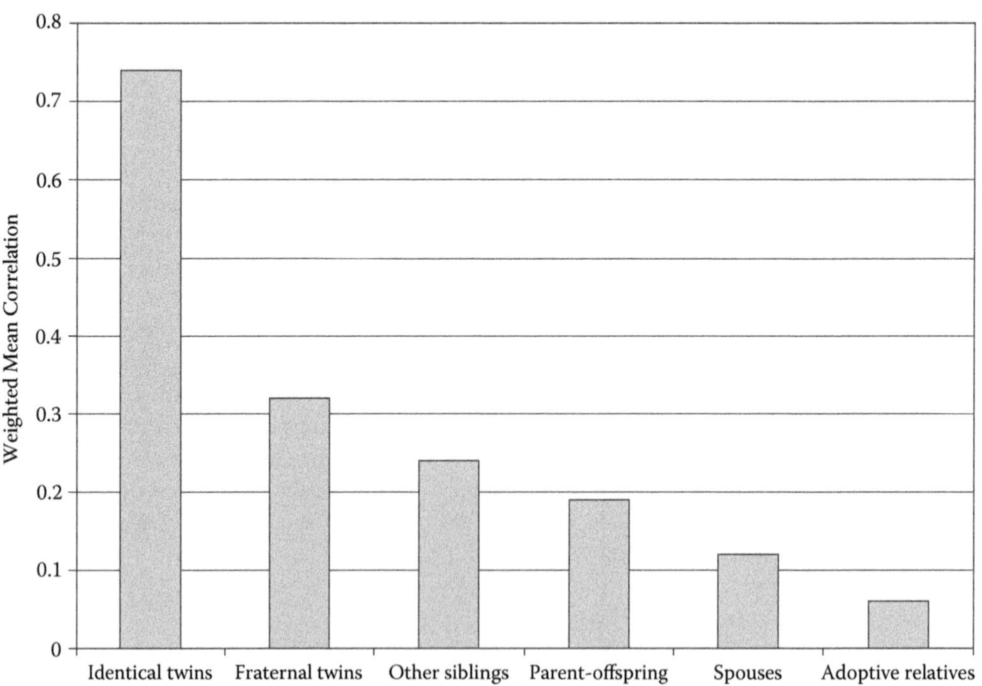

FIGURE 23.1 Pooled correlations of body mass index between various family pairs from multiple studies. Body mass index correlations pooled from multiple studies and weighted by study sample size. The number of studies contributing to each estimate is: 27 for identical (monozygotic) and fraternal (dizygotic) twins, 32 for nontwin siblings, 37 for parent–offspring, 24 for spouses, and 11 for adopted relatives. Correlations are highest for the most genetically similar pairs (i.e., identical twins), intermediate for moderately genetically similar pairs (i.e., fraternal twins, nontwin siblings, parent–offspring), and lowest for genetically unrelated pairs (i.e., spouses and adopted relatives) (From Maes, H.H. et al., *Behav Genet*, 1997. 27(4): 325–351.)

bility may decrease with increasing age [2]. In addition, overall and abdominal obesity appear to be mediated, in part, by similar genetic components [11,12]. Overwhelming, current research indicates that genetics are an important factor in the development of obesity.

Interaction between Genetics and the Environment

Although genetics contributes to overweight and obesity, this factor alone cannot explain the sharp increase in the worldwide prevalence of obesity over the last several decades. The current environment, promoting high caloric intake and low physical activity, is thought to be largely responsible for the recent epidemic. In 1962, Dr. James Neel hypothesized that the human genome evolved under conditions of low food availability and high physical activity requirements [13]. Evolutionary forces favored individuals with genotypes that had an increased survival rate during food shortages, such as those with a genetic propensity for storing fat [14]. Thus, the prevailing genetic characteristics of humans are particularly ill suited for the current environment and cannot accommodate the rapidly changing shift from conditions of low to high energy intake.

As such, the interplay between genetic predisposition and environmental factors is critical in understanding and reducing obesity. Several investigators [15–17] have suggested that the current population is characterized by individuals with differing genetic predispositions to obesity (Figure 23.2). As the environment changes from favoring low energy intake and high physical activity to high energy intake and low physical activity, individuals with a high genetic predisposition for obesity increase their BMI or fat mass more than those with a low predisposition. Individuals with genetic obesity, often characterized by a single genetic mutation (see the section on monogenic forms of obesity), have a high BMI in both environments. This model is supported by overfeeding studies. Among 12 pairs of identical male twins who participated in an overeating protocol for 100 days, the variability in weight and fat mass gain was three to six times greater between vs. within twin pairs [18]. Several genetic polymorphisms have also been associated with varying responses in overfeeding studies [19].

These data suggest that it is important to consider the environment and genetics in the study of obesity. Future research must focus on the genetic mutations underlying obesity (next section) and how these mutations may interact with interventions to reduce obesity (section on genetic variability and lifestyle interventions to reduce obesity and cancer risk).

GENETIC VARIABILITY AND OBESITY

Interest in and knowledge of the genetic influences of obesity have increased dramatically since the cloning of the mouse obese (*ob*) gene in 1994 [20]. Genetic determinants of individual variation in human adiposity are likely to be multiple and interacting; each genetic variant likely has only a small to modest effect. This section reviews monogenic and polygenic obesity disorders and obesity-related genes, highlighting the complexities and challenges involved in the search for susceptibility genes in human adiposity.

Animal Studies of Obesity

Recent findings have observed that mutations in rodent genes, which have human homologs, can cause similar phenotypes in humans, underscoring the highly conserved nature of the pathway regulating energy balance [15]. Spontaneous mutations causing obesity in mice have led to the cloning of the *ob* [20] and *db* [21] genes and the characterization of their human homolog gene products — leptin and the leptin receptor, respectively. Leptin is an endocrine hormone secreted by adipocytes that communicates information regarding long-term energy stores to the brain via its receptor. Mice carrying the *ob* or the *db* mutations are characterized by early onset obesity, hyperphagia, low core body temperature, insulin resistance, and susceptibility to diabetes mellitus

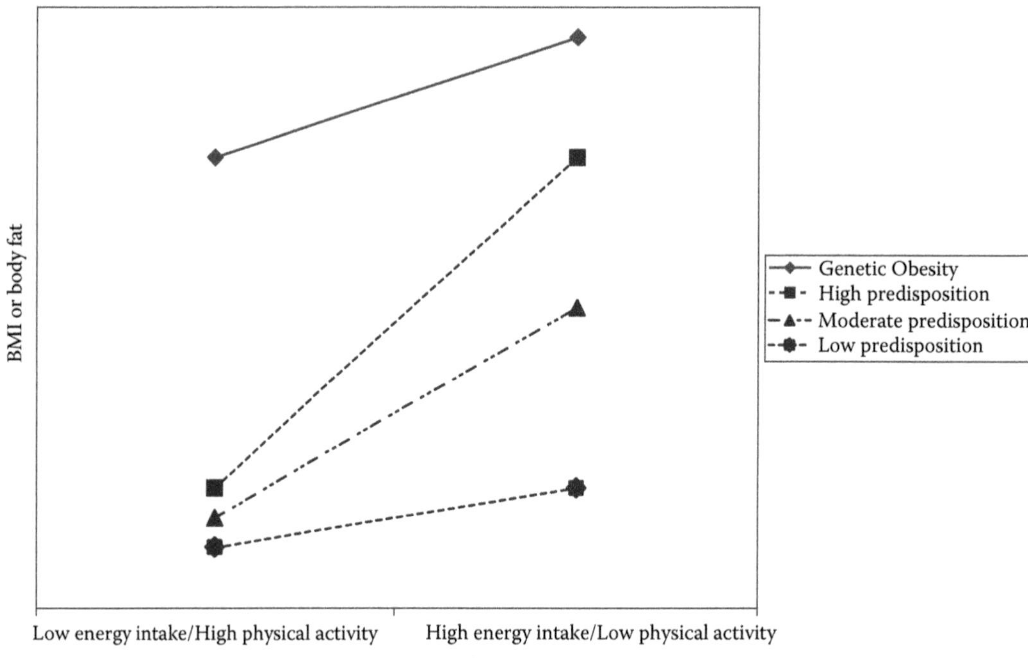

FIGURE 23.2 The interaction between genetic predisposition to obesity and the environmental milieu. Hypothetical response of four levels of genetic susceptibility toward obesity to changes in environmental conditions from a low energy intake/high physical activity to a high energy intake/low physical activity environment, in the presence of gene–environment interactions. —◆— indicates individuals with monogenic obesity (caused by a single genetic mutation); in both environments these individuals are obese. -■- indicates individuals who have a high genetic predisposition to obesity; in a low energy intake/high physical activity environment, these individuals may be normal to slightly overweight, but in a high energy intake/low physical activity environment, they become obese. –▲-- indicates individuals who have a moderate genetic predisposition to obesity and become overweight with an environmental shift toward high energy intake/low physical activity. -●- indicates individuals who are genetically resistant to obesity, so in both environments they are lean. (Adapted from Loos, R.J. and C. Bouchard, *J Intern Med*, 2003. 254(5): 401–425; Barsh, G.S. et al., *Nature*, 2000. 404(6778): 644–651; and Perusse, L. and C. Bouchard, *Nutr Rev*, 1999. 57(5 Pt 2): S31–37; discussion S37–368.)

[20,21]. The *ob* mutation results in a lack of leptin production, and the *db* mutation alters the normal splicing of the leptin receptor gene, creating a premature stop codon; both ultimately lead to decreased leptin signaling [22].

Additional single-gene mutations resulting in obesity-related phenotypes have also been identified in mice, all of which have been linked to relevant mutations in humans or have led to the identification of a genetic pathway in which other genes were mutated. Identified human homolog gene products include growth hormone, insulin-signaling protein, cholecystokinin receptor A, lipin, carboxypeptidase E, attractin, agouti signaling protein, and mahogunin [1]. Knockout and transgenic mouse models suggest that many other additional genes potentially affect the development of obesity-related phenotypes. The study of animal models allows for the identification and understanding of the behavioral, metabolic, and physiological pathways involved in obesity.

Monogenic Forms of Obesity

Monogenic forms of obesity are rare and are usually caused by a single mutation in a key regulatory gene, such as leptin. Pleiotropic obesity syndromes (e.g., obesity is one of multiple phenotypes)

— such as the autosomal dominant syndromes of Prader–Willi, Angelman, and Albright hereditary osteodystrophy; the autosomal recessive Alstrom, Cohen, and Bardet–Biedl syndromes; and the X-linked Wilson–Turner syndrome — also are extremely rare and follow a Mendelian pattern of inheritance. The human obesity gene map [1] has identified over 41 Mendelian syndromes relevant to human obesity. Obesity is a clinical manifestation of such syndromes but is not a dominant feature.

Single-gene disorders resulting in obesity appear to be largely independent of environmental factors (see Figure 23.2). Obesity-causing genes that are mutated include: leptin [23], leptin receptor [24], pro-opiomelanocortin [25], melanocortin 4 receptor (*MC4R*) [26], and proconvertase [27]. The *MC4R* gene has at least 42 different mutations associated with obesity, making it the most prevalent genetic cause of obesity identified to date. Elucidating the role of these rare mutations provides valuable insight into the complex physiological process of obesity and the critical genes involved in these processes; however, it cannot address the genetic influences involved in the etiology of polygenic obesity.

Identifying Genetic Components of Polygenic Obesity

Common forms of obesity arise from the complex interactions of genes (which remain relatively unknown), environmental factors, and lifestyle behaviors and do not display the typical Mendelian pattern of inheritance. Studies of candidate genes indicate that most obesity-related genes have important functions in adipose tissue or in pathways regulating energy expenditure and food intake. Two study designs, the candidate gene approach and genome-wide approach, have been widely used to identify obesity-susceptibility genes, e.g., genes that increase the risk of developing obesity, but are not sufficient or necessary to cause obesity.

The candidate gene approach identifies obesity-related genes *a priori* on the basis of data from animal or *in vitro* models, suggesting their involvement in a biochemical pathway related to energy balance regulation or adipose tissue biology. Such genes are usually assessed using population (association) studies, which are a powerful tool for detecting genetic variation contributing to common obesity. These studies compare the allele or genotype frequencies between cases (e.g., obese individuals) and controls (e.g., lean individuals) or compare a particular phenotype (e.g., BMI) to identify polymorphic markers that differ significantly between the two groups. Associations observed in such studies could be due to the following:

- The variant allele directly causes the phenotypic effect
- The allele is in linkage disequilibrium (i.e., the nonrandom association of alleles at linked loci) or the allele is closely associated with the true causal allele
- The observation is an artifact due to population stratification (differences in variant allele frequencies among diverse ethnic groups)
- Chance

Often, animal or *in vitro* studies are needed to determine whether the genetic variant is the likely cause of the obesity-related phenotype or is a marker for that phenotype. The candidate gene approach has successfully demonstrated that minor obesity genes contribute to the regulation of energy intake, energy expenditure, and nutrient partitioning [15]. For a comprehensive review of all the candidate gene studies conducted, see Snyder et al. [1] and Damcott et al. [28].

The genome-wide approach allows for the systematic survey of the entire genome to identify disease-related genes with no *a priori* assumptions about the potential importance of a particular gene or chromosomal region. Genome-wide scans are used to identify chromosomal regions showing linkage (or association) with obesity in large nuclear families and can potentially identify new or unsuspected candidate genes influencing human adiposity. In this approach, nonparametric linkage analysis is performed using a series of anonymous polymorphisms, spaced at constant intervals over the entire genome, to identify quantitative trait loci (QTLs) and, eventually, genes within these quantitative trait loci. Any locus that influences the variability of a quantitative trait (e.g., waist–hip ratio, BMI) may be classified as a quantitative trait loci.

The nonparametric linkage methods, often referred to as allele-sharing methods, identify the chromosomal regions that affected family members share more commonly than would be expected by chance; the statistical measure of linkage or the likelihood of genetic linkage between loci is the lod score (logarithm of the likelihood ratio for linkage). The regions identified from the scans will become the focus of more intensive follow-up analysis to determine the disease-predisposing allele. Parametric analytic techniques, which require *a priori* knowledge regarding the mode of inheritance, can also be used. However this approach may not be appropriate for complex phenotypes such as obesity and could result in spurious associations. A review of these methods can be found in Haines et al. [29]. Results from genome-wide scans have consistently suggested that obesity genes are located on chromosomes 2p, 3q, 5p, 6p, 7q, 10p, 11q, 17p, and 20q [15], which appear to contain one or more genes involved in body weight regulation. A third, more recent approach involves tissue-specific gene expression profiles comparing lean and obese individuals [15].

Specific Genetic Polymorphisms of Interest

More than 430 genes, markers, and chromosomal regions have been associated or linked with human obesity phenotypes [1]. The human obesity map reports that over 200 human quantitative trait loci for obesity phenotypes have been identified from genome-wide scans; 35 genomic regions harbor quantitative trait loci replicated among two to five studies [1]. All chromosomes except the Y chromosome have had putative loci identified in obesity-related phenotypes [1]. Over 270 studies have reported positive associations with 90 candidate genes; 15 are supported by at least 5 positive studies [1]. The human obesity gene map website: http://obesitygene.pbrc.edu provides a detailed description of all investigated genes and quantitative trait loci.

This section will focus on a few genes for which positive findings have been replicated in multiple independent study populations or that may be particularly relevant to cancer risk, including β_2- and β_3- adrenergic receptors (*ADR*s), hormone-sensitive lipase (*HSL*), tumor necrosis factor alpha (*TNF*-α), uncoupling protein-1 (*UCP-1*), leptin (*LEP*) and leptin receptor (*LEPR*), and perixosome proliferator activator receptor gamma-2 (*PPAR*γ*-2*) (Table 23.1).

The adrenergic system is a key regulator of energy balance through the stimulation of thermogenesis and lipid mobilization from fat stores [15,30,31]. Several coding and functional mutations have been described in the β_2-*ADR* gene, yet have been inconsistently associated with obesity [1,32–35]. The Trp64Arg polymorphism in the β_3-*ADR* has not been associated with obesity in meta-analyses [36–38]; however, the polymorphism may be important only among women [39]. The Trp64Arg polymorphism may also affect the susceptibility to colon cancer in obese subjects [40].

PPARγ-2 is a key regulator of adipocyte differentiation [41]. The Pro12Ala functional polymorphism is associated with decreased receptor activity [42] and has been examined in 30 independent studies with a total sample size of 19,136 subjects. Meta-analyses suggest that Ala12 homozygotes have a significantly higher BMI than heterozygotes and Pro12 homozygotes, particularly among overweight individuals [43]. However, the Ala12 allele has also been associated with a modest decreased risk of type-2 diabetes mellitus [44].

UCP-1 is expressed in brown adipose tissue and regulates the combustion of fatty acids. It has an important thermogenic effect by promoting heat production and enhancing energy expenditure [30]. The –3826 A/G promoter polymorphism may influence body weight regulation. Family-based and observational studies have observed associations between the variant allele and an increased gain in fat mass and a higher weight gain in adult life [45–47]. Weak or null associations between other *UCP-1* polymorphisms and obesity phenotypes have also been described [1,45,46,48–53].

TABLE 23.1
Selected Candidate Genes for Human Obesity

Gene	Chromosomal location	Gene function	Polymorphism	Reported polymorphism frequency[a]	Presumed polymorphism functional effect	Association with obesity phenotypes	Interaction with lifestyle interventions	Ref.
β_2-adreno-receptor	5q31–q32	Thermogenesis and lipolysis	Gln27Glu	7% J 40% C	Altered lipolytic response to catecholamines	Positive association with BMI, WHR, body weight	High-caloric diet on weight/fat gain; exercise on lipolysis	31–34
			Arg16Gly	50% J 55% C	Altered receptor function in fat cells	Inconclusive association with BMI, WHR, body weight	High-caloric diet on weight/fat gain	31,33,34
β_3-adreno-receptor	8p12–p11.1	Thermogenesis and lipolysis	Trp64Arg	20% J 12% A–A 8–12% C	Decreased receptor function and energy expenditure	Inconclusive association with BMI, obesity, fat mass, WHR	Low-fat diet or exercise on BMI change, weight/fat loss, insulin, glucose	28,35–39, 45, 76, 87–92
PPARγ-2	3p25.2	Adipocyte differentiation, glucose homeostatis, fat mass regulation	Pro12Ala	12–19% C 2% A–A 3% J	Decreased receptor activity	Positive association with BMI	Diet or exercise on weight/fat loss, BMI change, regain of weight	41–43, 80–86
UCP-1	4q31.1	Thermogenesis, fatty acid combustion, metabolic rate	−3826 A/G	25–27% C	Unknown	Inconclusive association with BMI, WHR, body weight, weight gain	Exercise on glucose	44–46, 76
Hormone-sensitive lipase	19q13.1–q13.2	Lipid metabolism, fatty acid mobilization	Multiple, including a CA repeat	NA	Decreased lipolysis	Positive association with increased fat accumulation	NA	54–58
TNF-α	6p21.3	Insulin sensitivity and lipolysis	−308 G/A	13–18% C	Altered gene transcription	Positive association with BMI, obesity	Diet plus exercise on developing diabetes	51,61–68
Leptin	7q32.2	Regulation of body weight	Multiple	NA	Altered leptin secretion	Positive association with body weight, BMI	Exercise on insulin	71
Leptin receptor	1p31.3	Receptor for leptin	Multiple	NA	Possibly altered receptor activity	Inconclusive association with BMI, fat mass, body weight	Diet or exercise on weight/fat loss, insulin	70,71

[a] J = Japanese, C = Caucasian, A–A = African–American, NA = not applicable.

HSL is a lipolysis-regulating protein that plays a critical role in energy homeostatis [54]. A noncoding dinucleotide (CA) repeat polymorphism may affect lipolysis regulation —subjects with five CA repeats are markedly resistant to lipolysis in subcutaneous fat cells [55], possibly leading to increased fat accumulation [56]. Additional polymorphisms in *HSL* also have been associated with obesity [57–59].

TNF-α is a cytokine that may modulate insulin sensitivity by inhibiting insulin signaling in fat cells [60] and stimulating lipolysis [61]. Increased levels of the cytokine have been linked to obesity and insulin resistance [62]. A –308 G/A promoter polymorphism increases gene transcription in adipocytes [63] and has been inconsistently associated with hip and waist circumference, insulin sensitivity, BMI, and body fat mass [52,64–68]. This promoter polymorphism is also associated with high rates of glucose oxidation in normal weight subjects and high rates of lipid synthesis in overweight subjects, suggesting an interaction between body weight and the functional promoter polymorphism [69].

Leptin and its receptor are involved in the long-term regulation of energy stores in the body, acting primarily in the hypothalamus [70]. Several polymorphisms in the coding region and the 5′ and 3′ untranslated regions of the leptin gene have been shown to be associated with leptin secretion, body weight, and BMI [1]. Polymorphisms in the leptin receptor have been inconsistently associated with obesity [1,71]. Recent evidence suggests that the association between obesity and non-Hodgkin's lymphoma may be mediated by leptin and the leptin receptor through their role in the regulation of immune function [72].

Challenges in Identifying Obesity-Related Genes

The principal methodological difficulties of addressing the gene–obesity associations in individual studies are:

- The modest nature of the expected associations
- The large number of gene variants that will likely lead to a large number of false positive and false negative results
- Population stratification, which can lead to false positive results

It is essential to create very large datasets of prospectively collected information to maximize the power to detect modest associations because effects in individual studies may not reach statistical significance due to insufficient power. It is necessary to analyze the genetic variation in functional genomic regions comprehensively and perform haplotype analysis, which takes into account multiple polymorphic variants across the entire gene. The functional significance of the polymorphisms on the corresponding protein must also be investigated in animal models and *in vitro* studies. False-positive findings are likely to occur, so it is essential to replicate results in multiple studies.

To avoid publication bias and the expenditure of resources on inappropriate areas, it is important that negative findings are published and that positive findings are followed up in a systematic fashion to determine whether the genetic variant is truly involved in the etiology of obesity. Because obesity is a complex phenotype, studies need to define the type of obese subjects studied clearly — i.e., upper body vs. lower body obesity or early vs. late onset — and to examine a variety of phenotypes, including BMI, body fat mass, percentage of body fat, abdominal fat, fat-free mass, skinfolds, resting metabolic rate, plasma leptin levels, and other components of fat distribution and energy balance. Correctly characterizing obesity-related phenotypes will increase power to detect genetic differences and aid in comparability across studies. For a review of the challenges in genetic studies of obesity, refer to Comuzzie et al. [73].

Gene–Gene Interactions

In the course of conducting genetic research of obesity, it will be important to identify synergistic relationships between different genetic mutations with respect to obesity [15]. Preliminary studies have suggested that additive and nonadditive genetic effects are important in obesity. In other words, allelic effects of some genetic polymorphisms may be amplified or diminished in the presence or absence of other genetic variants. Exploratory analyses have observed gene–gene interactions between polymorphisms in β_3-*ADR* and *UCP-1* with resting metabolic rate [74] and changes in body weight [75,76]. Similarly polymorphisms in β_3-*ADR* and *PPAR*γ-*2* may interact with respect to BMI, insulin, and leptin levels [77]. These findings reinforce the idea that specific polymorphism associations with obesity may be underestimated if only their individual and independent effects are considered. Thus, it is important to understand the underlying physiological pathways involved in obesity to better address possible gene–gene interactions.

GENETIC VARIABILITY AND LIFESTYLE INTERVENTIONS TO REDUCE OBESITY AND CANCER RISK

Gene–gene and gene–environment interactions are important in understanding the development of obesity. Of particular relevance to cancer is evidence suggesting that genetic predisposition may be important in the response of overweight and obese individuals to weight loss interventions. Much work has focused on behavioral and environmental barriers to intervention compliance; however less research has examined whether certain genetic mutations are linked with weight and fat loss resistance. An early study of seven identical male twin pairs who participated in twice daily exercise for 93 days reported that weight and fat loss were more similar within vs. between twin pairs [78]. Similarly, a family exercise intervention study reported that changes in waist circumference and abdominal fat measures were more similar within family groups than between families [79].

Several of the polymorphisms, including *PPAR*γ-*2* and β_3-*ADR*, discussed earlier also have been found to modify the effect of diet or exercise interventions on weight and fat loss. Prospective observational studies and intervention trials have been used to look at genetic modification of diet and exercise on BMI, weight, and fat. Multiple studies [80–86] suggest that the *PPAR*γ Pro12Ala polymorphism modifies the effect of dietary fat intake and/or exercise on obesity and weight and other intermediate biomarkers of obesity, such as insulin resistance (Table 23.1). This information lends biological credibility to the potential role of this polymorphism in obesity. Some [87–91] but not all [45,88,92] studies also suggest that polymorphisms in the β_3-*ADR* may slightly modify the effect of weight loss interventions (Table 23.1).

Two studies have reported that the combined effect of two or three polymorphisms may enhance resistance to weight loss. Phares et al. [91] reported that the combined genetic profile of α_2-, β_2-, and β_3-*ADR* polymorphisms and their respective interactions explained over 17% of variability in loss of fat mass and abdominal fat due to exercise among older adults. Another exercise intervention reported that polymorphisms in two different sex hormone metabolizing genes found in adipose tissue were associated with fat loss in older women; women with polymorphisms in both genes had a greater amount of fat loss than those with one or neither polymorphism, after accounting for adherence to the intervention [93] (Figure 23.3). These data suggest that it is important to understand how genetic predisposition may influence the success of weight loss interventions in the population. Focus on intermediate serum or plasma biomarkers is crucial to understanding the mechanisms underlying a possible interaction and how to better tailor interventions to individual patients.

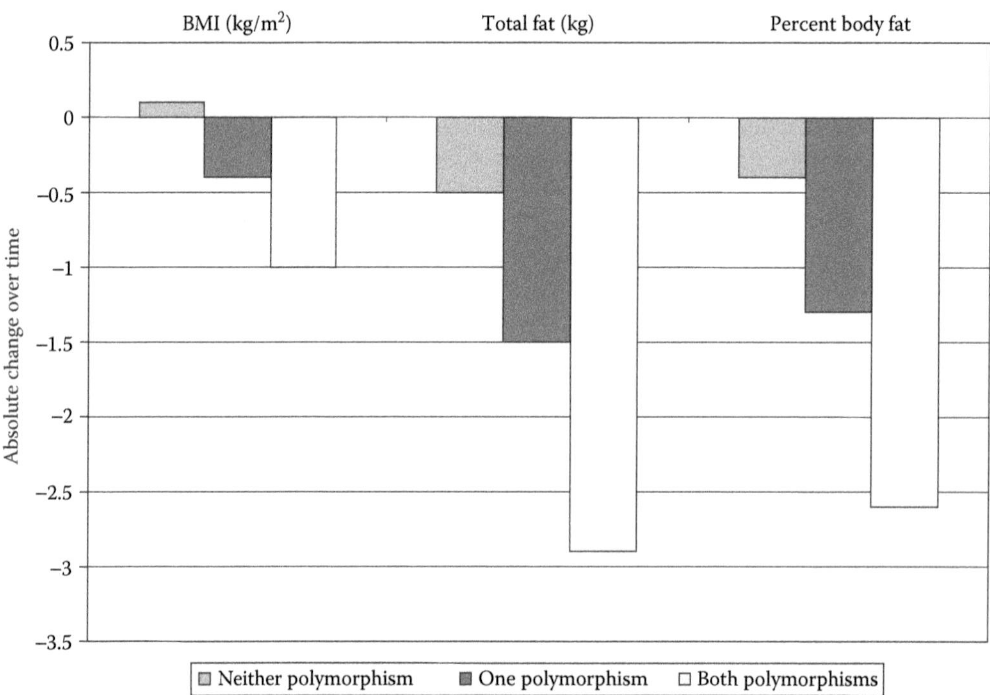

FIGURE 23.3 Change in body fat measures due to a 1-year exercise intervention among postmenopausal women with no, one, or both polymorphisms in two different sex hormone metabolizing genes. Change in body fat measures during a yearlong exercise intervention in postmenopausal women by genetic profile of the *CYP19* (TTTA) repeat and *COMT* Valine/Methionine polymorphisms. These genes are involved in the biosynthesis and metabolism of estrogens, which are involved in adipose tissue regulation. Women with 11 (TTTA) repeats or with the Val/Val genotype lost more fat than women of other genotypes in univariate analyses. The two polymorphisms appear to act synergistically, so women ▨ with neither the *CYP19* $(TTTA)_{11}$ repeat or the *COMT* Val/Val polymorphisms had the least amount of fat loss, after adjusting for age, caloric intake, and amount of exercise. Women ■ with the *CYP19* $(TTTA)_{11}$ repeat or the *COMT* Val/Val polymorphism had an intermediate amount of fat loss, and women □ with both polymorphisms had the most fat loss. (Adapted from Toworoger, S.S. et al. *Obesity Res.*, 2004. 12(6):972–981.)

CONCLUSIONS

Obesity is a complex multifactorial disease believed to be the result of an interaction between genetic and environmental factors. Family studies suggest that 40 to 65% of the variation in obesity is due to genetic factors. However, it is clear that the recent environmental shift promoting high energy intake and low physical activity contributes to the development of obesity in genetically predisposed individuals. To better understand the genetic components of obesity, research in animal models and individuals with monogenic obesity has provided a fundamental understanding of the physiological pathways involved in regulating adipose tissue and energy intake and expenditure. Focus on polygenic obesity, which is responsible for >95% of obese individuals, has identified few common polymorphisms that modestly affect obesity and likely account for a very small portion of the total variance of human adiposity.

Thus, it is important to identify more obesity-related polymorphisms and to better determine how gene–gene interactions are involved in the development of obesity. It is also critical to understand how genetic variability affects the ability of overweight and obese patients to lose weight and fat mass when participating in diet and exercise protocols. Intervention studies that have collected biological specimens from participants will be an invaluable resource in this effort. It is clear that the complex relationships among genes, environment, and behavioral variables on obesity-related phenotypes complicate the identification of susceptibility genes and create an incredible challenge for scientists investigating the genetics of obesity. However, advances in bioinformatics, the completion of the Human Genome Project, the advent of laboratory high-throughput genotyping techniques, and the introduction of robust analytical tools will allow the search for the identification of genes involved in common human obesity to continue.

REFERENCES

1. Snyder, E.E. et al., The human obesity gene map: the 2003 update. *Obesity Res*, 2004. 12(3): 369–439.
2. Maes, H.H., M.C. Neale, and L.J. Eaves, Genetic and environmental factors in relative body weight and human adiposity. *Behav Genet*, 1997. 27(4): 325–351.
3. Bouchard, C., Genetics of human obesity: recent results from linkage studies. *J Nutr*, 1997. 127(9): 1887S–1890S.
4. Ravussin, E. and C. Bouchard, Human genomics and obesity: finding appropriate drug targets. *Eur J Pharmacol*, 2000. 410(2–3): 131–145.
5. Bouchard, C. et al., The genetics of human obesity, in *Handbook of Obesity*, G.A. Bray, C. Bouchard, and W.P.T. James, Eds. 1998, Marcel Dekker: New York. 157–190.
6. Fabsitz, R.R., P. Sholinsky, and D. Carmelli, Genetic influences on adult weight gain and maximum body mass index in male twins. *Am J Epidemiol*, 1994. 140(8): 711–720.
7. Austin, M.A. et al., Genetic influences on changes in body mass index: a longitudinal analysis of women twins. *Obesity Res*, 1997. 5(4): 326–331.
8. Nelson, T.L., et al., Genetic and environmental influences on waist-to-hip ratio and waist circumference in an older Swedish twin population. *Int J Obesity Relat Metab Disord*, 1999. 23(5): 449–455.
9. Nelson, T.L. et al., Genetic and environmental influences on body fat distribution, fasting insulin levels and CVD: are the influences shared? *Twin Res*, 2000. 3(1): 43–50.
10. Nelson, T.L. et al., Genetic and environmental influences on body-fat measures among African–American twins. *Obesity Res*, 2002. 10(8): 733–739.
11. Faith, M.S. et al., Evidence for independent genetic influences on fat mass and body mass index in a pediatric twin sample. *Pediatrics*, 1999. 104(1 Pt 1): 61–67.
12. Cardon, L.R. et al., Genetic and environmental correlations between obesity and body fat distribution in adult male twins. *Hum Biol*, 1994. 66(3): 465–79.
13. Neel, J.V., Diabetes mellitus: a "thrifty" genotype rendered detrimental by "progress"? *Am J Hum Genet*, 1962. 14: 353–362.
14. Sharma, A.M., The thrifty-genotype hypothesis and its implications for the study of complex genetic disorders in man. *J Mol Med*, 1998. 76(8): 568–571.
15. Loos, R.J. and C. Bouchard, Obesity — is it a genetic disorder? *J Intern Med*, 2003. 254(5): 401–425.
16. Barsh, G.S., I.S. Farooqi, and S. O'Rahilly, Genetics of body-weight regulation. *Nature*, 2000. 404(6778): 644–651.
17. Perusse, L. and C. Bouchard, Genotype-environment interaction in human obesity. *Nutr Rev*, 1999. 57(5 Pt 2): S31–37; discussion S37–368.
18. Bouchard, C. et al., The response to long-term overfeeding in identical twins. *N Engl J Med*, 1990. 322(21): 1477–1482.
19. Ukkola, O. and C. Bouchard, Clustering of metabolic abnormalities in obese individuals: the role of genetic factors. *Ann Med*, 2001. 33(2): 79–90.
20. Zhang, Y. et al., Positional cloning of the mouse obese gene and its human homologue. *Nature*, 1994. 372(6505): 425–432.
21. Tartaglia, L.A. et al., Identification and expression cloning of a leptin receptor, OB-R. *Cell*, 1995. 83(7): 1263–1271.
22. Phillips, M.S. et al., Leptin receptor missense mutation in the fatty Zucker rat. *Nat Genet*, 1996. 13(1): 18–19.
23. Montague, C.T. et al., Congenital leptin deficiency is associated with severe early-onset obesity in humans. *Nature*, 1997. 387(6636): 903–908.

24. Clement, K. et al., A mutation in the human leptin receptor gene causes obesity and pituitary dysfunction. *Nature*, 1998. 392(6674): 398–401.
25. Krude, H. et al., Severe early onset obesity, adrenal insufficiency and red hair pigmentation caused by POMC mutations in humans. *Nat Genet*, 1998. 19(2): 155–157.
26. Vaisse, C. et al., A frameshift mutation in human MC4R is associated with a dominant form of obesity. *Nat Genet*, 1998. 20(2): 113–114.
27. Jackson, R.S. et al., Obesity and impaired prohormone processing associated with mutations in the human prohormone convertase 1 gene. *Nat Genet*, 1997. 16(3): 303–306.
28. Damcott, C.M., P. Sack, and A.R. Shuldiner, The genetics of obesity. *Endocrinol Metab Clin North Am*, 2003. 32(4): 761–786.
29. Haines, J. and M. Pericak–Vance, *Approaches to Gene Mapping in Complex Human Diseases*. 1998, New York: Wiley–Liss.
30. Arner, P., Hunting for human obesity genes? Look in the adipose tissue! *Int J Obesity Relat Metab Disord*, 2000. 24 Suppl 4: S57–62.
31. Katzmarzyk, P.T., L. Perusse, and C. Bouchard, Genetics of abdominal visceral fat levels. *Am J Human Biol*, 1999. 11(2): 225–235.
32. Large, V. et al., Human beta-2 adrenoceptor gene polymorphisms are highly frequent in obesity and associate with altered adipocyte beta-2 adrenoceptor function. *J Clin Invest*, 1997. 100(12): 3005–3013.
33. Echwald, S.M. et al., Gln27Glu variant of the human beta2-adrenoreceptor gene is not associated with early onset obesity in Danish men. *Diabetes*, 1998. 47(10): 1657–1658.
34. Ishiyama–Shigemoto, S. et al., Association of polymorphisms in the beta2-adrenergic receptor gene with obesity, hypertriglyceridaemia, and diabetes mellitus. *Diabetologia*, 1999. 42(1): 98–101.
35. Rosmond, R., Association studies of genetic polymorphisms in central obesity: a critical review. *Int J Obesity Relat Metab Disord*, 2003. 27(10): 1141–1151.
36. Allison, D.B. et al., Meta-analysis of the association of the Trp64Arg polymorphism in the beta3 adrenergic receptor with body mass index. *Int J Obesity Relat Metab Disord*, 1998. 22(6): 559–566.
37. Fujisawa, T. et al., Meta-analysis of the association of Trp64Arg polymorphism of beta 3-adrenergic receptor gene with body mass index. *J Clin Endocrinol Metab*, 1998. 83(7): 2441–2444.
38. Kurokawa, N. et al., Association of BMI with the beta3-adrenergic receptor gene polymorphism in Japanese: meta-analysis. *Obesity Res*, 2001. 9(12): 741–745.
39. Arner, P. and J. Hoffstedt, Adrenoceptor genes in human obesity. *J Intern Med*, 1999. 245(6): 667–672.
40. Takezaki, T. et al., Association of polymorphisms in the beta-2 and beta-3 adrenoceptor genes with risk of colorectal cancer in Japanese. *Int J Clin Oncol*, 2001. 6(3): 117–122.
41. Gurnell, M., PPARgamma and metabolism: insights from the study of human genetic variants. *Clin Endocrinol* (Oxf), 2003. 59(3): 267–277.
42. Deeb, S.S. et al., A Pro12Ala substitution in PPARgamma2 associated with decreased receptor activity, lower body mass index and improved insulin sensitivity. *Nat Genet*, 1998. 20(3): 284–287.
43. Masud, S. and S. Ye, Effect of the peroxisome proliferator activated receptor-gamma gene Pro12Ala variant on body mass index: a meta-analysis. *J Med Genet*, 2003. 40(10): 773–780.
44. Altshuler, D. et al., The common PPARgamma Pro12Ala polymorphism is associated with decreased risk of type-2 diabetes. *Nat Genet*, 2000. 26(1): 76–80.
45. Fumeron, F. et al., Polymorphisms of uncoupling protein (UCP) and beta 3 adrenoreceptor genes in obese people submitted to a low calorie diet. *Int J Obesity Relat Metab Disord*, 1996. 20(12): 1051–1054.
46. Oppert, J.M. et al., DNA polymorphism in the uncoupling protein (UCP) gene and human body fat. *Int J Obesity Relat Metab Disord*, 1994. 18(8): 526–531.
47. Cassard–Doulcier, A.M. et al., The Bcl I polymorphism of the human uncoupling protein (ucp) gene is due to a point mutation in the 5′-flanking region. *Int J Obesity Relat Metab Disord*, 1996. 20(3): 278–279.
48. Chagnon, Y.C. et al., The human obesity gene map: the 2002 update. *Obesity Res*, 2003. 11(3): 313–367.
49. Kogure, A. et al., Synergic effect of polymorphisms in uncoupling protein 1 and beta3-adrenergic receptor genes on weight loss in obese Japanese. *Diabetologia*, 1998. 41(11): 1399.

50. Heilbronn, L.K. et al., Association of -3826 G variant in uncoupling protein-1 with increased BMI in overweight Australian women. *Diabetologia*, 2000. 43(2): 242–244.
51. Ukkola, O. et al., Genetic variation at the uncoupling protein 1, 2 and 3 loci and the response to long-term overfeeding. *Eur J Clin Nutr*, 2001. 55(11): 1008–1015.
52. Herrmann, S.M. et al., Polymorphisms of the tumor necrosis factor-alpha gene, coronary heart disease and obesity. *Eur J Clin Invest*, 1998. 28(1): 59–66.
53. Schaffler, A. et al., Frequency and significance of the A→G (–3826) polymorphism in the promoter of the gene for uncoupling protein-1 with regard to metabolic parameters and adipocyte transcription factor binding in a large population-based Caucasian cohort. *Eur J Clin Invest*, 1999. 29(9): 770–779.
54. Holm, C. et al., Molecular mechanisms regulating hormone-sensitive lipase and lipolysis. *Annu Rev Nutr*, 2000. 20: 365–393.
55. Hoffstedt, J. et al., A common hormone-sensitive lipase i6 gene polymorphism is associated with decreased human adipocyte lipolytic function. *Diabetes*, 2001. 50(10): 2410–2413.
56. Arner, P., Genetic variance and lipolysis regulation: implications for obesity. *Ann Med*, 2001. 33(8): 542–546.
57. Magre, J. et al., Human hormone-sensitive lipase: genetic mapping, identification of a new dinucleotide repeat, and association with obesity and NIDDM. *Diabetes*, 1998. 47(2): 284–286.
58. Klannemark, M. et al., The putative role of the hormone-sensitive lipase gene in the pathogenesis of Type II diabetes mellitus and abdominal obesity. *Diabetologia*, 1998. 41(12): 1516–1522.
59. Lavebratt, C. et al., The hormone-sensitive lipase i6 gene polymorphism and body fat accumulation. *Eur J Clin Invest*, 2002. 32(12): 938–942.
60. Hotamisligil, G.S., Mechanisms of TNF-alpha-induced insulin resistance. *Exp Clin Endocrinol Diabetes*, 1999. 107(2): 119–125.
61. Gasic, S., B. Tian, and A. Green, Tumor necrosis factor alpha stimulates lipolysis in adipocytes by decreasing Gi protein concentrations. *J Biol Chem*, 1999. 274(10): 6770–6775.
62. Hotamisligil, G.S. et al., Increased adipose tissue expression of tumor necrosis factor-alpha in human obesity and insulin resistance. *J Clin Invest*, 1995. 95(5): 2409–2415.
63. Wilson, A.G. et al., Effects of a polymorphism in the human tumor necrosis factor alpha promoter on transcriptional activation. *Proc Natl Acad Sci USA*, 1997. 94(7): 3195–3199.
64. Fernandez–Real, J.M. et al., The TNF-alpha gene Nco I polymorphism influences the relationship among insulin resistance, percent body fat, and increased serum leptin levels. *Diabetes*, 1997. 46(9): 1468–1472.
65. Corbalan, M.S. et al., Influence of two polymorphisms of the tumoral necrosis factor-alpha gene on the obesity phenotype. *Diabetes Nutr Metab*, 2004. 17(1): 17–22.
66. Romeo, S. et al., The G-308A variant of the tumor necrosis factor-alpha (TNF-alpha) gene is not associated with obesity, insulin resistance and body fat distribution. *BMC Med Genet*, 2001. 2(1): 10.
67. Walston, J. et al., Tumor necrosis factor-alpha-238 and -308 polymorphisms do not associate with traits related to obesity and insulin resistance. *Diabetes*, 1999. 48(10): 2096–2098.
68. Brand, E. et al., Tumor necrosis factor-alpha–308 G/A polymorphism in obese Caucasians. *Int J Obesity Relat Metab Disord*, 2001. 25(4): 581–585.
69. Pihlajamaki, J. et al., The effect of the –308A allele of the TNF-alpha gene on insulin action is dependent on obesity. *Obesity Res*, 2003. 11(7): 912–917.
70. Jequier, E., Leptin signaling, adiposity, and energy balance. *Ann N Y Acad Sci*, 2002. 967: 379–388.
71. Heo, M. et al., A meta-analytic investigation of linkage and association of common leptin receptor (LEPR) polymorphisms with body mass index and waist circumference. *Int J Obesity Relat Metab Disord*, 2002. 26(5): 640–646.
72. Skibola, C.F. et al., Body mass index, leptin and leptin receptor polymorphisms, and non-Hodgkin's lymphoma. *Cancer Epidemiol Biomarkers Prev*, 2004. 13(5): 779–786.
73. Comuzzie, A.G. et al., Searching for genes underlying normal variation in human adiposity. *J Mol Med*, 2001. 79(1): 57–70.
74. Valve, R. et al., Synergistic effect of polymorphisms in uncoupling protein 1 and beta3-adrenergic receptor genes on basal metabolic rate in obese Finns. *Diabetologia*, 1998. 41(3): 357–361.
75. Clement, K. et al., Additive effect of A→G (–3826) variant of the uncoupling protein gene and the Trp64Arg mutation of the beta 3-adrenergic receptor gene on weight gain in morbid obesity. *Int J Obesity Relat Metab Disord*, 1996. 20(12): 1062–1066.

76. Fogelholm, M. et al., Additive effects of the mutations in the beta3-adrenergic receptor and uncoupling protein-1 genes on weight loss and weight maintenance in Finnish women. *J Clin Endocrinol Metab*, 1998. 83(12): 4246–4250.
77. Hsueh, W.C. et al., Interactions between variants in the beta3-adrenergic receptor and peroxisome proliferator-activated receptor-gamma2 genes and obesity. *Diabetes Care*, 2001. 24(4): 672–677.
78. Bouchard, C. et al., The response to exercise with constant energy intake in identical twins. *Obesity Res*, 1994. 2: 400–410.
79. Perusse, L. et al., Familial aggregation of amount and distribution of subcutaneous fat and their responses to exercise training in the HERITAGE family study. *Obesity Res*, 2000. 8(2): 140–150.
80. Robitaille, J. et al., The PPAR-gamma P12A polymorphism modulates the relationship between dietary fat intake and components of the metabolic syndrome: results from the Quebec Family Study. *Clin Genet*, 2003. 63(2): 109–116.
81. Luan, J. et al., Evidence for gene–nutrient interaction at the PPARgamma locus. *Diabetes*, 2001. 50(3): 686–689.
82. Franks, P.W. et al., Does peroxisome proliferator-activated receptor gamma genotype (Pro12ala) modify the association of physical activity and dietary fat with fasting insulin level? *Metabolism*, 2004. 53(1): 11–16.
83. Kahara, T. et al., PPARgamma gene polymorphism is associated with exercise-mediated changes of insulin resistance in healthy men. *Metabolism*, 2003. 52(2): 209–212.
84. Nicklas, B.J. et al., Genetic variation in the peroxisome proliferator-activated receptor-gamma2 gene (Pro12Ala) affects metabolic responses to weight loss and subsequent weight regain. *Diabetes*, 2001. 50(9): 2172–2176.
85. Lindi, V.I. et al., Association of the Pro12Ala polymorphism in the PPAR-gamma2 gene with 3-year incidence of type 2 diabetes and body weight change in the Finnish Diabetes Prevention Study. *Diabetes*, 2002. 51(8): 2581–2586.
86. Memisoglu, A. et al., Interaction between a peroxisome proliferator-activated receptor gamma gene polymorphism and dietary fat intake in relation to body mass. *Hum Mol Genet*, 2003. 12(22): 2923–2929.
87. Benecke, H. et al., A study on the genetics of obesity: influence of polymorphisms of the beta-3-adrenergic receptor and insulin receptor substrate 1 in relation to weight loss, waist to hip ratio and frequencies of common cardiovascular risk factors. *Exp Clin Endocrinol Diabetes*, 2000. 108(2): 86–92.
88. Garenc, C. et al., The Trp64Arg polymorphism of the beta3-adrenergic receptor gene is not associated with training-induced changes in body composition: The HERITAGE Family Study. *Obesity Res*, 2001. 9(6): 337–341.
89. Shiwaku, K. et al., Difficulty in losing weight by behavioral intervention for women with Trp64Arg polymorphism of the beta3-adrenergic receptor gene. *Int J Obesity Relat Metab Disord*, 2003. 27(9): 1028–1036.
90. Xinli, W. et al., Association of a mutation in the beta3-adrenergic receptor gene with obesity and response to dietary intervention in Chinese children. *Acta Paediatr*, 2001. 90(11): 1233–1237.
91. Phares, D.A. et al., Association between body fat response to exercise training and multilocus ADR genotypes. *Obesity Res*, 2004. 12(5): 807–815.
92. Rawson, E.S. et al., No effect of the Trp64Arg beta(3)-adrenoceptor gene variant on weight loss, body composition, or energy expenditure in obese, Caucasian postmenopausal women. *Metabolism*, 2002. 51(6): 801–805.
93. Tworoger, S.S. et al., The effect of CYP19 and COMT polymorphisms on exercise-induced fat loss in postmenopausal women. *Obesity Res*, 2004. 12(6): 972–981.

Section VI

Physical Activity and Cancer Prognosis

24 Quality of Life and Fatigue in Breast Cancer

Kerri Winters-Stone and Anna L. Schwartz

CONTENTS

Breast cancer is the second leading cause of cancer death for all women (after lung cancer) and the leading overall cause of cancer death in women between the ages of 40 and 59; the incidence of breast cancer is increasing. Fortunately, due to advances in treatment, women with early stage breast cancer have a high remission rate and even those with more aggressive disease may be afforded many additional years of life. Virtually all breast cancer patients undergo surgery and most receive some form or combination of adjuvant therapy, including radiation, chemotherapy, and/or hormone therapy.

Surgery and adjuvant treatments are associated with side effects that may have a significant impact on a survivor's quality of life (QOL) during treatment, although recent research indicates that QOL declines may persist into survivorship. A recent follow-up study on health-related QOL in breast cancer survivors reported that women treated with previous adjuvant therapy had a poorer QOL at an average of 6.3 years postdiagnosis compared to women who were not treated with adjuvant therapy [1]. In particular, past chemotherapy was a significant predictor of poorer current QOL. Thus, strategies that maintain or improve QOL from diagnosis into survivorship are important elements of the medical management and lifestyle of women with breast cancer.

QOL MEASUREMENT IN CANCER

Quality of life is a multidimensional concept that is described and assessed in many ways. Recommendations for QOL assessment in cancer clinical trials include physical, emotional, social, and self-perceptions of functioning [2–4]. In most settings, QOL is measured qualitatively through self-report, most often using one of any number of standardized instruments. Several cancer-specific QOL surveys have been developed and are useful when assessing the impact of issues unique to the cancer experience (e.g., diagnosis of a life-threatening illness and treatment), but may in turn omit more generalized QOL issues to minimize survey length and participant burden. Most QOL instruments attempt to assess the impact of disease and treatment on distinct, yet overlapping, domains of function including: physical, role, emotional and social, as well as a sum or weighted sum of these domains to yield a general QOL index. Because QOL is multidimensional and qualitative, and instruments are somewhat variable, reaching a conclusive evaluation of any strategy aimed at improving QOL, including exercise, can be rather challenging.

Including objective and quantifiable measures that may underpin the self-report QOL domains could aid in the evaluation of intervention strategies and could also lend insight as to the mechanism by which the intervention has its effect. Numerous studies have reported on QOL and associated changes in women with breast cancer during as well as following treatment. For the purposes of this chapter, when evaluating the efficacy of exercise to maintain or improve QOL during and after breast cancer treatment, descriptions of outcomes on self-report QOL and outcomes likely associated with QOL (i.e., anxiety, depression, body weight, functional ability) will be included.

EFFECT OF BREAST CANCER AND TREATMENT ON QOL

A breast cancer diagnosis can have obvious consequences on psychosocial aspects of QOL. Psychosocial domains of QOL affected by breast cancer and treatment include anxiety, depression, hostility, cognition, reduced social functioning, and body image concerns [5–8]. Treatment further affects psychosocial and physical aspects of QOL, regardless of the treatment regimen [9]. However, the magnitude and domains of QOL affected vary by treatment type and the accompanying side effects [10].

Surgical side effects often resolve during recovery, though scar tissue and persistent lymphedema can impair upper extremity function on the treated side and psychosocial concerns from mastectomy can persist beyond recovery [9]. Radiation side effects include fatigue, skin changes, lung fibrosis, and nausea. Side effects of chemotherapy tend to be more numerous and debilitating and include fatigue, nausea, vomiting, hair loss, weakness, cardiovascular declines, cognitive impairment, peripheral neuropathy, pain, diarrhea, insomnia, and ovarian failure in premenopausal patients that lead to consequences from abrupt estrogen depletion (e.g., early bone loss, hot flashes). Hormonal therapy with tamoxifen or anastrazole has notable side effects, including fatigue, hot flashes, night sweats, musculoskeletal pain/stiffness, vision changes, cognitive changes, and mood disorders depending on the medication. Side effects may contribute to the reduced physical domains of QOL reported by women treated for breast cancer, particularly those on adjuvant therapy [1,10,11].

The impact of breast cancer on certain domains of QOL may persist beyond the immediate post-treatment period and into survivorship. Prospective studies following women circa diagnosis through treatment and beyond indicate a persistent decline in domains of QOL up to 6.3 years postdiagnosis [9,12,13]. Specifically, using data from the Nurses' Health Study, Michael et al [13]. reported a higher risk of decline in functional health status among women with a breast cancer diagnosis compared to women never diagnosed with breast cancer, though the risks of decline decreased with time since diagnosis. Similarly, a long-term follow-up of women 3 to 6.3 years postdiagnosis reported a persistently lower self-report physical function compared to the general population and a higher risk of decline in physical function during survivorship in women who had a mastectomy and/or were treated with systemic adjuvant therapy, particularly chemotherapy [8,9]. Psychosocial QOL domains were similar between survivors and cancer-free controls.

The impact of breast cancer diagnosis and treatment on QOL may be most pronounced among women who are less healthy at diagnosis or have less social support. In general, younger and older women who have poorer mental and physical health at baseline tend to have poorer psychosocial and functional health into recovery [5,14,15]. Furthermore, women who are more socially isolated at diagnosis tend to be at a threefold greater risk of decline in social functioning after treatment

[13] and less social support at diagnosis is an independent predictor of lower long-term global QOL [1].

CANCER TREATMENT-RELATED FATIGUE

Fatigue is a significant problem in cancer care worth further description because it is a common side effect of all postsurgical treatments. Most cancer patients report fatigue during and after chemotherapy, radiotherapy, and hormonal therapy; some cite it as a reason for prematurely ending treatment [4,16–18]. Studies of breast cancer patients who have completed cancer treatment suggest that persistent fatigue negatively affects quality of life [18–20]. A comparison of fatigue experienced by women with breast cancer at least 1 year following the completion of treatment noted that patients who received adjuvant chemotherapy or bone marrow transplant experienced significantly greater fatigue than subjects who received only radiotherapy [19]. In a study of exercise in breast cancer patients receiving chemotherapy, a strong inverse relationship was observed between fatigue and QOL [21].

This cycle of fatigue with the related loss of self-esteem and inability to perform activities of daily living or maintain social relationships and employment may have a profound effect on patients' quality of life [20]. The relationship among the negative outcomes of fatigue and quality of life in women with breast cancer is clear. Strategies that reduce fatigue in the short and long term may have profound effects on quality of life.

HOW EXERCISE MAY IMPROVE QOL AND REDUCE FATIGUE IN BREAST CANCER

Exercise, in most cases, is a neglected area of the treatment plan for cancer patients. Most health care providers fail to advise patients about exercise and the benefits that can be gained from it [22], though evidence on physical activity benefits is accumulating and becoming recognized by the oncology community [23]. Inactivity may be the trigger for the marked fatigue, weakness, and declines in functional ability and quality of life experienced by cancer patients and survivors. Exercise improves physical condition and mood state in healthy people and those with a variety of physical diseases such as cardiovascular, metabolic, and rheumatic diseases [24]. Exercise may serve a restorative function and contribute to decreased attentional fatigue by shifting attention from the mundane tasks of daily life to a period of exercise, which stimulates neuromuscular function and produces hemodynamic changes [22], or it may simply reduce depression and anxiety [25]. Exercise in a group setting may also reduce social isolation — a reported risk factor for QOL decline in women with breast cancer [1,13]. Thus, physical and psychological benefits from exercise have the potential to reduce fatigue and improve functional status and QOL in women with breast cancer.

EVIDENCE FOR EXERCISE EFFECTS ON QOL AND FATIGUE IN BREAST CANCER

CROSS-SECTIONAL STUDIES

Due to greater feasibility, cross-sectional reports enjoy larger sample sizes. However, they are limited in the ability to establish cause and effect and most often rely on self-report activity, symptoms, and QOL. Despite these limitations, cross-sectional research can typically survey a broader demographic of the population and can generate hypotheses regarding the benefits of exercise.

Cross-sectional studies on breast cancer survivors using surveys and/or one-time physical assessments generally agree that exercise has a positive impact on the lives of breast cancer survivors during treatment. A retrospective survey of 71 early breast cancer survivors found that women who exercised throughout their treatment reported an increased quality of life [26]. A secondary analysis of data from a survey of physically active cancer patients to identify the most common symptoms experienced by women with breast cancer revealed that 45% of the sample returned to exercise within 24 hours after treatment, with no reported adverse effects [27]. The most frequently cited treatment-related symptoms improved with exercise were fatigue, general weakness, nausea, depression, and muscular weakness. A survey of 219 athletic cancer survivors' activity patterns demonstrated that patients with all types of cancer continue to exercise during treatment, albeit with reductions in the intensity and duration [22].

The majority of cross-sectional surveys of activity and QOL in breast cancer survivors are in those who completed treatment; most lend additional support for exercise benefits. Six of eight reports of post-treatment exercise participation detected significant differences in QOL and fatigue between survivors who exercised and those who did not. Sample sizes in these studies ranged from 54 to 119 and surveyed women undergoing various treatments. Exercisers reported better self-esteem [28], vigor [29,30], coping behavior [29], physical competence [28], body image [30,31], and general quality of life [26] and less confusion, distress, fatigue, depression, and mood disturbances [29–31] compared to nonexercising peers.

Only two of eight studies showed no differences between exercising and nonexercising survivors on measures of locus of control and psychosocial adjustment to cancer in 500 women who received various treatments and in 54 women treated with surgery only [32]. It should be noted that neither of these studies surveyed physical QOL domains or fatigue and thus they do not necessarily refute the positive effects cited in other reports.

Overall, cross-sectional surveys report a positive association among exercise, QOL and related psychosocial and physical factors, and fatigue. These studies cannot establish causality and include no objective measures of exercise or fitness. However, the consistency of findings generates sufficient reason to believe that exercise is feasible and beneficial for women with breast cancer during and following treatment and lends strong rationale for exercise intervention.

Quasiexperimental Studies

Quasiexperimental one-group pre–post test and observational exercise studies provide stronger evidence for exercise benefits, but are less generalizable and methodologically rigorous than randomized controlled trials. A limited number of studies have been conducted in women during and after treatment completion. In a study of exercise in breast cancer patients receiving chemotherapy, all women were prescribed an 8-week program of home-based, self-paced aerobic (mainly walking) exercise. In this study, subjects who adopted the exercise program experienced less fatigue and a higher quality of life (increased functional ability, reduced frequency and intensity of side effects, and improved positive and negative affect) [33–35].

Regression analyses showed that reductions in fatigue most likely mediated the positive effect of exercise on QOL [21]. Moreover, women who exercised longer experienced greater reductions in fatigue and the fatigue-reducing effect of exercise persisted for the next 24 hours, suggesting dose–response and carry-over effects of exercise on fatigue [36]. A 16-week structured, supervised, multimodal exercise program (aerobic + strength + flexibility exercise) also improved fitness (aerobic capacity, strength, flexibility) and QOL (increased positive affect, well-being and function, decreased distress) among 45 women treated for primary breast cancer [37].

Studies in breast cancer survivors post-treatment are mixed, but are also less methodologically rigorous because half observed exercise responses to intact community-based or self-reported exercise vs. an experimental program. Pinto et al. [38] followed exercise levels over 12 months in 69 women who had recently completed treatment for early stage breast cancer. Though average exercise participation did not change over time and was below recommended levels for health, exercising was associated with improved physical function. Exercise was not associated with overall mood or cancer-related symptoms.

Twenty breast cancer survivors who volunteered to train for dragon-boat racing were followed over a 6-month period that included 2 months of aerobic and upper body strength training followed by 4 months of competition. Only lymphedema was monitored and was neither exacerbated nor improved by exercise [39]. A small study of ten breast cancer survivors participating in an 8-week multimodal, low–moderate-intensity program reported a trend toward fatigue reduction and improved quality of life and no effect on lymphedema [38]. Peters et al. [40] reported improved satisfaction with life among 24 early breast cancer survivors participating in a 7-month program that was initially supervised (first 5 weeks) then turned to self-directed, moderate-intensity cycle ergometry.

Quasiexperimental and observation studies of exercise in breast cancer lend modest support for exercise benefits on QOL improvement and fatigue reduction. Studies in women undergoing active treatment reported positive effects on QOL and fatigue. Post-treatment studies struggled to find a significant effect of exercise on QOL [38,40] and fatigue [39], but were generally of limited design. Randomized controlled trials will provide the strongest evidence for exercise benefits.

Randomized Controlled Trials

True randomized controlled trials (RCTs) are more challenging to execute, but provide the strongest evidence for exercise benefits. Several exercise RCTs have been conducted in breast cancer survivors in active treatment or post-treatment.

Randomized controlled exercise trials have been conducted in women undergoing active treatment with radiation or chemotherapy. Only one study focused strictly on women with early stage breast cancer receiving radiation therapy [41]. Subjects randomized to the 6-week home-based, self-paced walking program experienced fewer and less intense symptoms, less fatigue, and improved functional ability measured by 12-minute walk. The same research group attempted a similar RCT in women undergoing active chemo- or radiation therapy, but had some problems with exercise compliance and contamination when 50% of the control group self-initiated walking exercise [42]. Participants were recategorized as walkers or nonwalkers and data reanalyzed. Women who walked reported less fatigue, less decline in physical function, and increased functional ability, quality of life, vigor, and mood.

Most RCTs in actively treated women were in those undergoing chemotherapy for early stage disease. Two of the first studies examined the effects of supervised moderate-intensity cycle ergometry exercise. MacVicar and colleagues [43] demonstrated a 40% increase in functional capacity among women with stage II breast cancer receiving chemotherapy without steroids. No such changes were observed in the control or placebo (stretching) groups. Exercising subjects increased their exercise time and intensity, demonstrating a training effect that may improve patients' QOL and ability for self-care. In a separate report, the same exercise program was found to attenuate weight gain and body fat increases compared to inactive controls [44].

These studies were among the first to demonstrate the safety and feasibility of an ambitious exercise intervention in women with breast cancer receiving chemotherapy. Later, Mock and colleagues [45] combined a home-based, self-paced walking program and support group intervention for women with breast cancer. Subjects in the intervention group reported increased exercise time, less fatigue, less nausea, less depression, and lower emotional distress than subjects in the control group. However, it is impossible to determine which intervention affected specific outcomes.

Perhaps the most ambitious study to date in actively treated women was conducted by Segal and colleagues [46], who studied the effects of 26 weeks of walking exercise on QOL and aerobic capacity in 124 women treated with radiation or chemotherapy for early stage disease. Women were randomly assigned to a usual care group or to one of two exercise groups that performed the same low–moderate intensity walking program in a supervised or self-directed (i.e., at home, in community) setting. Women in the self-directed group reported improved physical function compared to declines reported by the usual care group. The supervised exercise group reported a slight increase in physical function that was not significantly different from controls.

The authors speculate that chemotherapy may have moderated the failure of the supervised group to improve because separate group comparisons among women not on chemotherapy showed trends for an exercise effect in supervised participants. Exercise did not affect other QOL domains or aerobic capacity in self-directed or supervised groups, suggesting that improved physical function may occur in the absence of measurable fitness improvements. This study was the largest RCT thus far; it suggests that home-based exercise has a beneficial effect on QOL in women undergoing treatment and that chemotherapy may moderate the effectiveness of group exercise.

A similar number of RCTs have been conducted in women who were, on average, 3 years post-treatment completion, usually on small samples. A cross-over design to test the effects of 10 weeks of supervised moderate-intensity aerobic exercise on psychological factors in breast cancer survivors ($N = 24$) found that exercise significantly reduced depression and anxiety but not self-esteem [25]. Similarly, breast cancer survivors ($n = 24$) randomly assigned to a 12-week supervised aerobic exercise program reported improved body image and less emotional distress compared to wait-list controls [31,47].

McKenzie et al. [47] conducted a small RCT in women with early stage disease and post-treatment lymphedema ($n = 14$). Women performed upper extremity light-intensity resistance and arm ergometry exercise for 8 weeks. No changes in arm volume or circumference occurred, indicating neither a positive or negative effect of exercise on lymphedema. Exercisers reported improved physical function, general health, and vitality compared to decreases reported by controls, but group differences were not statistically different. A small study that focused on physical performance and immune cell function reported that 8 weeks of supervised aerobic plus resistance exercise modestly improved aerobic performance and leg strength, but had no effect on immune factors. Improvements in physical performance are likely to improve physical functioning, though this was not specifically investigated.

To date, the largest exercise trial in long-term survivors was conducted in 53 postmenopausal women who completed treatment for early stage disease; some were on hormone therapy [48]. Women were randomly assigned to usual care or supervised moderate-intensity cycle ergometry exercise three times/week for 15 weeks. Exercisers significantly improved their aerobic capacity, quality of life, happiness, self-esteem, and physical well-being, and lowered fatigue compared to usual care. Body weight and body composition were unaffected.

Results from RCTs provide promising evidence for the feasibility and beneficial effects of exercise in women currently treated or who have completed treatment for breast cancer. Importantly, these trials have established that exercise, even of moderate intensity, is tolerable during treatment and can attenuate treatment-related symptoms, particularly fatigue, physical changes, and QOL declines. Though sample sizes tended to be small, significant effects of exercise were detected. A handful of studies in women who completed treatment suggest that exercise is beneficial into survivorship. Because physical function may not fully recover following treatment [1,13], it is important to establish that long-term survivors can improve physical functioning and physical performance well after their treatment has ended — perhaps to prediagnosis levels, though this hypothesis has not been specifically studied.

SUMMARY

In general, exercise studies of varying design support the hypothesis that exercise can improve quality of life and associated physical and psychosocial factors and can lower fatigue. Cross-sectional and quasiexperimental studies are mostly in support of this hypothesis, although a few, limited studies failed to establish a positive effect of exercise training. Randomized controlled trials are relatively few in number and are difficult to compare due to differences in exercise protocols and samples. However, all showed some evidence for exercise benefits and, importantly, these studies determined that exercise is feasible for and acceptable by most women during and after treatment and that women in active treatment for breast cancer can adapt to exercise similarly to the general population.

The ability to improve functional ability and quality of life of women during and after treatment has tremendous personal and societal impact. Women are surviving breast cancer in record numbers, in part due to more aggressive treatment that can compromise QOL. As discussed, exercise is a low-cost, broadly effective approach that can maintain or improve QOL for women during treatment and for those likely to lead many productive years post-treatment. Furthermore, the utility of exercise may even prove to have economic implications in that patients who maintain function may be able to continue to work and may remain functionally independent longer than their counterparts who may be experiencing more limits in functional ability due to conditions associated with inactivity and disuse.

Limitations of the current research are important to mention. Relatively few RCTs were conducted and most were on relatively small samples. Despite the small sample sizes, significant benefits of exercise were detected, though the largest trial in actively treated women failed to detect a significant benefit of exercise in women participating in a supervised program compared to self-directed (i.e. home based) exercise. In contrast, most studies of home-based or supervised programs suggest either setting can be effective. Most interventions were of limited duration, so long-term effectiveness of exercise training on QOL and fatigue in breast cancer survivors is unknown.

Currently, a specific exercise prescription for improving QOL and reducing fatigue in breast cancer survivors cannot be derived from this literature. Most studies followed the general recommendations for reducing mortality and morbidity from chronic disease for 30 minutes of moderate-intensity activity most days of the week and used aerobic exercise as the sole or central mode of exercise [49]; they show that this public health prescription benefits women with breast cancer. However, it is not clear what minimal or optimal effective dose of exercise significantly improves QOL and reduces fatigue.

FUTURE DIRECTIONS

The current literature on exercise effects on QOL and fatigue in breast cancer survivors is promising and has generated exciting avenues for further study. Future studies need to be of longer duration, or participants who continue to exercise after trials are completed should be followed so that it can be determined whether women will adhere to exercise long term. Because exercise benefits are known to reverse when training is discontinued [50,51], the types of programs and approaches that promote long-term adherence must be explored. Likewise, because the most feasible setting to promote long-term adherence may be community or home-based programs [52], further and more rigorous study of these settings is warranted.

Additionally, the minimal or optimal effective exercise prescription cannot be determined from current studies. None compared varying doses of exercise intensity (low vs. moderate vs. high), time (short vs. long) or frequency (< 3 vs. > 3 days/week) or compared different modes of activity (i.e., aerobic vs. resistance). Only direct comparisons within a particular sample can determine the minimum amount of exercise necessary to produce significant benefits, whether more exercise produces greater benefits, and whether different modes of exercise are equally effective or have specific benefits.

It is also important to attempt to address the mechanisms through which exercise affects QOL and fatigue. One study suggests that physical fitness improvements may not underpin QOL and symptom improvement [46]. Because women more socially isolated and in poorer health at diagnosis are more likely to experience declines in QOL and physical health through treatment and beyond and are less likely to exercise, it would also behoove the research community to develop interventions that could be employed in these populations and later implemented in the community. The current research has led to recommendations to include exercise as part of the long-term treatment plan for breast cancer patients [53]. Excitingly, important work is yet to be done in order to develop effective exercise prescriptions and programs sustainable long term and accessible by all.

REFERENCES

1. Ganz PA, Desmond KA, Leedham B, Rowland JH, Meyerowitz BE, Belin TR 2002 Quality of life in long-term, disease-free survivors of breast cancer: a follow-up study. *J Natl Cancer Inst* 94(1):39–49.
2. Rejeski WJ, Brawley LR, Shumaker SA 1996 Physical activity and health-related quality of life. *Exercise Sport Sci Rev* 24:71–108.
3. Nayfield SG, Ganz PA, Moinpour CM, Cella DF, Hailey BJ 1992 Report from a National Cancer Institute (USA) workshop on quality of life assessment in cancer clinical trials. *Qual Life Res* 1(3):203–210.
4. King CR, Haberman M, Berry DL, Bush N, Butler L, Dow KH, Ferrell B, Grant M, Gue D, Hinds P, Kreuer J, Padilla G, Underwood S 1997 Quality of life and the cancer experience: the state of the knowledge. *Oncol Nursing Forum* 24(1):27–41.
5. Ganz PA, Guadagnoli E, Landrum MB, Lash TL, Rakowski W, Silliman RA 2003 Breast cancer in older women: quality of life and psychosocial adjustment in the 15 months after diagnosis. *J Clin Oncol* 21(21):4027–4033.
6. Ganz PA, Coscarelli A, Fred C, Kahn B, Polinsky ML, Petersen L 1996 Breast cancer survivors: psychosocial concerns and quality of life. *Breast Cancer Res Treat* 38(2):183–199.
7. Ganz PA, Hirji K, Sim MS, Schag CA, Fred C, Polinsky ML 1993 Predicting psychosocial risk in patients with breast cancer. *Med Care* 31(5):419–431.
8. Ganz PA, Schag AC, Lee JJ, Polinsky ML, Tan SJ 1992 Breast conservation vs. mastectomy. Is there a difference in psychological adjustment or quality of life in the year after surgery? *Cancer* 69(7):1729–1738.
9. Ganz PA, Kwan L, Stanton AL, Krupnick JL, Rowland JH, Meyerowitz BE, Bower JE, Belin TR 2004 Quality of life at the end of primary treatment of breast cancer: first results from the moving beyond cancer randomized trial. *J Natl Cancer Inst* 96(5):376–387.
10. Ganz PA, Rowland JH, Meyerowitz BE, Desmond KA 1998 Impact of different adjuvant therapy strategies on quality of life in breast cancer survivors. *Recent Results Cancer Res* 152:396–411.
11. Ganz PA 2001 Impact of tamoxifen adjuvant therapy on symptoms, functioning, and quality of life. *J Natl Cancer Inst Monogr* (30):130–134.
12. Ganz PA 2001 Menopause and breast cancer: symptoms, late effects, and their management. *Semin Oncol* 28(3):274–283.
13. Michael YL, Kawachi I, Berkman LF, Holmes MD, Colditz GA 2000 The persistent impact of breast carcinoma on functional health status: prospective evidence from the Nurses' Health Study. *Cancer* 89(11):2176–2186.
14. Ganz PA, Greendale GA, Petersen L, Kahn B, Bower JE 2003 Breast cancer in younger women: reproductive and late health effects of treatment. *J Clin Oncol* 21(22):4184–4193.
15. McBride CM, Clipp E, Peterson BL, Lipkus IM, Demark–Wahnefried W 2000 Psychological impact of diagnosis and risk reduction among cancer survivors. *Psychooncology* 9(5):418–427.
16. Blesch KS, Paice JA, Wickham R, Harte N, Schnoor DK, Purl S, Rehwalt M, Kopp PL, Manson S, Coveny SB, et al. 1991 Correlates of fatigue in people with breast or lung cancer. *Oncol Nursing Forum* 18(1):81–87.
17. Winningham ML, Nail LM, Burke MB, Brophy L, Cimprich B, Jones LS, Pickard–Holley S, Rhodes V, St Pierre B, Beck S, et al. 1994 Fatigue and the cancer experience: the state of the knowledge. *Oncol Nursing Forum* 21(1):23–36.
18. Curt GA, Breitbart W, Cella D, Groopman JE, Horning SJ, Itri LM, Johnson DH, Miaskowski C, Scherr SL, Portenoy RK, Vogelzang NJ 2000 Impact of cancer-related fatigue on the lives of patients: new findings from the Fatigue Coalition. *Oncologist* 5(5):353–360.

19. Respini D, Jacobsen PB, Thors C, Tralongo P, Balducci L 2003 The prevalence and correlates of fatigue in older cancer patients. *Crit Rev Oncol Hematol* 47(3):273–279.
20. Jacobsen PB, Stein K 1999 Is fatigue a long-term side effect of breast cancer treatment? *Cancer Causes Control* 6(3):256–263.
21. Schwartz AL 1999 Fatigue mediates the effects of exercise on quality of life. *Qual Life Res* 8(6):529–538.
22. Schwartz AL 1998 Patterns of exercise and fatigue in physically active cancer survivors. *Oncol Nursing Forum* 25(3):485–491.
23. Brown JK, Byers T, Doyle C, Coumeya KS, Demark–Wahnefried W, Kushi LH, McTieman A, Rock CL, Aziz N, Bloch AS, Eldridge B, Hamilton K, Katzin C, Koonce A, Main J, Mobley C, Morra ME, Pierce MS, Sawyer KA 2003 Nutrition and physical activity during and after cancer treatment: an American Cancer Society guide for informed choices. *Calif Cancer J Clin* 53(5):268–291.
24. Durstine JL, Painter P, Franklin BA, Morgan D, Pitetti KH, Roberts SO 2000 Physical activity for the chronically ill and disabled. *Sports Med* 30(3):207–219.
25. Segar ML, Katch VL, Roth RS, Garcia AW, Portner TI, Glickman SG, Haslanger S, Wilkins EG 1998 The effect of aerobic exercise on self-esteem and depressive and anxiety symptoms among breast cancer survivors. *Oncol Nursing Forum* 25(1):107–113.
26. Young–McCaughan S, Sexton DL 1991 A retrospective investigation of the relationship between aerobic exercise and quality of life in women with breast cancer. *Oncol Nursing Forum* 18(4):751–757.
27. Schwartz AL, Winningham ML 1995 Problems related to exercise reported by athletic breast cancer survivors. *Oncol Nursing Forum* 22:351.
28. Baldwin M, Courneya KS 1997 Exercise and self-esteem in breast cancer survivors: an application of the exercise and self-esteem model. *J Sport Exercise Psychol* 19:347–359.
29. Pinto BM, Maruyama NC 1998 Exercise in the rehabilitation of breast cancer survivors. *Psychooncology* 8:191–206.
30. Pinto BM, Trunzo JJ 2004 Body esteem and mood among sedentary and active breast cancer survivors. *Mayo Clin Proc* 79(2):181–186.
31. Pinto BM, Clark MM, Maruyama NC, Feder SI 2003 Psychological and fitness changes associated with exercise participation among women with breast cancer. *Psychooncology* 12(2):118–126.
32. Bremer BA, Moore CT, Bourbon BM, Hess DR, Bremer KL 1997 Perceptions of control, physical exercise, and psychological adjustment to breast cancer in South African women. *Ann Behav Med* 19(1):51–60.
33. Schwartz AL, Nail LM, Chen S, Meek P, Barsevick AM, King ME, Jones LS 2000 Fatigue patterns observed in patients receiving chemotherapy and radiotherapy. *Cancer Invest* 18(1):11–19.
34. Schwartz AL 2000 Daily fatigue patterns and effect of exercise in women with breast cancer. *Cancer Pract* 8(1):16–24.
35. Schwartz AL 2000 Exercise and weight gain in breast cancer patients receiving chemotherapy. *Cancer Pract* 8(5):231–237.
36. Schwartz AL, Mori M, Gao R, Nail LM, King ME 2001 Exercise reduces daily fatigue in women with breast cancer receiving chemotherapy. *Med Sci Sports Exercise* 33(5):718–723.
37. Kolden GG, Strauman TJ, Ward A, Kuta J, Woods TE, Schneider KL, Heerey E, Sanborn L, Burt C, Millbrandt L, Kalin NH, Stewart JA, Mullen B 2002 A pilot study of group exercise training (GET) for women with primary breast cancer: feasibility and health benefits. *Psychooncology* 11(5):447–456.
38. Pinto BM, Trunzo JJ, Reiss P, Shiu SY 2002 Exercise participation after diagnosis of breast cancer: trends and effects on mood and quality of life. *Psychooncology* 11(5):389–400.
39. Turner J, Hayes S, Reul–Hirche H 2004 Improving the physical status and quality of life of women treated for breast cancer: a pilot study of a structured exercise intervention. *J Surg Oncol* 86(3):141–146.
40. Peters C, Lotzerich H, Niemeier B, Schule K, Uhlenbruck G 1994 Influence of a moderate exercise training on natural killer cytotoxicity and personality traits in cancer patients. *Anticancer Res* 14(3A):1033–1036.
41. Mock V, Dow KH, Meares CJ, Grimm PM, Dienemann JA, Haisfield–Wolfe ME, Quitasol W, Mitchell S, Chakravarthy A, Gage I 1997 Effects of exercise on fatigue, physical functioning, and emotional distress during radiation therapy for breast cancer. *Oncol Nursing Forum* 24(6):991–1000.

42. Mock V, Pickett M, Ropka ME, Muscari Lin E, Stewart KJ, Rhodes VA, McDaniel R, Grimm PM, Krumm S, McCorkle R 2001 Fatigue and quality of life outcomes of exercise during cancer treatment. *Cancer Pract* 9(3):119–127.
43. MacVicar MG, Winningham ML, Nickel JL 1989 Effects of aerobic interval training on cancer patients' functional capacity. *Nursing Res* 38(6):348–351.
44. Winningham ML, MacVicar MG, Bondoc M, Anderson JI, Minton JP 1989 Effect of aerobic exercise on body weight and composition in patients with breast cancer on adjuvant chemotherapy. *Oncol Nursing Forum* 16(5):683–689.
45. Mock V, Burke MB, Sheehan P, Creaton EM, Winningham ML, McKenney–Tedder S, Schwager LP, Liebman M 1994 A nursing rehabilitation program for women with breast cancer receiving adjuvant chemotherapy. *Oncol Nursing Forum* 21(5):899–907; discussion, 908.
46. Segal R, Evans W, Johnson D, Smith J, Colletta S, Gayton J, Woodard S, Wells G, Reid R 2001 Structured exercise improves physical functioning in women with stages I and II breast cancer: results of a randomized controlled trial. *J Clin Oncol* 19(3):657–665.
47. McKenzie DC, Kalda AL 2003 Effect of upper extremity exercise on secondary lymphedema in breast cancer patients: a pilot study. *J Clin Oncol* 21(3):463–466.
48. Courneya KS, Mackey JR, Bell GJ, Jones LW, Field CJ, Fairey AS 2003 Randomized controlled trial of exercise training in postmenopausal breast cancer survivors: cardiopulmonary and quality of life outcomes. *J Clin Oncol* 21(9):1660–1668.
49. Pate RR, Pratt M, Blair SN, Haskell WL, Macera CA, Bouchard C, Buchner D, Ettinger W, Heath GW, King AC, et al. 1995 Physical activity and public health. A recommendation from the Centers for Disease Control and Prevention and the American College of Sports Medicine. *JAMA* 273(5):402–407.
50. Winters KM, Snow CM 2000 Detraining reverses positive effects of exercise on the musculoskeletal system in premenopausal women. *J. Bone Miner Res* 15:2495–2503.
51. Dalsky G, Stocke KS, Ehsani AA 1988 Weight-bearing exercise training and lumbar bone mineral content in postmenopausal women. *Ann Intern Med* 108:824–828.
52. King AC, Haskell WL, Taylor B, Kraemer HC, DeBusk RF 1991 Group- vs. home-based exercise training in healthy older men and women: a community based clinical trial. *JAMA* 266:1535–1542.
53. Neff MJ 2004 ACS releases guidelines on nutrition and physical activity during and after cancer treatment. *Am Fam Phys* 69(7):1803–1805.

25 Exercise and Quality of Life in Survivors of Cancer Other Than Breast

Kerry S. Courneya, Kristin L. Campbell, Kristina H. Karvinen, and Aliya B. Ladha

CONTENTS

This chapter summarizes evidence regarding the effects of exercise on quality of life (QOL) in survivors of cancers other than breast cancer. It begins by providing a brief overview of the incidence and survival rates for the most common nonbreast cancers and then briefly reviews the major medical treatments for these cancers and discusses their implications for QOL. Next, the concept of QOL and how it has been defined and measured in the cancer field is examined. After that, the published research on exercise and QOL in nonbreast cancer survivors is summarized. For this purpose, the literature review is divided into studies that included: (1) mixed site cancer survivors (i.e., survivors from more than one cancer site) and (2) single site cancer survivors (i.e., survivors from a single cancer site). Then, the two largest randomized controlled trials conducted in single site cancer survivors are reviewed. Finally, future research directions are discussed. Parenthetically, throughout this chapter, the term "cancer survivor" is used — as suggested by the National Coalition for Cancer Survivorship — to refer to any individual diagnosed with cancer, from the time of discovery and for the balance of life.

NONBREAST CANCER INCIDENCE AND SURVIVAL RATES

Although breast cancer is by far the most common cancer diagnosed in American women, it still accounts for only about one third of cancers in this population [1]. The obvious converse of this fact is that nonbreast cancers account for about two thirds of all cancers diagnosed in American women (Table 25.1). After breast cancer, the most common cancers in American women are lung, colorectal, uterine corpus (endometrium), ovarian, non-Hodgkin's lymphoma, and skin melanoma [1]. These six cancers account for about 40% of all the cancers diagnosed in American women (a combined total more than breast) and about 60% of all the nonbreast cancers. For American men, the most common cancers are prostate, lung, colorectal, urinary bladder, skin melanoma, and non-Hodgkin's lymphoma [1]. These six cancers account for over 70% of all the cancers diagnosed in American men (Table 25.1).

Many of the most common cancers in men and women have good survival rates. For example, prostate, colorectal, urinary bladder, skin melanoma, uterine corpus, and ovarian cancers all have 5-year relative survival rates of over 90% if they are detected early (Table 25.2). The high incidence rates and good survival rates for nonbreast cancers have resulted in over 7 million Americans who are survivors of these cancers.

MEDICAL TREATMENTS FOR CANCER

Although the prognosis for surviving many of the most common cancers is very good, medical treatments are usually needed. The most common treatments for cancer are surgery, radiation therapy, and systemic (i.e., drug) therapy such as chemotherapy, endocrine or hormone therapy, and biological or immunotherapy. These medical interventions reduce the risk of recurrence and improve survival, but they can also negatively affect QOL. For example, depending on the location and extent of the operation, surgery can result in significant morbidities such as wound complications, infections, loss of function, decreased range of motion, diarrhea, dyspnea, pain, numbness, lymphedema, fatigue, and anxiety [2]. Similarly, depending on the dose and the site that is irradiated, radiation therapy can cause acute toxicities and late effects, including pain, blistering, reduced elasticity, decreased range of motion, nausea, fatigue, dry mouth, diarrhea, lung fibrosis, and cardiomyopathy [3].

TABLE 25.1
Estimated New Cancer Cases and Deaths for the Most Common Cancer Sites by Sex[a]

	Estimated new cases			Estimated new deaths		
Site	Total	Male	Female	Total	Male	Female
All sites	1,368,030	699,560	668,470	563,700	290,890	272,810
Prostate	230,110	230,110	—	29,900	29,900	—
Breast	217,440	1,450	215,990	40,580	470	40,110
Lung	173,770	93,110	80,660	160,440	91,930	68,510
Colorectal	146,940	73,620	73,320	56,730	28,320	28,410
Urinary bladder	60,240	44,640	15,600	12,710	8,780	3,930
Melanoma	55,100	29,900	5,200	7,910	5,050	2,860
Non-Hodgkin's lymphoma	54,370	28,850	25,520	19,410	10,390	9,020
Uterine corpus	40,320	—	40,320	7,090	—	7,090
Ovarian	25,580	—	25,580	16,090	—	16,090

[a]U.S., 2004.

Note: Excludes basal and squamous cell skin cancers and *in situ* carcinomas, except urinary bladder.

Source: Adapted from the American Cancer Society. *Cancer Facts & Figures 2004*. Atlanta: American Cancer Society, 2004.

TABLE 25.2
Five-Year Relative Survival Rates for the Most Common Cancers Other than Breast by Stage at Diagnosis[a]

Site	All stages %	Local %	Regional %	Distant %
Prostate	97.5	100.0	100.0	34.0
Lung	14.9	48.7	16.0	2.1
Colorectal	62.3	90.1	65.5	9.2
Urinary bladder	81.8	94.4	48.2	5.8
Melanoma	89.6	96.7	60.1	13.8
Non-Hodgkin's lymphoma	56.0	—	—	—
Uterine corpus	84.4	96.2	64.7	26.0
Ovarian	53.0	94.7	72.0	30.7

[a]U.S., 1992–1999.

Note: Rates are adjusted for normal life expectancy and are based on cases diagnosed from 1992–1999 followed through 2000.

Source: Adapted from the American Cancer Society. *Cancer Facts & Figures 2004*. Atlanta: American Cancer Society, 2004.

Chemotherapy may cause significant side effects including fatigue, anorexia, nausea, anemia, neutropenia, thrombocytopenia, peripheral neuropathies, ataxia, alopecia, and cardiotoxicity [4]. The incidence and severity of these side effects depends on the types of drugs, mechanisms of action, drug dosage, administration schedule, presence of other comorbidities, and the use of supportive care interventions [4]. The side effects from chemotherapy can appear immediately, within a few weeks or months, or even years after treatment has been completed (i.e., late effects). Hormone therapy can have significant side effects, such as weight gain, muscle loss, proximal muscle weakness, fat accumulation in the trunk and face, osteoporosis, fatigue, hot flashes, and increased susceptibility to infection. Finally, although biological therapies tend to be better tolerated than chemotherapy, they can still produce flu-like symptoms that can be quite severe [5].

For many cancers, multimodal treatment (i.e., surgery, radiotherapy, and systemic therapy) is the standard of care. The timing and sequence of the multimodal treatments vary, depending on many factors including the type of cancer and its stage. It is possible, however, that some cancer survivors may be treated on multiple occasions with multiple modalities, concurrently or sequentially, for many months or years. Consequently, it is easy to see that such prolonged and intensive medical treatments may take a heavy toll on the QOL of cancer survivors.

QUALITY OF LIFE IN CANCER SURVIVORS

The concept of QOL is very important to cancer survivors. Gains made in survival from medical treatments must be judged against any potential decrements in QOL. In fact, QOL has become a standard endpoint in clinical trials of cancer survivors and in cancer care practice [6]. Perhaps not surprisingly, QOL is a difficult concept to define. Farquhar [7] has noted that most definitions can be categorized as global definitions or component definitions. Global definitions focus on overall happiness and satisfaction with life without making reference to any particular component of life. Component definitions, on the other hand, break down QOL into a series of component parts thought to be essential to QOL; most cancer researchers have adopted this latter definition [6]. Although no consensus has been reached on the number and nature of QOL components relevant for cancer survivors, the most commonly mentioned components include physical, functional, emotional, cognitive, spiritual, and social. Farquhar [7] has noted that such component definitions most likely contribute to the global evaluations of QOL.

Despite the difficulties in defining QOL, there is good agreement that it is personal and subjective [6]. Consequently, QOL is primarily measured by self-report. Some cancer researchers have used generic QOL measures such as the Short Form 36 Health Survey [8], but most have used one of the cancer-specific QOL measures, such as the Cancer Rehabilitation Evaluation System [9], the European Organization for Research and Treatment of Cancer Quality of Life Questionnaire [10], the Functional Living Index — Cancer [11], and the Functional Assessment of Cancer Therapy scale [12]. These scales assess multiple components of QOL such as physical, functional, and emotional well-being, using items relevant to cancer survivors.

EXERCISE AND QUALITY OF LIFE IN CANCER SURVIVORS

Previous reviews have noted that about 50% of studies on exercise in cancer survivors have focused *exclusively* on breast cancer survivors [13] and that even studies open to mixed site cancer survivors have recruited a disproportionate number of breast cancer survivors. Consequently, knowledge about exercise in cancer survivors is based largely on research in breast cancer survivors. However, breast cancer accounts for only 16% of the total cancers diagnosed in the U.S. The disproportionate focus of exercise researchers on breast cancer may have arisen for several reasons:

- Breast cancer is the most common cancer in women, which allows for an adequate sample size to conduct a single-center study on a single cancer site.
- The generally good prognosis of the disease makes QOL an important issue and exercise interventions feasible.
- The greater abundance of funding for breast cancer-specific research may have enticed exercise researchers into this area.

In any case, in this chapter we review studies that have examined exercise and QOL in any group of cancer survivors other than breast.

A literature search was conducted in May, 2004, using the CD-ROM databases CancerLit, CINAHL, HERACLES, MEDLINE, PsycINFO, and SPORT Discus. Key words that related to cancer (i.e., cancer, oncology, tumor, neoplasm, carcinoma); the postdiagnosis time period (i.e., rehabilitation, therapy, adjuvant therapy, treatment, intervention, palliation); and exercise (i.e., exercise, physical activity, physical therapy, sport, weight training) were combined and searched. Relevant articles were then hand-searched for further pertinent references. To be included in the review, a study must have been published in a peer-reviewed journal and to have examined aerobic or resistance exercise. Studies had to include at least some nonbreast cancer survivors and a QOL endpoint. Studies that included a multiple intervention package (e.g., exercise combined with diet, social support, counseling, etc.) were excluded.

The search located 26 studies consisting of 1816 nonbreast cancer survivors from over 20 different cancer sites (Table 25.3). The studies were reviewed in two separate categories: (1) those that included survivors from mixed cancer sites (i.e., had more than one cancer site in a single study) and (2) those that were restricted to survivors of a single cancer site (e.g., prostate, colorectal). This review begins by providing an overall summary of the samples, methods, and results from the mixed cancer site studies. It then presents an ancillary analysis comparing breast to nonbreast cancer survivors from one of the previous trials involving mixed site cancer survivors [14]. Finally, an overall summary of the single site cancer studies is provided, followed by a detailed review of the two largest exercise trials in single site cancer survivors.

TABLE 25.3
Number of Single and Mixed Cancer Site Studies in the Exercise Domain (Excluding Breast)

	Single cancer site studies		Mixed cancer site studies		Total	
Cancer site	No. studies	Total N	No. studies	Total N	No.	N
Prostate	2	575	1	12	3	587
Lung			5	14	5	14
Colorectal	3	276			3	276
Urinary bladder					0	0
Skin melanoma	1	12	2	5	3	17
Non-Hodgkin's lymphoma	1	438	6	53	7	491
Hodgkin's disease	1	9	5	40	6	49
Uterine corpus (endometrium)					0	0
Colon			2	13	2	13
Sarcoma			4	11	4	11
Ovarian			1	6	1	6
Multiple myeloma	2	104	2	9	4	113
Leukemia	1	12	4	30	5	42
Head and neck	1	20			1	20
Other			11	177	11	177
Total						
Nonbreast	12	1446	14	370	26	1816
Breast			9	197		2013

STUDIES INVOLVING MIXED SITE CANCER SURVIVORS

Table 25.4 lists the 14 studies located that examined exercise and QOL in mixed site cancer survivors. Three studies were observational and 11 were interventions. Of the three observational studies, two were cross-sectional and one was prospective. One survey was completed during treatment and the other two were completed post-treatment. Of the 11 intervention studies, 5 were uncontrolled trials (i.e., one group pre–post-test designs), 4 were nonrandomized controlled trials, and 2 were randomized controlled trials. Two initiated the exercise program during treatment, four included survivors during and after treatment, and five initiated the exercise intervention after treatment. The 14 studies contained 567 participants — 156 in the observational studies (about 52 per study) and 411 in the intervention studies (about 37 per study). The most common cancer diagnoses among the 567 participants were:

Breast (37.0%)
Non-Hodgkin's lymphoma (9.9%)
Hodgkin's disease (7.6%)
Prostate (4.2%)
Colorectal (3.9%)
Testicular (3.5%)
Lung (2.8%)
Leukemia (2.7%)
Central nervous system (2.3%)
Germ cell (2.3%)
Ovarian (2.1%)
Multiple myeloma (1.6%)
Melanoma (1.4%)
Sarcoma (1.1%)

TABLE 25.4
Summary of Studies Examining Exercise in Mixed Cancer Sites

Sample/treatment	Design	Exercise intervention/measures	QOL outcomes/measures	QOL results	Ref.
Observational studies					
78 consecutive cancer patients (34 breast, 21 non-Hodgkin's, 11 testicular, 6 Hodgkin's, 3 sarcoma, 2 multiple myeloma, 1 lung) admitted for chemotherapy and bone marrow transplantation	Cross-sectional	Maximal performance assessed by treadmill test	Profile mood states and symptom checklist–90 revised	Maximal performance significantly associated with distress and fatigue in a negative direction	14
53 adolescent cancer survivors (17 Hodgkin's or lymphoma, 12 leukemia, 8 central nervous system); 85% had completed treatment	Cross-sectional	Self-reported exercise, prediagnosis, during, and after treatment	Depression and multiple self-concept indices	Patients active at all three timepoints had best psychosocial status	15
25 cancer patients (8 breast, 7 multiple myeloma, 7 non-Hodgkin's lymphoma, 2 Hodgkin's disease, 1 other) who had just completed chemotherapy and bone marrow transplantation	Prospective	Self-reported cycle ergometry and walking during hospital stay	Functional Assessment of Cancer Therapy Fatigue Scale	Cycling duration per day correlated significantly with fatigue and QOL at discharge	16
Intervention studies					
70 mixed cancer patients (46 breast, 13 germ cell, 5 sarcoma, 4 lung, 1 adrenocarcinoma, 1 neuroblastoma) undergoing autologous peripheral blood stem cell transplant; patients with solid tumors	Nonrandomized controlled trial	Supervised "biking" using a bed ergometer seven/week for 30 min at 50% of cardiac reserve (220 age-resting HR) from time of HDC until discharge	Medical records	Experimental group showed lower severity of pain and incidence of diarrhea	17
32 cancer patients (17 breast, 12 non-Hodgkin's lymphoma, 1 non–small cell lung, 1 sarcoma, 1 seminola) who underwent high-dose chemotherapy and autologous peripheral blood stem cell transplantation	Nonrandomized controlled Trial	Supervised treadmill walking five times/week for 6 weeks, 15–30 min at 80% HR max using interval training	Reported feeling of fatigue and limitation in activities of daily living (by interview)	25% of controls reported fatigue with usual daily activities; none reported in exercise group	18
Five cancer patients who reported fatigue (one medulloblastoma, one non-Hodgkin's lymphoma, one Hodgkin's lymphoma, one lung, one breast); three were on treatment	Uncontrolled trial (pre–post-test)	Daily supervised treadmill walking for 6 weeks, 15–30 min at 80% HR max	Clinical observation of fatigue	Clear decrease in fatigue	19
20 cancer survivors (17 general carcinoma, 1 lymphoma, 2 leukemia) who had just completed adjuvant therapy (M = 14 months postdiagnosis)	Uncontrolled trial (pre–post-test)	Supervised aerobic and weight training two times/week at own RPE for 10 weeks	Modified Rotterdam Quality of Life Survey	Significant increase in quality of life	20

12 prostate and 13 leukemia/general carcinoma survivors (84% had completed treatment)	Uncontrolled trial (pre–post test)	Supervised aerobic and weight training two/week at own RPE for up to 20 weeks	Modified Rotterdam Quality of Life Survey	Increased quality of life, but only for leukemia patients	21
59 cancer patients (31 breast, 6 seminoma, 2 sarcoma, 4 lung carcinoma, 7 Hodgkin's disease, 9 non-Hodgkin's lymphoma) who had just completed high-dose chemotherapy and bone marrow transplantation	Nonrandomized controlled trial	Daily supervised bed ergometer biking during hospitalization (about 2 weeks) for 30 min at 50% HR reserve	Profile of mood states and the symptom checklist–90 revised	Exercise group showed decrease in psychological distress; controls showed increase in fatigue and decrease in vigor	22
Three children aged 13–14 successfully treated for acute lymphoblastic leukemia and other neoplasms with 11 healthy controls	Nonrandomized controlled Trial	Supervised 12 weeks of aerobic exercise three/week for 30 min at 70–85% of the child's HR max	Mood state (Piers–Harris Self-Concept Scale)	High anxiety was reduced with exercise training	23
Nine cancer patients (four bowel, two pancreas, one breast, one oral, one melanoma)	Uncontrolled trial	Home-based individualized program (walking and stretching) of daily activity for 28 days	Multidimensional Fatigue Inventory (MFI), Symptom Distress Scale (SDS), Hospital Anxiety and Depression Scale (HADS), and Quality of Life Scale (QOLS)	Improved QOL in all participants and increase in activity with no increase in fatigue	24
18 cancer survivors (15 breast, 3 colon) post-treatment	Randomized controlled trial	Supervised low intensity (25–35% HRR) or moderate intensity (40–50% HRR) aerobic exercise program, three times/week, for 10 weeks	QOL Index for Cancer Patients and the Linear Analog Self-Assessment (LASA) measuring fatigue, anxiety, confusion, depression, energy, and anger	Significant increase in quality of life and energy in exercise groups compared to controls; fatigue and anxiety significantly decreased in exercise group pre and post	25
62 men and women diagnosed with various cancers; some undergoing treatment	Uncontrolled trial	Supervised aerobic exercise 2 days/week for 12 weeks with 3–5 days/week of exercise at home	Cancer Rehabilitation Evaluation System — Short Form (CARES-SF)	Significant improvement in quality of life	26
108 cancer patients (44 breast, 10 colon, 6 ovarian, 4 stomach, 4 melanoma, 3 Hodgkin's, 3 non-Hodgkin's, 3 lung, 3 brain, 3 lymphoma, 17 other, 8 unknown)	Randomized controlled trial (group pyschotherapy ± exercise intervention)	Home-based, moderate-intensity walking program for 20–30 min., 3–5 days/week at 65–75% estimated max HR	Functional Assessment of Cancer Therapy — General (Fact-G), Satisfaction with Life Scale (SWLS), Centre for Epidemiological Studies Depression (CES-D), State-Trait Anxiety Inventory (STAI), Fatigue Scale (FS)	Exercise group showed improvements in physical and functional well-being, life satisfaction, and fatigue compared with controls	27

Notes: HR = heart rate; HDC = high-dose chemotherapy; RPE = rate of perceived exertion.

The rest of the cancer sites had less than 1%, except those categorized as "other" (6.0%), "general carcinoma" (5.3%), or "unknown" (1.4%).

In the three observational studies, exercise was assessed by self-report (two studies) and a maximal treadmill performance. In the 11 intervention studies, supervised exercise was used in 7 studies, 2 used home-based protocols, and 2 used a combination of supervised and home-based sessions. Exercise frequencies ranged from two sessions per week (two studies), to three to five sessions per week (four studies) and five to seven sessions per week (five studies). Exercise intensity was prescribed as 65 to 85% of measured or estimated heart rate maximum in four studies; 25 to 50% of heart rate reserve or cardiac reserve in three studies, an unspecified rating of perceived exertion in two studies and less conventional techniques in two other studies. Exercise mode included a mix of aerobic exercise (five studies), walking or treadmill walking (four studies), or cycle ergometer (two studies). The lengths of the interventions were 2 weeks (two studies), 4 weeks (one study), 6 weeks (two studies), 10 weeks (three studies), 12 weeks (two studies), or 20 weeks (one study).

The QOL variables assessed in the studies were

Fatigue (seven studies)
QOL (five studies)
Pain and symptoms (three studies)
Anxiety (three studies)
Depression (three studies)
General mood states (three studies)
Self-concept (two studies)
Ability to perform activities of daily living (one study)
Distress (one study)
Satisfaction with life (one study)

Most studies assessed more than one QOL endpoint. Overall, the results of these 14 studies showed many QOL improvements with exercise. More specifically, improvements with exercise were reported for

Fatigue (six studies)
QOL (five studies)
Anxiety (two studies)
Pain and symptoms (one study)
Activities of daily living (one study)
Distress (one study)
Improved life satisfaction (one study)

The findings were consistent across intervention study design.

Although the findings for the studies in mixed site cancer survivors were primarily positive, important limitations need to be highlighted

- Only 2 of the 14 studies were randomized controlled trials.
- Because the inclusion of mixed cancer sites makes it difficult to comment on any single cancer site, the clinical utility of these studies may be limited.
- Breast cancer was by far the most common cancer site in these studies (37%), which means that the information generated from these studies is still primarily applicable to breast cancer survivors.
- The sample sizes were quite small and spread among many different cancer sites. Consequently, it was not feasible to conduct subanalyses based on cancer sites (i.e., examine cancer site as a moderator of exercise effects).

To explore this issue here, the authors report an ancillary subanalysis based on cancer site from one of their previously published trials — the *Group* Psychotherapy and *Home*-Based *P*hysical *E*xercise (GROUP-HOPE) trial. This trial was a randomized controlled trial that examined whether a home-based exercise program could improve QOL in mixed site cancer survivors attending group psychotherapy classes. About 41% of the participants were breast cancer survivors. Significant effects in favor of the exercise group for functional well-being, fatigue, and sum of skinfolds have been previously reported [14]. The data were also analyzed by cancer site (breast vs. nonbreast) using an overall multivariate analysis of variance that contained all 13 outcomes. Such an analysis was significantly underpowered and, not surprisingly, no significant interaction was reported.

Here, analyses of variance are presented only for the three endpoints with significant effects (functional well-being, fatigue, and sum of skinfolds). These unplanned post hoc analyses revealed no cancer site by group interaction for functional well-being [$F(1,92) = 0.3$; $p = 0.604$], but borderline significant interactions for fatigue [$F(1,92) = 3.7$; $p = 0.057$] and sum of skinfolds [$F(1,92) = 3.7$; $p = 0.058$]. Independent t-tests on change scores within each cancer site category suggested that exercise had a larger effect on sum of skinfolds in breast compared to nonbreast cancer survivors (Table 25.5; Figure 25.1) and a larger effect on fatigue in nonbreast compared to breast cancer survivors (Table 25.5; Figure 25.2). These data should be interpreted with caution, however, given the post hoc nature of these analyses and relatively small sample sizes. Nevertheless, they are suggestive of a differential response to exercise between breast and nonbreast cancer survivors.

STUDIES INVOLVING SINGLE SITE CANCER SURVIVORS

Table 25.6 lists the 12 studies located that examined exercise and QOL in single site cancer survivors. Five studies were observational and seven were interventions. Of the five observational studies, three were retrospective, one was prospective, and one was cross-sectional. Of the seven intervention studies, four were randomized controlled trials and three were uncontrolled trials. A total of 1446 participants were involved in the studies, including 1129 participants in the observational studies (approximately 226 per study) and 317 in the intervention studies (approximately 45 per study). The cancer sites examined in these studies included three colorectal, two prostate, two multiple myeloma, and one each for non-Hodgkin's lymphoma, acute leukemia, skin melanoma, Hodgkin's disease, and head and neck.

The five observational studies measured exercise with self-report scales. The three retrospective studies had cancer survivors recall exercise at three time points: prediagnosis, during treatment, and post-treatment. The prospective study obtained reports of exercise for 4 months after surgery and the cross-sectional study obtained current exercise for cancer survivors after completion of various treatments. Of the seven intervention studies, four initiated the exercise program during treatment, two after treatment, and one included survivors during and after treatment.

Four of the intervention studies consisted of supervised exercise and three examined home-based exercise. Exercise frequency was reported as three sessions per week (five studies), three to five sessions per week (one study), or four sessions per week (one study). Four of the intervention programs consisted of aerobic exercise, two involved resistance training, and one combined aerobic and resistance exercise. In the four aerobic exercise interventions, the exercise modality was chosen by the participants in two studies, not specified in one study, and consisted of walking or another preferred activity in one study. The prescribed exercise intensities consisted of 85% of measured heart rate maximum (one study), 65 to 75% of measured heart rate maximum (one study), 65 to 80% of measured heart rate maximum (one study), or was self-selected by the participants (one study). Durations of aerobic exercise sessions were 15 to 30 minutes (one study), 20 to 30 minutes (one study), 30 minutes (one study), and 40 to 60 minutes (one study).

The resistance exercise studies consisted of total body exercises involving major muscle groups in one study and upper body exercises designed to enhance scapular stability and restoring/main-

TABLE 25.5
Effects of Home-Based Exercise on Physical Fitness and Quality of Life in Mixed-Site Cancer Survivors by Cancer Site (Breast vs. Nonbreast)[a]

	Baseline	P value[b]	Post-test	Mean change	Difference between groups in mean change (95% CI)	P value[c]
Breast cancer (*n* = 39)						
Functional well-being (0–28)						
Exercise group (n = 19)	15.4 (4.2)	0.210	17.4 (5.0)	2.0 (4.0)	1.5 (−1.1 to 4.0)	0.245
Control group (n = 20)	17.2 (4.4)		17.7 (5.2)	0.5 (3.8)		
Fatigue (0–52)						
Exercise group (*n* = 19)	21.6 (10.0)	0.840	21.4 (13.6)	−0.2 (12.5)	1.2 (−5.6 to 8.1)	0.719
Control group (*n* = 20)	22.2 (9.1)		20.8 (9.9)	−1.4 (8.3)		
Sum of skinfolds (mm)						
Exercise group (*n* = 19)	111.0 (33.0)	0.883	102.7 (39.4)	−8.3 (24.9)	−20.6 (−4.6 to −36.5)	0.013
Control group (*n* = 20)	112.8 (42.6)		125.1 (40.5)	12.3 (24.2)		
Nonbreast cancer (*n* = 57)						
Functional well-being (0–28)						
Exercise group (*n* = 32)	15.1 (5.4)	0.262	16.1 (5.5)	1.0 (4.7)	2.4 (0.0 to 4.8)	0.047
Control group (*n* = 25)	16.8 (5.6)		15.3 (5.5)	−1.4 (4.0)		
Fatigue (0–52)						
Exercise group (*n* = 32)	23.3 (11.0)	0.464	18.7 (9.8)	−4.6 (11.0)	−7.1 (−1.7 to −12.5)	0.012
Control group (*n* = 25)	21.2 (10.3)		23.7 (9.8)	2.5 (9.0)		
Sum of skinfolds (mm)						
Exercise group (*n* = 32)	96.4 (44.5)	0.672	92.1 (40.5)	−4.4 (9.6)	−6.1 (0.4 to −12.5)	0.064
Control group (*n* = 25)	101.8 (50.8)		103.5 (49.6)	1.7 (14.6)		

[a]Data are from the Group Psychotherapy and Home-Based Physical Exercise (GROUP-HOPE) trial [14].
[b]P-value for difference between groups at baseline.
[c]P-value for differences in change scores between groups from baseline to post-test.

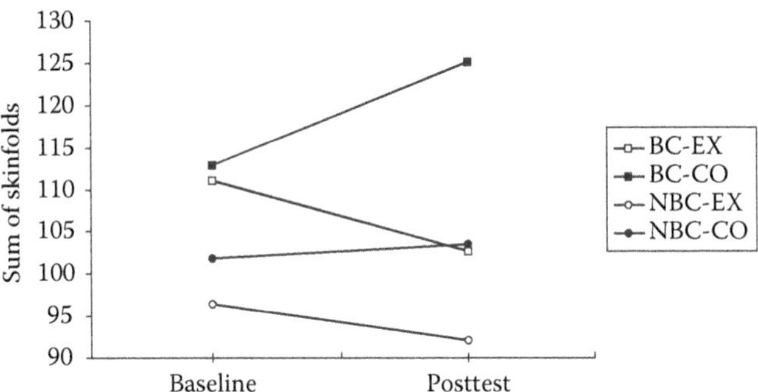

FIGURE 25.1 Borderline significant interaction between experimental group and cancer site on sum of skinfolds from the GROUP-HOPE Trial. BC = breast cancer; NBC = nonbreast cancer; EX = exercise; CO = control [14].

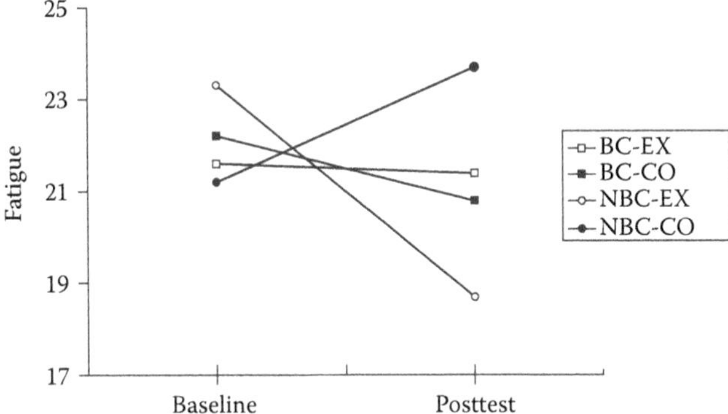

FIGURE 25.2 Borderline significant interaction between experimental group and cancer site on fatigue from the GROUP-HOPE Trial. BC = breast cancer; NBC = nonbreast cancer; EX = exercise; CO = control [14].

taining strength in the other. One of the studies involving resistance exercise consisted of two sets of eight to ten repetitions of nine exercises at an intensity of 60 to 70% of one maximum repetition. The other consisted of one to two sets of 15 to 20 repetitions of six exercises at a rate of perceived exertion of "somewhat hard." The lengths of the interventions were 10 weeks (one study), 12 weeks (two studies), 4 months (two studies), 20 weeks (one study), and 6 months (one study).

A variety of quality of life endpoints were measured in the studies, including:

QOL (eight studies)
Fatigue (seven studies)
Mood states (three studies)
Life satisfaction (two studies)
Psychological impact of cancer (one study)
Depression (one study)
Cognition (one study)
Sleep (one study)
Pain and disability (one study)

Most studies had more than one QOL endpoint. Overall, the results of these 12 studies showed many QOL improvements with exercise. More specifically, improvements with exercise were reported for

TABLE 25.6
Summary of Studies Examining Exercise in Single-Cancer Sites Other than Breast

Sample/treatment	Design	Exercise intervention/measures	QOL outcomes/measures	QOL results	Ref.
Observational studies					
130 colorectal cancer survivors who were post-treatment	Retrospective	Self-reported exercise prediagnosis, during treatment, and post-treatment	Functional Assessment of Cancer Therapy Fatigue (FACT fatigue) Scale and Satisfaction with Life Scale (SWL)	Survivors who permanently relapsed from exercise reported lowest quality of life	28
53 postsurgical colorectal cancer patients	Prospective	Self-reported exercise over 4 months	Functional Assessment for Cancer Therapy-Fatigue (FACT-F)	Increase in frequency of light exercise from pre- to postsurgery correlated with better quality of life and life satisfaction	29
420 prostate cancer survivors who had completed various treatments	Cross-sectional	Self-reported exercise frequency, duration, length of time, and intentions using stage-of-change measure	Psychological impact of cancer (impact of events scale)	Prostate cancer survivors who reported exercising regularly had significantly lower impact scores than those who were not exercising	30
88 multiple myeloma cancer survivors	Retrospective	Self-reported exercise prediagnosis, active treatment, and off-treatment	FACT-G, the Centre for Epidemiological Studies Depression (CES-D) scale	Significant positive correlations between total exercise and all QOL outcomes except physical well-being	31
438 non-Hodgkin's lymphoma survivors from provincial cancer registry	Retrospective	Self-reported exercise prediagnosis, active treatment, and off treatment	FACT-Anemia	Survivors meeting ACSM exercise guidelines had less fatigue, better physical and functional well-being, and better overall QOL during and off treatment	32
Intervention studies					
12 patients with acute leukemia who underwent bone marrow transplants	Uncontrolled trial (pre–post-test)	Home-based exercise program for 30 min, three times/week, at 85% of HR max starting 1 week before BMT and lasting 4 months	Beck's Depression Inventory	Patients found exercise program "worthwhile"	33

12 melanoma patients prescribed to take methylphenidate	Uncontrolled trial	Aerobic exercise 15–30 min/session, 4 days/week, duration of 4 months	Medical Outcomes Study (36 Short Form), Schwartz Cancer Fatigue Scale, Trail Maker Forms A and B (cognitive function)	Improved fatigue, decreased quality of life and cognition in exercise alone group compared to exercise + methylphenidate group	34
93 postsurgical colorectal cancer survivors; 66% were receiving adjuvant therapy	Randomized controlled trial	Home-based exercise program, three to five times/week, moderate intensity for 20–30 mins	FACT-G, CES-D, anxiety, STAI	ITT analysis revealed no significant differences; ancillary analyses (↑ vs. ↓ fitness) shared differences on overall QOL and multiple subdomains in favor of high-fitness group	35
Nine post-treatment fatigued Hodgkin's cancer survivors	Uncontrolled trial (pre–post-test)	Home-based aerobic exercise training program three times/week, 40–60 mins for 20 weeks at 65–80% intensity	Fatigue Questionnaire (FQ), SF-36	Decrease in total fatigue by 43.7%	36
155 men with prostate cancer receiving androgen deprivation	Randomized controlled trial	Supervised resistance exercise; two sets of 8–12 reps at 60–70% one RM, 3 days/week for 12 weeks	FACT-Fatigue	Fatigue decreased and quality of life increased in exercisers compared to controls	37
16 multiple myeloma cancer survivors receiving HDC and BMT	Randomized controlled trial	Home-based combined aerobic and upper and lower strength training program, three times/week for 30–60 min for 6 months, walking or other preferred	Mood states, sleep	Trends toward a difference for multiple QOL outcomes in exercise training	38
20 patients with squamous cell carcinoma of the head and neck following radical neck dissection	Randomized controlled trial	Supervised progressive 12-week resistance program for the shoulder; three times/week; six exercises; one to two sets of 15–20 reps	Shoulder Pain and Disability Index (SPADI) and Functional Assessment of Cancer Therapy — Head & Neck (FACT-H&N)	Exercise group showed a significant decrease in pain and disability	39

QOL (seven studies)
Fatigue (five studies)
Pain (one study)
Psychological impact of cancer (one study)
Sleep (one study)
Improved life satisfaction (one study)

The findings were consistent across intervention study design.

Although the findings for the studies in single site cancer survivors were also primarily positive, they too suffered from methodological limitations. First, only 4 of the 13 studies were randomized controlled trials. Second, the methodology of most studies was not well described (e.g., enrollment, randomization, blinding, analytical plan). Third, the sample sizes in the intervention studies were very small, with two exceptions [37,40]. Fourth, follow-up of participants was limited. Here, a more detailed review of the two largest exercise trials in single site cancer survivors other than breast is provided.

In the largest randomized controlled trial to date, Segal et al. [37] examined the effects of supervised resistance exercise training on muscular fitness and QOL in prostate cancer survivors treated with androgen deprivation therapy (a common drug treatment for prostate cancer survivors that depletes testosterone to castrate levels). Participants (n = 155) were randomly assigned to an exercise (n = 82) or control (n = 73) group. The exercise group performed nine resistance exercises three times per week at 60 to 70% of one repetition maximum for a 12-week period. The primary endpoints were fatigue and QOL (assessed by self-report scales) and the secondary endpoints were upper- and lower-body muscular strength (assessed by standard load tests for the chest press and leg press).

The researchers reported a 13% loss to follow-up (20/155) and a 79% adherence rate among all participants randomized to the exercise arm (including dropouts). Intention to treat analyses using "last observation carried-forward" for missing data showed statistically significant differences in change scores favoring the exercise group for fatigue, QOL, and upper- and lower-body muscular fitness. The fatigue change was 3.0 points and the QOL change was 5.3 points, both of which may be considered clinically meaningful changes for the particular self-report scales that were used. In terms of muscular strength, the exercise group increased upper-body strength by 41% and lower-body strength by 32% compared to the control group's decline in these measures by 8 and 4%, respectively. Moreover, subgroup analyses showed that these favorable effects were present for men who were treated with palliative vs. curative intent and for men who had been treated with the therapy for shorter vs. longer than 1 year.

Courneya et al. (2003) examined the effects of a home-based exercise program on QOL in colorectal cancer survivors who had recently completed surgery [35]. About 55% of participants were receiving adjuvant therapy at the time of the exercise intervention. Participants (n = 102) were randomly assigned in a 2:1 ratio to an exercise (n = 69) or control (n = 33) group. The exercise group was asked to exercise on their own three to five times per week for 16 weeks at a moderate intensity (60 to 80% of estimated maximum heart rate) for at least 20 to 30 minutes each time. The primary endpoints were QOL (assessed by self-report scales) and cardiovascular fitness (assessed by a submaximal treadmill test).

The authors reported a 9% loss to follow-up (9/102) and a 76% adherence rate among those who completed the trial (excluding dropouts). The authors also reported that 52% of the control group reported regular exercise. Intention to treat analyses on those who had completed the trial showed no statistically significant differences between the two arms. In an "as treated" ancillary analyses, the authors reported that participants who increased their fitness over the course of the intervention had more favorable changes in anxiety, depression, overall QOL, and satisfaction with life compared to those whose fitness decreased over the course of the intervention. The QOL change score difference was 6.5 points, which may be considered clinically meaningful for the self-report scale that was used.

MECHANISMS OF ENHANCED QUALITY OF LIFE FROM EXERCISE IN CANCER SURVIVORS

Overall, the results of 26 studies to date suggest that exercise may improve QOL in survivors of nonbreast cancers. Several biopsychosocial mechanisms may explain the QOL improvements in cancer survivors that result from exercise training. Courneya (2001) has proposed a simple organizational model on how exercise might enhance QOL during cancer treatment (Figure 25.3) [41]. First, exercise may alter one of the many hypothesized biopsychosocial mechanisms thought to underlie improved coping and adjustment to cancer (e.g., fitness, self-efficacy, social interaction). In turn, changes in these biopsychosocial mechanisms may alleviate or prevent the occurrence of many of the common symptoms and side effects associated with cancer and its treatments (e.g., fatigue, insomnia, pain, anorexia). Amelioration of these effects may then reduce their impact on the ability to perform activities of daily living, leisure activities, interactions with others, and so on. Finally, enhanced physical and social activities may improve psychological distress/well-being (e.g., anxiety, depression) thereby improving overall QOL. No studies have examined the potential mechanisms of change for exercise and QOL in nonbreast cancer survivors.

FUTURE RESEARCH DIRECTIONS

Given the paucity of research on exercise in nonbreast cancer survivors, it is rather obvious that a significant amount of work needs to be completed in these populations. In general, randomized controlled trials are needed that focus explicitly on nonbreast cancer populations. It is clear from past research that exercise trials targeting multiple cancer survivor groups will likely attract a significant number of breast cancer survivors. Consequently, such studies will not likely recruit

Quality of Life	General (i.e., noncontent-specific) happiness and satisfaction with life
↑	
Symptom Distress	Psychological/Emotional well-being (e.g., anxiety, depression, anger, hope, pride)
↑	
Symptom Interference	Functional well-being (e.g., activities of daily living, leisure activities, work), social well-being (i.e., interaction with others), spiritual well-being (e.g., meaning, purpose)
↑	
Symptom Occurrence	Physical well-being (e.g., nausea, pain, fatigue, dyspnea, insomnia, poor appetite, constipation, diarrhea, weight change, asthenia, cachexia), cognitive well-being (e.g., attention, confusion)
↑	
Mechanisms	Biologic (e.g., hemoglobin, physical fitness), psychologic (e.g., self-efficacy, distraction), social (e.g., interaction, support)
↑	
Exercise	Type, amount (frequency, intensity, duration), progression, context (i.e., physical and social environment)

FIGURE 25.3 Model of exercise and quality of life in cancer survivors during treatment [41].

sufficient numbers of any nonbreast cancer group to be able to comment on the utility of exercise in these populations.

Moreover, even if such studies were to exclude breast cancer survivors explicitly, problems with mixing multiple cancer sites in a single study would still be present (i.e.,"apples and oranges"). The main concern is that each cancer site is unique in terms of its demographic and behavioral profile, its disease pathophysiology, its prognosis and standard medical treatments, and its physical and psychosocial sequelae. Thus, different cancer survivor groups may respond differently to different exercise interventions.

The obvious solution to the "apples and oranges" problem is simply to conduct exercise trials in single site cancer groups. Such research may be a challenge, however, given the smaller number of persons diagnosed with nonbreast cancers. Nevertheless, a starting point would be to conduct studies in single site cancers that have sufficient numbers to warrant such a study — namely, prostate, lung, and colorectal. Prostate cancer actually has a higher incidence than breast cancer (see Table 25.1), so single center studies of this cancer group should be feasible. To date, however, only one study has examined exercise in prostate cancer survivors [37]. Similarly, colorectal cancer has a relatively high incidence rate and single center studies of this cancer should also be feasible in major centers. Once again, however, only one exercise trial has been conducted in this population [35]. Finally, although lung cancer is very common, the safety, feasibility, and efficacy of exercise in this population may be tenuous for obvious reasons. Nevertheless, clinical trials of exercise in selected lung cancer survivors may be warranted.

It may also be possible to conduct multicenter trials of single site cancers. This option may be useful for the most common cancers but may be particularly valuable for cancers with moderately high incidence rates, such as urinary bladder, skin melanoma, non-Hodgkin's lymphoma, and endometrial (see Table 25.1). This approach has the added strength of increasing the generalizability of the findings. One limitation of this approach, however, is the difficulty of standardizing exercise interventions across different centers. Nevertheless, as more research groups become involved in this type of research, the capacity for such multicenter trials will become greater.

Other options for facilitating exercise studies in single site cancers include:

- Keeping the eligibility criteria very broad (e.g., not restricting the sample based on age, comorbidities, disease stage, etc.)
- Focusing on prevalent cancer cases (e.g., all survivors > 5 years post-treatment) rather than incident cancer cases (i.e., only newly diagnosed survivors)
- Testing home-based rather than center-based exercise interventions (which tends to exclude a large number of participants based on location alone)

Other creative strategies may be needed to conduct adequately powered exercise studies in all cancer survivor groups that may potentially benefit.

For studies that do not target nonbreast cancer survivor groups specifically, it may be possible to conduct subgroup analyses in the sample. Such analyses may help determine whether other cancer survivors respond to an exercise training intervention to the same extent as breast cancer survivors. The secondary analyses conducted in this chapter suggest that breast and nonbreast cancer survivors may respond differently to exercise, although the study was not designed or powered to answer such a question. If possible, it would be ideal to power the study *a priori* to conduct such a subgroup analysis by stratifying on cancer site prior to randomization and attempting to recruit equal numbers of breast and nonbreast cancer survivors.

In addition to starting research programs in nonbreast cancer survivor groups, research will be needed that examines the effects of exercise interventions on all aspects of QOL in these cancer survivors, including physical, functional, emotional, cognitive, spiritual, and social well-being. It will also be important to determine whether exercise can help control some of the common side effects of cancer treatments including nausea, pain, fatigue, weakness, and/or depression. Moreover, for all of the preceding questions, it will be important to determine the optimal type (e.g., aerobic vs. resistance training), volume (i.e., frequency, intensity, and duration), progression, and context (e.g., center-based vs. home-based, individual vs. group formats) of exercise for all cancer survivor groups. Finally, studies are needed to elucidate further the mechanisms of change in QOL and to compare and integrate exercise with other currently accepted QOL interventions for cancer survivors. This information will allow for evidence-based guidelines for a given endpoint of interest in a given cancer survivor group.

SUMMARY

Interest in the possible role of exercise in enhancing QOL in cancer survivor groups other than those surviving breast cancer is growing. Preliminary research suggests that exercise may be an effective QOL intervention for prostate, colorectal, and other nonbreast cancer survivors; however, the evidence is still sparse — even for the most common cancers (e.g., prostate, colorectal). Encouragingly, recent research on nonbreast cancer survivor groups has been increasing in quantity and quality.

ACKNOWLEDGMENTS

Kerry S. Courneya is supported by the Canada Research Chairs Program and a Research Team Grant from the National Cancer Institute of Canada with funds from the Canadian Cancer Society and the Sociobehavioral Cancer Research Network. Kristin L. Campbell and Kristina H. Karvinen are supported by a Health Research Studentship from the Alberta Heritage Foundation for Medical Research.

REFERENCES

1. American Cancer Society. (2004). *Cancer Facts and Figures 2004*. Atlanta: American Cancer Society.
2. Frogge, M.H. & Cunning, S.M. (2000). Surgical therapy. In C.H. Yarbro, M. Goodman, M.H. Frogge & S.L. Groenwald (Eds.), *Cancer Nursing: Principles and Practice*. Sudbury, MA: Jones & Bartlett Publishers.
3. Maher, K.E. (2000). Radiation therapy: toxicities and management. In C.H. Yarbro, M. Goodman, M.H. Frogge, & S.L. Groenwald (Eds.), *Cancer Nursing: Principles and Practice* (pp. 323–351). Sudbury, MA: Jones & Bartlett Publishers; Mc Bride, C.M., Clipp, E., Peterson, B.L., Lipkus, I.M., & Demark–Wahnefried, W. (2000). Psychological impact of diagnosis and risk reduction among cancer survivors. *Psychooncology*, 9:418–427.
4. Camp–Sorrell, D. (2000). Chemotherapy: toxicity management. In C.H. Yarbro, M. Goodman, M.H. Frogge, & S.L. Groenwald (Eds.), *Cancer Nursing: Principles and Practice* (pp. 444–486). Sudbury, MA: Jones & Bartlett Publishers.
5. Battiato, L.A. & Wheeler, V.S. (2000). Biotherapy. In C.H. Yarbro, M. Goodman, M.H. Frogge, & S.L. Groenwald (Eds.), *Cancer Nursing: Principles and Practice* (pp. 543–579). Sudbury, MA: Jones & Bartlett Publishers.
6. Ferrans, C.E. (2000). Quality of Life as an outcome of cancer care. In C.H. Yarbro, M. Goodman, M.H. Frogge, and S.L. Groenwald (Eds.) *Cancer Nursing: Principles & Practice*. (pp. 243–258). Sudbury, MA: Jones and Bartlett Publishers.
7. Farquhar, M. (1995). Definitions of quality of life: a taxonomy. *J Adv Nursing*, 22, 502–508.
8. Ware, J.E., Sherbourne, C., et al. (1992). The MOS 36-Item Short-Form Health Survey (SF-36): 1. Conceptual framework and item selection. *Med Care*, 30, 473–483.
9. Schag, C.A. & Heinrich, R.L. (1990). Development of a comprehensive quality of life measurement tool: CARES. *Oncology*, 4, 135–138.

10. Aaronson, N.K., Ahmedzai, S., Bergman, B., et al. (1993). The European Organization for Research and Treatment of Cancer QLQ-C30: a quality-of-life instrument for use in international clinical trials in oncology. *J Natl Cancer Inst*, 85, 365–376.
11. Schipper, H., Clinch, J., McMurray, A., & Levitt, M. (1984). Measuring the quality of life of cancer patients: the Functional Living Index — Cancer: development and validation. *J Clin Oncol*, 2, 472–483.
12. Cella, D.F., Tulsky, D.S., Gray, G., Sarafian, B., Linn, E., Bonomi, A., Silberman, M., Yellen, S.B., Winicour, P., Brannon, J., Eckberg, J., Lloyd, S., Purl, S., Blendowski, C., Goodman, M., Barnicle, M., Stewart, I., McHale, M., Bonomi, P., Kaplan, E., Taylor, S., Thomas, C.R., & Harris, J. (1993). The functional assessment of cancer therapy scale: development and validation of the general measure. *J Clin Oncol*, 11, 570–579.
13. Courneya, K.S. (2003). Exercise in cancer survivors: an overview of research. *Med Sci Sports Exercise*, 35, 1846–1852.
14. Courneya, K.S., Friedenreich, C.M., Sela, R.A., Quinney, H.A., Rhodes, R.E., & Handman, M. (2003). The Group Psychotherapy and Home-Based Physical Exercise (GROUP-HOPE) Trial in cancer survivors: physical fitness and quality of life outcomes. *Psychooncology*, 12, 357–374.
15. Dimeo, F., Stieglitz, R.D., Novelli–Fischer, U., Fetscher, S., Mertelsmann, R., & Keul, J. (1997) Correlation between physical performance and fatigue in cancer patients. *Ann Oncol*, 8:1251–1255.
16. Keats, M.R., Courneya, K.S., Danielsen, S., & Whitsett, S.F. (1999). Leisure-time physical activity and psychosocial well-being in adolescents after cancer diagnosis. *J Pediatr Oncol Nursing*, 16:180-188.
17. Courneya, K.S. Keats, M.R., and Turner, R.A. (2000). Physical exercise and quality of life in cancer patients following high dose chemotherapy and autologous bone marrow transplantation. *Psychooncology*. 9:127–136.
18. Dimeo, F., Fetscher, S., Lange, W., Mertelsmann, R., & Keul, J. (1997) Effects of aerobic exercise on the physical performance and incidence of treatment-related complications after high-dose chemotherapy. *Blood*, 90:3390–3394.
19. Dimeo, F.C., Tilmann, M.H., Bertz, H., et al. (1997). Aerobic exercise in the rehabilitation of cancer patients after high dose chemotherapy and autologous peripheral stem cell transplantation. *Cancer*. 79:1717–1722.
20. Dimeo, F., Rumberger, B.G., & Keul, J. (1998) Aerobic exercise as therapy for cancer fatigue. *Med Sci Sports Exerc*, 30:475–478.
21. Durak, E.P. & Lilly PC. (1998) The application of an exercise and wellness program for cancer patients: a preliminary outcomes report. *J Strength Cond Res*, 12:3–6.
22. Durak, E.P, Lilly, P.C., & Hackworkth, J.L. (1999). Physical and psychosocial reponses to exercise in cancer patients: a 2-year follow-up survey with prostate, leukemia, and general carcinoma. *JEPonline*, 2.
23. Dimeo, F.C., Stieglitz, R.D., Novelli–Fischer, U., Fetscher, S., & Keul, J. (1999). Effects of physical activity on the fatigue and psychologic status of cancer patients during chemotherapy. *Cancer*, 85:2273–2277.
24. Shore, S. & Shepard, R.J. (1999). Immune responses to exercise in children treated for cancer. *J Sports Med Phys Fitness*, 39:240–243.
25. Porock, D., Kristjanson, L.J., Tinnelly, K., Duke, T., & Blight, J. (2000). An exercise intervention for advanced cancer patients experiencing fatigue: a pilot study. *J Palliat Care*, 16:30–36.
26. Burnham, T.R. & Wilcox, A. (2002). Effects of exercise on physiological and psychological variables in cancer survivors. *Med Sci Sports Exercise*, 34, 1863–1867.
27. Young–McCaughan, S., Mays, M.Z., Arzola, S.M., Yoder, L.H., Dramiga, S.A., Leclerc, K.M., et al. (2003). Research and commentary: change in exercise tolerance, activity and sleep patterns and quality of life in patients with cancer participating in a structured exercise program. *Oncol Nursing Forum*, 30, 441–454.
28. Courneya, K.S. & Friedenreich, C.M. (1997). Relationship between exercise pattern across the cancer experience and current quality of life in colorectal cancer survivors. *J Alternative Complementary Med*, 3, 215–226.

29. Courneya, K.S., Friedenreich, C.M., Arthur, K., & Bobick, T.M., (1999). Understanding exercise motivation in colorectal cancer pateints: a prospective study using the theory of planned behavior. *Rehabil Psychol,* 44:68–84.
30. McBride, C.M., Clipp, E., Peterson, B.L., Lipkus, I.M., & Denmark–Wahnerfried W. (2000) Psychological impact of diagnosis and risk reduction among cancer survivors. *Psychooncology*, 9(5), 418–427.
31. Jones, L.W., Courneya, K.S., Vallance, J.K.H., et al. (2004). Association between exercise and quality of life in multiple myeloma cancer survivors, *Supp Care Cancer.* 12:780–788.
32. Vallance J.K.H., Courneya, K.S., Jones, L.W., and Reiman, A.R. (in press). Differences in quality of life between non-hodgkins lymphoma survivors meeting and not meeting public health exercise guidelines. *Psychooncology.*
33. Decker, W.A., Turner–McGlade, J., & Fehir, K.M., (1989). Psychological aspects and the Physiological effects of a cardiopulmonary exercise program in patients undergoing bone marrow transplantation (BMT) for acute leukemia (AL). *Transplant Proc*, 21:3068–3069.
34. Schwartz, A.L., Thompson, J.A., & Masood, N. (2002). Interferon-induced fatigue in patients with melanoma: a pilot study of exercise and methylphenidate. *Oncol Nursing Forum*, 29:E85–90.
35. Courneya, K.S., Friedenreich, C.M., Quinney, H.A., Fields, A.L.A., Jones, L.W., & Fairey, A.S. (2003). A randomized trial of exercise and quality of life in colorectal cancer survivors. *Eur J Cancer Care*, 12, 347–357.
36. Oldervoll, L.M., Kaasa, S., Knobel, H., & Loge, J.H. (2003). Interferon-induced fatigue in patients with melanoma: a pilot study of exercise and methylphenidate. *Oncol Nursing Forum*, 39, 57–63.
37. Segal, R., Reid, R.D., Courneya, K.S., Malone, S.C., Parliament, M.B., Scott, C.G., et al. (2003). Resistance exercise in men receiving androgen deprivation therapy for prostate cancer. *J Clin Oncol*, 21, 1653–1659.
38. Coleman, E.A., Coon, S., Hall-Barrow, J., et al. (2003). Feasability of exercise during treatment for multiple myeloma. *Cancer Nurs.* 26:410-419.
39. McNeely, M.L., Parliament, M.B., Courneya, K.S., & Haykowsky, M. (2004). Resistance exercise for post neck dissection shoulder pain: three case reports. *Physiother Theory Pract*, 20:41–56.
40. Corneya, K.S., Mackey, J.R., Bell, G.J., et al. (2003). Randomized controlled trial of exercise training in postmenopausal breast cancer survivors: cardiopulmonary and quality of life outcomes. *J Clin Oncol.* 21:1660–1668.
41. Courneya, K.S. (2001). Exercise interventions during cancer treatment: biopsychological outcomes. *Exerc Sport Sci Rev.* 29:60–64.

26 Physical Activity and Physiological Effects Relevant to Prognosis

Page E. Abrahamson and Marilie D. Gammon

CONTENTS

INTRODUCTION

Although physical activity has been consistently shown to reduce the risk of cancers of the colon and breast [1], little is known about whether physical activity also influences cancer recurrence or mortality. Much of the previous research among cancer survivors has successfully identified many clinical factors, such as treatment modalities and tumor characteristics, that enhance survival. However, given that modifiable lifestyle factors such as physical activity decrease the risk of cancer development, it is plausible that these factors could also have a favorable impact on cancer prognosis. Most research addressing physical activity among cancer survivors, however, has focused on exercise as a means to improve quality of life issues (i.e., sleep, fatigue, anxiety, depression, etc.) during and following cancer treatment [2].

Long-term survival rates for cancer patients have largely improved over the past 20 years due to advanced approaches in early detection techniques and adjuvant treatment [3]. More than 9 million cancer survivors currently live in the U.S. [4], and survivors are quite interested in identifying behaviors that they can undertake in an effort to alter the course of their disease. Recreational activity is a prime candidate to consider because of the opportunity for behavioral modification and the many noncancer health benefits of exercise. Identifying any beneficial prognostic effects of exercise on cancer survival might allow for recommendations to be made regarding its use as a clinical prognostic indicator and provide a basis for intervention strategies aimed at helping cancer patients make lifestyle changes to improve prognosis. Interventions among survivors are under way to promote increased physical activity [5] to test the effect of activity on general well-being or alleviate treatment-related symptoms [2,6], but little is known of whether it can actually help to reduce a person's chance of dying.

Factors such as physical activity that play a role in preventing cancer occurrence could also affect subsequent survival. The biological mechanisms suspected to mediate the relationship between physical activity and cancer development may continue to influence prognosis. Regular moderate activity has been hypothesized to affect cancer onset by altering endogenous sex hormones (particularly for hormone-related cancers such as breast or prostate), prostaglandins (mainly colon cancer, but perhaps breast or prostate as well), immune function, insulin or insulin-like growth factors (IGF), and body weight [7].

Few studies have investigated the various physiological responses of exercise among cancer survivors to gain further understanding of potential mechanisms related to recurrence, the presence of metastases, or mortality. The effect of exercise on hormone changes has been examined in one small pilot study of breast cancer survivors in which a slight, nonsignificant decrease in hormone levels associated with activity was reported [8]. One randomized controlled trial addressed exercise training on changes in insulin, insulin resistance, IGF, and IGF-binding protein (IGFBP) among post-treatment breast cancer survivors [9]. In this study, exercise had significant physiological effects on IGF-1, IGFBP-3, and the IGF–IFGBP-3 molar ratio, but no difference was observed between the treatment and control groups for fasting insulin, glucose, insulin resistance, IGF-II, or IGFBP-1.

Several interventions conducted among breast cancer patients have shown physical activity programs to result in weight loss [10]. Among cancer survivors, the potential mechanism most studied in relation to exercise is immune function. A recent review of six small experimental studies of activity during or after treatment found that four studies reported statistically significant improvements in cancer-related immune system function [11]. Although literature regarding the physiological response to exercise among survivors is beginning to emerge, it is still unclear how and whether any of these changes relate to cancer survival because none of the studies described earlier included cancer recurrence or mortality as an outcome.

METHODS

A comprehensive literature search was performed to identify epidemiological studies that examined recreational or occupational physical activity in relation to cancer survivorship, excluding those focused on quality of life issues. A computerized search of English language publications up to June 2004 was conducted using the PubMed online database (National Library of Medicine, Bethesda, MD) as well as manual searches of abstract lists for recent cancer or epidemiology conferences and the reference lists of all relevant articles. This search revealed pertinent articles for three distinct areas of research.

In this chapter, studies evaluating the relationship between physical activity and survival endpoints among cohorts of cancer survivors are reviewed. Next, studies addressing the association between physical activity and the risk of cancer mortality among apparently healthy noncancer cohorts are discussed. Finally, studies of physical activity prevalence in cancer survivors are examined to understand the effects of a cancer diagnosis on exercise patterns. No studies were found that explored whether cancer prognosis was associated with occupational physical activity.

RESULTS

Studies of Physical Activity and Prognosis among Cancer Survivors

Table 26.1 outlines three studies (one published article [12] and two conference abstracts [13,14]) that examined the effect of physical activity on survival within cohorts of cancer survivors. All three studies were limited to examining the effects of recreational exercise among breast cancer survivors. Two recent reports based on large numbers of women with breast cancer — one using data from population-based cohort studies in New Jersey and Atlanta [14] and the other from the Nurse's Health Study [13] — provide evidence for a reduced risk of death associated with higher levels of activity. In contrast, the smallest study, based on data from a population-based study in

TABLE 26.1
Epidemiological Studies of Physical Activity and Survival among Cancer Patient Cohorts

Study population	Study size (no. deaths)	Year of diagnosis	Years of follow-up	Physical activity measure	Main results	Adjusted factors	Author, year, ref.
Breast cancer patients aged < 55 years at diagnosis in Atlanta and New Jersey	1264 (292)	1990–1992	8–10	Intensity and frequency used to calculate relative units for year prior to diagnosis	All-cause mortality, high 4th vs. low 4th (reference): HR = 0.78 (95% CI = 0.56–1.08) p-value for linear trend = 0.10	Stage, income (BMI did not confound)	Abrahamson, 2004, 14
Breast cancer patients from the Nurses Health Study	2296 (230)	1984–1996	6–16	MET-h/week at least 2 years after diagnosis	Breast cancer mortality: <3 MET-h/week: reference 3–8.9: RR = 0.81 (95% CI = 0.59–1.13) 9–14.9: RR = 0.46 (95% CI = 0.26–0.82) 15–23.9 RR = 0.58 (95% CI = 0.38–0.90) 24: RR = 0.71 (95% CI = 0.46–1.09) p-value for the linear trend = 0.05. Similar results for breast cancer recurrence	Stage, BMI, and “other factors”	Holmes, 2004, 13
Breast cancer patients; aged 20–74 years at diagnosis in Australia	412 (112)	1982–1984	5–7	Kcal/week in the year prior to diagnosis	Breast cancer mortality by kcal/week: 0: HR = reference >0 – ≤2000: HR = 1.42 (95% CI = 0.78–2.60) >2000 – ≤4000: HR = 0.73 (95% CI = 0.37–1.42) >4000: HR = 0.98 (95% CI = 0.50–1.94) P for trend: 0.80	Age, ER and PR status, tumor size, education, history of benign breast disease, age at menarche, age at first birth, height, BMI, energy intake, menopausal status	Rohan, 1995, 12

Australia, found no association [12]. The effect estimates were adjusted for different factors in each study, but each controlled for tumor stage or for size; this is important because mortality rates differ significantly by stage of disease [3].

There were some important differences among these studies that could explain in part the lack of consistency between these results. Accurately and comprehensively assessing physical activity levels is a challenge in epidemiological studies. As is often the case, the methods of measuring activity varied tremendously. The assessment tools used in each study included different types of activities and none took into account all three of the important components of activity (frequency, duration, and intensity), which is considered critical for a comprehensive assessment. The timing of the physical activity measurement should also be taken into consideration because important time periods of physical activity (for example, before or after diagnosis and treatment) may enhance survival, although no specific critical time period has yet been identified. Two studies [12,14] measured recreational activity in the year prior to diagnosis and reported conflicting results; the other [13] evaluated the effect of exercise at least 2 years following diagnosis and reported a decrease in mortality. Thus, it remains unclear whether the timing of the physical activity is critical in influencing survival.

Mortality rates varied among these three survivorship studies from as low as 10% [13] to a high of 27% [12]. This variation could be due to differences in the outcome (breast cancer mortality vs. all-cause mortality), distribution of disease stage, and the amount of follow-up time since diagnosis, which ranged from 5 to 16 years. The study populations also varied considerably with respect to age at diagnosis, geographic location, and year of diagnosis; these factors could affect results if mortality or physical activity level is related to any of them. For instance, the average 5-year survival was 78% overall for women diagnosed during 1983 to 1985 compared with 87% for those diagnosed later in 1992 to 1999 [15].

It is inappropriate to draw any strong conclusions regarding the relationship between physical activity and breast cancer survival, given the limited number of studies. However, the two most recently reported studies [13,14] are very promising. This points to a great need for further research among breast cancer survivors, as well as survivors of other cancers, among whom no studies have been conducted.

Studies of Physical Activity and Risk of Cancer Mortality among Noncancer Cohorts

Table 26.2 lists the epidemiological cohort studies investigating the relationship between recreational physical activity and risk of all-cancer or cancer-specific mortality among adults who were free of cancer at study entry. In each of these cohorts, healthy adults were assessed for physical activity at the time of enrollment and followed for assorted lengths of time to assess cancer-related deaths. Studies with all-cause mortality as the end-point were excluded because, among noncancer survivors, a large portion of those deaths are assumed to be attributable to cardiovascular or other noncancer diseases.

Interpretation of the results found in the studies shown in Table 26.2 is difficult. In cohort studies in which the outcome under study is mortality and cancer incidence is not assessed, the results are clouded. Because it is known that physical activity reduces the incidence of several of the most common cancers (breast and colon, for example), any association noted with cancer mortality in these studies may simply reflect the association between activity and the development of cancer. Alternatively, these results could indicate that exercise reduces the incidence and mortality of all but the most severe cases of cancer.

Despite the ambiguity in interpreting them, the cohort studies shown in Table 26.2 may be informative, given the few available studies of exercise and prognosis among cohorts comprised entirely of cancer survivors. The results from these general population studies are mixed. With respect to all-cancer mortality, three investigations reported a statistically significant inverse rela-

TABLE 26.2
Epidemiological Studies of Physical Activity (PA) and Cancer Mortality in Noncancer Cohorts

Study population	Study size and year of PA assessment	Years/date of follow-up since PA assessment	Physical activity measure	Main results	Adjusted factors	Author, year, ref.
Women aged ≥ 65 at baseline, Study of Osteoporotic Fractures	1. Baseline: n = 9518 (1986–1988) 2. To assess PA changes, measured again 4–7.7 years later (1992–1994): n = 7553	1. Up to 12.5 years 2. Up to 6.7 years	Walking; frequency and duration of leisure activities in past year; k-cal/week	1. Cancer mortality (633 deaths) by quintile: 1: reference 2: HR = 0.77 (95% CI = 0.60–0.97) 3: HR = 0.90 (95% CI = 0.71–1.13) 4: HR = 0.62 (95% CI = 0.48–0.81) 5: HR = 0.85 (95% CI = 0.67–1.09) No association with walking. 2. PA changes: PA at time 1, PA at time 2 Cancer mortality (264 deaths) Sedentary, sedentary: reference Sedentary, active: HR = 0.49 (0.29–0.84) Active, sedentary: HR = 0.61 (0.42–0.90) Active, active: HR = 0.82 (0.58–1.16)	1. Age, smoking, BMI, stroke, diabetes, hypertension, self-rated health 2. Same as no. 1, plus coronary heart disease, cancer, chronic obstructive pulmonary disease, hip fracture, baseline physical activity	Gregg, 2003, 19
College Alumni Health Study, mean age = 47 at baseline, 93% men	N = 32,687 (Baseline in 1962 or 1966; updated again in 1977, 1980, 1988, or 1993)	Until 1995	Frequency and duration of walking, stair climbing, sports and recreational activities in past week	Pancreatic cancer mortality (212 deaths): < 2100 kJ/week: RR = 1.0 2100–4199: RR = 0.98 (95% CI = 0.65–1.49) 4200–10,499: RR = 0.92 (0.62–1.35) ≥10,500: RR = 1.31 (0.69–1.92) p for trend = 0.24 Similar pattern for walking, stairs climbed, or broken down by light, moderate, or vigorous activity.	Age, gender, smoking, diabetes mellitus	Lee, 2003, 29
Swedish men aged 48.6–51.1 years at baseline	N = 2285 (1970–1973)	Up to 25.7 years	Three questions: Sedentary, walking or cycling, and active sport or heavy gardening	Cancer mortality (n = 216 deaths): Low PA: RR 1.09 (95% CI = 0.73–1.64) Medium PA: 0.96 (0.70–1.33) High PA: reference	Age, height, BMI, serum fatty acids, blood pressure, serum triglycerides, cholesterol, serum glucose, smoking	Kilander, 2001, 23

– *(continued)*

TABLE 26.2 (CONTINUED)
Epidemiological Studies of Physical Activity (PA) and Cancer Mortality in Noncancer Cohorts

Study population	Study size and year of PA assessment	Years/date of follow-up since PA assessment	Physical activity measure	Main results	Adjusted factors	Author, year, ref.
Nurses Health Study, women aged 30–55 years at first baseline	N = 80,348 (1980, 1982, 1986, 1988, and 1992 combined to obtain cumulative PA level)	Until 1996	1980: single question of average hours/week spent on a variety of activities listed; 1982: hours/week engaged in activity strenuous enough to build up a sweat; 1986, 1988, 1992: average time/week during previous year spent on a variety of activities	Cancer mortality (4746 deaths): <1 h/week: reference 1–1.9: RR = 0.92 (0.83–1.02) 2–3.9: RR = 0.85 (0.76–0.94) 4–6.9: RR = 0.95 (0.85–1.07) ≥7: RR = 0.87 (0.72–1.04) p for trend = 0.25	Age at baseline, smoking, alcohol, height, BMI, postmenopausal hormone use	Rockhill, 2001, 21
Whitehall Study, British men aged 40–64 years at baseline	N = 11,663 (1967–1969)	Until 1995	Minutes walking or bicycling to and from work each day	Cancer mortality (1151 deaths) in men without disease at study entry: 0–9 min/day: RR = 1.05 (0.9–1.2) 10–19: RR = 0.99 (0.9–1.1) ≥20: reference; p for trend = 0.62 Lung cancer mortality (308 deaths): 0–9 min/day: RR = 1.30 (1.0–1.8) 10–19: RR = 1.03 (0.8–1.3) ≥20: reference; p for trend = 0.12 No association for mortality from prostate, colon, hematopoietic, stomach, rectal, or pancreas cancers	Age, employment grade, BMI, smoking, forced expiratory volume in 1 sec	Batty, 2001, 24

Whitehall Study, British men aged 40–64 years at baseline	N = 6619 (1969–1970)	Until 1995	Participation in sports or hobbies; classified as active (vigorous sports), moderately active (active hobbies), or inactive (no physical exertion)	Cancer mortality (636 deaths) in men without disease at study entry: Inactive: RR = 1.34 (1.1–1.7) Moderately active: RR = 1.19 (1.0–1.5) Active: RR = reference; p for trend < 0.01 Stronger pattern for hematopoietic, cancers, but no statistically significant association for mortality from lung or colorectal cancer	Age, employment grade, BMI, smoking, forced expiratory volume in 1 sec	Davey Smith, 2000, 16
Honolulu Heart Program, men aged 61–81 of Japanese ancestry	N = 707 (1980–1982)	12 years	Average miles walked per day	Cancer mortality (62 deaths): 0–0.9 vs. 2.1–8 miles/day: RR = 2.4 (1.1–5.4) 0.0–0.9 vs. 1.0–2.0: RR = 1.5 (0.9–2.7) 1.0–2.0 vs. 2.1–8.0: RR = 1.6 (0.8–3.4) p for trend = 0.02	Age, cholesterol, alcohol use, overall physical activity, hypertension, diabetes, % Japanese diet	Hakim, 1998, 17
Iowa Women's Health Study, aged 55–69 at baseline	N = 32,763 (1986)	7 years	Frequency of participation in (1) moderate or (2) vigorous activity	Cancer mortality (1101 deaths): 1. Frequency of moderate activity: Rarely/never: RR = 1.0 1/week to few/month: RR = 0.79 (0.60–1.03) 2–4 times/week: RR = 0.80 (0.61–1.05) >4 times/week: RR = 0.85 (0.63–1.15) p for trend = 0.33 2. Frequency of vigorous activity: Rarely/never: RR = 1.0 1/week to few/month: RR = 1.09 (0.77–1.53) 2–4 times/week: RR = 0.83 (0.52–1.33) >4 times/week: RR = 0.69 (0.31–1.54) p for trend = 0.28 No association using physical activity index (low, medium, high) created from combining moderate and vigorous	Ages at baseline, menarche, first live birth, menopause, parity; alcohol use; total energy intake; smoking; estrogen use; BMI at baseline and age 18; waist-to-hip ratio, education; marital status; family history of cancer	Kushi, 1997, 25

(continued)

TABLE 26.2 (CONTINUED)
Epidemiological Studies of Physical Activity (PA) and Cancer Mortality in Noncancer Cohorts

Study population	Study size and year of PA assessment	Years/date of follow-up since PA assessment	Physical activity measure	Main results	Adjusted factors	Author, year, ref.
Adults aged 20–88 years old (22% women) at baseline from the Cooper Clinic in Texas	*N* = 29,903 (1975–1989)	Average of ~8 years	Sedentary (no activity); category I–II (1–10 miles/week of walk, jog, run, or other activities); category III (11–20 miles/week of walk, jog, or run); category IV–V (>20 miles/week of walk, jog, or run)	Cancer mortality in men (139 deaths): Sedentary: RR = 1.0 I–II: RR = 0.71 (0.49–1.03) III: RR = 0.42 (0.18–0.97) IV–V: RR = 0.15 (0.02–1.12) P for trend = 0.002 Cancer mortality in women (31 deaths): Sedentary: RR = 1.0 I–II: RR = 0.84 (0.38–1.88) III: RR = 0.95 (0.21–4.37) IV–V: RR = 2.85 (0.62–13.16) P for trend = 0.56	Age at baseline, examination year, smoking, chronic illnesses, and electrocardiogram abnormalities	Kampert, 1996, 20
Framingham Heart Study, women only, aged 50–74 at baseline	*N* = 1404 (1969–1973)	16 years	Time spent sleeping, resting, or engaged in light, moderate, or vigorous activity	Cancer deaths by activity quartile, no. (%): 1 (lowest): 35 (32%) 2: 35 (32%) 3: 21 (19 %) 4 (highest): 17 (16%)	None	Sherman, 1994, 22
German vegetarians ≥ 10 years at baseline (55% female)	*N* = 1904 (1978)	11 years	Self-evaluation of physical activity level (high, medium, or low)	Cancer mortality: Low: reference Medium or high: RR = 0.95 (0.30–3.03)	None	Chang–Claude, 1993, 27
British Regional Heart Study, men aged 40–59 at baseline	*N* = 7496 (1978–1980)	9.5 years	Frequency of regular walking or cycling, recreational activity, or sporting (vigorous) activity	Cancer mortality (217 deaths): Inactive/occasional: RR = 1.0 Light/moderate: RR = 0.84 (0.63–1.15) Vigorous: RR = 0.59 (0.38–0.92) Similar pattern when limiting to lung or digestive cancers, but not "other sites"	Age, systolic blood pressure, BMI, smoking, social class, alcohol use, blood cholesterol, ischemic heart disease	Wannamethee, 1993, 18

Canada Health Survey, men and women aged 30–69 at baseline	N = 9486 (1978–1979)	7 years	Physical activity index based on frequency, duration, and intensity of different activities	Cancer mortality (165 deaths): Very active: RR = 1.0 Active: RR = 1.4 (0.8–2.3) Moderate: RR = 0.8 (0.4–1.4) Inactive: RR = 1.2 (0.7–1.9)	Age, sex, smoking, alcohol use	Arraiz, 1992, 26
Multiple Risk Factor Intervention Trial, men aged 35–57 at baseline	N = 12,138 (1974)	10.5 years	Minutes/day of activity	Cancer mortality (265 deaths) by tertiles: 0–29 min/day: HR = 1.0 30–69 min/day: HR = 1.22 (0.91–1.63) 70–359 min/day: HR = 1.06 (0.78–1.44)	Age, treatment vs. control group of intervention, blood cholesterol, blood pressure, smoking	Leon, 1991, 28

tionship between activity level and risk of cancer death [16–18], four others found an inverse association that was not statistically significant [19–22], and no association was observed for the remaining six studies [23–28]. The majority of these studies were able to control for potential confounding factors. However, it is possible that assessment of these factors may have been inadequate if these changed over the course of the follow-up period.

Few studies examined the relationship between physical activity and risk of death from specific cancers. One of the studies with a statistically significant relationship for all-cancer mortality observed similar results for lung or digestive cancer mortality, but no such relationship for "other cancers" [18]. In the Whitehall Study, which is a cohort of British middle-aged men, among those who were physically inactive, a worse prognosis was observed for all-cancer or hematopoietic cancer mortality, but no significant association was found for mortality from lung or colorectal cancer [16]. Another analysis from the Whitehall Study observed an inverse relationship between the number of minutes walking or bicycling to work each day and lung cancer mortality, but no association for all-cancer mortality or death from prostate, colon, hematopoietic, stomach, rectal, or pancreatic cancers [24]. One study looked exclusively at pancreatic cancer mortality and found no association with physical activity level [29].

Many possible explanations can be offered for the equivocal results. There was tremendous heterogeneity between these cohorts with regard to gender, age, study size, period of enrollment, geographic location, number of years of follow-up, and the year of study enrollment when physical activity was assessed. As with the studies in the preceding section, the physical activity assessment was seldom consistent and few measured all three major components of exercise: frequency, duration, and intensity. A big concern with long-term cohorts is the potential for misclassification of the physical activity exposure if the activity level measured at baseline is not reflective of average levels prior to the time of study entry or changes in activity during the follow-up period.

Most of these studies measured physical activity only once at baseline and none attempted to assess lifetime activity. One study combined 5 years of physical activity assessments over a 12-year period to obtain a cumulative average activity level [21]. Another study assessed activity at baseline and again 4.7 to 7 years later to assess the effect of changes in activity level. In this study, no association was present for the baseline measure alone, but those who were sedentary at baseline and then considered active at the second interval had a significantly lower risk of cancer death compared to those who were sedentary at both points in time [19].

Although the relationship between physical activity and risk of cancer death remains inconclusive, a small majority of the studies listed in Table 26.2 point in the direction of a preventive role of physical activity on cancer mortality. More research with better assessment methods for physical activity among cohorts of cancer survivors is clearly needed.

Prevalence of Physical Activity among Cancer Survivors

Studies examining the prevalence of recreational physical activity among cancer survivors are described in Table 26.3. These employ several different types of study designs. Several studies simply reported the prevalence of activity. A study of prostate and breast cancer survivors found the majority (62 and 56%, respectively) reported being active ("activity that gets your heart thumping or causes you to sweat for periods > 30 minutes") on a routine weekly basis [30]. However, another small study [31] of breast cancer patients found most women to exercise below American College of Sports Medicine [32] guidelines (vigorous exercise at least ≥ three times/week for ≥20 minutes per day or moderate exercise ≥ five times per week for ≥30 minutes per day). A report on survivors of childhood cancers found that those who were still under age 18 remained relatively active, but that survivors over 18 were active much less frequently [33].

Activity levels of long-term cancer survivors (mean of 10 to 12 years following diagnosis) were compared to controls in two of the most recent studies. One Norwegian study reported higher levels of activity for the testicular cancer survivors compared to controls sampled from the general

TABLE 26.3
Epidemiological Studies Reporting Prevalence of Physical Activity (PA) among Cancer Survivors

Cancer type	Study population	Physical activity measure	Time between diagnosis and PA measure	Main results	Author, year, ref.
Breast	335 cases and 16,880 noncases aged ≥ 18 years from the 1998 National Health Interview Study	Frequency and duration of light, moderate, or vigorous activity	Mean = 10.1 years	Similar proportion of survivors (22.8%)[a] were active compared to controls (24.1%);[a] survivors were more likely than controls to meet American College of Sports Medicine guidelines [32] for vigorous activity (OR^b = 1.42, 95% CI = 0.97–2.10) and total activity (OR^b = 1.28, 95% CI = 0.91–1.80), but not light/moderate activities (OR^b = 0.95, 95% CI = 0.62–1.46)	Blanchard, 2003, 35
Adult cancers	352 cases with mean age of 59.6 from seven U.S. states	"Has the amount you exercise changed since you were diagnosed with cancer?"	43.1% ≤ 1 year since diagnosis; 56.9% > 1 year	15.7% exercised more, 53.6% exercised the same, and 30.6% exercised less; increasing exercise was related to older age (≥55 vs. <55), African American ethnicity (vs. white), >1 year since diagnosis (vs. ≤1 year), and not currently in treatment after adjusting for age, gender, race, marital status, income, education, living arrangement, cancer site, stage, time since diagnosis, treatment status	Blanchard, 2003, 36
Breast, prostate, and colorectal (diagnosed 1997–1998)	356 adults aged 20–79 years in Washington state	Patients asked if he or she had begun physical activities in the past 12 months aimed at coping with cancer or reducing risk of spreading or recurrence	Maximum of 2 years	20.8% reported adding a new physical activity	Patterson, 2003, 41
Testicular (diagnosed 1980–1994)	1276 male cases aged 20–59 years and 20,391 control men aged 18–59 in the general Norwegian population	Duration and frequency of low- and high-level PA	Mean = ~12 years	More survivors were "highly active" (43%) compared with the general population (37%), $p < 0.0001$ Likelihood of being "physically active" in survivors vs. general population: OR^c = 1.32 (95% CI = 1.10–1.58)	Thorsen, 2003, 34

(continued)

TABLE 26.3 (CONTINUED)
Epidemiological Studies Reporting Prevalence of Physical Activity (PA) among Cancer Survivors

Cancer type	Study population	Physical activity measure	Time between diagnosis and PA measure	Main results	Author, year, ref.
Breast (diagnosed 1996–1999)	812 cases in New Mexico (≥18 years old) and Washington (40–64 years old)	Type, duration, and frequency of activities for the year prior to diagnosis and the month prior to interview	4–12 months since diagnosis	Activity decreased by 2 h/week (11%, $p < 0.05$) from pre- to postdiagnosis; decreases in activity were greatest for women treated with radiation and chemotherapy compared to surgery only or radiation only and for obese women compared to normal weight women	Irwin, 2003, 37
Breast (diagnosed 1995–1997)	175 cases with mean age of 52.3 years in Alberta, Canada	Any exercise of at least moderate intensity done ≥ three times/week at prediagnosis, during treatment, and post-treatment	Mean = 20.2 months	Prediagnosis / Treatment / Post-Treatment / % Active / Active / Active / 13 Active / Active / Inactive / 2 Active / Inactive / Active / 19 Active / Inactive / Inactive / 9 Inactive / Active / Active / 2 Inactive / Active / Inactive / 3 Inactive / Inactive / Active / 9 Inactive / Inactive / Inactive / 43	Rhodes, 2001, 40
Breast and prostate (diagnosed 1992–1997)	978 cases aged 28–91 years at interview, Duke Hospital	Frequency, duration, intensity, and length of time participating in exercise since diagnosis	0.4–6.3 years since diagnosis	Prostate: 62% exercising routinely with 85% of those practicing behavior for ≥6 months for a mean of 4.6 sessions/week with sessions lasting a mean of 44.7 min Breast: 56% exercising routinely with 76% of those practicing behavior for ≥6 months for a mean of four sessions/week with sessions lasting a mean of 41.2 minutes	Demark-Wahnefried, 2000, 30
Breast	71 cases with mean age of 57.4 years in Rhode Island	Frequency, type, duration, and length of time participating in vigorous or moderate exercise since diagnosis	Mean = 248 days (range = 27–483)	20 (28%) met American College of Sports Medicine recommendations (32), 37 (52%) exercised below recommended levels, 14 (20%) did not exercise at all	Pinto, 1998, 31

Breast (diagnosed 1994–1995)	167 cases with mean age of 53.1 years in Alberta, Canada	Frequency of mild, moderate, or strenuous exercise for ≥15 min in a typical week prior to diagnosis, during treatment, and following treatment	Mean = 17.4 months	Prediagnosis	Treatment	Post-Treatment	%	Courneya, 1997, 38
				Active	Active	Active	25	
				Active	Active	Inactive	1	
				Active	Inactive	Active	28	
				Active	Inactive	Inactive	12	
				Inactive	Active	Active	2	
				Inactive	Active	Inactive	1	
				Inactive	Inactive	Active	6	
				Inactive	Inactive	Inactive	26	
Colorectal (diagnosed 1992–1995)	130 cases aged 26 to 81 years in Alberta, Canada	Frequency of mild, moderate, or strenuous exercise for ≥15 min in a typical week prior to diagnosis, during treatment, and following treatment	Mean = 27.2 months (range = 9–51)	Prediagnosis	Treatment	Post-Treatment	%	Courneya, 1997, 39
				Active	Active	Active	31	
				Active	Active	Inactive	1	
				Active	Inactive	Active	16	
				Active	Inactive	Inactive	14	
				Inactive	Active	Active	3	
				Inactive	Active	Inactive	2	
				Inactive	Inactive	Active	3	
				Inactive	Inactive	Inactive	30	
Childhood cancers	160 patients aged 9.8–29.5 years at interview in Memphis, Tennessee	Frequency of exercise habits	Age range at diagnosis = 0.2–19.9 years	Hours/week	<18 at Interview	>18 at Interview		Mulhern, 1995, 33
				<1	6.4%	17.5%		
				1–2	12.7%	35.0%		
				3–4	24.6%	22.5%		
				5–6	15.5%	7.5%		
				>6	40.9%	17.5%		

[a] Age-adjusted

[b] Adjusted for age, obesity, race, education, income, smoking, and co-morbidity

[c] Adjusted for age, BMI, education, living as a couple, co-morbidity, and smoking.

population [34]. The other study, based on the National Health Interview Study cohort, found a comparable proportion of breast cancer survivors and noncases to be active overall [35]. However, the survivors in this study were more likely to meet the American College of Sports Medicine [32] guidelines for vigorous activity or total activity, but had a similar likelihood of meeting the guidelines for light or moderate activity.

Two studies retrospectively measured pre- and postdiagnosis exercise levels. A study of adult cancer survivors found 15.7% exercised more, 53.6% exercised the same amount, and 30.6% exercised less after diagnosis compared with the earlier prediagnostic period [36]. The survivors were more likely to increase their exercise levels following diagnosis if not currently undergoing treatment and if interviewed more than a year since their diagnosis. In a similar study of breast cancer survivors interviewed 4 to 12 months following diagnosis, activity levels decreased by 2 hours/week from pre- to postdiagnosis [37]. Decreases were greatest for women treated with radiation and chemotherapy compared to surgery or radiation alone as well as for those who were obese compared to normal weight women.

Two studies of breast cancer survivors and one with colorectal cancer survivors examined physical activity participation before diagnosis, during cancer treatment, and post-treatment [38–40]. These studies generally found one quarter to one third of survivors remained consistently active or inactive at all three periods. Another large group was found to be inactive only during the treatment period; a significant proportion of those who were active prior to diagnosis never resumed an active lifestyle following treatment.

These studies provide some insight into the impact of a cancer diagnosis on physical activity behaviors. In particular, cancer patients undergo special challenges associated with treatment, such as fatigue and weight change, that may affect ability or interest in maintaining or initiating exercise. Although activity appears to diminish in the treatment phase, the studies of longer term survivors suggest that perhaps activity levels eventually resume to prediagnosis levels for most people or, at least, levels comparable to the general population. However, it is unclear how quickly activity increases during the post-treatment period.

From a methodological standpoint, it may not be sufficient to assess only prediagnosis activity in studies of physical activity and survival if prediagnosis levels are not reflective of postdiagnosis levels. To clarify whether pre- and/or postdiagnosis exercise influences survival, future studies will need to include comprehensive assessment of activity through the life course as well as the postdiagnostic period.

FUTURE DIRECTIONS

This review exposes the scarcity of research on whether survival is enhanced among those who are physically active, occupationally or recreationally, before or after cancer diagnosis. There is a strong need for further identification of new prognostic factors to improve the prediction of women at increased risk for recurrence or mortality. Physical activity is particularly noteworthy because it is a modifiable factor that could provide an opportunity for patients to enhance their survival. In addition to studying the impact of exercise on survival outcomes (mortality, recurrence, secondary cancers, and metastasis) among cohorts of survivors, intervention studies of the physiological effects of activity among cancer patients are warranted in order to better understand the potential underlying mechanisms.

Most studies reviewed here were conducted among breast cancer survivors. Future studies should include patients of different cancer sites and stages because of considerable variation in pathogenesis, mortality rates, and treatment-related problems. More thorough and comprehensive physical activity assessments that incorporate measures of intensity, duration, frequency, and timing of the activity would aid in determining the true relationship between physical activity and prognosis.

REFERENCES

1. Lee IM. Physical activity and cancer prevention: data from epidemiologic studies. *Med Sci Sports Exercise* 2003; 35(11):1823–1827.
2. Courneya KS. Exercise in cancer survivors: an overview of research. *Med Sci Sports Exercise* 2003; 35(11):1846–1852.
3. Reis LAG, Eisner MP, Kosary CL, Hankey BF, Miller BA, Clegg L, Edwards BK (Eds.) *SEER Cancer Statistics Review, 1973–1999.* 2002, Bethesda, MD: National Cancer Institute.
4. American Cancer Society. *Cancer Facts and Figures 2004.* 2004, Atlanta: American Cancer Society.
5. Demark–Wahnefried W, Clipp EC, McBride C, Lobach DF, Lipkus I, Peterson B, Clutter Snyder D, Sloane R, Arbanas J, Krause WE. Design of FRESH START: a randomized trial of exercise and diet among cancer survivors. *Med Sci Sports Exercise* 2003; 35(3):415–424.
6. Irwin ML, Ainsworth BE. Physical activity interventions following cancer diagnosis: methodologic challenges to delivery and assessment. *Cancer Invest* 2004; 22(1):30–50.
7. Westerlind KC. Physical activity and cancer prevention: mechanisms. *Med Sci Sports Exercise* 2003; 35(11):1834–1840.
8. McTiernan A, Ulrich C, Kumai C, Bean D, Schwartz R, Mahloch J, Hastings R, Gralow J, Potter J. Anthropometric and hormone effects of an eight-week exercise-diet intervention in breast cancer patients: results of a pilot study. *Cancer Epidemiol Biomarkers Prev* 1998; 7(6):477–481.
9. Fairey AS, Courneya KS, Field CJ, Bell GJ, Jones LW, Mackey JR. Effects of exercise training on fasting insulin, insulin resistance, insulin-like growth factors, and insulin-like growth factor binding proteins in postmenopausal breast cancer survivors: a randomized controlled trial. *Cancer Epidemiol Biomarkers Prev* 2003; 12(8):721–727.
10. McTiernan A. Physical activity after cancer: physiologic outcomes. *Cancer Invest* 2004; 22(1):68–81.
11. Fairey AS, Courneya KS, Field CJ, Mackey JR. Physical exercise and immune system function in cancer survivors. *Cancer* 2002; 94:539–551.
12. Rohan TE, Fu W, Hiller JE. Physical activity and survival from breast cancer. *Eur J Cancer Prev* 1995; 4(5):419–424.
13. Holmes MD, Chen WY, Feskanich D, Colditz GA. Physical activity and survival after breast cancer diagnosis. American Association of Cancer Research, Orlando, FL, March 2004.
14. Abrahamson PE, Gammon MD, Lund MJ, Britton JA, Eley W, Porter P, Brinton LA, Flagg EW, Coates RJ. Physical activity and breast cancer survival among young women. American Society of Preventive Oncology, Bethesda, MD, March 2004.
15. Surveillance, Epidemiology, and End Results Program, 1973–2000. Division of Cancer Control and Population Sciences, National Cancer Institute, Bethesda, MD, 2003.
16. Davey Smith G, Shipley MJ, Batty GD, Morris JN, Marmot M. Physical activity and cause-specific mortality in the Whitehall Study. *Public Health* 2000; 114(5):308–315.
17. Hakim AA, Petrovitch H, Burchfiel CM, Ross GW, Rodriguez BL, White LR, Yano K, Curb JD, Abbott RD. Effects of walking on mortality among nonsmoking retired men. *N Engl J Med* 1998; 338(2):94–99.
18. Wannamethee G, Shaper AG, Macfarlane PW. Heart rate, physical activity, and mortality from cancer and other noncardiovascular diseases. *Am J Epidemiol* 1993; 137(7):735–748.
19. Gregg EW, Cauley JA, Stone K, Thompson TJ, Bauer DC, Cummings SR, Ensrud KE. Relationship of changes in physical activity and mortality among older women. *JAMA* 2003; 289(18):2379–2386.
20. Kampert JB, Blair SN, Barlow CE, Kohl HW. Physical activity, physical fitness, and all-cause and cancer mortality: a prospective study of men and women. *Ann Epidemiol* 1996; 6(5):452–457.
21. Rockhill B, Willett W, Manson J, Leitzmann M, Stampfer M, Hunter D, Colditz G. Physical activity and mortality: a prospective study among women. *Am J Public Health* 2001; 91(4):578–583.
22. Sherman S, D'Agostino R, Cobb J, Kannel W. Physical activity and mortality in women in the Framingham Heart Study. *Am Heart J* 1994; 83:879–884.
23. Kilander L, Berglund L, Boberg M, Vessby B, Lithell H. Education, lifestyle factors and mortality from cardiovascular disease and cancer. A 25-year follow-up of Swedish 50-year-old men. *Int J Epidemiol* 2001; 30(5):1119–1126.
24. Batty GD, Shipley MJ, Marmot M, Smith GD. Physical activity and cause-specific mortality in men: further evidence from the Whitehall Study. *Eur J Epidemiol* 2001; 17(9):863–869.

25. Kushi LH, Fee RM, Folsom AR, Mink PJ, Anderson KE, Sellers TA. Physical activity and mortality in postmenopausal women. *JAMA* 1997; 277(16):1287–1292.
26. Arraiz GA, Wigle DT, Mao Y. Risk assessment of physical activity and physical fitness in the Canada Health Survey mortality follow-up study. *J Clin Epidemiol* 1992; 45(4):419–428.
27. Chang-Claude J, Frentzel-Beyme R. Dietary and lifestyle determinants of mortality among German vegetarians. *Int J Epidemiol* 1993; 22(2):228–236.
28. Leon AS, Connett J. Physical activity and 10.5 year mortality in the Multiple Risk Factor Intervention Trial (MRFIT). *Int J Epidemiol* 1991; 20(3):690–697.
29. Lee IM, Sesso HD, Oguma Y, Paffenbarger RS. Physical activity, body weight, and pancreatic cancer mortality. *Br J Cancer* 2003; 88(5):679–683.
30. Demark-Wahnefried W, Peterson B, McBride C, Lipkus I, Clipp EC. Current health behaviors and readiness to pursue lifestyle changes among men and women diagnosed with early stage prostate and breast carcinomas. *Cancer* 2000; 88(3):674–684.
31. Pinto BM, Maruyama NC, Engebretson TO, Thebarge RW. Participation in exercise, mood, and coping in survivors of early stage breast cancer. *J Psychosoc Oncol* 1998; 16(2):45–58.
32. Pate RR, Pratt M, Blair SN, Haskell WL, Macera CA, Bouchard C, Buchner D, Ettinger W, Heath GW, King AC, Kriska A, Leon AS, Marcus BH, Morris J, Paffenbarger RS, Patrick K, Pollock M, Rippe JM, Sallis J, Wilmore JH. Physical activity and public health. A recommendation from the Centers for Disease Control and Prevention and the American College of Sports Medicine. *JAMA* 1995; 273:402–407.
33. Mulhern RK, Tyc VL, Phipps S, Crom D, Barclay D, Greenwald C, Hudson M, Thompson EI. Health-related behaviors of survivors of childhood cancer. *Med Pediatr Oncol* 1995; 25(3):159–165.
34. Thorsen L, Nystad W, Dahl O, Klepp O, Bremnes RM, Wist E, Fossa SD. The level of physical activity in long-term survivors of testicular cancer. *Eur J Cancer* 2003; 39(9):1216–1221.
35. Blanchard CM, Cokkinides V, Courneya KS, Nehl EJ, Stein K, Baker F. A comparison of physical activity of posttreatment breast cancer survivors and noncancer controls. *Behav Med* 2003; 28(4):140–149.
36. Blanchard CM, Denniston MM, Baker F, Ainsworth SR, Courneya KS, Hann DM, Gesme DH, Reding D, Flynn T, Kennedy JS. Do adults change their lifestyle behaviors after a cancer diagnosis? *Am J Health Behav* 2003; 27(3):246–256.
37. Irwin ML, Crumley D, McTiernan A, Bernstein L, Baumgartner R, Gilliland FD, Kriska A, Ballard-Barbash R. Physical activity levels before and after a diagnosis of breast carcinoma. *Cancer* 2003; 97:1746–1757.
38. Courneya KS, Friedenreich CM. Relationship between exercise during treatment and current quality of life among survivors of breast cancer. *J Psychosoc Oncol* 1997; 15:35–57.
39. Courneya KS, Friedenreich CM. Relationship between exercise pattern across the cancer experience and current quality of life in colorectal cancer survivors. *J Altern Complement Med* 1997; 3:215–226.
40. Rhodes RE, Courneya KS, Bobick TM. Personality and exercise participation across the breast cancer experience. *Psycho-Oncology* 2001; 10:380-388.
41. Patterson RE, Neuhouser ML, Hedderson MM, Schwartz SM, Standish LJ, Bowen DJ. Changes in diet, physical activity, and supplement use among adults diagnosed with cancer. *J Am Diet Assoc* 2003; 103:323–328.

Section VII

Energy Balance and Cancer Prognosis

27 Energy Balance and Cancer Prognosis, Breast Cancer

Pamela J. Goodwin

CONTENTS

INTRODUCTION

Energy balance, as reflected by body size, has received considerable attention as a potential prognostic factor in breast cancer. In 1976, Abe [1] first reported an association of obesity with poor outcome in early stage breast cancer. As of early 2004, over 50 studies [1–51] examining this association had been published (a smaller body of research has investigated body size in metastatic breast cancer). The majority of the studies in locoregional breast cancer have identified an adverse prognostic effect of obesity, leading to a growing consensus that obesity is a significant and independent adverse prognostic factor in breast cancer. One recent review [52] concluded that "the current evidence relating increased body weight to breast cancer outcome and the documented favorable effects of weight loss on clinical outcome in other comorbid conditions support consideration of programs for weight loss in breast cancer patients." Thus, there is interest in the development of weight loss programs targeting women with breast cancer and, more importantly, in studying the effect of such programs on the outcomes of these women.

In parallel to this research examining prognostic effects of weight in breast cancer, additional work has investigated the phenomenon of weight gain after diagnosis of locoregional breast cancer [53–90]. This research has demonstrated that weight gain in this situation is common and is associated with a variety of factors (reviewed later). Some evidence indicates that large amounts of weight gain postdiagnosis may contribute to poor breast cancer outcomes. These observations have enhanced interest in the development of weight management programs for women with breast cancer.

More recently, research has increasingly focused on understanding the underlying physiological basis for an adverse prognostic effect of obesity in breast cancer [49,52,91]. Several potential mechanisms for this effect have been hypothesized; the majority focus on alterations in hormone levels (notably estrogen) in obese individuals. Recent research has suggested that insulin, a member of the insulin/IGF family of growth factors, may also play an important role. Alternate explanations include suggestions that obesity is associated with presentation of breast cancer at more advanced stages or that it may lead to undertreatment, particularly in those receiving chemotherapy. These potential mechanisms will be discussed.

Despite the growing consensus that obesity is associated with breast cancer outcome, a detailed review of the evidence supporting this potential association is necessary. The 51 published studies of obesity and locoregional breast cancer prognosis [1–51] will be reviewed in the next section, followed by a discussion of weight gain postdiagnosis. Potential pathophysiological mechanisms for an adverse prognostic effect of obesity will be discussed in subsequent sections.

OBESITY AND BREAST CANCER PROGNOSIS

Published studies examining the association of a measure of body size (weight, or an index of obesity such as body mass index (wt/ht^2, BMI) or percent ideal weight) are outlined in Table 27.1. Studies published as full reports are included; studies published in abstract form only are not included. Furthermore, only studies that focused on women with locoregional breast cancer or reported on results in locoregional breast cancer separately are included. A small number of studies in which less than 10% of the study population had advanced disease is also included, as long as the stage was considered in the analysis [14,15,20,23,31]. Studies conducted solely in advanced breast cancer are excluded because mechanisms for prognostic effects of obesity might differ significantly in the metastatic setting — for example, metastatic disease may lead to weight loss. These studies will be summarized briefly at the end of this section. Table 27.1 lists studies in chronological order, and information is provided on study design, including:

- Calendar years of recruitment
- Whether the study was single or multiple institutions
- The number of subjects with locoregional breast cancer studied
- The method used to obtain measurements of body size (typically abstraction from medical records; occasionally self-report or direct measurement)
- The measure of body size studied (typically weight, or an index of obesity such as Quetelet index or BMI)
- The menopausal status of the women studied
- The use of systemic adjuvant therapy (many studies involved women diagnosed before the widespread use of systemic adjuvant therapy and did not address this issue)
- The main results with respect to prognostic effects of obesity
- When relevant, additional comments

It can be seen that studies included in Table 27.1 span more than a quarter of a century, from 1976 to 2004. The majority were retrospective cohort studies, with patients identified through hospital records, government registries, screening programs, or, occasionally, randomized clinical trials. Most studies used measures of body size that were obtained for nonresearch proposes (usually taken from clinical records or registry databases). Approaches such as this could lead to increased measurement error, especially if factors such as the amount of clothing worn were not controlled (potentially increasing type II error) or to systematic underestimation of body size in studies in which weight was self-reported (potentially introducing bias). The size of the studies varied considerably: from 25 [7] to over 8000 [20] participants; the average size was 942 subjects.

Body size was measured for study purposes in only 12 studies [14,20,26,29,33,35, 37,38,42,44,46,49]; in the majority of these studies, it was measured many years prior to breast cancer diagnosis as part of screening or etiological studies. In the remaining studies, body size was usually obtained from medical records; occasionally, it was obtained by self-report. In several studies, subjects were recruited years prior to diagnosis for research into risk factors or screening programs [20,26,29,33,35–37,42,43,48]. By design, these studies capture the effect of body size (and other factors) on breast cancer risk and prognosis. All entries in Table 27.1 (apart from time period of recruitment) relate to the impact of body size on breast cancer prognosis. However, because body size was measured years prior to diagnosis in these studies, the relationship between

TABLE 27.1
OBESITY AND PROGNOSIS IN LOCOREGIONAL BREAST CANCER

Design (period of recruitment)	n	Body size: Method	Body size: Measure	Menopausal status	Systemic adjuvant Rx	Results	Comments	Author (ref.), year
Case-control (hospital) (1966–1976)	134	NS	Standard weight[a]	NS	NS	Reduced 5-yr. OS in obese vs. nonobese (56 vs. 80%)		Abe (1), 1976
Retrospective cohort (hospital) (1940–1965)	962	Medical records	Weight	All	None	Decreased 5-yr. DFS with increasing W (p-trend 0.025) Decreased 5-yr. DFS if W > 130 lb. (RR 1.44, $p < 0.001$ overall; RR 2.65, $p < 0.005$ N0; RR 1.27, $p > 0.10$ N1) Decreased 5-yr. BCS in N0	Women dying of non-breast cancer causes withdrawn at death Results independent of year of diagnosis	Donegan (2), 1978
Retrospective cohort (hospital) (1971–1976)	83	Medical records	Obesity index[b]	All	None	Decreased DFS if OI > 2.45 (all, trend in N0, N+) RR monthly recurrence 3× ↑ in obese women W not prognostic in N1		Donegan (3), 1978
Retrospective cohort (hospital) (1968–1974)	106	Medical records	Quetelet index[b]	All	NS	$Q > 2.45$ not associated with recurrence (all, N0, N+)		Sohrabi (4), 1980
RCT (hospital) (1965–1972)	749	Trial records	Weight Quetelet index[b]	Pre/post	(1) None (2) Ovarian radiation (<45 yrs.) (3) Ovarian radiation plus prednisone (>45 yrs.)	Decreased DFS if weight ≥ 64 kg (all, postmenopausal, trend in premenopausal) Similar findings for weight, Q, body surface area	Significant interaction of W with effectiveness of adjuvant hormone therapy Adverse effect of W greatest in tumors with favorable prognostic factors Results adjusted for stage, N, grade, menopausal status	Boyd (5), 1981

(continued)

TABLE 27.1 (CONTINUED)
OBESITY AND PROGNOSIS IN LOCOREGIONAL BREAST CANCER

Design (period of recruitment)	n	Body size		Menopausal status	Systemic adjuvant Rx	Results	Comments	Author (ref.), year
		Method	Measure					
Retrospective cohort (hospital) (prior to 1979)	374	Medical records	Weight Quetelet index[b]	All	NS	Decreased 5-yr. DFS in women ≥ 150 lb (49 vs. 67%, $p = 0.026$) ($Q \geq 3.5$ produced similar results) — overall stages 2 and 3	Greatest adverse effect of W in women with high cholesterol	Tartter (6), 1981
Case-control (hospital) (recruitment period NS)	25	Medical records	Weight % Ideal weight[c]	Pre/post	NS	W, obesity significantly associated with 10-yr. OS		Zumoff (7), 1982
Retrospective cohort (hospital) (since 1971 some earlier)	231	Medical records	Weight Quetelet index[b]	Pre/post	74 CXT	Decreased DFS, OS if weight ≥ 64 kg or Q ≥ 3.5	Significance of W (but not Q) for DFS lost with adjustment for # nodes, age — significance of both lost for OS	Eberlein (8), 1985
Retrospective cohort (hospital) (1975–1981)	237	Medical records	Weight Quetelet index[b]	Pre/post	All CXT	Decreased DFS and OS in heavier women (log rank but not Cox model significant) Similar results with Q	Similar results when N, T, ER, menopausal status included in Cox models	Heasman (9), 1985
Cohort (hospital) (1957–1965)	518	NS	Quetelet index[b]	Pre/post	NS	Obesity not associated with OS (HR 0.98–1.00)	Adjusted for age, stage	Gregorio (10), 1985
Retrospective cohort (hospital) (1975–1983)	1078	Medical records	Quetelet index[b]	Pre/post	NS	Obesity not associated with OS, BCS	Black women more likely to be obese	Ownby (11), 1985
Case-control study of OC use — follow-up of BC patients (multihospital) (1968–1977)	582	Self-report	Usual weight Quetelet index[b]	Pre	NS	Decreased OS in heavier women (RR 1.7 if weight ≥ 155 lb. vs. ≤ 112 lb., $p = 0.011$) No significant effect of Q ($p = 0.12$)	Adjusted for stage, nodes	Greenberg (12), 1985

Follow-up of BC cases in a multicity case-control study of diet and BC (1973–1975)	100	NS	Weight	Pre/post	NS	Decreased BCS with W > 63 kg vs. ≤ 63 kg. (HR = 1.68, $p = 0.023$)	Non-breast cancer deaths censored Independent of type of surgery	Newman (13), 1986
Retrospective cohort (population) (1976–1983)	1281	Measured preop weight, recalled height	BMI[b]	Pre/post	NS	No effect of BMI on recurrence after consideration of T, N Earlier recurrence if BMI ≥ 28 when T < 5 cm. or < 2 cm or N0, or ER+, PgR+	107 subjects had metastases and were not included in recurrence analyses	McNee (14), 1987
SEER registry (1973–1982)	838	Self-report	Weight BMI[b]	Pre/post	NS	Reduced OS in premenopausal women if W > 140 lbs. (HR vs. ≤ 140 = 1.7, $p = 0.04$) or BMI > 30.5 (HR vs. < 30.5 = 1.6, $p = 0.08$) No effect in postmenopausal women	16 patients were stage IV Results adjusted for stage	Mohle–Boetani (15), 1988
Retrospective cohort (hospital) (1960–1984)	637	Medical records	Weight	Pre/post	191 CXT	W not associated with RFS, OS		Goodwin (16), 1988
Retrospective cohort (hospital) (1982–1984)	472	Medical records	Weight BMI[b]	Pre/post	Induced menopause in some	BMI > 28, W > 73 kg associated with worse prognosis in stage I (HR 4.17, 3.21); nonsignificant in stage II W significantly associated with poor prognosis multivariately	Results adjusted for stage, ER, PgR, menopausal status, cholesterol, therapy Deaths and recurrence combined as prognostic outcome	Hebert (17), 1988
Historical cohort (hospital) in RCT (1971–1973)	68	Trial and hospital records	Weight/ideal weight Quetelet index[b]	Pre/post	None	Significantly decreased OS with high Quetelet index (curvilinear association)	Adjusted for stage, treatment, menopausal status	Suissa (18), 1989
Provincial cancer registry (1971–1974)	1121	NS	Weight	Pre/post	NS	Significantly decreased 10-yr. relative survival if W ≥ 66kg overall ($p = 0.39$), premenopausal ($p = 0.043$) but not postmenopausal	Adjusted for stage, N, and non-breast cancer deaths	Lees (19), 1989
National TB screening program (1963–1975)	8427	Measured years prediagnosis	Quetelet index	Pre/post	NS	Significantly reduced BCS with high Q (highest vs. lowest quintile) in stages I, II but not III, IV (age adjusted) (HR stage I 1.70, stage II 1.42)	Non-breast cancer deaths censored 636 subjects were stage IV at diagnosis	Tretli (20), 1990

(continued)

TABLE 27.1 (CONTINUED)
OBESITY AND PROGNOSIS IN LOCOREGIONAL BREAST CANCER

Design (period of recruitment)	n	Body size		Menopausal status	Systemic adjuvant Rx	Results	Comments	Author (ref.), year
		Method	Measure					
Retrospective cohort (cases in case-control study at 7 hospitals) (1975–1978)	213	Self-report	Weight Quetelet index[b] BSA	Pre/post	87 CXT; 130 hormones	Significantly reduced relative OS with high Q (adjusted for histological and clinical [stage] variables)		Kyogoku (21), 1990
Retrospective cohort (hospital) (1972–1988)	593	NS	BMI[b]	Pre/post	NS	Decreased 10-yr. (but not 5-yr.) OS in obese overall and in postmenopausal (but not premenopausal)		Kimura (22), 1990
Tumor registries (multiple hospitals) (1975–1979)	1960	NS	BMI[b]	Pre/post	82 CXT; 22 hormones	Decreased BCS with BMI ≥ 24.6 (stage III, all stages)	120 were stage IV BMI < 21.5 also associated with decreased BCS Blacks heavier but obesity effect similar to whites	Coates (23), 1990
National registry (1983–1984)	1744	Self-report	Weight BMI[b]	Pre/post	Some	No significant association of W, BMI with OS in early stage BC Low W associated with reduced OS in advanced BC	Adjusted for *T* size, number of nodes, grade, skin invasion Early BC: *T* < 4 cm., N0, grade I, no skin invasion	Ewertz (24), 1991
Cases in multihospital case-control study (1975-1980)	343	Self-report	Weight Obesity index[d]	Pre/post	NS	Obesity associated with BCS in Japanese, not Caucasians; HR 3.53 (95% CI 1.25–10.00)	Non-breast cancer deaths censored Adjusted for stage, menopausal status, fat intake	Nomura (25), 1991

National screening program (1974–1978)	242	Measured years prediagnosis	BMI[b]	Pre/post	NS	Decreased OS with high BMI (HR 2.1, 95% CI 1.2–3.8 for BMI ≥ 27 vs. < 22)	High cholesterol associated with decreased OS Adjusted for age, stage, cholesterol Attributable risk of death due to BMI: 50%	Vatten (26), 1991
Two RCTs (multihospital) (1974–1985)	1392	NS	BMI[b]	Pre/post	Some	Obesity not associated with DFS; obesity associated with BCS, OS in univariate and multivariate analyses (adjusted for ER+, nodes, *T*)	Blacks had higher BMI than whites Effect of obesity not independent of poverty	Gordon (27), 1992
Retrospective cohort (hospital) (1976–1978)	923	Medical records	Weight % Optimal weight[c]	Pre/post	NS	Decreased DFS if % optimal W $\geq 125\%$ (HR 1.45, $p = 0.003$) overall and in N0 (HR 1.93, $p = 0.001$) Decreased BCS after local but not distant recurrence in obese	Effect greatest in N0 patients Adjusted for age, stage, *T* size, CXT Similar results for BMI	Senie (28), 1992
Follow-up of BC cases developing in a population-based general health screening (1963–1965)	1170	Measured years prediagnosis	Weight	Pre/post	NS	Decreased BCS with high Q ($p = 0.0006$); HR 1.7 BMI ≥ 28 vs. ≤ 22 overall and in women 50–59 ($p = 0.009$)	Beta lipoprotein inversely associated with survival in < 50 y.o.; opposite association in ≥ 60 y.o.	Tornberg (29), 1993
Retrospective cohort —women enrolled on three adjuvant CXT protocols (hospital) (1974–1982)	735	Medical records	Ideal weight[f] Quetelet index[b]	Pre/post	All received chemotherapy	Decreased DFS and OS with higher Q ($p = 0.01$) or obesity ($> 120\%$ ideal weight) ($p \leq 0.02$)	Association of obesity with DFS, OS not linear but quadratic model did not improve fit over linear model Adjusted for stage, *N*, menopausal status	Bastarrachea (30), 1994

(continued)

TABLE 27.1 (CONTINUED)
OBESITY AND PROGNOSIS IN LOCOREGIONAL BREAST CANCER

Design (period of recruitment)	n	Body size: Method	Body size: Measure	Menopausal status	Systemic adjuvant Rx	Results	Comments	Author (ref.), year
Retrospective cohort (hospital) (1977–1985)	301	Medical records	BMI[b]	Post	112 received CXT or XRT	BMI not associated with DFS or BCS	Women with non-BC deaths excluded 18 had stage IV BC Adjusted for age, stage, *T*, *N*, ER, PgR, treatment	Katoh (31), 1994
Cases in a national case-control study (1984–1995)	422	NS	BMI[b]	Pre	NS	Increased BMI significantly associated with increased risk of death (8% increase per unit BMI, HR 5.93 for BMI $\geq$ 29 vs. < 19)	All but 2 women died of BC Adjusted for several BC risk factors, including age	Holmberg (32), 1994
Cases in RCT of mammographic screening (1980–1985)	1268	Measured years prediagnosis (mean 2.5 years)	Weight BMI[b] Triceps skinfold Weight/height	Pre/post	NS	BMI, W not associated with 5-yr. BCS	Triceps skinfold associated with 5-yr. BCS (adjusted for W, *N*, age) Non-BC death considered a withdrawal	Jain (33), 1994
Retrospective cohort — patients on CXT protocols (hospital) (1983–1989)	473	Medical records	Weight % Ideal weight[g]	Pre/post	300 received CXT; 283 (ER positive) received tamoxifen	W, % ideal weight not associated with DFS	Adjusted for *N*, *T* size, grade, ER, PgR, menopausal status	Obermair (34), 1995
Cases in population-based screening program (1974–1988)	241	Measured years prediagnosis	Weight Quetelet index[b]. Triceps and subscapular skinfold thickness	Post	NS	Q not associated with BCS	Similar findings for other body size variables	den Tonkelaar (35), 1995

Cases in population-based Iowa Women's Health Study Cohort (1986–1991)	698	Self-report years prediagnosis	Weight BMI[b] Waist/hip ratio	Post	NS	1.9 fold increased crude fatality rate in upper tertile of BMI or W (not significant after adjustment for age, stage ER)	Waist/hip ratio not associated with fatality High-calorie intake associated with increased fatality	Zhang (36), 1995
National Tuberculosis Screening Program (hospital) (1963–1975)	1238	Measured years prediagnosis	Quetelet index[b]	Pre/post	Approximately one-third of ER positive received tamoxifen	Obesity (upper quintile of Q) associated with decreased BCS at 6 yrs. ($p = 0.04$) (adjusted for T size, N, nuclear area) (HR 1.49 crude, 1.37 adjusted)	Obesity associated with decreased BCS in ER/PgR positive, increased BCS in ER/PgR negative patients Non-BC deaths censored	Maehle (37), 1996
RCT (CALGB 8541) (multihospital) (NS)	1435	Measured	BMI[b] % Ideal weight[b]	?Pre/post	All received CXT (FAC at three dose levels)	Obesity not associated with failure (death from any cause or relapse)	Dosing according to actual W may be associated with reduced risk of death or relapse	Rosner (38), 1996
Population-based cancer registry (1976–1985)	1164	Medical records	BMI[b]	Pre/post	92 CXT or tamoxifen	BMI not associated with OS or BCS in pre- or postmenopausal women		Lethaby (39), 1996
Prospective cohort (multihospital) (1970–1975)	2455	Cohort study records	Weight	Pre/post	NS	Improved OS, BCS in women ≤ 60 kg ($p = 0.002$) – effect confined to postmenopausal women (adjusted for age, *T*, stage)	Effect mainly on BC related deaths	Haybittle (40), 1997
Provincial cancer registry (1978–1989)	1169	Registry records	BMI[b]	Pre/post	Some received CXT, tamoxifen	Decreased BCS if BMI > 22.8 in *N* but not *N* + BC	Adjusted for *T* size, number of nodes, ER, age, treatment	Newman (41), 1997

(continued)

TABLE 27.1 (CONTINUED) OBESITY AND PROGNOSIS IN LOCOREGIONAL BREAST CANCER

Design (period of recruitment)	n	Body size: Method	Body size: Measure	Menopausal status	Systemic adjuvant Rx	Results	Comments	Author (ref.), year
Cases in RCT of mammographic screening (1980–1985)	676	Measured prediagnosis	Weight BMI[b]	Pre/post	NS	W, BMI not associated with BCS	Some subset analyses showed adverse prognostic effects of high triceps skinfold thickness Non-BC deaths considered withdrawals	Jain[i] (42), 1997
Population-based random survey (1975–1980)	378	Self-report prediagnosis	BMI[b] Height	Pre/post	NS	Decreased BCS with increasing BMI (HR 1.1 per unit BMI, $p < 0.05$)	Adjusted for age, stage, ethnicity Non-BC deaths censored	Galanis (43), 1998
Prospective cohort (hospital) (1982–1984)	472	Measured	Weight Relative weight BMI[b]	Pre/post	NS	Decreased DFS, BCS with increasing BMI overall (HR 1.04, 1.06 respectively) and in premenopausal women (HR 1.09, 1.12 respectively) but not postmenopausal women Similar results for OS	Adjusted for age, stage, ER	Hebert (44), 1998
Retrospective cohort (patients enrolled onto three trials) (hospital) (NS)	448	Medical records	BMI[b] Height Weight	Pre/post (93% post)	NS	BMI, W not associated with OS, DFI	Univariate and adjusted for T size, nodal status	Menon (45), 1999
Prospective cohort (hospital) (≥ 10 years earlier)	166	Measured and reported	Weight Height Quelelet index[b] Skinfold Waist/hip circumference	Pre/post	None	Decreased BCS with higher BMI (HR BC death 1.00 per unit) Android obesity, adult W gain associated with reduced BCS High BMI associated with reduced risk of BC death ($p < 0.01$)	Adjusted for stage	Kumar (46), 2000

Retrospective cohort (hospital) (1976–1988)	605	Medical records	BMI[b]	Pre/post	126 CXT; 46 tamoxifen; 29 both	High BMI associated with decreased risk local recurrence (HR 0.88 per unit BMI) BMI not associated with distant recurrence	Adjusted for age, *N*, intraduct cancer, multifocality	Marret (47), 2001
SEER registry (Washington State) (1992–1993)	1177	Self-reported weight 1 year prediagnosis	Weight BMI[b]	< 45 yrs. old	446 CXT; 177 hormone	High BMI associated with reduced OS (HR 2.5 for BMI ≥ 25.8 vs. ≤ 20.6, $p < 0.05$)	BMI risk absent in those receiving adjuvant doxorubicin Adjusted for *T* size, *N*, ER, PgR, c-erb B-2, BCL-2, p53, p27	Daling (48), 2001
Prospective cohort (multihospital) (1989–1996)	525	Measured	Weight BMI[b]	Pre/post	147 CXT only; 151 tamoxifen only; 46 both	Decreased OS, DFS with increased BMI (HR 1.72, 1.78 respectively, $p < 0.01$ for BMI > 27.8 vs. < 21.9) (similar for BCS)	Insulin identified as a potential physiologic mediator Adjusted for age, *T* stage, *N* stage, ER, PgR, grade Curvilinear associations of BMI with outcome	Goodwin (49), 2002
RCT (prospective) with registration arm (NSABP B-14) (1982–1988)	3385	Trial records	BMI[b]	Pre/post	2198 tamoxifen	BMI not associated with BC recurrence or BCS High BMI associated with increased risk of contralateral breast primary (HR 1.52), other second primary cancers (HR 1.45), overall mortality and non-BC mortality (HR 1.49) (HRs for BMI > 30 vs. 18.5–24.9)	All tumors ER positive, node negative Underweight women (BMI < 18.5 had reduced OS (vs. BMI 18.5–24.9) Effect of tamoxifen did not differ by BMI	Dignam (50), 2003
Prospective cohort (hospital) (1963–1999)	1579	Registry records	BMI[b]	Pre/post	NS	Obesity not significantly associated with DFS ($p = 0.13$) or OS ($p = 0.06$) (BMI ≥ 30 vs. < 30 kg/m^2)		Carmichael (51), 2004

(continued)

TABLE 27.1 (CONTINUED)
OBESITY AND PROGNOSIS IN LOCOREGIONAL BREAST CANCER

[a]Standard weight (kg) = (height in centimeters – 100) × 0.9.
[b]Quetelet index = weight (pounds)/height (inches)^2; BMI = weight (kg)/height (cm)^2; obesity index = weight (pounds)/height (in.).
[c]Calculated from U.S. Air Force table of standard weights.
[d]Obesity index = weight (kg)/height (m)$^{1.5182}$
[e]Optimal weight = midpoint of weight range for height recommended for women with medium frame.
[f]Ideal weight = upper limit of range for height recommended for women with a medium frame.
[g]Ideal weight = Broca's index = (height [cm] – 100) – 10%.
[h]Ideal weight = 100 + 5 (height [in.] – 60).
[i]Cases are a subset of those reported in Jain, 1994.

Notes:
CALGB = Cancer and Leukemia Group B
OS = overall survival
DFS = disease-free survival
BCS = breast cancer specific survival
RR = relative risk
HR = hazard ratio
N0 = uninvolved axillary nodes
N1 = involved axillary nodes
N+ = positive axillary nodes
N– = negative axillary nodes
BMI = body mass index
RFS = recurrence free survival
FAC = 5-fluorouracil, doxorubicin, cyclophosphamide
NS = not stated
OI = obesity index
W = weight
Q = Quetelet index
CXT = chemotherapy
N = nodal stage
T = tumor stage
ER = estrogen receptor
BC = disease-free interval
RCT = randomized clinical trial
XRT = radiation therapy
CXT = chemotherapy
DFI = disease free interval

obesity and prognosis may differ from the relationship when body size was measured at breast cancer diagnosis.

The majority of studies calculated a measure of obesity, usually BMI (weight/height^2, also known as Quetelet index), to analyze prognostic effects. Because such measures take the relationship of weight to height into consideration, they may provide information that is more biologically meaningful than weight alone.

Only 21 studies reported on the use of systemic adjuvant therapy (chemotherapy, hormonal therapy or ovarian ablation) in their study population [5,8,9,16,17,21,23,24,27,30, 31,34,37–39,41,46–50]; many of these included the effects of such treatment in adjusted prognostic analyses. However, the majority of studies did not address the issue of systemic adjuvant therapy, descriptively or in their analyses. Often this was because subjects were diagnosed prior to the widespread use of systemic adjuvant therapy; however, many studies of women diagnosed after 1980 did not consider this potentially important factor. Furthermore, although most studies attempted to consider effects of other prognostic factors (e.g., age, stage, grade) by analyzing effects of obesity in subsets of women or by conducting multivariate prognostic analyses, few studies considered effects of all potentially important confounders.

As can be seen from Table 27.1, the majority of studies identified an adverse prognostic effect of obesity in women with locoregional breast cancer. In total, 36 studies, representing 35,103 women (73.1% of those studied), identified a significant adverse effect of weight or obesity overall or in a subset of women. In contrast, 15 studies involving 12,949 women (26.9% of all women studied) failed to identify a significant adverse effect of body size. The magnitude of the prognostic effect was not always reported and, when it was, comparison groups were not consistent. Some authors reported hazard ratios (HRs) for subjects above and below an average weight (or BMI) [5]; others reported HRs for subjects above a specific BMI cutpoint compared to those with a "normal" BMI (20 to 25 kg/m^2) [29] or per unit BMI [44]. In general, when effect sizes were reported, they were moderate, obese women having an increased risk of recurrence or death in the range of 1.5 to 2.5.

In some studies, when extremes were examined, they were associated with larger risk (fourfold or greater) [32]. These observations are in keeping with an earlier meta-analysis [92] in which over 30 studies were included. The HRs for distant recurrence and death in overweight women were 1.91 (95% CI 1.52 to 2.40) and 1.56 (95% CI 1.38 to 1.76), respectively. Vatten et al. [26] calculated the attributable risk of death in breast cancer due to BMI > 27 kg/m^2 to be approximately 50% in their study, suggesting that the contribution of obesity to breast cancer outcome may be of considerable clinical relevance.

Some evidence indicates that the association of obesity with breast cancer outcome may not be linear. Curvilinear (quadratic) associations were reported in two studies [18,49] but not confirmed in another study [30]. Body size was treated as an ordinal variable in many studies (often as a dichotomous variable in earlier studies); in these studies, the linear (or nonlinear) nature of the association could not be examined. Nonetheless, it appears that prognostic effects of BMI are probably greatest in the most overweight women and that underweight women may also have poor outcomes.

No characteristics of study design consistently distinguished studies identifying significant adverse effects of obesity from those that did not. Early as well as recent studies have identified, or failed to identify, significant adverse effects. Mean sample size in "positive" studies was 981 women and, in "negative" studies, it was 831 — a difference unlikely to account for the observed variability in results. The smallest study [7], involving 25 women, identified a significant adverse prognostic effect of overweight and obesity at 10 years. The measure of body size investigated also did not predict results; significant adverse effects were identified when body size was measured as weight, percent ideal weight, or an obesity index and when body size was treated continuously or ordinally in analyses. As noted previously, some studies measured body size years prior to diagnosis;

many of these studies identified significant adverse prognostic effects of obesity, although effects of body size on breast cancer risk may confound these results.

The results reported by Dignam et al. [50] suggest that obesity may increase risk of new primary cancers and non-breast cancer related mortality but not breast cancer recurrence or death. That is, it may not actually have an effect on breast cancer progression. However, results of the full range of studies suggest that this is not the case. Of the studies listed in Table 27.1, 27 reported associations of obesity with overall survival (or all cause mortality); 17 of these (63.0%) identified significantly increased risk in obese women. Breast cancer-specific mortality was examined in 25 studies; 17 of these (68.0%) identified significant adverse effects of obesity. The effect of obesity on breast cancer recurrence was evaluated in 20 studies; 13 (65.0%) identified adverse effects. Finally, 40 studies considered effects of obesity on at least one breast cancer-specific outcome (recurrence or breast cancer-specific survival). Of these, 28 (70%) identified significant adverse effects.

Thus, there is little evidence that adverse prognostic effects of obesity in breast cancer are due to effects on non-breast-cancer deaths; on the contrary, a slightly greater proportion of studies that evaluated breast cancer-specific outcomes identified adverse prognostic effects when compared to studies evaluating all-cause mortality. Dignam et al. [50] studied women with low-risk breast cancer (hormone receptor positive, node negative), many of whom received tamoxifen. Failure to identify effects of obesity on breast cancer outcomes may reflect low breast cancer event rates, and a greater relative contribution of competing (i.e., not breast cancer) causes of deaths in this good prognosis population.

One possible explanation for the inconsistent prognostic effects of obesity reported is that obesity exerts a prognostic effect present only in a subgroup of women. Differential effects according to menopausal status or hormone receptor (estrogen, progesterone) status have been most commonly postulated. Studies investigating these subsets are summarized in Table 27.2 and Table 27.3.

Given that the association of obesity with breast cancer risk varies according to menopausal status, it is plausible that prognostic effects of obesity might differ with respect to menopausal status. Obesity is associated with an increased breast cancer risk in postmenopausal women and a decreased risk in premenopausal woman (see Chapter 14 [93]). In Table 27.2, results of studies that reported prognostic effects of obesity in premenopausal and postmenopausal women separately are summarized. Prognostic effects of obesity in premenopausal women were evaluated in 13 studies. Eight of these (61.5%) identified significant adverse effects, despite the fact that sample sizes were considerably smaller than in the full studies listed in Table 27.1. Six (42.9%) of the 14 studies that evaluated prognostic effects in postmenopausal women identified significant adverse effects of obesity. Once again, these analyses were usually conducted in subsets of the overall study population, leading to reduced power.

These results suggest that an adverse prognostic effect of obesity is present in pre- and postmenopausal women and, in contrast to the impact of obesity on breast cancer risk, its impact on prognosis may be greatest in premenopausal women. As will be discussed later, this observation has implications for understanding potential pathophysiological mechanisms for prognostic effects of obesity.

Prognostic effects of obesity in hormone receptor-positive and hormone receptor-negative breast cancer have been reported in a smaller number of studies (Table 27.3). Two early studies [14,37] provide evidence that the prognostic effect of obesity may be greatest in estrogen and/or progesterone receptor-positive individuals. As noted earlier, a recent study by Dignam et al. [50] analyzed prognostic effects of obesity in the NSABP-B14 study conducted in estrogen receptor-positive, node negative-breast cancer. This study failed to identify an effect of obesity on breast cancer recurrence or breast cancer death, despite the finding of an increased risk of contralateral breast cancer and increased all-cause mortality in obese individuals. The majority of women in that study received tamoxifen, and it is possible that administration of tamoxifen to women with estrogen receptor-positive breast cancer may abrogate the adverse prognostic effects of obesity.

TABLE 27.2
Prognostic Effects of Obesity in Premenopausal vs. Postmenopausal Women

Premenopausal			Postmenopausal			
n	Prognostic effect seen?	Comment	n	Prognostic effect seen?	Comment	Author (ref.), year
	—		295	Significantly increased risk of recurrence (RR 2.4, $p < 0.02$) if W < 130 lb		Donegan (2), 1978
235	HR 1.13 for weight ≥ 64 kg vs. < 64 kg, $p = 0.28$	Interaction of treatment with weight in < 45 y.o.	218	HR 1.27 for weight ≥ 64 kg, $p = 0.002$	Similar results for *Q*	Boyd (5), 1981
226	W, BMI adversely associated with OS (HR 1.7 for W > 140 and 1.6 for BMI > 30.5)				No significant association of W, BMI with OS	Mohle–Boetani (15), 1988
309	Significant adverse effect of weight (adjusted for stage, nodes), $p = 0.043$		544	Weight not significantly associated with survival $p = 0.33$ (adjusted for stage, nodes)	Adverse effect of weight in overall study population	Lees (19), 1989
NS	Adverse effect of Q similar in all age groups (30–49, 50–64, ≥65)	Adverse effect in stage I, II but not III, IV	NS	Adverse effect of *Q* similar in all age groups (30–49, 50–64, ≥65)	Adverse effect in stage I, II but not III, IV	Tretli (20), 1990
332	No difference in survival for BMI > 23.1 vs. < 21.0		261	Decreased survival in BMI > 23.1 vs. < 21.0 ($p < 0.05$)		Kimura (22), 1990
196	HR 2.4 (cancer death) for Q ≥ 28 vs. ≤ 22, $p = 0.10$	Age ≤ 49	287 (50–59); 687 (≥60)	HR 2.1 (cancer death) for Q ≥ 28 vs. ≤ 22 $p = 0.0009$ for age 50–59 (comparable HR for ≥ 60 y.o = 1.2, $p = 0.39$)		Tornberg (29), 1993
422	Reduced OS with BMI ≥ 29 vs. < 19 (HR 5.93, 95% CI 1.98–17.8)	< 45 y.o.		—		Holmberg (32), 1994
	—		301	BMI not associated with recurrence or BC death		Katoh (31), 1994
363	Weight, BMI not associated with BC death	Mixed pre, peri, unknown menopausal status	537	Weight, BMI not associated with BC death		Jain (33), 1994
	—		241	Q not associated with OS		den Tonkelaar (35), 1995

(continued)

TABLE 27.2 (CONTINUED)
Prognostic Effects of Obesity in Premenopausal vs. Postmenopausal Women

Premenopausal			Postmenopausal			
N	Prognostic effect seen?	Comment	n	Prognostic effect seen?	Comment	Author (ref.), year
	—		698	BMI, weight associated with death (HR 1.9) — effect nonsignificant after adjustment for age, stage, ER		Zhang (36), 1995
275	No significant association of BMI ≥ 28 vs. < 28 with OS ($p = 0.29$)	< 50 y.o.	555	No significant association of BMI ≥ 28 vs. < 28 on OS ($p = 0.13$)	≥ 50 y.o.	Lethaby (39), 1996
980	No adverse effect of weight ≤ 60 kg vs. > 60 kg on OS	Pre + perimenopausal	1475	HR 1.27 (1.12–1.45) $p = 0.002$ if weight ≥ 60 kg vs. < 60 kg (OS)		Haybittle (40), 1997
222	Higher BMI associated with increased risk of recurrence — HR 1.09, 95% CI 1.02–1.17, $p = 0.01$ per kg/m^2 — HR BC death 1.12 (1.03–1.22, $p = 0.007$)		250	Effects of BMI not significant		Hebert (44), 1998
	—		375	No effect of W or BMI on DFI or OS		Menon (45), 1999
1177	High BMI an independent predictor of mortality (HR 1.7, 95% CI 1.0–2.9, $p < 0.05$) for highest vs. lowest quartile	< 45 y.o.		—		Daling (48), 2001
1035	No effect of BMI on recurrence or BC death Increased contralateral BC in obese (HR 1.52) Increased overall mortality in obese ("similar" in pre, post)	Pre + perimenopausal	2350	No effect of BMI on recurrence or BC death Increased contralateral BC in obese HR 1.63, 95% CI 1.07–2.51 Increased total mortality in obese ("similar" in pre, post)		Dignam (50), 2003

Notes:
BMI = body mass index
HR = hazard ratio
Q = Quetelet index
BC = breast cancer
OS = overall survival
DFI = disease-free interval
RR = relative risk
W = weight
ER = estrogen receptor

TABLE 27.3
Prognostic Effects of Obesity According to Hormone Receptor Status

Hormone receptor positive		Hormone receptor negative		
n	**Prognostic effect of obesity**	**n**	**Prognostic effect of obesity**	**Author (ref.), year**
432	ER+ — increased risk	247	ER− — no effect	McNee (14), 1987
357	PgR+ — increased risk	255	PgR− — no effect	
399	ER+ — increased risk, $p = 0.03$ (adjusted HR 2.18)	233	ER− — reduced risk, $p = 0.02$ (adjusted HR 0.36)	Maehle (37), 1996
272	PgR+ — non-significant increased risk, $p = 0.18$ (adjusted HR 1.91)	272	PgR− — no effect	
230	ER and PgR+ — increased risk, $p = 0.04$ (adjusted HR 3.16)	157	ER and PgR− — reduced risk, $p = 0.02$ (adjusted HR 0.17)	
3385	ER^+, N0 — obesity associated with increased risk of contralateral BC and all cause mortality but not BC recurrence or death			Dignam (50) 2003

Notes:
ER = estrogen receptor
PgR = progesterone receptor
HR = hazard ratio for highest vs. lowest quintile
N0 = node negative
BC = breast cancer

A second study [37] reported a reduced risk of death in obese vs. nonobese women who were estrogen receptor negative. Unfortunately, the small number of studies that have investigated prognostic effects of obesity according to estrogen receptor status, coupled with the small numbers of subjects with receptor-negative tumors, make it difficult to draw conclusions about the potential for differential effects of obesity in receptor-positive and -negative breast cancer. Additional research in this area, which also examines interactions with hormonal adjuvant therapies (estrogen receptor blockers, aromatase inhibitors), is needed to resolve this issue.

The question of whether prognostic effects of obesity differ according to the presence or absence of other tumor characteristics was addressed in the 13 studies summarized in Table 27.4. With some exceptions, these studies identified effects that were greatest in tumors with favorable prognostic factors — usually defined as small tumor size, less advanced tumor stage, or uninvolved axillary lymph nodes. Taken together with results in hormone receptor-positive cancers summarized in Table 27.3, these results suggest that adverse prognostic effects of obesity may be greatest in lower risk breast cancers, but they are not absent in higher risk cancers

This observation contrasts to some extent with growing evidence, summarized in Table 27.5, that obese women are more likely to have breast cancers that have unfavorable prognostic characteristics. In the majority of studies that examined this relationship, obesity was associated with advanced stage, larger tumor size, and/or greater axillary nodal involvement. Inconsistent associations of obesity with estrogen receptor status have been reported. Because of these observations, it has been suggested that adverse prognostic effects of obesity may not be independent of traditional prognostic factors — that is, obese women may present with more advanced stage breast cancer, possibly due to delayed diagnosis.

TABLE 27.4
Prognostic Effects of Obesity According to Prognostic Factors Other Than Hormone Receptors

Effect	Author (ref.), year
Effect greatest in N0	Donegan (2), 1978a
Effect greatest in N0	Donegan (3), 1978 b
Effect greatest in tumors with favorable prognostic factors (clinical stage I, N0) but not low grade	Boyd (5), 1981
Effect greatest in stage II, III	Tartter (6), 1981
Effect greatest with one to three nodes involved (vs. 0 or ≥4 nodes)	Eberlein (8), 1985
Effect greatest with $T \leq 5$ cm, N0, ER positive, PgR positive	McNee (14), 1987
Effect greatest in stage I cancer	Hebert (17), 1988
Effect greatest in stage I and II but not III cancer	Tretli (20), 1990
Effect greatest in stage III	Coates (23), 1991
Effect greatest in N0	Senie (28), 1992
Effect greatest in stage III (vs. II)	Bastarrachea (30), 1994
Effect greatest in N0	Newman (41), 1997
Effect greatest in those not receiving adjuvant chemotherapy (especially doxorubicin-based chemotherapy)	Daling (48), 2001

Notes:
ER = estrogen receptor
N0 = node negative
PgR = progesterone receptor
T = tumor

TABLE 27.5
Association of Obesity with Prognostic Factors

Favorable factors associated with obesity	Unfavorable factors associated with obesity	Author (ref.), year
Lower nuclear grade	Advanced clinical stage, larger *T* size, higher *N* stage, vessel involvement	Abe (1), 1976
	Greater axillary nodal involvement	Eberlein (8), 1985
	Advanced stage (white, but not black, patients) (no association with ER or grade)	Ownby (11), 1985
	Positive axillary nodes	Greenberg (12), 1985
	T size > 5 cm	McNee (14), 1987
	Advanced stage	Mohle–Boetani (15), 1988
	Larger *T* size	Tretli (20), 1990
	≥ Four involved nodes	Ewertz (24), 1991
	Advanced stage	Nomura (25), 1991
	Larger *T* size (not *N* stage or ER)	Senie (28), 1992
	Advanced stage, larger *T* size	Bastarrachea (30), 1994
	Larger *T* size	Obermair (34), 1995
	More advanced stage	Zhang (36), 1995
	Larger *T* size, ER negativity	Lethaby (39), 1996
Lower stage (I)	> 2 cm *T* size	Haybittle (40), 1997
ER positive	Advanced stage, larger *T* size, more involved nodes	Newman (41), 1997
	Positive axillary nodes	Jain (42), 1997
	ER negative, high S-phase fraction, high histologic grade, high cell count, large *T* size	Daling (48), 2001
	Advanced *T* stage	Goodwin (49), 2002
	Higher levels of ER, PgR, larger *T* size	Dignam (50), 2003
	Larger *T* size, worse Nottingham prognostic index	Carmichael (51), 2004

Notes:
ER = estrogen receptor
N = nodal stage
PgR = progesterone receptor
T = tumor

However, this appears to be unlikely as the sole explanation for an adverse prognostic effect of obesity, given that the adverse prognostic effect of obesity identified in studies listed in Table 27.1 persisted after adjustment for many prognostic factors, notably tumor stage and nodal status, and, at times, hormone receptor status and tumor grade in the majority of studies that conducted such analyses. In at least one study [27], an adverse effect of obesity was seen only after adjustment for such factors.

As noted earlier, only a minority of the studies listed in Table 27.1 reported use of adjuvant systemic therapy — chemotherapy or hormonal therapy. Furthermore, in most of the studies that did report use of systemic adjuvant therapy, not all women received such therapy and prognostic effects of obesity were rarely reported after adjustment for adjuvant therapy or only in those receiving adjuvant therapy. Nonetheless, two recent studies conducted in the context of randomized clinical trials of systemic therapy failed to identify adverse prognostic effects of obesity on breast cancer recurrence or death in those receiving chemotherapy [38] or tamoxifen [50]. As noted previously, adverse effects of obesity on contralateral breast cancer and on all-cause mortality were noted in the latter study.

Daling et al. [48] reported that adverse effects of obesity present in the overall study population and in those receiving non-anthracycline-based chemotherapy were not present in those who received doxorubicin-based adjuvant chemotherapy. These observations raise the question of whether modern adjuvant systemic adjuvant therapies abrogate prognostic effects of obesity in locoregional breast cancer. This is an area that should be an urgent focus for future research because this would influence the design of future intervention studies.

The preceding discussion has focused on locoregional breast cancer. A small number of studies has investigated prognostic effects of obesity in recurrent or metastatic breast cancer [8,10,94,95]. An adverse effect of obesity was seen in only one of these studies [8]. However, the available data are insufficient to draw firm conclusions about effects of obesity on outcomes in metastatic breast cancer.

In summary, the prognostic effects of obesity in locoregional breast cancer have been extensively studied. The preponderance of evidence supports an adverse effect on breast cancer outcomes (although the effect may not be linear). The effect is moderate in size and may be most pronounced, but not exclusive to, tumors with characteristics that are usually associated with favorable outcomes. Obesity influences prognosis in pre- and postmenopausal women. However, despite this extensive body of research, important questions remain. These include whether effects of obesity differ according to hormone receptor status and, more importantly, whether obesity influences prognosis in women receiving current adjuvant therapies, including anthracyclines, taxanes, tamoxifen, and aromatase inhibitors.

WEIGHT GAIN AFTER BREAST CANCER DIAGNOSIS

Weight gain after diagnosis of locoregional breast cancer was first reported by Dixon et al. in 1978 [54]. Since that time, over 35 studies [55–90] have examined this phenomenon. All but two [78,80] of these studies have found evidence of weight gain during the first year or two after breast cancer diagnosis. This weight gain has been shown to be associated with anxiety over appearance [55] and with reduced quality of life [96]. The weight gain reported has been of variable magnitude with averages ranging from more than 10 kg over 1 year [55,56] to approximately 1 kg [65]. Some studies have reported weight gain to occur in almost 100% of women [9]; others have reported lower prevalence. Weight gain in the range of 1 to 3 kg during the first year after diagnosis has been most commonly reported, particularly in recent studies. Earlier studies (prior to 1990) tended to identify greater weight gain than more recent studies, likely reflecting changes in adjuvant therapy (see later sections) and, perhaps, greater clinician and patient awareness that weight gain is a potential problem.

It was initially hypothesized that this postdiagnosis weight gain was related to overeating, possibly in an attempt to relieve chemotherapy-associated nausea. However, evidence supporting that hypothesis is weak and a number of other factors have emerged as being associated with weight gain. Summarized in Table 27.6, these factors can be grouped into several categories. The first relates to menopausal status. Young age, premenopausal status, and onset of menopause (as evidenced by cessation of menses or reduction in serum estradiol levels) have been fairly consistently associated with greater weight gain. The second factor that has been most consistently associated with weight gain is systemic adjuvant therapy. The use of chemotherapy (as opposed to no chemotherapy) has been associated with the greatest degree of weight gain (most studies focused only on those receiving chemotherapy).

Two studies have demonstrated that anthracycline-based chemotherapy is associated with less weight gain than non-anthracycline-based chemotherapy [85,97]. Longer duration of adjuvant chemotherapy (1 or more years) in earlier studies may have contributed to the larger weight gain reported prior to the 1990s; older chemotherapy protocols that included prednisone and ovarian ablation [9,18] were also associated with greater degrees of weight gain, as were multiagent (vs. single agent) chemotherapy regimens. Chemotherapy combined with hormonal interventions such

TABLE 27.6
Factors Associated with Weight Gain after Breast Cancer Diagnosis

Age/menopause	Young age (68,71)
	Premenopausal status (59,69,70)
	Onset of menopause (69)/reduction estradiol (60)
Adjuvant therapy	Any chemotherapy (68,69)
	Multiagent (vs. single) (9)
	CMF (vs. anthracycline) (85,96)
	Ovarian ablation ± prednisone (vs. other) (9,18)
	Tamoxifen vs. no tamoxifen (63,65,69,73)
Initial BMI	Lower (68)
Psychological/HRQOL	Distress/depression (60,70)
	Altered eating behavior (61)
Caloric intake	High intake (74)/no effect (60,69,80)
Physical activity	Low activity (68,81,83)/no effect (60,69,78,80,87)
Resting energy expenditure	Reduced expenditure (60,72,78,87)/no effect (80)

as medroxyprogesterone acetate [64] or leuprorelin [84] has also been associated with greater weight gain. There is some controversy as to whether tamoxifen is associated with weight gain. Two studies have identified significant weight gain [63,69] in women receiving tamoxifen and two have not [65,73]. Regardless, weight gain in women on tamoxifen is minor and may be comparable to that seen in the general population [65].

Weight gain has been reported to be greatest in women who have lower (as opposed to higher) BMI when initially diagnosed [68]. Psychological distress and/or a disinhibited pattern of eating (i.e., eating in response to factors other than hunger) have also been associated with greater weight gain [60,61,70]. High caloric intake has been inconsistently associated with weight gain; the majority of studies have failed to find an association [60,69,74,80]. Similarly, reduced physical activity has been inconsistently associated with weight gain [60,68,69,78,80,81,83,87]. Several studies have reported reduced resting metabolic rate in women receiving adjuvant chemotherapy [60,72,78,87], suggesting that reduced resting energy expenditure that is not balanced by reduced energy intake may contribute to the weight gain seen in these patients. Subclinical hypothyroidism has also been postulated as a potential underlying cause of postdiagnosis weight gain [97].

The nature of the weight gain that occurs during adjuvant chemotherapy has been investigated in several studies. Demark–Wahnefried et al. have provided evidence that this weight gain is associated with an increase in fat mass accompanied by a decrease in lean body mass, a pattern seen with sarcopenic obesity [83]. Sarcopenic obesity has been observed with chronic use of corticosteroids, prolonged physical inactivity, or hypopituitartism or hypogonadism, as well as increasing age and menopause. Additional studies have shown that weight gain after breast cancer diagnosis is associated with increased fat mass (although there is some inconsistency as to whether the increased fat mass is visceral or nonvisceral) and/or decreased fat-free or lean mass [66,72,79,80,86,87]. This suggests that weight gain during adjuvant chemotherapy is due to positive energy balance resulting from reduced energy expenditure (reduced resting energy expenditure likely compounded by reduced physical activity) with no compensatory reduction in energy intake.

Taken together, these observations suggest that interventions involving physical activity that would result in direct increases in energy expenditure, as well as secondary increases in resting energy expenditure as a result of increases in lean body mass (i.e., muscle mass), might be most useful in preventing weight gain after breast cancer diagnosis. In this regard, our group has conducted a phase II intervention study of a multidisciplinary weight management intervention in locoregional breast cancer. The intervention included physical activity and dietary intervention

TABLE 27.7
Prognostic Effects of Weight Gain

n	Weight gain (kg)	Prognostic effect	Author (ref.), year
67	8.2	Adverse	Bonomi (99), 1984
62	>10	Adverse	Chlebowski (58), 1986
545	5.9 (premenopausal)	Adverse (premenopausal)	Camoriano (59), 1990
237	4.3	None	Heasman (9), 1985
62	<10	None	Chlebowski (58), 1986
637	1.21–5.55	None	Goodwin (16), 1988
445	1.6	None	Goodwin (69), 2001
106	0.5%/month	None	Costa (71), 2002

(reduced calories) as well as psychosocial support. The most important predictor of successful weight management was physical activity; the likelihood of successful weight management increased 78% with every 30 additional minutes of physical activity weekly [98]. Furthermore, Winningham [75] has demonstrated that increases in physical activity during chemotherapy are associated with increases in lean mass.

Prognostic effects of weight gain have been examined in seven studies [9,16,58,59,69,71,99] (see Table 27.7). The average weight gain reported in these studies has varied from 1.21 kg over 1 year to more than 10 kg over 1 year. Three of these studies have identified adverse prognostic effects of postdiagnosis weight gain [58,59,99]. These three studies were those in which average weight gain was the largest, varying from 5.9 to more than 10 kg. These observations suggest that weight gain postdiagnosis contributes to the adverse prognostic effect of obesity at diagnosis, but that the degree of weight gain must be considerable before this adverse prognostic effect can be identified. These observations provide support for the use of interventions to prevent weight gain after breast cancer diagnosis and strengthen the rationale for research to investigate the impact of interventions designed to promote weight loss after breast cancer diagnosis.

PATHOPHYSIOLOGY OF ADVERSE PROGNOSTIC EFFECTS OF OBESITY

A number of factors have been proposed as potential mediators of an adverse prognostic effect of obesity. The first of these, presentation of breast cancer at a more advanced stage in obese women, was discussed earlier. Although breast cancers developing in obese women are more likely to have unfavorable prognostic characteristics, available evidence suggests that adverse prognostic effects of obesity are independent of those prognostic factors. It has also been suggested that chemotherapy underdosing in obese women — a practice that may have been more common in the past than it is currently — may contribute to adverse prognostic effects of obesity [100]. It is possible that this has played a role in women receiving chemotherapy in the past; however, such underdosing (or dosing for ideal as opposed to actual body weight) is less common today. Furthermore, the majority of studies that identified adverse prognostic effects of obesity involved women who were not receiving chemotherapy, suggesting that this is not a primary mechanism for an adverse prognostic effect of obesity.

Hormonal factors have received the most attention as potential mediators of adverse prognostic effects of obesity in breast cancer [52,53,91]. Obesity is associated with higher circulating levels of estrogens in postmenopausal women, due to increased peripheral aromatization of androstenedione to estriol, which is subsequently converted to estradiol, coupled with reduced circulating levels of sex hormone-binding globulin (SHBG), leading to increased levels of free estrogen. This may contribute to adverse prognostic effects of obesity in postmenopausal breast cancer. Some evidence indicates that obese postmenopausal women with advanced breast cancer experience a significantly reduced response rate when treated with the aromatase inhibitor letrozole [101]. However, increased estrogen levels are unlikely to be a central explanation for prognostic effects of obesity in premenopausal women in whom the ovaries (and not adipose tissue) are the major source of estrogen production. Furthermore, in one study [49], circulating estradiol levels were not strongly associated with obesity, were not associated with outcome, and did not mediate adverse prognostic effects of obesity in women with locoregional breast cancer; this suggests that other factors play important roles.

Recent research has focused on the role of insulin and other members of the insulin/IGF family of growth factors in mediating adverse prognostic effects of obesity [49,53]. Obesity is associated with the insulin resistance syndrome (also known as the metabolic syndrome) [102,103]. The relative resistance of insulin receptors in skeletal muscle and other tissues to metabolic effects of insulin leads to compensatory hyperinsulinemia in an attempt to maintain normal glucose homeostasis. However, insulin and IGF-I receptors are overexpressed in breast cancer cells [104] and are not insulin resistant [105,106]. Activation of these tyrosine kinase receptors results in activation of insulin response substrate-I (IRS-I) [107] and downstream activation of the mitogen-activated protein (MAP) kinase pathway (important in cell proliferation) and the phosphoinositidyl-3 kinase/akt (P13k-Akt) pathway (involved in anchorage independent growth and inhibition of apoptosis), leading to proliferation and growth [108–110]. The role of the insulin resistance syndrome in cancer risk is discussed in Chapter 20 [111].

Insulin not only interacts with its own receptor in breast cancer cells, but also contributes to regulation of IGF-I and IGF binding proteins. These entities, in turn, interact in a complex fashion with the receptors of this growth factor family, leading to further activation of the signaling pathways described previously. The relative contribution of insulin and the IGFs and their cognate receptors in these mitogenic signaling pathways remains an area of intense research interest [112].

Empiric evidence for an important role of insulin in mediation of adverse prognostic effects of obesity has been provided [49]. In a cohort of 535 women with newly diagnosed locoregional breast cancer, fasting insulin levels were strongly correlated with BMI ($r = 0.59$, $p < 0.001$). High fasting insulin levels were significantly associated with an increased risk of distant recurrence and death, independent of effects of BMI and other prognostic factors. Women whose insulin levels were in the upper quartile had a 2.1-fold increased risk of distant recurrence and a 3.3-fold increased risk of death compared to women whose insulin levels were in the lowest quartile. In the same cohort, circulating levels of IGF-I, IGF-II, IGFBP-1, and IGFBP-3 were not convincingly associated with outcome [113]. Rose et al.[114] have recently suggested that leptin, an adipocytokine associated with cell growth, migration, and invasion as well as angiogenesis, may play a role in prognostic effects of obesity, perhaps in association with insulin. However, in the cohort study described above, leptin did not make independent contributions to breast cancer outcome [115].

It is unlikely that any of these mechanisms act alone. Insulin and IGFs contribute to regulation of aromatase activity and SHBG levels [116,117], and cross-talk exists between insulin/IGF signaling pathways and estrogen signaling pathways within breast cancer cells (this interaction may be mediated by the progesterone receptor [118–120]), leading to the possibility that these mechanisms act in concert to affect prognosis adversely). One potential schema for such interaction is shown in Figure 27.1.

Further research to enhance understanding of factors mediating adverse prognostic effects of obesity is urgently needed. Such research is expected to contribute to development of targeted therapies to reverse adverse effects of obesity. These interventions should be pursued in parallel to research that directly addresses obesity through a variety of lifestyle and possibly pharmacological interventions.

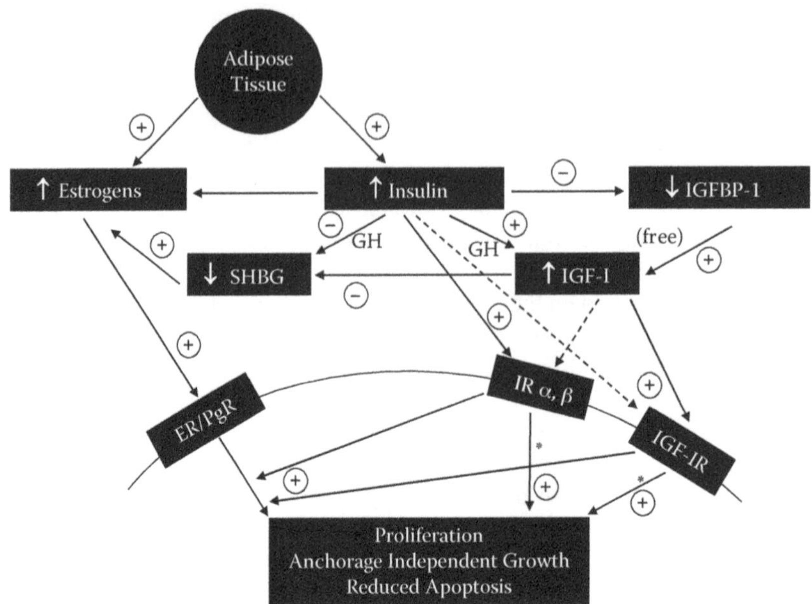

FIGURE 27.1 Interaction of estrogen and insulin/IGF mechanisms.

CONCLUSIONS

A large body of research has investigated prognostic effects of obesity in breast cancer. This research conclusively demonstrates that obesity exerts an adverse prognostic effect on disease-free survival, breast cancer-specific survival, and overall survival. The effect is moderate in size, with hazard ratios for obese compared to nonobese women in the range of 2. This corresponded to an approximate attributable risk of 50% in one study [26], an effect that is highly relevant clinically. The adverse prognostic effect of obesity appears to be independent of stage at presentation and of other prognostic factors and to be present in both pre- and postmenopausal women. Some evidence suggests that it is probably present in women receiving modern adjuvant chemotherapy; however, further research to confirm this is needed.

Weight gain is common after breast cancer diagnosis; the magnitude of this weight gain has become smaller in recent years, likely reflecting increasing awareness of the phenomenon, as well as more widespread use of shorter term, anthracycline-based chemotherapy, which is associated with less weight gain. A growing consensus is that weight gain during adjuvant chemotherapy is due to reduced energy expenditure (reduced resting energy expenditure, probably compounded by reduced physical activity) in the absence of reduction in caloric intake. It is likely that interventions focusing on physical activity will be effective in preventing this weight gain.

The situation with respect to obesity at breast cancer diagnosis is somewhat more complex. It is likely that this obesity is due to a complex group of factors, similar to those seen in the general population — including excess caloric intake and excess dietary fat intake, as well as reduced physical activity — that have resulted in imbalances in energy balance. The positive energy balance that results in obesity at breast cancer diagnosis (and that may have contributed to breast cancer in postmenopausal women) is probably long term. In this situation, multifactorial interventions will likely be necessary. Such interventions should target energy intake and energy expenditure and may require psychosocial components to address motivational issues. Considerable work has been done to develop interventions targeting obesity in women with breast cancer. This work has shown that physical activity and dietary modification are feasible and that modest weight loss is possible. These issues will be discussed in greater detail in Chapter 34 and Chapter 35.

In parallel to this observational work regarding obesity and weight gain in breast cancer, there has been enhanced understanding of the pathophysiological basis for a contribution of obesity to breast cancer outcome. A number of hormonal mechanisms have been postulated, and empiric evidence supports the role of the insulin/IGF family of growth factors, which likely act in concert with estrogenic mechanisms.

Although much is known about obesity and breast cancer outcome, additional research is needed. Observational research to examine the effect of obesity as a prognostic factor in women receiving modern adjuvant therapies, including anthracyclines, taxanes, and aromatase inhibitors, is recommended. This research could be most efficiently conducted in the context of ongoing and completed randomized clinical trials. Additionally, research to understand the pathophysiology of prognostic effects of obesity will likely yield important information that can be used to develop targeted therapies in women unable or unwilling to lose weight. Such interventions could potentially include insulin or IGF receptor blockers. Finally, research will be needed to ascertain the benefits of weight loss after breast cancer diagnosis. Demonstration of a probable link between obesity and poor prognosis does not mean that reversal of obesity will result in improved outcomes; this must be demonstrated in well designed, randomized clinical trials. Furthermore, it is likely that a single intervention to promote weight loss will not work for all women with breast cancer, so evaluation of a variety of interventions and motivational approaches is warranted.

REFERENCES

1. Abe R, Kumagai N, Kimura M, Hirosaki A, Nakamura T. Biological characteristics of breast cancer in obesity. *Tohoku J Exp Med* 1976; 120:351–359
2. Donegan WL, Hartz AJ, Rimm AA. The association of body weight with recurrent cancer of the breast. *Cancer* 1978; 41:1590–1594.
3. Donegan WL, Jayich S, Koehler MR, Donegan JH. The prognostic implications of obesity for the surgical cure of breast cancer. *Breast Dis Breast*. 1978; 4:14–17.
4. Sohrabi A, Sandoz J, Spratt JS, Polk HC Jr. Recurrence of breast cancer. Obesity, tumor size, and axillary lymph node metastases. *JAMA* 1980; 244:264–265.
5. Boyd NF, Campbell JE, Germanson T, Thomson DB, Sutherland DJ, Meakin JW. Body weight and prognosis in breast cancer. *J Natl Cancer Inst* 1981; 67:785–789.
6. Tartter PI, Papatestas AE, Ioannovich J, Mulvihill MN, Lesnick G, Aufses AH Jr. Cholesterol and obesity as prognostic factors in breast cancer. *Cancer* 1981; 47:2222–2227.
7. Zumoff B, Gorzynski JG, Katz JL, Weiner H, Levin J, Holland J, Fukushima DK. Nonobesity at the time of mastectomy is highly predictive of 10-year disease-free survival in women with breast cancer. *Anticancer Res* 1982; 2:59–62.
8. Eberlein T, Simon R, Fisher S, Lippman ME. Height, weight, and risk of breast cancer relapse. *Breast Cancer Res Treat* 1985; 5:81–86.
9. Heasman KZ, Sutherland HJ, Campbell JA, Elhakim T, Boyd NF. Weight gain during adjuvant chemotherapy for breast cancer. *Breast Cancer Res Treat* 1985; 5:195–200.
10. Gregorio DI, Emrich LJ, Graham S, Marshall JR, Nemoto T. Dietary fat consumption and survival among women with breast cancer. *J Natl Cancer Inst* 1985; 75:37–41.
11. Ownby HE, Frederick J, Russo J, Brooks SC, Swanson GM, Heppner GH, Brennan MJ. Racial differences in breast cancer patients. *J Natl Cancer Inst* 1985; 75:55–60.
12. Greenberg ER, Vessey MP, McPherson K, Doll R, Yeates D. Body size and survival in premenopausal breast cancer. *Br J Cancer* 1985; 51:691–697.
13. Newman SC, Miller AB, Howe GR. A study of the effect of weight and dietary fat on breast cancer survival time. *Am J Epidemiol* 1986; 123:767–774.
14. McNee RK, Mason BH, Neave LM, Kay RG. Influence of height, weight, and obesity on breast cancer incidence and recurrence in Auckland, New Zealand. *Breast Cancer Res Treat* 1987; 9:145–150.

15. Mohle-Boetani JC, Grosser S, Whittemore AS, Malec M, Kampert JB, Paffenbarger RS Jr. Body size, reproductive factors, and breast cancer survival. *Prev Med* 1988; 17:634–642.
16. Goodwin PJ, Panzarella T, Boyd NF. Weight gain in women with localized breast cancer — a descriptive study. *Breast Cancer Res Treat* 1988; 11:59–66.
17. Hebert JR, Augustine A, Barone J, Kabat GC, Kinne DW, Wynder EL. Weight, height and body mass index in the prognosis of breast cancer: early results of a prospective study. *Int J Cancer* 1988; 42:315–318.
18. Suissa S, Pollak M, Spitzer WO, Margolese R. Body size and breast cancer prognosis: a statistical explanation of the discrepancies. *Cancer Res* 1989; 49:3113–3116.
19. Lees AW, Jenkins HJ, May CL, Cherian G, Lam EW, Hanson J. Risk factors and 10-year breast cancer survival in northern Alberta. *Breast Cancer Res Treat* 1989; 13:143–151.
20. Tretli S, Haldorsen T, Ottestad L. The effect of premorbid height and weight on the survival of breast cancer patients. *Br J Cancer* 1990; 62:299–303.
21. Kyogoku S, Hirohata T, Takeshita S, Nomura Y, Shigematsu T, Horie A. Survival of breast-cancer patients and body size indicators. *Int J Cancer* 1990; 46:824–831.
22. Kimura M. Obesity as prognostic factors in breast cancer. *Diabetes Res Clin Pract* 1990; 10(suppl 1):S247–S251.
23. Coates RJ, Clark WS, Eley JW, Greenberg RS, Huguley CM Jr, Brown RL. Race, nutritional status, and survival from breast cancer. *J Natl Cancer Inst* 1990; 82:1684–1692.
24. Ewertz M, Gillanders S, Meyer L, Zedeler K. Survival of breast cancer patients in relation to factors which affect the risk of developing breast cancer. *Int J Cancer* 1991; 49:526–530.
25. Nomura AM, Marchand LL, Kolonel LN, Hankin JH. The effect of dietary fat on breast cancer survival among Caucasian and Japanese women in Hawaii. *Breast Cancer Res Treat* 1991; 18(suppl 1):S135–S141.
26. Vatten LJ, Foss OP, Kvinnsland S. Overall survival of breast cancer patients in relation to preclinically determined total serum cholesterol, body mass index, height and cigarette smoking: a population-based study. *Eur J Cancer* 1991; 27:641–646.
27. Gordon NH, Crowe JP, Brumberg DJ, Berger NA. Socioeconomic factors and race in breast cancer recurrence and survival. *Am J Epidemiol* 1992; 135:609–618.
28. Senie RT, Rosen PP, Rhodes P, Lesser ML, Kinne DW. Obesity at diagnosis of breast carcinoma influences duration of disease-free survival. *Ann Intern Med* 1992; 116:26–32.
29. Tornberg S, Carstensen J. Serum beta-lipoprotein, serum cholesterol and Quetelet's index as predictors for survival of breast cancer patients. *Eur J Cancer* 1993; 29A:2025–2030.
30. Bastarrachea J, Hortobagyi GN, Smith TL, Kau SW, Buzdar AU. Obesity as an adverse prognostic factor for patients receiving adjuvant chemotherapy for breast cancer. *Ann Intern Med* 1994; 120:18–25.
31. Katoh A, Watzlaf VJ, D'Amico F. An examination of obesity and breast cancer survival in postmenopausal women. *Br J Cancer* 1994; 70:928–933.
32. Holmberg L, Lund E, Bergstrom R, Adami HO, Meirik O. Oral contraceptives and prognosis in breast cancer: effects of duration, latency, recency, age at first use and relation to parity and body mass index in young women with breast cancer. *Eur J Cancer* 1994; 30A:351–354.
33. Jain M, Miller AB. Premorbid body size and the prognosis of women with breast cancer. *Int J Cancer* 1994; 59:363–368.
34. Obermair A, Kurz C, Hanzal E, Bancher-Todesca D, Thoma M, Bodisch A, Kubista E, Kyral E, Kaider A, Sevelda P, Gitsch G. The influence of obesity on the disease-free survival in primary breast cancer. *Anticancer Res* 1995; 15:2265–2269.
35. den Tonkelaar I, de Waard F, Seidell JC, Fracheboud J. Obesity and subcutaneous fat patterning in relation to survival of postmenopausal breast cancer patients participating in the DOM-project. *Breast Cancer Res Treat* 1995; 34:129–137.
36. Zhang S, Folsom AR, Sellers TA, Kushi LH, Potter JD. Better breast cancer survival for postmenopausal women who are less overweight and eat less fat. The Iowa Women's Health Study. *Cancer* 1995; 76:275–283.
37. Maehle BO, Tretli S. Premorbid body mass index in breast cancer: reversed effect on survival in hormone receptor negative patients. *Breast Cancer Res Treat* 1996; 41:123–130.

38. Rosner GL, Hargis JB, Hollis DR, Budman DR, Weiss RB, Henderson IC, Schilsky RL. Relationship between toxicity and obesity in women receiving adjuvant chemotherapy for breast cancer: results from cancer and leukemia group B study 8541. *J Clin Oncol* 1996; 14:3000–3008.
39. Lethaby AE, Mason BH, Harvey VJ, Holdaway IM. Survival of women with node negative breast cancer in the Auckland region. *NZ Med J* 1996; 109:330–333.
40. Haybittle J, Houghton J, Baum M. Social class and weight as prognostic factors in early breast cancer. *Br J Cancer* 1997; 75:729–733.
41. Newman SC, Lees AW, Jenkins HJ. The effect of body mass index and estrogen receptor level on survival of breast cancer patients. *Int J Epidemiol* 1997; 26:484–490.
42. Jain M, Miller AB. Tumor characteristics and survival of breast cancer patients in relation to premorbid diet and body size. *Breast Cancer Res Treat* 1997; 42:43–55.
43. Galanis DJ, Kolonel LN, Lee J, Le Marchand L. Anthropometric predictors of breast cancer incidence and survival in a multi-ethnic cohort of female residents of Hawaii, United States. *Cancer Causes Control* 1998; 9:217–224.
44. Hebert JR, Hurley TG, Ma Y. The effect of dietary exposures on recurrence and mortality in early stage breast cancer. *Breast Cancer Res Treat* 1998; 51:17–28.
45. Menon KV, Hodge A, Houghton J, Bates T. Body mass index, height and cumulative menstrual cycles at the time of diagnosis are not risk factors for poor outcome in breast cancer. *Breast* 1999; 8:328–333.
46. Kumar NB, Cantor A, Allen K, Cox CE. Android obesity at diagnosis and breast carcinoma survival: evaluation of the effects of anthropometric variables at diagnosis, including body composition and body fat distribution and weight gain during life span, and survival from breast carcinoma. *Cancer* 2000; 88:2751–2757.
47. Marret H, Perrotin F, Bougnoux P, Descamps P, Hubert B, Lefranc T, Le Floch O, Lansac J, Body G. Low body mass index is an independent predictive factor of local recurrence after conservative treatment for breast cancer. *Breast Cancer Res Treat* 2001; 66:17–23.
48. Daling JR, Malone KE, Doody DR, Johnson LG, Gralow JR, Porter PL. Relation of body mass index to tumor markers and survival among young women with invasive ductal breast carcinoma. *Cancer* 2001; 92:720–729.
49. Goodwin PJ, Ennis M, Pritchard KI, Trudeau ME, Koo J, Madarnas Y, Hartwick W, Hoffman B, Hood N. Fasting insulin and outcome in early-stage breast cancer: results of a prospective cohort study. *J Clin Oncol* 2002; 20:42–51.
50. Dignam JJ, Wieand K, Johnson KA, Fisher B, Xu L, Mamounas EP. Obesity, tamoxifen use, and outcomes in women with estrogen receptor-positive early-stage breast cancer. *J Natl Cancer Inst* 2003; 95:1467–1476.
51. Carmichael AR, Bendall S, Lockerbie L, Prescott RJ, Bates T. Does obesity compromise survival in women with breast cancer? *Breast* 2004; 13:93–96.
52. Chlebowski RT, Aiello E, McTiernan A. Weight loss in breast cancer patient management. *J Clin Oncol* 2002; 20:1128–1143.
53. Boyd DB. Insulin and cancer. *Integr Cancer Ther* 2003; 2:315–329.
54. Dixon JK, Moritz DA, Baker FL. Breast cancer and weight gain: an unexpected finding. *Oncol Nursing Forum* 1978; 5:5–7.
55. Knobf MK, Mullen JC, Xistris D, Moritz DA. Weight gain in women with breast cancer receiving adjuvant chemotherapy. *Oncol Nursing Forum* 1983; 10:28–33.
56. Bonomi P, Bunting N, Fishman D, Wolter J, Hernandez A, Foltz W, Shorey A, Straus A, Anderson K, Roseman D, Economou S. Weight gain during adjuvant chemotherapy or hormono-chemotherapy for stage II breast cancer evaluated in relation to disease free survival (DFS) (abstr.). *Breast Cancer Res Treat* 1984; 4:339.
57. Huntington MO. Weight gain in patients receiving adjuvant chemotherapy for carcinoma of the breast. *Cancer* 1985; 56:472–474.
58. Chlebowski RT, Weiner JM, Reynolds R, Luce J, Bulcavage L, Bateman JR. Long-term survival following relapse after 5-FU but not CMF adjuvant breast cancer therapy. *Breast Cancer Res Treat* 1986; 7:23–30.
59. Camoriano JK, Loprinzi CL, Ingle JN, Therneau TM, Krook JE, Veeder MH. Weight change in women treated with adjuvant therapy or observed following mastectomy for node-positive breast cancer. *J Clin Oncol* 1990; 8:1327–1334.

60. Foltz AT. Weight gain among stage II breast cancer patients: a study of five factors. *Oncol Nursing Forum* 1985; 12:21–26.
61. DeGeorge D, Gray JJ, Fetting JH, Rolls BJ. Weight gain in patients with breast cancer receiving adjuvant treatment as a function of restraint, disinhibition, and hunger. *Oncol Nursing Forum* 1990; 17:23–28.
62. Levine EG, Raczynski JM, Carpenter JT. Weight gain with breast cancer adjuvant treatment. *Cancer* 1991; 67:1954–1959.
63. Hoskin PJ, Ashley S, Yarnold JR. Weight gain after primary surgery for breast cancer — effect of tamoxifen. *Breast Cancer Res Treat* 1992; 22:129–132.
64. Hupperets PS, Wils J, Volovics L, Schouten L, Fickers M, Bron H, Schouten HC, Jager J, Smeets J, de Jong J, Blijham GH. Adjuvant chemohormonal therapy with cyclophosphamide, doxorubicin and 5-fluorouracil (CAF) with or without medroxyprogesterone acetate for node-positive breast cancer patients. *Ann Oncol* 1993; 4:295–301.
65. Kumar NB, Allen K, Cantor A, Cox CE, Greenberg H, Shah S, Lyman GH. Weight gain associated with adjuvant tamoxifen therapy in stage I and II breast cancer: fact or artifact? *Breast Cancer Res Treat* 1997; 44:135–143.
66. Cheney CL, Mahloch J, Freeny P. Computerized tomography assessment of women with weight changes associated with adjuvant treatment for breast cancer. *Am J Clin Nutr* 1997; 66:141–146.
67. Sitzia J, Huggins L. Side effects of cyclophosphamide, methotrexate, and 5-fluorouracil (CMF) chemotherapy for breast cancer. *Cancer Pract* 1998; 6:13–21.
68. Rock CL, Flatt SW, Newman V, Caan BJ, Haan MN, Stefanick ML, Faerber S, Pierce JP. Factors associated with weight gain in women after diagnosis of breast cancer. Women's Healthy Eating and Living Study Group. *J Am Diet Assoc* 1999; 99:1212–1221.
69. Goodwin PJ, Ennis M, Pritchard KI, McCready D, Koo J, Sidlofsky S, Trudeau M, Hood N, Redwood S. Adjuvant treatment and onset of menopause predict weight gain after breast cancer diagnosis. *J Clin Oncol* 1999; 17:120–129.
70. McInnes JA, Knobf MT. Weight gain and quality of life in women treated with adjuvant chemotherapy for early-stage breast cancer. *Oncol Nursing Forum* 2001; 28:675–684.
71. Costa LJ, Varella PC, del Giglio A. Weight changes during chemotherapy for breast cancer. *Sao Paulo Med J* 2002; 120:113–117.
72. Del Rio G, Zironi S, Valeriani L, Menozzi R, Bondi M, Bertolini M, Piccinini L, Banzi MC, Federico M. Weight gain in women with breast cancer treated with adjuvant cyclophosphomide, methotrexate and 5-fluorouracil. Analysis of resting energy expenditure and body composition. *Breast Cancer Res Treat* 2002; 73:267–273.
73. Lankester KJ, Phillips JE, Lawton PA. Weight gain during adjuvant and neoadjuvant chemotherapy for breast cancer: an audit of 100 women receiving FEC or CMF chemotherapy. *Clin Oncol (R Coll Radiol)* 2002; 14:64–67.
74. Grindel CG, Cahill CA, Walker M. Food intake of women with breast cancer during their first six month of chemotherapy. *Oncol Nursing Forum* 1989; 16:401–407.
75. Winningham ML, MacVicar MG, Bondoc M, Anderson JI, Minton JP. Effect of aerobic exercise on body weight and composition in patients with breast cancer on adjuvant chemotherapy. *Oncol Nursing Forum* 1989; 16:683–689.
76. Boyar AP, Rose DP, Loughridge JR, Engle A, Palgi A, Laakso K, Kinne D, Wynder EL. Response to a diet low in total fat in women with postmenopausal breast cancer: a pilot study. *Nutr Cancer* 1988; 11:93–99.
77. Nordevang E, Ikkala E, Callmer E, Hallstrom L, Holm LE. Dietary intervention in breast cancer patients: effects on dietary habits and nutrient intake. *Eur J Clin Nutr* 1990; 44:681–687.
78. Demark–Wahnefried W, Hars V, Conaway MR, Havlin K, Rimer BK, McElveen G, Winer EP. Reduced rates of metabolism and decreased physical activity in breast cancer patients receiving adjuvant chemotherapy. *Am J Clin Nutr* 1997; 65:1495–1501.
79. Aslani A, Smith RC, Allen BJ, Pavlakis N, Levi JA. Changes in body composition during breast cancer chemotherapy with the CMF-regimen. *Breast Cancer Res Treat* 1999; 57:285–290.
80. Kutynec CL, McCargar L, Barr SI, Hislop TG. Energy balance in women with breast cancer during adjuvant treatment. *J Am Diet Assoc* 1999; 99:1222–1227.

81. Schwartz AL. Exercise and weight gain in breast cancer patients receiving chemotherapy. *Cancer Pract* 2000; 8:231–237.
82. Rock CL, McEligot AJ, Flatt SW, Sobo EJ, Wilfley DE, Jones VE, Hollenbach KA, Marx RD. Eating pathology and obesity in women at risk for breast cancer recurrence. *Int J Eat Disord* 2000; 27:172–179.
83. Demark-Wahnefried W, Peterson BL, Winer EP, Marks L, Aziz N, Marcom PK, Blackwell K, Rimer BK. Changes in weight, body composition, and factors influencing energy balance among premenopausal breast cancer patients receiving adjuvant chemotherapy. *J Clin Oncol* 2001; 19:2381–2389.
84. Schmid P, Untch M, Wallwiener D, Kosse V, Bondar G, Vassiljev L, Tarutinov V, Kienle E, Luftner D, Possinger K. Cyclophosphamide, methotrexate and fluorouracil (CMF) vs. hormonal ablation with leuprorelin acetate as adjuvant treatment of node-positive, premenopausal breast cancer patients: preliminary results of the TABLE-study (Takeda Adjuvant Breast Cancer Study with Leuprorelin Acetate). *Anticancer Res* 2002; 22:2325–2332.
85. Martin M, Villar A, Sole-Calvo A, Gonzalez R, Massuti B, Lizon J, Camps C, Carrato A, Casado A, Candel MT, Albanell J, Aranda J, Munarriz B, Campbell J, Diaz–Rubio E. Doxorubicin in combination with fluorouracil and cyclophosphamide (i.v. FAC regimen, day 1, 21) vs. methotrexate in combination with fluorouracil and cyclophosphamide (i.v. CMF regimen, day 1, 21) as adjuvant chemotherapy for operable breast cancer: a study by the GEICAM group. *Ann Oncol* 2003; 14:833–842.
86. Freedman RJ, Aziz N, Albanes D, Hartman T, Danforth D, Hill S, Sebring N, Reynolds JC, Yanovski JA. Weight and body composition changes during and after adjuvant chemotherapy in women with breast cancer. *J Clin Endocrinol Metab* 2004; 89:2248–2253.
87. Harvie MN, Campbell IT, Baildam A, Howell A. Energy balance in early breast cancer patients receiving adjuvant chemotherapy. *Breast Cancer Res Treat* 2004; 83:201–210.
88. Bonadonna G, Valagussa P, Rossi A, Tancini G, Brambilla C, Zambetti M, Veronesi U. Ten-year experience with CMF-based adjuvant chemotherapy in resectable breast cancer. *Breast Cancer Res Treat* 1985; 5:95–115.
89. De Conti RC. Weight gain in the adjuvant chemotherapy of breast cancer. *Proc Am Soc Clin Oncol* 1982; 1:73.
90. Kumar N, Allen KA, Riccardi D, Bercu BB, Cantor A, Minton S, Balducci L, Jacobsen PB. Fatigue, weight gain, lethargy and amenorrhea in breast cancer patients on chemotherapy: is subclinical hypothyroidism the culprit? *Breast Cancer Res Treat* 2004; 83:149–159.
91. Stephenson GD, Rose DP. Breast cancer and obesity: an update. *Nutr Cancer* 2003; 45:1–16.
92. Goodwin PJ, Esplen MJ, Winocur J, Butler K, Pritchard KI. Development of a weight management program in women with newly diagnosed locoregional breast cancer. In: Bitzer J. and Stauber M. Eds. *International Society of Psychosomatic Obstetrics and Gynaecology: Psychosomatic Obstetrics and Gynecology*. Italy: Monduzzi Editore, International Proceedings, 1995:491–496.
93. Ballard-Barbash R. Chap. 14, this volume.
94. Williams G, Howell A, Jones M. The relationship of body weight to response to endocrine therapy, steroid hormone receptors and survival of patients with advanced cancer of the breast. *Br J Cancer* 1988; 58:631–634.
95. Kamby C, Ejlertsen B, Andersen J, Birkler NE, Rytter L, Zedeler K, Rose C. Body size and menopausal status in relation to the pattern of spread in recurrent breast cancer. *Acta Oncol* 1989; 28:795–799.
96. Kornblith AB, Hollis DR, Zuckerman E, Lyss AP, Canellos GP, Cooper MR, Herndon JE, Phillips CA, Abrams J, Aisner J, Norton L, Henderson C, Holland JC. Effect of megestrol acetate on quality of life in a dose–response trial in women with advanced breast cancer. The Cancer and Leukemia Group B. *J Clin Oncol* 1993; 11:2081–2089.
97. Shepherd L, Parulekar W, Day A, Ottaway J, Bramwell V, Levine M, Pritchard K. Weight gain during adjuvant therapy in high-risk pre/perimenopausal breast cancer patients: Analysis of a National Cancer Institute of Canada Clinical Trials Group (NCIC CTG) phase II study (abstr.). *Proc Am Soc Clin Oncol* 2001; 20:36a.
98. Goodwin P, Esplen MJ, Butler K, Winocur J, Pritchard K, Brazel S, Gao J, Miller A. Multidisciplinary weight management in locoregional breast cancer: results of a phase II study. *Breast Cancer Res Treat* 1998; 48:53–64.

99. Bonomi P, Bunting N, Fishman D, Wolter J, Hernandez B, Foltz A, Shorey W, Straus A, Anderson K, Roseman D, Economou S. Weight gain during adjuvant chemotherapy or hormono-chemotherapy for stage II breast cancer evaluated in relation to disease free survival (DFS) (abstr.). *Br Cancer Res Treat* 1984; 4:339.
100. Madarnas Y, Sawka CA, Franssen E, Bjarnason GA. Are medical oncologists biased in their treatment of the large woman with breast cancer? *Breast Cancer Res Treat* 2001; 66:123–133.
101. Schmid P, Possinger K, Bohm R, Chaudri H, Verbeek A, Grosse Y, Luftner D, Petrides P, Sezer O, Wischnewsky M. Body mass index as predictive parameter for response and time to progression (TTP) in advanced breast cancer patients treated with letrozole or megestrol acetate (abstr.). *Proc Am Soc Clin Oncol* 2000; 19:103a.
102. Reaven GM. Banting lecture 1988. Role of insulin resistance in human disease. *Diabetes* 1988; 37:1595–1607.
103. Shen BJ, Todaro JF, Niaura R, McCaffery JM, Zhang J, Spiro A, III, Ward KD. Are metabolic risk factors one unified syndrome? Modeling the structure of the metabolic syndrome X. *Am J Epidemiol* 2003; 157:701–711.
104. Papa V, Pezzino V, Costantino A, Belfiore A, Giuffrida D, Frittitta L, Vannelli GB, Brand R, Goldfine ID, Vigneri R. Elevated insulin receptor content in human breast cancer. *J Clin Invest* 1990; 86:1503–1510.
105. Hwang DL, Papoian T, Barseghian G, Josefsberg Z, Lev-Ran A. Absence of down-regulation of insulin receptors in human breast cancer cells (MCF-7) cultured in serum-free medium: comparison with epidermal growth factor. *J Recept Res* 1985; 5:27–43.
106. Mountjoy KG, Finlay GJ, Holdaway IM. Abnormal insulin-receptor down regulation and dissociation of down regulation from insulin biological action in cultured human tumor cells. *Cancer Res* 1987; 47:6500–6504.
107. Jackson JG, White MF, Yee D. Insulin receptor substrate-1 is the predominant signaling molecule activated by insulin-like growth factor-I, insulin, and interleukin-4 in estrogen receptor-positive human breast cancer cells. *J Biol Chem* 1998; 273:9994–10003.
108. Zong CS, Zeng L, Jiang Y, Sadowski HB, Wang LH. Stat3 plays an important role in oncogenic Ros- and insulin-like growth factor I receptor-induced anchorage-independent growth. *J Biol Chem* 1998; 273:28065–28072.
109. Grimberg A, Cohen P. Role of insulin-like growth factors and their binding proteins in growth control and carcinogenesis. *J Cell Physiol* 2000; 183:1–9.
110. Resnicoff M, Baserga R. The role of the insulin-like growth factor I receptor in transformation and apoptosis. *Ann NY Acad Sci* 1998; 842:76–81.
111. Blackburn G, Waltman B. Chap. 20, this volume.
112. Sandhu MS, Dunger DB, Giovannucci EL. Insulin, insulin-like growth factor-I (IGF-I), IGF binding proteins, their biologic interactions, and colorectal cancer. *J Natl Cancer Inst* 2002; 94:972–980.
113. Goodwin PJ, Ennis M, Pritchard KI, Trudeau ME, Koo J, Hartwick W, Hoffma B, Hood N. Insulin-like growth factor binding proteins 1 and 3 and breast cancer outcomes. *Breast Cancer Res Treat* 2002; 74:65–76.
114. Rose DP, Gilhooly EM, Nixon DW. Adverse effects of obesity on breast cancer prognosis, and the biological actions of leptin (review). *Int J Oncol* 2002; 21:1285–1292.
115. Goodwin PJ, Ennis M, Fantus IG, Pritchard KI, Trudeau ME, Koo J, Hood N. Is leptin a mediator of adverse prognostic effects of obesity in breast cancer? *J Clin Oncol*. (in press).
116. Peiris AN, Sothmann MS, Aiman EJ, Kissebah AH. The relationship of insulin to sex hormone-binding globulin: role of adiposity. *Fertil Steril* 1989; 52:69–72.
117. Nestler JE, Powers LP, Matt DW, Steingold KA, Plymate SR, Rittmaster RS, Clore JN, Blackard WG. A direct effect of hyperinsulinemia on serum sex hormone-binding globulin levels in obese women with the polycystic ovary syndrome. *J Clin Endocrinol Metab* 1991; 72:83–89.
118. Oesterreich S, Zhang P, Guler RL, Sun X, Curran EM, Welshons WV, Osborne CK, Lee AV. Re-expression of estrogen receptor alpha in estrogen receptor alpha-negative MCF-7 cells restores both estrogen and insulin-like growth factor-mediated signaling and growth. *Cancer Res* 2001; 61:5771–5777.
119. Dupont J, Le Roith D. Insulin-like growth factor 1 and oestradiol promote cell proliferation of MCF-7 breast cancer cells: new insights into their synergistic effects. *Mol Pathol* 2001; 54:149–154.

120. Dupont J, Karas M, LeRoith D. The potentiation of estrogen on insulin-like growth factor I action in MCF-7 human breast cancer cells includes cell cycle components. *J Biol Chem* 2000; 275:35893–35901.

28 Energy Balance and Cancer Prognosis: Colon, Prostate, and Other Cancers

Cheryl L. Rock

CONTENTS

INTRODUCTION

Overweight and obesity are clinical indicators of energy imbalance or, specifically, excess energy intake relative to expenditure. Overweight and obesity are clearly associated with increased risk for several chronic diseases and conditions, including type-2 diabetes mellitus, coronary heart disease, high blood cholesterol, high blood pressure, gallbladder disease, and osteoarthritis [1]. In the general population, excess body weight also has been observed to be significantly associated with increased mortality from all cancers combined and for cancers of several specific sites [2].

Based on fairly consisting findings from numerous studies, obesity appears to be an important negative prognostic factor for women who have been diagnosed and treated for breast cancer [3] (also, see Chapter 27, Chapter 34, and Chapter 35). Fewer studies have examined the associations between energy imbalance (as indicated by overweight or obesity) and recurrence or survival after the diagnosis of other types of cancer. However, this is an area of current interest, particularly in view of the increasing rates of obesity in the U.S., and studies that can address this issue are ongoing.

Several mechanisms to explain the association between overweight or obesity and prognosis following the diagnosis of cancer have been suggested. Alterations in metabolic and hormonal factors that may affect cancer progression, such as gonadal reproductive hormones, insulin, and other growth factors, are possible mediating factors [4,5], but other factors also may explain how obesity affects survival. For example, optimal surgical procedures for accurate diagnosis and initial treatment may be compromised by excess adiposity [6]. Chemotherapy regimens have generally been developed and tested in clinical studies involving mainly normal-weight individuals; the obese patient presents with altered body composition (e.g., increased proportion of fat to total body weight) and altered pharmokinetics due to obesity-related differences in hepatic and renal function [7–9].

In the studies that have examined associations between overweight or obesity and survival following the diagnosis of cancer, the subjects originate from different potential sources or pools, which influences the nature of the available data and the characteristics of the sample. They may be cases originally identified for case-control studies, cases that occur in clinical trials or ongoing cohort studies, or cases identified through hospital-based care and evaluated as a clinical series report (or retrospective chart review). In the reported studies, the effect of obesity on prognosis is typically examined using premorbid weight or weight at diagnosis. Thus, the issue of whether postdiagnosis weight reduction through diet and/or increased physical activity can modify the relationship usually cannot be addressed.

Also, overweight or obesity is not uniformly defined across these studies, and approaches used include calculating relative weight (weight for height compared with previously published optimal weight data) or comparing across subgroups using an arbitrary cut-point. The most common approach to defining overweight or obesity is based on the calculated body mass index (BMI, weight [kg]/height [m^2]). BMI should be considered an indicator rather than a specific measure of adiposity; in adults, this index correlates better with total body fat at the ends of the spectrum than in the midrange [10].

COLON AND RECTAL CANCER

The relationship between overweight or obesity and prognosis following the diagnosis of colon cancer has been examined in a few studies. In an early study, Tartter et al. [11] examined cumulative 5-year recurrence-free rates in 279 stage II to stage III colon cancer patients identified over a 3-year period at a medical center in relation to weight, height, and an index of obesity (weight × 100/height^2). Overall, patients above the median weight were found to be at significantly increased risk of recurrence (76 vs. 54%, $p < 0.01$), and women (but not men) above the median obesity index score were at significantly greater risk of recurrence (74 vs. 52%, $p < 0.01$). Slattery et al. [12] subsequently examined the relationships among BMI, selected dietary factors, and survival in 411 colon cancer cases identified through two population-based case-control studies, with a median follow-up of 56 months. After underweight patients were excluded, increasing BMI was associated with a nonsignificant increase in overall mortality, although energy intake was found to be associated directly with survival.

Relevant findings were reported in a more recent study of survival in relation to dietary factors (but not obesity) in 171 cases of colorectal cancer identified through another case-control study [13]. In this study, high energy intake was again associated with increased likelihood of survival: 5-year relative risk of death for the highest vs. the two lowest tertiles of energy intake was 0.18 (95% confidence interval [CI] 0.07, 0.44). However, accurate estimates of energy intake are difficult to obtain with the dietary assessment approaches used in epidemiological studies, so the interpretation of these findings is constrained.

Within a large, randomized adjuvant chemotherapy trial, the relationships between BMI and outcomes over a median follow-up of 9.4 years were recently examined in 3759 patients with stage II to stage III colon cancer [14]. Compared with normal-weight women (BMI < 25 kg/m^2), obese women (BMI ≥ 30 kg/m^2) experienced significantly worse overall mortality (hazard ratio [HR] 1.34, 95% CI 1.07, 1.67) and a nonsignificant increase in risk for recurrence (HR 1.24, 95% CI 0.98, 1.59). BMI was unrelated to mortality or risk for recurrence in men in that study.

In another study that focused specifically on rectal cancer and used the same cut-points for defining obesity, the relationships between BMI and outcomes were examined in a target group of 1688 participants in a randomized adjuvant chemotherapy clinical trial [15]. In that study, obese men with rectal cancer were more likely than normal-weight men to have a local recurrence (HR

1.61, 95% CI 1.00, 2.59). However, obesity was unrelated to risk for recurrence in women, and BMI was not associated with overall mortality in men or women.

Based on the few studies reported to date, some evidence, although not conclusive or consistent, indicates that energy imbalance resulting in overweight or obesity may influence risk for recurrence and survival following the diagnosis of colon or rectal cancer. However, this is not an established relationship.

PROSTATE CANCER

Results of two studies that examined several dietary and nutritional factors, including obesity, and survival after the diagnosis of prostate cancer have been reported, both based on cases identified through population-based case-control studies. Meyer et al. [16] prospectively followed 384 men diagnosed with prostate cancer, with a median duration of follow-up of 5.2 years. When adjusted for known prognostic factors, BMI was not found to be related to mortality in that study. In a group of 408 men diagnosed with prostate cancer who were followed for a median of 4.9 years, Kim et al. [17] similarly observed no relationship between BMI and survival.

The relationship between obesity (defined by relative weight) and 5-year tumor-specific mortality also was examined in a clinical series of 235 men identified at a community hospital [18]. In that study, men who were at least 10% overweight were less likely to have advanced tumors. When they were subgrouped and examined by obesity and smoking status, tumor-specific mortality was lower in obese than nonobese nonsmokers, and in obese nonsmokers compared to all other subgroups (10 vs. 30%, $p < 0.001$); this reflects lower mortality in those with tumors of identical stages and a larger percent with less advanced tumors. In contrast, in a multi-institutional retrospective analysis of clinical and pathological data from 860 patients, Amling et al. [19] found that obese (BMI ≥ 30 kg/m^2) vs. nonobese (BMI < 30 kg/m^2) patients with prostate cancer present for radical prostatectomy at a younger age with higher grade and more pathologically advanced cancers.

The relationship between obesity and risk for biochemical recurrence (i.e., increasing circulating prostate-specific antigen) following radical prostatectomy was examined in one study involving data from 1106 men identified through a multi-institutional database, with a median follow-up of 33 months [20]. Moderate and severe obesity (defined as BMI ≥ 35 kg/m^2), relative to lower BMI levels, was significantly associated with risk for biochemical recurrence (HR 1.99, 95% CI 1.21, 3.27). Controlled for all preoperative clinical variables and year of surgery, BMI ≥ 35 kg/m^2 was found to be significantly associated with increased likelihood of biochemical recurrence ($p < 0.01$); however, differences across categories of lower ranges of BMI (e.g., <25, 25 to <30, 30 to <35 kg/m^2) were not observed.

Clearly, the divergent results from studies to date that have examined whether overweight or obesity influences survival after the diagnosis and treatment of prostate cancer preclude well-supported conclusions at this time. Data from a large, ongoing randomized controlled trial testing the effect of supplemental micronutrients on the incidence of primary prostate cancer are expected to provide some additional insight relating to energy imbalance and survival [21]. Although incident prostate cancer is the primary endpoint for that trial, secondary endpoints will include prostate cancer-free survival and all-cause mortality. Extensive data on nutritional factors (including weight and height) are being collected as well.

GYNECOLOGICAL CANCERS

OVARIAN CANCER

To date, only one epidemiological study has examined the relationship between nutritional factors, including selected dietary intakes and obesity, and survival following the diagnosis of ovarian cancer [22]. In a cohort of 609 women with invasive ovarian cancer, 5-year survival was examined in relation to intakes and BMI, adjusted for known prognostic factors. When compared across tertiles (<22.2, 22.3 to 25.8, and >25.8 kg/m^2), BMI was unrelated to survival. However, the investigators noted that women with BMI < 20 kg/m^2 had a somewhat better likelihood of survival than the rest of the women, although this difference was not statistically significant (HR 0.8, 95% CI 0.48, 1.35).

Endometrial Cancer

The relationships among overweight or obesity, tumor characteristics, and survival following the diagnosis of endometrial cancer have been examined in three retrospective studies. Anderson et al. [23] analyzed data from 492 women with endometrial carcinoma who were identified through a medical center database, with a mean follow-up of 4.2 years. Analyzed as a continuous variable, BMI was directly related to time to recurrence ($p < 0.02$), and a marginally significant protective effect was found for survival ($p = 0.0645$). Notably, the heavier patients were more likely to have less aggressive disease, indicated by a higher incidence of better differentiated, less invasive adenocarcinomas in those women in that study.

Similar findings were reported by Everett et al. [24] in 396 patients who also were identified through a single medical center database and had a median 27-month follow-up period [24]. No differences in survival were observed across three categories of BMI (<30, 30 to 40, and >40 kg/m^2). Similar to the study by Anderson et al. [23], a beneficial effect of obesity (BMI > 40 vs. BMI < 30 kg/m^2) on risk for recurrence was marginally significant in this study ($p = 0.065$), when adjusted for covariates such as grade, nodes, myometrial invasion, and stage. Also, patients with BMI > 40 kg/m^2 were more likely to have endometrioid histology, lower stage disease, and lower grade tumors than women with BMI < 30 kg/m^2. However, 23% of the women with BMI > 40 kg/m^2 who had complete surgical staging with lymphadenectomy were found to be stage II and higher, indicating evidence for cervical or extrauterine disease.

In a retrospective analysis of data from 121 women treated for endometrial carcinoma at a Polish hospital [25], obese patients (presumably those with BMI ≥ 25 kg/m^2) had a longer 5-year survival compared to nonobese patients (87.4 vs. 73.4%, $p = 0.05$). When examined across BMI categories, patients with "mild obesity" (defined as BMI 25 to 29 kg/m^2) had the longest 5-year survival rate, and patients with "morbid obesity" had the same survival rate as normal-weight patients as defined by being in an appropriate BMI category.

Although only a few relevant studies have been reported, current evidence suggests that obesity may not be a negative prognostic factor for endometrial cancer. However, there are complicating issues in fully describing risk for recurrence or cancer progression in this patient population. Complete surgical staging via lymphadenectomy is sometimes not performed if the pathologic findings suggest that the patient is at low risk of recurrence [24]. In both of the two studies that addressed the issue, obesity was found to be associated with more favorable tumor characteristics, which suggests that the available data and the accurate interpretation of findings are complicated.

Cervical Cancer

The relationship between overweight or obesity and survival following the diagnosis of cervical cancer has been examined in two retrospective studies. Based on data from 175 patients diagnosed with advanced squamous cell cervical cancer at a medical center, 5-year survival was observed to be unrelated to obesity [26]. Although the definition of obesity in that study was not provided, obese patients reportedly had a 39% survival compared to 35% survival for nonobese patients.

In a retrospective review of 302 cases of primary cervical adenocarcinoma (stages I, II, and III/IV) at a Taiwanese hospital, the relationships between various prognostic factors and 5-year survival were examined for a median follow-up period of 63 months [27]. Obesity (although not defined) was tested for effect as a dichotomous variable (obese vs. nonobese) and was not significantly independently related to survival in that study.

Thus, both of the studies that have addressed the question of whether obesity affects risk for recurrence or survival in women who have been diagnosed with invasive cervical cancer found no relationship. However, the approaches used to examine this issue were crude, and more data and analysis relating to this area are needed prior to drawing conclusions.

Vulvar Cancer

Contrasting findings have been reported in two retrospective studies of the relationship between obesity and survival in women who have been diagnosed with invasive squamous cell vulvar carcinoma. Based on data from 50 cases identified at a Greek hospital, with a median follow-up of 61 months, Kouvaris et al. [28,29] found that overall survival was lower in women defined as obese (25.8 vs. 40.7 months for BMI ≥ 27 and < 27 kg/m^2, respectively, $p < 0.02$). In contrast, Kirschner et al. [30] found no relationship between obesity (defined as BMI ≥ 27 kg/m^2) and survival in 136 cases identified at a medical center, with a median follow-up of 69.3 months. Given the limited available data and divergent results from these studies, conclusions regarding a possible relationship between energy imbalance and survival in vulvar cancer would be premature at this time.

OTHER CANCERS

Whether overweight or obesity is associated with risk for recurrence or survival in patients with renal cell carcinoma has been addressed in one study. Yu et al. [31] examined data from 360 renal cell carcinoma patients identified at multiple institutions; the majority of the cases had been identified in a prior case-control study. Obesity (defined as BMI ≥ 120% of standard BMI) was associated with later recurrence and longer survival in that study. Adjusted for other potentially prognostic factors, the hazard ratio for disease recurrence between the obese and nonobese patients was 0.43 (95% CI 0.19, 0.98) and the adjusted death hazard ratio was 0.68 (95% CI 0.38, 1.22).

Data from 787 patients diagnosed and treated for gastric carcinoma at a Japanese hospital were examined to address whether obesity was associated with recurrence-free 5-year survival rates [6]. Investigators found that significantly fewer lymph nodes were removed in D2 and D3 dissections in patients identified as obese (BMI > 24.7 kg/m^2 for men and > 22.6 kg/m^2 for women) ($p < 0.03$). Furthermore, obesity was independently associated with shorter recurrence-free survival in T2/T3 cases in multivariate analysis (median 50 months vs. 69 months for high BMI vs. low BMI, respectively, $p < 0.03$), adjusted for other potentially influencing factors.

Some clinical data in the scientific literature have suggested that overweight or obese (vs. nonobese) patients are at increased risk for chemotherapy-related toxicity and adverse side effects, although the findings are not consistent. For example, examination of the clinical course of 262 patients treated for small-cell lung cancer with standard dose chemotherapies revealed no consistent associations of significance between increasing BMI levels and toxicity from therapy [7]. In contrast, risk of death associated with high-dose chemotherapy and autograph treatment has been found to be substantially higher in patients with higher vs. lower BMI in a few studies.

In a retrospective analysis of 121 patients administered this treatment, patients with BMI ≥ 28 kg/m^2 exhibited a risk of death of 2.9 (95% CI 1.3, 6.2) compared to patients with lower BMI, adjusted for other influencing factors [8]. In another similar study that focused on clinical data from 54 patients who underwent autologous stem cell transplantation, treatment-related toxicity and mortality, overall survival, and disease-free survival were all observed to be significantly adversely affected by obesity [9]. In that study, patients were grouped as obese (BMI ≥ 27.8 kg/m^2 in men and ≥ 27.3 kg/m^2 in women), underweight (BMI ≤ 20.7 kg/m^2 in men and ≤ 19.1 kg/m^2 in women), and normal weight or nonobese, and the underweight subgroup was excluded from the analysis of outcomes.

SUMMARY AND CONCLUSIONS

Evidence relating to the effect of energy imbalance, as indicated by overweight or obesity, and risk for recurrence or survival following the diagnosis of cancers other than breast cancer is rather limited. For colorectal cancer, available evidence does suggest the possibility of an unfavorable effect of overweight or obesity on survival, but some inconsistencies have been found in the results of the studies reported to date. Even more divergent results have been found in studies relating overweight or obesity to recurrence or survival following the diagnosis of prostate cancer.

For cancers of other types, the current evidence is even more meager, with the evidence available consisting of very mixed results. Notably, the few studies relating to endometrial cancer that have published to date even suggest the possibility of a protective effect of obesity. Available data relating to cervical cancer are limited but consistently suggest a lack of effect of obesity on survival.

Given the established relationship between overweight and obesity and risk for other chronic diseases, such as cardiovascular disease and type-2 diabetes mellitus, achieving and maintaining a healthy weight is an appropriate recommendation for cancer survivors [32]. Regardless of a specific association with cancer progression, the well-established relationship of overweight and obesity, disease burden, and overall mortality provides a compelling reason to encourage energy balance in this target population [1].

REFERENCES

1. Must A, Spandano J, Coakley EH, Field AE, Colditz G, Dietz WH. The disease burden associated with overweight and obesity. *JAMA* 1999; 282:1523–1529.
2. Calle EE, Rodriguez C, Walker–Thurmond K, Thun MJ. Overweight, obesity, and mortality from cancer in a prospectively studied cohort of U.S. adults. *N Engl J Med* 2003; 348:1625–1638.
3. Rock CL, Demark-Wahnefried W. Nutrition and survival after the diagnosis of breast cancer: a review of the evidence. *J Clin Oncol* 2002; 20:3302–3316.
4. Chlebowski RT, Aiello E, McTiernan A. Weight loss in breast cancer patient management. *J Clin Oncol* 2002; 20:1128–1143.
5. McTiernan A, Ulrich C, Slate S, Potter J. Physical activity and cancer etiology: associations and mechanisms. *Cancer Causes Control* 1998; 9:487–509.
6. Dhar DK, Kubota H, Tachibana M, Kotoh T, Tabara H, Masunaga R, Kohno H, Nagasue N. Body mass index determines the success of lymph node dissection and predicts the outcome of gastric carcinoma patients. *Oncology* 2000; 59:18–23.
7. Georgiadis MS, Steinberg SM, Hankins LA, Ihde DC, Johnson BE. Obesity and therapy-related toxicity in patients treated for small-cell lung cancer. *J Natl Cancer Inst* 1995; 87:361–366.
8. Tarella C, Caracciolo D, Gavarotti P, Argentino C, Zallio F, Corradini P, Novero D, Magnani C, Pileri A. Overweight as an adverse prognostic factor for non-Hodgkin's lymphoma patients receiving high-dose chemotherapy and autograft. *Bone Marrow Transplantation* 2000; 26:1185–1191.
9. Meloni G, Proia A, Capria S, Romano A, Trape G, Trisolini SM, Vignetti M, Mandelli F. Obesity and autologous stem cell transplantation in acute myeloid leukemia. *Bone Marrow Transplantation* 2001; 28:365–367.
10. Curtin F, Morabia A, Pichard C, Slosman DO. Body mass index compared to dual-energy x-ray absorptiometry: evidence for a spectrum bias. *J Clin Epidemiol* 1997; 50:837–843.
11. Tartter PI, Slater G, Papatestas AE, Aufses AH. Cholesterol, weight, height, Quetelet's index, and colon cancer recurrence. *J Surg Oncol* 1984; 27:232–235.
12. Slattery ML, Anderson K, Samowitz W, Edwards SL, Curtin K, Caan B, Potter JD. Hormone replacement therapy and improved survival among postmenopausal women diagnosed with colon cancer. *Cancer Causes Control* 1999; 10:467–473.
13. Dray X, Boutron-Ruault MC, Bertrais S, Sapinho D, Benhamiche–Bouvier AM, Faivre J. Influence of dietary factors on colorectal cancer survival. *Gut* 2003; 52:868–873.

14. Meyerhardt JA, Tepper JE, Niedzweicki D, Hollis DR, McCollum AD, Brady D, O'Connell MJ, Mayer RJ, Cummings B, Willett C, Macdonald JS, Benson AB, Fuchs CS. Impact of body mass index on outcomes and treatment-related toxicity in patients with stage II and III rectal cancer: findings from Intergroup Trial 0114. *J Clin Oncol* 2004; 22:648–657.
15. Meyerhardt JA, Catalano PJ, Haller DG, Mayer RJ, Benson AB, Macdonald JS, Fuchs CS. Influence of body mass index on outcomes and treatment-related toxicity in patients with colon carcinoma. *Cancer* 2003; 98:484–495.
16. Meyer F, Bairati I, Shadmani R, Fradet Y, Moore L. Dietary fat and prostate cancer survival. *Cancer Causes Control* 1999; 10:245–251.
17. Kim DJ, Gallagher RP, Hislop TG, Holowaty EJ, Howe GR, Jain J, McLaughlin JR, The CZ, Rohan TE. Premorbid diet in relation to survival from prostate cancer. *Cancer Causes Control* 2000; 11:65–77.
18. Daniell HW. A better prognosis for obese men with prostate cancer. *J Urol* 1996; 155:220–225.
19. Amling CL, Kane CJ, Riffenburgh RH, Ward JF, Roberts JL, Lance RS, Friedrichs PA, Moul JW. Relationship between obesity and race in predicting adverse pathologic variables in patients undergoing radical prostatectomy. *Urology* 2001; 58:723–728.
20. Freedland SJ, Aronson WJ, Kane CJ, Presti JC, Amling CL, Elashoff D, Terris MK. Impact of obesity on biochemical control after radical prostatectomy for clinically localized prostate cancer: a report by the Shared Equal Access Regional Cancer Hospital Database Study Group. *J Clin Oncol* 2004; 22:446–453.
21. Klein EA, Lippman SM, Thompson IM, Goodman PJ, Albanes D, Taylor PR, Coltman C. The Selenium and Vitamin E Cancer Prevention Trial. *World J Urol* 2003; 21:21–27.
22. Nagle CM, Purdie DM, Webb PM, Green A, Harvey PW, Bain CJ. Dietary influences on survival after ovarian cancer. *Int J Cancer* 2003; 106:264–269.
23. Anderson B, Connor JP, Andrews JI, Davis CS, Buller RE, Sorosky JI, Benda JA. Obesity and prognosis in endometrial cancer. *Am J Obstet Gynecol* 1996; 174:1171–1178.
24. Everett E, Tamimi H, Greer B, Swisher E, Paley P, Mandel L, Goff B. The effect of body mass index on clinical/pathologic features, surgical morbidity, and outcome in patients with endometrial cancer. *Gynecol Oncol* 2003; 90:150–157.
25. Studzinski Z, Zajewski W. Factors affecting the survival of 121 patients treated for endometrial carcinoma at a Polish hospital. *Arch Gynecol Obstet* 2003; 267:145–147.
26. Hopkins MP, Morley GW. Prosnostic factors in advanced stage squamous cell cancer of the cervix. *Cancer* 1993; 72:2389–2393.
27. Chen RJ, Chang DY, Yen ML, Lee EF, Huang SC, Chow SN, Hsieh CY. Prognostic factors of primary adenocarcinoma of the uterine cervix. *Gynecol Oncol* 1998; 69:157–164.
28. Kouvaris J, Kouloulias V, Loghis C, Sykiotis C, Balafouta M, Vlahos L. Prognostic factors for survival in invasive squamous cell vulvar carcinoma: a univariate analysis. *Gynecol Obstet Invest* 2001; 51:262–265.
29. Kouvaris JR, Kouloulias VE, Loghis CD, Balafouta EJ, Miliadou AC, Vlahos LJ. Minor prognostic factors in squamous cell vulvar carcinoma. *Eur J Gynaec Oncol* 2001; 22:305–308.
30. Kirschner CV, Yordan EL, De Geest K, Wilbanks GD. Smoking, obesity, and survival in squamous cell carcinoma of the vulva. *Gynecol Oncol* 1995; 56:79–84.
31. Yu ML, Asal NR, Geyer JR. Later recurrence and longer survival among obese patients with renal cell carcinoma. *Cancer* 1991; 68:1648–1655.
32. Brown JK, Byers T, Doyle C, Courneya KS, Demark-Wahnefried W, Kushi LH, McTiernan A, Rock CL, Aziz N, Bloch A, Eldridge B, Hamilton K, Katzin C, Koonce A, Main J, Mobley C, Morra ME, Pierce MS, Sawyer K. Nutrition and physical activity during and after cancer treatment: an American Cancer Society guide for informed choices. *Calif Cancer J Clin* 2003; 53:268–291.

Section VIII

Implementation

29 Physical Activity and Energy Balance

Mikael Fogelholm

CONTENTS

COMPONENTS OF DAILY ENERGY EXPENDITURE

In energy balance, daily energy intake equals energy expenditure, and body weight and energy content (body composition) are unchanged. The daily energy expenditure can be divided into the following components (Figure 29.1):

- Basal (or resting) energy expenditure (BEE or REE)
- Diet-induced thermogenesis (DIT)
- Energy expenditure (EE) caused by physical activity (PAEE)

The basic unit for energy expenditure is the kilojoule (megajoule = 1000 kJ) per time unit (usually MJ/day). 1 kJ = 0.24 kcal (or 1 kcal = 4.18 kJ), which is still often used in the literature.

Daily energy expenditure is strongly related to body mass and particularly to fat-free mass (FFM = body mass – fat mass) [1]. Also, fat mass shows a positive correlation with daily energy expenditure, but the slope (increase of energy expenditure per kilogram of fat mass) is less steep than for fat-free mass [1]. Daily energy expenditure is also higher in men than in women, but the difference disappears after adjustment for the higher proportion of fat-free mass in men. Very cold or hot environments, genetic differences, hormonal status (e.g., concentrations of thyroid and growth

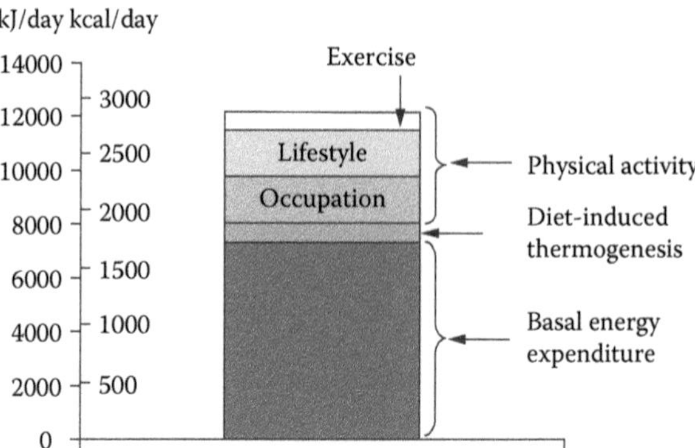

FIGURE 29.1 Components of daily energy expenditure.

hormone), sympathetic activity, psychological state, pharmacological agents, and several disease states may increase or decrease daily energy expenditure, mainly by affecting resting energy expenditure [2,3].

Factors associated with basal energy expenditure and diet-induced thermogenesis are described briefly next. The remaining part of this chapter deals with components and determinants of daily physical activity and the relation among physical activity, weight management, and health.

Basal Energy Expenditure

Basal energy expenditure or basal metabolic rate (BMR) is defined as the energy expenditure of an individual lying at physical and mental rest in a thermoneutral environment, about 12 hours after the previous meal. Resting energy expenditure is measured in less rigorous conditions than basal energy expenditure is. Therefore, resting energy expenditure is considered to be approximately 5% higher than basal energy expenditure. The mean energy expenditure during sleep is slightly lower than during arousal [1] and sleeping energy expenditure is about 10% lower than basal energy expenditure. However, despite small systematic differences, sleeping energy expenditure, basal energy expenditure, and resting energy expenditure are very strongly intercorrelated and the terms are often used interchangeably.

The strongest determinant of basal energy expenditure is fat-free mass, which explains up to 80% of interindividual variation [1]. The relationship seems to be linear, at least within a normal range of adult fat-free mass (40 to 100 kg). The maximal interindividual variation at a given fat-free mass is about 2.1 MJ, indicating the possible magnitude of difference in resting energy expenditure between two individuals with a similar fat-free mass. Genetic variation, body composition, variation of hormone concentration, energy balance and physical fitness are factors that have been found to explain the variations of basal energy expenditure, after adjustment for fat-free mass [2–5]. Physical activity, mainly strength training, may also increase absolute basal energy expenditure by increasing muscle mass.

Basal energy expenditure is measured in the laboratory by using the ventilated hood method [6]. This method is based on indirect calorimetry, that is, measurement of oxygen consumption, carbon dioxide production, and ventilation [7]. Measurement of resting energy expenditure is carried out in the morning after an overnight fast. Strenuous physical activity and alcohol consumption are not allowed on the day preceding the measurement. Smoking is not allowed and any physical activity should be restricted between waking up and resting energy expenditure measurement. The measurements are taken while the subject is in a lying or half-sitting position, with a typical duration between 30 and 60 min. Basal energy expenditure can be calculated from the calorimetry data in several ways. We have used a 45-min measurement. The first 15 min data are not used. The mean

TABLE 29.1
Prediction Equations for Basal Energy Expenditure (MJ/day)

Age (years)	Males	Females
<3	0.249 × weight − 0.13	0.244 × weight + 0.13
4–10	0.095 × weight + 2.11	0.085 × weight + 2.03
11–18	0.074 × weight + 2.75	0.056 × weight + 2.90
19–30	0.064 × weight + 2.84	0.0615 × weight + 2.08
31–60	0.0485 × weight + 3.67	0.0364 × weight + 3.47
61–75	0.0499 × weight + 2.93	0.0386 × weight + 2.88
>75	0.035 × weight + 3.43	0.0410 × weight + 2.61

Note: To obtain the result as kilocalories per day, divide the result by 0.004184.

Source: WHO. WHO Technical Report Series; 724. Geneva: WHO, 1985.

energy expenditure (kJ or kcal/min) is calculated separately from 16- to 30-min and 31- to 45-min data, and the lower of these values is used as basal energy expenditure.

Because of the technical constraints of basal energy expenditure measurements, determinations of energy requirements are usually based on predicted basal energy expenditure. Table 29.1 shows prediction equations for basal energy expenditure, as given by WHO/FAO/UNU [8]. Several prediction equations use fat-free mass, with or without fat mass, as the independent variable. However, because most individuals do not know their fat-free mass and accurate assessment of body composition is difficult and time consuming, it may be equally acceptable to use prediction equations with body weight as the independent variable, and age (group) and sex as classifying variables.

Oxygen consumption at rest is approximately 3.5 ml/kg per minute [9]. Therefore, a "quick and dirty" method to estimate resting energy expenditure is to use 1 kcal or 4.2 kJ per kilogram of body weight per minute. This is a very rough estimation, but gives an indication of the magnitude of resting energy expenditure.

Diet-Induced Thermogenesis

Diet-induced thermogenesis or diet-induced energy expenditure can be defined as the increase in energy expenditure above basal energy expenditure divided by the energy content of the food ingested [10]. The postprandial rise in energy expenditure lasts for several hours, but about 90% of diet-induced thermogenesis is observed within 4 h of the meal. Diet-induced thermogenesis is assumed to be 10% of daily energy expenditure in individuals consuming an average mixed diet and being in energy balance. However, the diet-induced thermogenesis of fats is only 5% of their energy content, whereas diet-induced thermogenesis of proteins amounts to approximately 20%. Diet-induced thermogenesis of carbohydrates is normally around 10%, but may be up to 20%, if carbohydrates are directly converted to fat (*de novo* lipogenesis); however, the latter does not normally occur in individuals consuming diets typical of European and North American countries [11].

Physical Activity — Definitions and Classifications

Physical activity is defined as any bodily movement achieved by contraction of skeletal muscles that increases energy expenditure above resting levels [12]. The daily physical activity level (PAL) is defined as total energy expenditure divided by basal energy expenditure (or resting energy expenditure). This way of quantifying physical activity assumes that the variation of daily energy expenditure is based on physical activity and body size.

TABLE 29.2
Classification of Physical Activity by Intensity

Intensity	Example	METs[a]	Heart rate	% HR_{res}[b]	% HR_{max}[c]
Inactivity	Laying, sitting	1–2	50–70	0–15	25–40
Light	Slow walking	2–3	70–90	15–30	40–50
Moderate	Brisk walking	3–6	90–120	30–55	50–70
Vigorous	Jogging	6–10	120–160	55–85	70–90
Very strenuous	Competitive running	11–20	160–180	85–100	90–100

[a]Metabolic equivalents, activity energy expenditure divided by resting energy expenditure.
[b]Percent of heart rate reserve = 100 × (exercise HR – resting HR/(max HR – resting HR)). This is approximately equal to percent of VO_2 max.
[c]Percent of max heart rate = 100 × (exercise HR/max HR).
Note: The MET values and heart rates are only meant to be used as an approximate description. HR = heart rate.

Daily physical activity (and physical activity-induced energy expenditure) may be classified by using intensity (energy expenditure) or type of physical activity. Intensity is categorized from total inactivity to extremely vigorous physical activity (Table 29.2). Absolute energy expenditure is determined by body weight (basal energy expenditure) and intensity of physical activity, so heavier individuals may reach quite high energy expenditures with only moderate-intensity activities. Therefore, the intensity of physical activity is usually expressed as metabolic equivalents or MET values [9]. The MET value of an activity is obtained by dividing activity energy expenditure by resting energy expenditure. METs therefore show the magnitude of increased energy expenditure in relation to resting energy expenditure.

Inactivity is defined as physical activity with energy expenditure very close to resting energy expenditure. Many daily activities, such as slow walking, watering flowers, making food, washing dishes, etc., are light, without any noticeable increases in breathlessness or sweating. Moderate activities, such as brisk walking, vigorous cleaning of the house, bicycling, golf, and stretching, may induce a little sweating and an increase in the heart rate. Vigorous activities, such as running, swimming, ball games, and gym training, lead to heavy perspiration and breathlessness.

It should be noted that the individual feeling of strenuousness depends on training history and fitness. Therefore, an elite marathon runner may run 2 h at an intensity of 15 METs and regard this as "moderate," whereas an untrained individual would be totally exhausted after running 5 min of the same intensity. An exercise intensity level of 10 METs is already subjectively very strenuous for a nonathlete. It may be read from Table 29.1 that energy expenditure for a 70-kg man during 1 h varies between approximately 70 kcal (290 kJ) and 700 kcal (2900 kJ) , but that the consumption may even reach 1300 kcal/h (5400 kJ/h) for an elite long-distance runner.

Another classification of physical activity is based on the type of activity (Figure 29.2). The gross classification uses three subcategories — namely, occupational and leisure activities (excluding exercise) and physical exercise. *Occupational physical activity* varies between light (<2 METs) and heavy (5 to 8 METs) [9]. Although it is fairly easy to characterize some occupations as light (office work, predominantly requiring sitting) or moderate (waiter/waitress, predominantly requiring walking), most occupations are a mixture of all kinds of activities. For instance, although loading and unloading a truck are heavy physical activities, a major part of a truck driver's day is often spent driving — that is, in a sitting position with energy expenditure close to the resting levels. Recent trends indicate that physical activity and energy expenditure have decreased in all kinds of occupations [13].

Occupational physical activity
- light (sitting)
- light/moderate (standing)
- moderate (walking)
- heavy (walking, carrying heavy objects)

Leisure activity
- non-exercise activities
- commuting by walking etc.
- playing, informal games
- household chores
- garden work
- picking berries/mushrooms
- nature (bird watching etc.)

Exercise activity
- aerobic (running etc.)
- strength (gym training)
- flexibility, skills (ball games)
- other

FIGURE 29.2 Components of physical activity.

Exercise is a subcategory of physical activity: it is voluntary, deliberate physical activity performed because of anticipated positive consequences on physical, psychological, and/or social well-being [12]. Exercise may be divided into several subcategories (Figure 29.2):

- Aerobic exercise refers to activities such as running, very brisk walking, bicycling, cross-country skiing, swimming, rowing, and paddling. The intensity is typically between 5 and 10 METs for nonathletes.
- Strength training, typically done at a gym, refers to a wide variation of training protocols. Training with light weights (in relation to one's maximal load) and high number of repetitions result in improved aerobic capacity, rather than strength per se. However, heavy loads and fewer repetitions improve strength by neural adaptation and muscle hypertrophy [14]. Although the subjective feeling of strain may be quite heavy during a strength training session, the average energy expenditure is usually lower than for aerobic training (3 to 7 METs) [9].
- Some types of exercise require more skills than physical fitness (e.g., playing golf, shooting) and the mean intensity during these activities remains often below 5 METs.
- Ball games (e.g., soccer, basketball, badminton, tennis) are a combination of aerobic and anaerobic activity, strength, and skills. The mean intensity may be quite high (7 to 14 METs), but not necessarily comparable to very intense endurance sports.

Leisure physical activity is defined in this chapter as all physical activity outside occupational hours, but excluding physical exercise. Therefore, leisure physical activity comes close to the term *lifestyle activity* [15,16]. One of the main differences between exercise and other leisure activities is motivation: the main motive for exercise is usually exercise by itself or the anticipated physical, psychological, and/or social consequences of exercise. However, lifestyle physical activities are carried out in order to achieve something else, such as going from home to work, shopping, cleaning the house or garden, or enjoying nature. Lifestyle activity is often incorporated into one's daily schedule, but exercising may require a "spare" hour or even more [15]. The intensity of leisure physical activity is usually low to moderate, typically between 2 and 5 METs.

Inactivity means a state with energy expenditure close to resting energy expenditure. In everyday life, inactivity means sitting and lying while awake. However, the difference between resting energy expenditure and energy expenditure during inactive waking hours is not always the same. Some individuals have an unconscious habit of spontaneous, involuntary muscle movements, such as fidgeting. This is sometimes referred to as nonexercise activity thermogenesis. Although the increase in energy expenditure due to fidgeting and other small movements is not large in absolute terms, some studies have related this kind of an activity to improved weight control [17]. Because of limited data, more studies are needed to confirm the potential importance of nonexercise activity thermogenesis.

An important question is how much energy expenditure can be increased by physical activity. This is illustrated by calculations presented in Table 29.3. The example uses a hypothetical person with resting energy expenditure of 1500 kcal/day (6.3 MJ) — that is, a very lean man (55 to 60 kg) or a heavier woman (70 to 75 kg). The daily activities are classified as sleep, occupation, leisure (inactivity and light activities), walking, and running. In the "basic" column, the individual is assumed to be involved in very light occupation (mostly sitting throughout the day), without any leisure activities. The daily physical activity level (PAL) is obtained by summing the products of intensity (as METs) and duration of all daily activity types and then dividing this sum by 24. Total daily energy expenditure is then obtained by multiplying the daily physical activity level by the resting energy expenditure. The basic example shows a very low daily physical activity level (PAL < 1.4).

The next column illustrates a situation with 30 min of brisk walking instead of leisure inactivity. This amount is close to the basic recommendation for health-enhancing physical activity [18]. According to the calculation, this adds about 6% or 120 kcal to the daily energy expenditure. Running for 30 min, instead of walking, leads to a 13% increase in daily energy expenditure. However, if running substitutes light activities — not complete inactivity — the increase in daily energy expenditure is slightly less. When walking and running are performed for 30 min daily, the increase in energy expenditure is 18% or 380 kcal. The last column shows the effect of slightly increased occupational activity: if half of the working day requires easy walking, instead of sitting (mean MET increases from 1.5 to 2.0), the daily energy expenditure is increased by 12%. This shows that small changes in occupational activity may lead to considerable changes in daily energy requirements.

As shown in Table 29.3, increased physical activity rarely increases daily energy expenditure by more than 20% or 400 kcal. This should be related to dietary changes that may induce an energy deficit of 500 to 1000 kcal/day. Although approximately 400 kcal/day or 3000 kcal/week may be regarded as a practical upper limit for leisure physical activity and exercise energy expenditure in nonathletes, higher values are obviously possible. Some randomized trials have achieved considerable energy expenditures (e.g., 700 to 1000 kcal/day) even in untrained and obese individuals, but the sustainability of this kind of an activity is questionable. Athletes, on the other hand, may use from 1000 to 5000 kcal in daily training [19–21].

INTENSITY OF PHYSICAL ACTIVITY AND USE OF ENERGY SUBSTRATES

The previous part of this chapter was related to physical activity and total energy expenditure. Although muscle work always increases total energy expenditure, the use of energy substrates depends on the intensity level. Figure 29.3 illustrates the relative contribution of fats and carbohydrates during activities of different intensities [22]. As the intensity is increased from light levels to above 30 to 40% VO_2 max (i.e., shift from light to moderate), two changes take place: the muscle starts to use more intramuscular substrates (fats and carbohydrates) and, especially, the use of muscle glycogen is increased. It is possible that the use of intramuscular substrates is a prerequisite for metabolic adaptations and many health benefits of physical activity (see the section on physical

TABLE 29.3
Hypothetical Example of Effects of Physical Activity on Daily Energy Expenditure for a Person with Resting Energy Expenditure of 1500 kcal (6.3 MJ) per Day

Activity	MET	Basic, h	Walker[a]	Jogger 1[b]	Jogger 2[c]	Walk + jog[d]	Occupation 2[e]
Sleep	1	8	8	8	8	8	8
Work	1.5	8	8	8	8	8	8
Leisure:							
Inactivity	1.3	4	3.5	3.5	4	3.5	4
Light	2	4	4	4	3.5	3.5	4
Walking	5	0	0.5	0	0	0.5	0
Jogging	10	0	0	0.5	0.5	0.5	0
MET h[f]		33.2	35.0	37.6	37.2	39.0	37.2
PAL[g]		1.38	1.46	1.56	1.55	1.63	1.55
EE, kcal[h]		2075	2190	2346	2325	2440	2325
EE, kJ		8682	9166	9819	9728	10212	9728
difference, %[i]			5.6	13.1	12.0	17.6	12.0

[a] 30 min walking instead of leisure inactivity.
[b] 30 min jogging instead of leisure inactivity.
[c] 30 min jogging instead of leisure light activity.
[d] 30 min walking and 30 min jogging instead of leisure inactivity and light activity.
[e] Occupational energy expenditure = 2 METs.
[f] MET hours = daily sum of the product of duration and MET.
[g] Daily physical activity level = product of MET hours divided by 24 (MET hours of resting energy expenditure).
[h] Energy expenditure = product of PAL and resting energy expenditure (assumed to be 1500 kcal or 6.3 MJ).
[i] Difference in energy expenditure (in percentage) from the basic model.

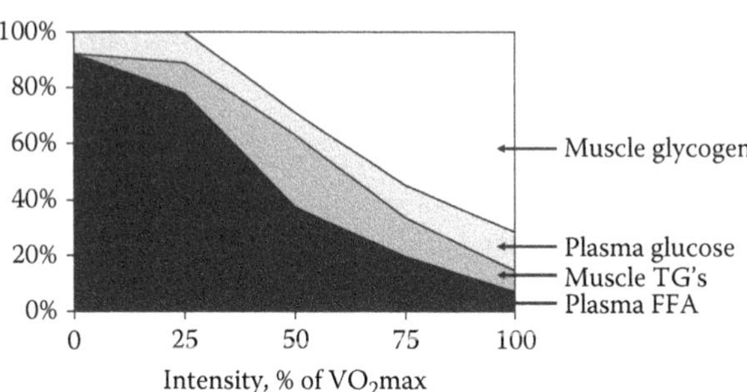

FIGURE 29.3 The proportional whole-body substrate oxidation rates when exercising with different intensities. (Adopted from Romijn, J.A. et al., *Am J Physiol* 1993; 265:E380–E391.)

activity and metabolic health in this chapter). When the intensity reaches 65 to 75% VO_2 max (i.e., shift from moderate to vigorous), muscle glycogen becomes the predominant energy source. It is conceivable that the oxidation of fat cannot cover the total energy needs during vigorous activity and that intramuscular carbohydrates are needed when the activity level is high [23].

In addition to fats and carbohydrates, protein is also used as an energy source [24,25]. In normal circumstances, the share of proteins is less than 5% of total energy expenditure. Deaminated amino acids are oxidized, some directly in the mitochondria (e.g., branched-chain amino acids) and some after gluconeogenetic transformation to glucose. However, if muscle glycogen stores are depleted or if protein intake is much higher than the daily protein needs, the contribution of proteins may be much higher [25].

Although the use of energy substrates clearly depends on the intensity of physical activity, many other factors may also contribute. The duration of physical activity is one important factor, particularly when the intensity is between 40 and 80% VO_2 max — that is, when intramuscular substrates are used for energy [22]. Studies show a gradual shift from predominantly carbohydrate use (60 to 70% of total energy expenditure in the beginning) to use of fats (the share of carbohydrates decreases to 30 to 40% after 2 to 3 h). The use of muscle glycogen and intramuscular triglycerides decreases as the exercise duration increases [22]. Other factors affecting muscle substrate use are nutritional status (carbohydrate use increases after consumption of carbohydrates), training history, and muscle fiber composition (fat oxidation increases after endurance training and in individuals with a predominantly type I ["slow twitch"] muscle fibers [26–28]).

Some people believe that low-intensity exercise, with increased proportional oxidation of fat, could be optimal for weight reduction and maintenance. In contrast, some studies have found higher postexercise energy expenditure after high-intensity exercise [29–31]. Despite lay beliefs, the use of muscle substrate during physical activity has no relevance to 24-h substrate oxidation, energy expenditure, weight management, or body composition [32]. High-intensity exercise depletes muscle glycogen stores and leads to higher postexercise fat oxidation [28,33]. Conversely, low-intensity exercise with high fat oxidation is followed by increased postexercise carbohydrate oxidation, compared with a high-intensity exercise condition. This means that high fat oxidation during exercise is followed by low postexercise fat oxidation and vice versa. Total physical activity energy expenditure, regardless of the intensity, is therefore the important factor for weight management. However, intensity and the mode of exercise have some important consequences for health, which are briefly described in later sections on physical activity and metabolic health and on recommendations for physical activity and exercise.

PHYSICAL ACTIVITY AND WEIGHT MANAGEMENT

Physical Activity and Primary Prevention of Weight Gain

Exercise and leisure lifestyle activities are not necessarily associated. An individual may be an active exerciser but otherwise passive, or a nonsporty but lifestyle-active individual. Some individuals are active, or passive, in both behavioral domains. Unfortunately, only a few studies have analyzed the interactions among exercise, lifestyle activity, and obesity. Figure 29.4 shows the association between the two main domains of physical activity (leisure lifestyle and exercise) and the prevalence of obesity in 15 European Union countries [34]. About 15,000 adults were divided into five groups (quintile classification) according to the time spent in vigorous exercise and according to their leisure inactivity (the time spent sitting or lying down). Quintile 1 (EX1 or IN1) refers to those with the lowest levels of exercise or lifestyle inactivity, respectively.

The most active combination (high exercise activity, EX5, low inactivity, IN1) was used as the reference category (prevalence of obesity = 1). As can be seen from the figure, those with no exercise activity (EX1) and very high leisure inactivity (IN5) had a fourfold increased prevalence of obesity. Low leisure inactivity (IN1), together with low exercise activity (EX1), was only associated with a doubling of obesity risk, compared to the fourfold increase in the extreme situation. In summary, the message of this cross-sectional study [34] is that a combination of low lifestyle inactivity (= high leisure activity) and high exercise activity is optimal for weight control. Being active in one of these domains is, however, clearly better than total inactivity.

The main problem with cross-sectional evaluations is their inability to infer causality. Although randomized, controlled interventions are needed to show a cause–effect relationship, these kinds of designs are rarely practical in studying primary prevention of obesity. However, cohort studies or prospective follow-ups may bring additional insight to the role of individual health behavior or environment on weight change. A systematic analysis on the associations between physical activity and weight change has been carried out [35]. This review identified 16 prospective, observational

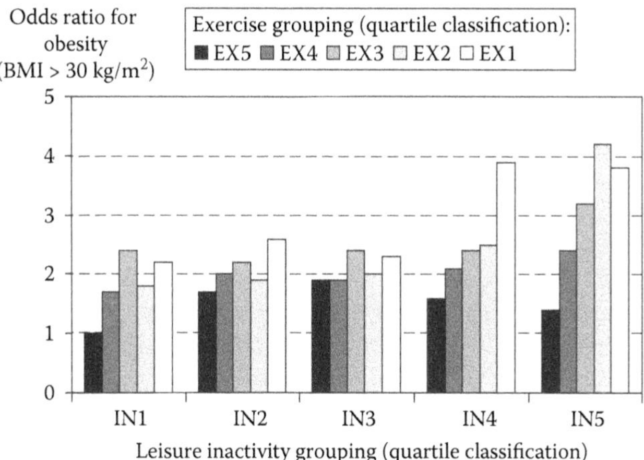

FIGURE 29.4 The risk (odds ratio) for obesity among 15,000 EU citizens, divided according to their leisure inactivity (quintile classification) and exercise activity (quintile classification). (Data from Martinez–Gonzalez, M.A. et al., *Int J Obes* 1999; 23:1192–1201.)

studies. The mean duration of the follow-up was approximately 7 years, with a range from 2 to 21 years.

The outcomes were grouped according to when physical activity data were collected — that is, whether baseline, follow-up, or change (from baseline to follow-up) in physical activity was compared against change in weight. Results from the studies using baseline physical activity data were inconsistent. Three studies [36–38] reported that a large volume of physical activity predicted smaller weight change. High baseline work activity was associated with less weight gain in one study [36]. In contrast, two studies reported that a large volume of vigorous physical activity at baseline was associated with greater weight gains [36,39]. Finally, three studies did not find a significant association between baseline total physical activity [40,41] or TV/VCR watching [42] and the magnitude of weight change.

The results with physical activity data at follow-up were more consistent: Four studies found that a large volume of physical activity or exercise [38,40,43,44] at follow-up was associated with less weight gain. Only one study [45] did not find such an association. Many studies used data on physical activity from baseline and follow-up. About half of the studies reported that an increase in physical activity was associated with less weight gain [37,38,40,46–49]. In summary, this systematic analysis indicated that those who maintain or increase their physical activity also show the best weight control over a period of several years. Physical activity at baseline does not consistently predict weight change, perhaps because of changes in physical activity during the follow-up. Unfortunately, the prospective studies did not allow a two-dimensional analysis (lifestyle and exercise activity) of physical activity [34].

Physical Activity during Weight Reduction

The effects of physical activity on weight reduction, without a concomitant low-energy diet, have been evaluated in a considerable number of studies (for reviews, see references 50 through 53). A meta-analysis [51] identified 53 papers, published between 1950 and 1988, with randomized, controlled trials and with data on physical activity and changes in body composition. Dietary weight reduction programs were excluded. The average study length was approximately 17 weeks, except for studies with weight training (average duration 10 weeks in males and 12 weeks in females). Males lost 1.3 kg body weight in trials with running or walking and 1.1 kg in trials with cycling. The respective fat-mass losses were greater for running/walking (1.6 or 0.12 kg/week) and cycling

(1.9 or 0.11 kg/week) trials. Weight training resulted in a mean increase in body weight (1.2 kg), but a reduction in fat mass (1.0 kg). Results for females were more modest: Body mass or fat mass changed significantly only after running/walking (–0.6 and –1.3 kg, respectively), but not after cycling.

Another systematic review [52] identified ten studies, published between 1983 and 1995, with comparisons of exercise alone with no treatment in obese subjects. A third systematic review [53] included studies with obese subjects, who were randomized into exercise and control (no diet) groups. Combining these two reviews [52,53] yields 18 studies. In short-term interventions (<26 weeks; $n = 8$), the mean weight reduction was 0.24 kg/week in exercising subjects and 0.05 kg/week in control groups (mean difference 0.19 kg/week favoring exercise). Long-term studies (≥26 weeks, $n = 10$) found only a 0.03 kg body mass reduction in exercising subjects and a 0.01 kg body mass increase in control groups (mean difference 0.04 kg/week favoring exercise).

A reduction in energy intake may be regarded as a core method during weight reduction. The additional effects of a concomitant physical activity program (most typically, aerobic exercise three to four times weekly, total training duration of 2 to 4 h/week, expected increase in weekly energy expenditure about 1500 kcal or 6.3 MJ) on weight loss has been studied in several randomized, controlled interventions (for reviews, see Garrow and Summerbell [50] and Wing [52]). A majority of the 19 studies identified by Wing [52] did not find any statistically significant differences between exercise + diet vs. diet only. Nevertheless, when all short-term (<26 weeks) studies are pooled, the average weight loss was 0.1 kg/week greater in exercising subjects. In long-term studies (≥26 weeks), the mean difference was 0.02 kg/week favoring exercising subjects.

Figure 29.5 combines the preceding two reviews [52,53]. The open triangles represent studies using a diet only vs. exercise + diet design. The filled triangles indicate studies with exercise vs. control (no treatment) design. It is clearly visible that physical exercise leads to a beneficial outcome, but that the difference to the no-exercise group is modest in studies with a longer duration. The apparent reason for this discrepancy is poor long-term adherence to exercise programs.

The largest improvement in weight reduction was achieved in studies with a rather high prescribed exercise level [53]. However, a clear dose–response relationship was only observed for short term (<16 weeks) studies. It seems that the enhancement in weight loss is linear up to a prescribed energy expenditure of 2000 kcal (8.4 MJ) per week. This energy expenditure level is achieved by walking briskly for 50 to 60 min/day or by jogging for approximately 30 min/day. Beyond this exercise level, the slope gets weaker. An apparent reason for this is that it becomes increasingly difficult to adhere to high-volume exercise prescriptions. In fact, it has been shown

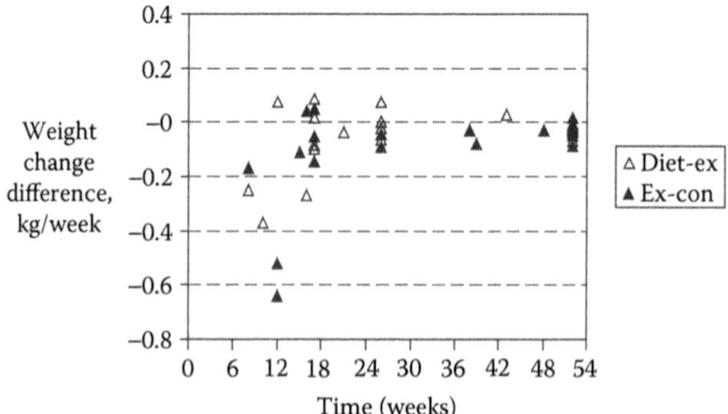

FIGURE 29.5 Difference in weight change (kg/week) between exercise vs. control (black triangles) or between diet + exercise vs. diet only (white triangles), as a function of duration of the intervention. (Data from Wing, R.R. *Med Sci Sports Exerc* 1999; 31(11 suppl):S547–S552 and Ross, R. and Janssen, I. *Med Sci Sports Exerc* 2001; 33(6 suppl):S521–S527.)

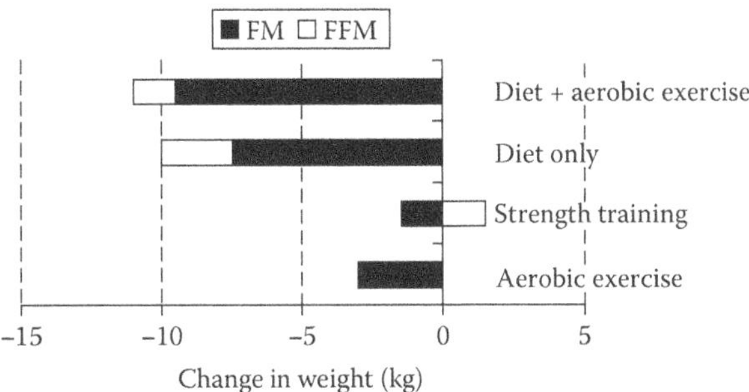

FIGURE 29.6 Change in body composition during weight reduction with or without physical exercise: meta-analytic findings. (Data from Garrow, J.S. and Summerbell, C.D. *Eur J Clin Nutr* 1995; 49:1–10.)

[54] that less than 50% of the subjects with a target of 10 MJ/week or 2500 kcal/week (corresponding to 480 min/week) energy expenditure during walking reached this goal. Similarly, less than 70% of the subjects with a 4.2 MJ/week (1000 kcal/week) goal reached this level [54]. Other possible explanations are a reduction in physical activities other than the prescribed exercise program [55] or an increase in the controls' physical activity [56].

Figure 29.6 summarizes the results from a meta-analysis [50] on the effects of exercise, with or without diet, on weight and body composition. The results concerning weight compare well with those presented previously [51–53]. The inclusion of studies with body composition data brings some additional insight, however. It can be seen from the figure that the contribution of fat loss during diet-induced weight reduction is approximately 75% of the total weight loss. When aerobic exercise is used as the only means for weight reduction, the magnitude of weight reduction is modest but almost all is fat mass. Compared to diet, exercise improves the loss of visceral and subcutaneous fat [57]. Moreover, when added to a weight-reducing diet, exercise spares about 1 kg of fat-free mass, but cannot prevent a loss of fat-free mass [50].

Because the amount of energy expenditure is related to the total work done, it can be assumed that fractionization (dividing the daily activity dose into multiple, shorter periods) has no effect on weight change. Several studies have compared different kinds of walking prescriptions (long vs. short bouts; walking integrated freely into daily routines vs. structured and planned walking; at home or group based) (for reviews, see Hardman [58] and Fogelholm [59]). The prescribed duration for physical activity was 90 to 200 min/week. As expected, fractionization had a similar effect on weight loss to that of exercising one longer bout daily.

Physical Activity and Maintenance of Reduced Body Weight

Weight maintenance after weight reduction is more difficult than initial weight loss [60]. The effects of physical activity during weight reduction on weight loss maintenance have been examined in a systematic review [35]. Eight studies were accepted as randomized interventions with a prospective follow-up of at least 1 year's duration. The duration of weight reduction varied between 8 weeks and 12 months. Three studies used very low energy diet during the weight reduction phase; the other studies used a more conventional diet with restricted energy intake. All studies used aerobic exercise (walking or ergometer cycling) with a target duration of approximately 90 to 180 min/week.

Only one study [61] found clearly that exercise training during weight reduction led to less weight gain during the follow-up compared to nonexercising groups. In another study [62], weight regain was smallest in exercising subjects randomized to supportive telephone contacts during the follow-up. However, exercising subjects who were randomized to no extended support showed a tendency to regain even more weight than the diet-only subjects did. A third study [63] reported better weight maintenance in one physical exercise group (n = 5), but the finding was apparently caused by one outlier. In contrast to these results, four studies did not find exercise training to improve maintenance of reduced body weight [64–67]. The weighed mean results of these eight studies suggested that exercise during weight reduction slowed weight regain by approximately 0.02 kg/week [35].

The idea of introducing physical activity immediately after weight reduction as a maintenance intervention came originally from the group of Professor Michael Perri. In one of their studies [68], they used several weight-maintenance techniques, including aerobic exercise, in two groups. All groups participating in the 6-month weight-maintenance intervention had less weight gain, compared with the controls who were not contacted after the weight reduction. Nevertheless, the exercise groups did not succeed any better or worse than the other weight-maintenance groups.

In another weight-maintenance intervention [69], 67 participants were randomized into exercise-focused and weight-focused groups after a 6-month weight-reduction period. The exercising subjects met biweekly in supervised exercise sessions and were also trained in relapse prevention strategies to avoid or cope with lapses in exercise. The weight-focused group learned problem-solving of weight-related difficulties, without emphasis on physical activity. During the unsupervised follow-up (6 months), the exercise-group gained more weight than the weight-focused group.

In our study [70], weight-reduced, but still overweight or obese, women were randomized into control, moderate-walking (target activity energy expenditure 4.2 MJ/week), and heavy-walking (8.4 MJ/week) groups for a 9-month intervention period. All groups received diet counseling. Compared with the end of weight reduction, weight regain at the 2-year follow-up was 3.5 kg (95% confidence interval 0.2 to 6.8) less in the moderate-walking group vs. control subjects. The heavy-walking group did not differ from the controls.

A more recent study investigated whether walking or resistance training after weight reduction prevents weight regain in males [56]. A 2-month weight reduction by very low energy diet was followed by a 6-month weight-maintenance intervention and 23 months' unsupervised follow-up. Resistance training attenuated the regain of body fat mass during the intervention, but not during the follow-up. The walking subjects did not differ from controls.

Several observational studies and post hoc analyses have shown a positive dose–response between the amount (energy expenditure or duration) of physical activity and weight-loss maintenance (for a systematic review, see Fogelholm and Kukkonen–Harjula [35]). Some observational studies have estimated the amount of total exercise [71–73] or walking [56], which is associated with improved weight-loss maintenance. The results are surprisingly similar: an average exercise energy expenditure of 9 to 10 MJ/week (2200 to 2400 kcal/week), corresponding to walking 70 to 80 min/day, seems to be associated with stable weight (±1 kg for more than 1 year) after substantial weight reduction. These estimates concur with a recent expert panel recommendation [74]. However, it should be noted that a smaller amount of walking may slow down, although not prevent, weight regain [54,69,70].

In summary, the expected weight loss with 150 to 200 min/week of moderate-intensity exercise should be 2 to 3 kg in studies with 3 to 6 months' duration. The enhanced weight reduction when this exercise level is added to a weight-reduction diet is slightly less. Thus, 250 to 300 min/week (or 35–45 min daily) seems more suitable for weight reducing purposes. This recommendation is close to the 45 min moderate-intensity exercise per day recommended in a recent report from an expert panel [74]. Splitting the daily walking into multiple, shorter (10 to 20 min) periods leads to a similar weight loss compared with walking an identical daily duration in one single period. For maintenance of reduced body weight, more than 60 min of moderate exercise per day after weight reduction might be needed.

PHYSICAL ACTIVITY AND METABOLIC HEALTH

Physical activity has several beneficial effects on health [75,76]. The general relationship among physical activity, obesity, and health is outlined in Figure 29.7. It is remarkable that most benefits of physical activity are also obtained through successful weight control. This means that physical activity may prevent cancer, cardiovascular heart diseases, hypertension, type-2 diabetes, and several musculoskeletal disorders by improving weight control. However, as clearly stated in the preceding part of this chapter, many individuals may find it difficult to increase their physical activity to levels that are clearly related to improved weight control. Therefore, it is extremely important to appreciate other health benefits of physical activity. Another way of putting it: physical activity can prevent major chronic diseases by improved weight control and by other metabolic responses, independent of body weight.

The next part of this chapter summarizes the most important dose–response issues related to physical activity and metabolic health. Those who want a deeper insight may read, for instance, the American College of Sports Medicine evidence-based dose–response symposium report [76]. In many cases, "dose" refers to the total volume, or energy expenditure, of physical activity. However, energy expenditure is a function of training mode, intensity, frequency, and duration. Some of these subcomponents of total physical activity dose may be important for the health benefits.

The American College of Sports Medicine dose–response report [77], together with another recent review [78], examined the long-term (at least 12 weeks) effects of aerobic exercise training and blood lipids. Both concluded that the effects of exercise training on LDL-cholesterol and triglycerides are small. About half of the studies cited in these reviews reported a 5 to 20% (mean 7%) [77] increase in HDL-cholesterol concentration. A dose–response association between the prescribed volume of exercise and change in HDL-cholesterol concentration was not clear [77]; however, a threshold of 4.2 MJ/week (1000 kcal/week) [77] and 5 MJ/week (1200 kcal/week) [78] for a significant effect was suggested.

A meta-analysis [79] examined, among other factors, the effects of different exercise intensities (below or above 70% VO_2 max) on blood lipids. The intensity category had no effect on triglycerides or HDL-cholesterol concentration. In contrast, the exercise-related decrease in LDL-cholesterol concentration was more marked after high-intensity (mean: –0.16 mmol/L) than after moderate-intensity (–0.07 mmol/L) training. The results of the Studies on Targeted Risk Reduction Interven-

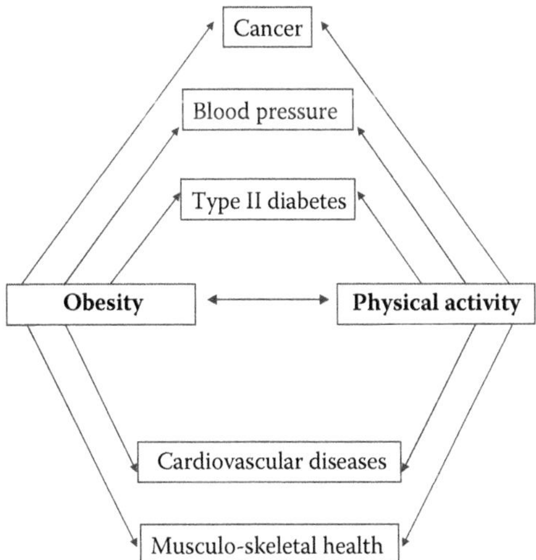

FIGURE 29.7 Relationships among physical activity, obesity, and chronic diseases.

tions through Defined Exercise (STRRIDE) support this conclusion [80]: higher training volume (distance covered: 32 vs. 19 km/week) was clearly related to beneficial effects on 12 indicators of lipid profile (including, for example, concentrations of LDL particles, small LDL particles, large HDL particles, and very low density lipoproteins). Intensity (moderate = 40 to 55% VO_2 max vs. high = 65 to 80% VO_2 max) had no clear effect on HDL-cholesterol, VLDL-cholesterol, or triglycerides; the high-intensity protocol was more beneficial on LDL-related measures.

Judged from the preceding results, vigorous aerobic activities may be superior in decreasing LDL-cholesterol concentration, whereas intensity is not equally important for HDL-cholesterol and triglycerides. A minimum intensity is much more difficult to identify. One recent study [81] reported on the effects of an acute exercise bout on postprandial metabolism. The researchers had earlier found that a higher amount (duration) of moderate-intensity exercise was positively related to postprandial triglyceride clearance and insulin sensitivity. This time they used two exercise protocols with equal energy expenditure (1100 kcal), but varying intensity (light = 25% vs. moderate = 65% VO_2 max). The subjects cycled for 90 (moderate intensity) or 240 (light intensity) min. Despite remarkable exercise energy expenditure and duration, the light-intensity bout did not have any effects on triglyceride clearance or insulin response to a fatty meal. In contrast, the moderate-intensity exercise had a clear positive effect on both variables. These and some other data suggest that very light physical activities may not be effective in improving the metabolic profile, despite an increase in energy expenditure. However, more research is needed to clarify this important issue.

Physical activity, even without weight loss, improves insulin sensitivity in individuals with impaired glucose tolerance [82]. A meta-analysis of the effects on exercise, with or without diet, on type-2 diabetics [83] included 12 aerobic training studies with duration between 8 to 52 weeks. The amount of prescribed exercise (mostly cycling or walking) was 90 to 210 min/week in 11 studies, and 300 min/week in the remaining study. Exercise intensity was moderate. Using postintervention HbA_{1c} as the main outcome variable, the combined result was 0.66% units lower (= better) in the exercise groups compared with the nonexercise groups. Therefore, a clinically significant and positive response was observed. Weight loss in exercise groups was on average 1.7 kg larger in studies without dietary treatment and 0.9 kg larger in studies combining diet with or without exercise. These differences were not statistically significant. Although epidemiological data suggest that higher amounts of physical activity are related to lower incidence of type-2 diabetes, the data from controlled trials are insufficient to confirm a dose–response relationship [82]. Exercise intensity is probably not very important for glucose tolerance, but the answer to this question is still unclear [84].

Physical activity lowers blood pressure immediately after an aerobic exercise session [85] and as a response to long-term training [86]. The response is associated with initial blood pressure; the blood-pressure-lowering effects of exercise are clearer in individuals with (mild) hypertension. Two recent reviews [86,87] analyzed the effect of different exercise intensities on blood pressure. Both reviews concluded that the blood pressure response to moderate, in contrast to vigorous, physical activity may be more favorable. However, the data are not very conclusive and even vigorous physical activity is clearly better than inactivity.

Obesity and high body weight have a beneficial effect on bone mineral mass and density. In contrast, obesity has a negative effect on many other musculoskeletal disorders, including muscle fitness and function, especially at older ages [88]. Nevertheless, the potential importance of strength (resistance) training in improving the general health and well-being of individuals with obesity has been undervalued. One reason for this could be the very small effects of strength training on body weight [50] and the belief that strength training does not have a positive effect on metabolic health. The latter belief can be disputed. A meta-analysis of randomized clinical trials [89] has shown that strength training leads to a 3-mm Hg decrease of systolic blood pressure in normo- and hypertensive individuals. Moreover, other studies have confirmed that muscle hypertrophy improves insulin sensitivity, even in subjects with normal glucose tolerance [90].

The final issue is related to splitting the daily exercise dose, i.e., fractionization. Studies on fractionization have mostly used moderate-intensity physical activity [58,59]. Based on the available data, splitting the daily dose into shorter (10 to 20 min) segments has no apparent effect on blood lipids, blood pressure, or glucose metabolism. It is unclear whether the segments could be shorter than 10 min.

Several mechanisms explain why physical activity is beneficial to metabolic health. Figure 29.8 outlines the best known effects of physical activity on short-term and long-term metabolism [26,27,91]. Short-term responses include changes in transporter proteins (e.g., GLUT-4), enzymes, and peripheral vascular resistance. Changes in oxygen delivery and utilization and in muscle cross-sectional area are achieved only after several weeks of training. The loss of adaptation follows an inverse order: transporter protein and enzyme activities are lost rapidly, whereas improved vascularization and muscle size remain for some weeks even during inactivity [92,93].

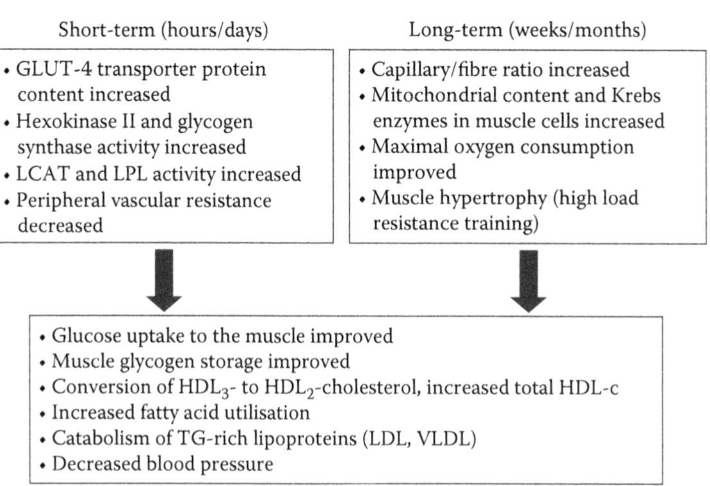

Exercise training, metabolic responses and health benefits
Short-term (hours/days)
• GLUT-4 transporter protein content increased
• Hexokinase II and glycogen synthase activity increased
• LCAT and LPL activity increased
• Peripheral vascular resistance decreased
Long-term (weeks/months)
• Capillary/fibre ratio increased
• Mitochondrial content and Krebs enzymes in muscle cells increased
• Maximal oxygen consumption improved
• Muscle hypertrophy (high load resistance training)
• Glucose uptake to the muscle improved
• Muscle glycogen storage improved
• Conversion of HDL_3- to HDL_2-cholesterol, increased total HDL-c
• Increased fatty acid utilisation
• Catabolism of TG-rich lipoproteins (LDL, VLDL)
• Decreased blood pressure

FIGURE 29.8 A summary of short- and long-term metabolic responses to increased physical activity.

RECOMMENDATION FOR PHYSICAL ACTIVITY AND EXERCISE

How Much Physical Activity Is Efficacious for Management of Obesity?

The recommended amount of physical activity for the management of obesity depends on several issues, such as the magnitude of desired outcome, recent history of weight change, and present individual physical activity level. The minimal amount of 150 to 200 min/week (25 to 30 min daily) moderate-intensity activity may improve cardiorespiratory fitness (in unfit individuals) and insulin sensitivity; however, a marked effect on weight, body composition, or fat distribution should not be expected. Increasing the total duration of physical activity to about 250 to 300 min/week (35 to 45 min daily) should bring about beneficial changes in weight, body composition, and HDL-cholesterol. Possibly much more than 300 min/week of moderate physical activity may be needed to prevent weight regain after substantial weight loss.

All of the preceding recommendations should be interpreted as the desired *increase* in physical activity. This is well illustrated with the number of daily steps taken by individuals with different activity levels. Several studies show that individuals (normal weight and obese) without volitional physical activities (but excluding totally inactive individuals) take about 5000 to 7000 steps/day [70,94,95]. This corresponds to walking 4 to 5 km or 40 to 50 min. Thus, the "30 min/day" or "150 to 200 min/week" recommendation means an increase above the basic activity — that is, to approximately 8000 to 10,000 steps/day (rough equivalents: 30 min = 3 km = 3500 steps). Furthermore, "45 min/day walking" is roughly equivalent to 10,000 to 12,000 steps/day and "60 min/day" to 12,000 to 14,000 daily steps.

What Is a Sustainable Prescription?

An interesting question is whether the set target level of walking (or any exercise) should be higher than the actual target. The justification for this question is that the actual completed amount of physical activity is often lower than the prescribed amount. For instance, in one study [54], the "high physical activity group" had a target of exercise energy expenditure 10 MJ/week (2500 kcal/week) or walking approximately 70 min/day. Out of this group, less than 50% reached the target. In fact, 22% failed even to reach the "low physical activity group" target of 4.2 MJ/week (1000 kcal/week) or 30 min/day. Perhaps the prescribed amount could be 20 to 25% higher than the actual target. However, the individual should increase his or her exercise levels only gradually toward these goals.

It has been suggested that the number of daily steps can be increased by 10% every 2 weeks, if the basic level is less than 8000 steps/day [94]. It is not known how fast the amount of walking can be increased, but perhaps the change should not be more than 2000 to 2500 steps/day or 15 to 20 min/day during 2 months. An increase of twice this magnitude is needed for clear health benefits, so an efficacious and sustainable walking program may not produce significant results until several months have passed. It should be noted that the data are inadequate to tell whether, because of injury risks and/or poor physical fitness, obese individuals need to progress more slowly in increasing their levels of exercise.

Is Moderate Physical Activity Enough for Management of Obesity?

An important question is whether moderate physical activity is enough or whether more vigorous activity is needed for better weight control and health. As already discussed, the added impact of high-intensity activity (vs. moderate intensity) on weight and insulin sensitivity seems negligible (as long as energy expenditure is kept constant) [84]. High-intensity activity may have an additional positive effect on LDL-lipoproteins [79,80]. Nevertheless, some cross-sectional studies show that a combination of high duration of walking activity (or low duration of leisure inactivity) and vigorous exercise activity is optimal for weight control [34] and prevention of cardiovascular heart diseases [96]. Moreover, individuals who are successful at long-term maintenance of substantial body weight loss expend almost 30% of their weekly physical activity energy in vigorous activities, such as running [97]. Some high-intensity activities might simply be needed to increase the total energy expenditure up to efficacious levels. Perhaps walking or other moderate-intensity activities as the only mode of physical activity are too time consuming.

What Kind of Support and Monitoring Is Needed?

Self-monitoring is a way to get immediate feedback. Pedometers (step counters) are quite inexpensive and simple devices for monitoring the number of daily steps. Unfortunately, some pedometers give an unacceptably biased result, from an underestimation of 25% to an overestimation of 45% [98]. Although systematic biases between pedometers are not very likely to affect monitoring of changes, it is important to be aware of potentially poor comparability between different devices. Accelerometers (movement counters) and heart-rate monitors with built-in equations for energy expenditure assessment are other possibilities for monitoring. However, a simple activity log (diary) may be as useful as these technical methods. Self-reporting is a potential weakness of an activity log, but the strength is that all kinds of activities are easily recorded. Cycling and gym training, for instance, are not accurately assessed by pedometers and accelerometers, and a heart-rate monitor is less precise in assessing light and very intense activities [99].

Poor adherence to prescribed exercise is a great problem in weight-reduction interventions. After 4 to 6 months, increased physical activity levels typically return toward baseline. This is observed in studies with an unsupervised follow-up [70], as well as during biweekly group meetings [100]. There is no panacea to increase long-term adherence to increased physical activity in obese (or weight-reduced) individuals [35]. Compared with group-based exercise, home-based exercise may improve long-term adherence [101]. However, Andersen et al. [71] did not find a difference in 1-year adherence between lifestyle activity (walking and other activities integrated freely into daily routines) vs. aerobics class groups. At present, the only advice would be to listen to the patient: some may find regular group meetings supportive, but others may prefer the time saved when walking from home. Moreover, it is important to tell the patient about difficulties in maintaining new activity habits.

CONCLUSIONS AND RECOMMENDATIONS

This chapter has outlined the main relationships among physical activity, weight control, and metabolic health. It is assumed that physical activity has a cancer-preventing effect by improving weight maintenance, as well as by metabolic effects independent of weight change. A recommendation for leisure physical activity and exercise must consider volume (energy expenditure during physical activity), as well as intensity, frequency, duration of a single exercise session, and exercise type. The following conclusions are therefore a basis for the recommendation:

- Volume, duration, energy expenditure:
  - It is apparent that a positive linear or curvilinear dose–response between physical activity and health exists, at least up to a energy expenditure during physical activity of 2500 kcal/week (10.5 MJ).
  - The first clinically (and statistically) significant results on body weight and metabolic health are observed with a weekly energy expenditure during physical activity of 1000 kcal (4.2 MJ). Smaller amounts of physical activity may be beneficial (compared to total inactivity), but the results are difficult to show and they may be clinically insignificant.
  - A 1000 kcal/week dose is equal to 150 to 200 min of moderate or 100 to 120 min of vigorous physical activity weekly.
- Intensity:
  - Vigorous intensity exercise (>70% VO_2 max) may be needed to improve the LDL-cholesterol profile.
  - Moderate- and vigorous-intensity exercises are equally effective in improving HDL-cholesterol and triglyceride concentration.
  - Moderate-intensity exercise may reduce blood pressure even better than vigorous exercise; however, the difference is not large.
  - The intensity of physical activity should perhaps be at least moderate (>30 to 40% VO_2 max) to cause metabolic health benefits.
  - Total energy expenditure and 24-h substrate oxidation are related to the amount of work performed, not to the intensity per se.
  - Some studies indicate that a combination of lifestyle (moderate) physical activity and (vigorous) exercise is related to the highest activity energy expenditure and to the best health outcome. Perhaps a combination is the most sustainable approach on a long-term basis.
- Frequency and duration of a single exercise session:
  - A suitable frequency for moderate-intensity physical activity seems to be daily and, for vigorous activity, every other day. This frequency means that a new physical activity session starts before all acute health benefits (e.g., decreased blood pressure,

improved insulin sensitivity, decreased HDL-cholesterol) have returned to their initial levels.
  - A preferred daily dose — within the frame of a recommended weekly amount — is 20 to 60 min.
  - The daily dose can be split into shorter (10- to 20-min) segments without a loss of metabolic health responses.
- Mode of physical activity:
  - The majority of studies have used moderate or vigorous structured aerobic exercise, such as brisk walking, jogging, or bicycling.
  - Strength (resistance) training improves muscle fitness without compromising metabolic health. Therefore, strength training is a natural component of a health-enhancing physical activity recommendation.
  - Lifestyle activity leads, when performed at sufficient intensity, to similar effects on weight and metabolic health as more structured (aerobic) exercise with the same intensity and volume.

The old American College of Sports Medicine recommendation (aerobic exercise greater than or equal to five times, 20 to 60 min, per week) for physical activity was based on vigorous activity and improvement of cardiovascular fitness [102]. The new paradigm from 1995 emphasizes moderate intensity and daily frequency [18]:

- Every (U.S.) adult should accumulate 30 min or more of moderate-intensity physical activity on most, preferably all, days of the week.
- The recommended 30 min of activity can be accumulated in short bouts of activity.
- People who already meet the recommendation are also likely to derive some additional health and fitness benefits from becoming more physically active.

Some ongoing walking promotion projects are using the number of daily steps as the main message and pedometers as the recommended technique to monitor the progress ("10,000 Steps Rockhampton" and "Colorado on the Move") [103,104]. In the latter project, the aim is to increase the number of daily steps by 2000. Although the "30 minutes daily" and the "10,000 steps" approaches are very straightforward and easy to remember, they may be criticized for being too simple. People may concentrate too much on lifestyle activity and walking; thus, the benefits of occasional vigorous activity and strength training may be forgotten.

The UKK Institute's physical activity pie was designed in 2004 as a new graphical presentation of the physical activity recommendations (Figure 29.9). The pie is strongly based on the consensus statement of Pate et al. [18] and other data on the relationships between physical activity and health (discussed earlier in this chapter). The pie is divided into two halves, each representing an energy expenditure of 1000 kcal/week (4.2 MJ). The bottom half describes lifestyle, daily, moderate-intensity physical activities. The upper half describes more structured, moderate or vigorous exercise. These are divided into two subcategories, depending on whether the main outcomes are improvements in cardiorespiratory health or musculoskeletal function.

The recommendation is that either "half of the pie" (1000 kcal/week) is enough to offset most, if not all, of the diseases related to physical inactivity. For most individuals, the bottom half (lifestyle activity) may be the most sustainable approach. However, the "whole pie" (2000 kcal/week) is clearly optimal for weight control and metabolic health benefits. No special recommendations are offered for physical activity in prevention of cancer — prevention of all chronic metabolic diseases is achieved by approximately similar physical activity doses.

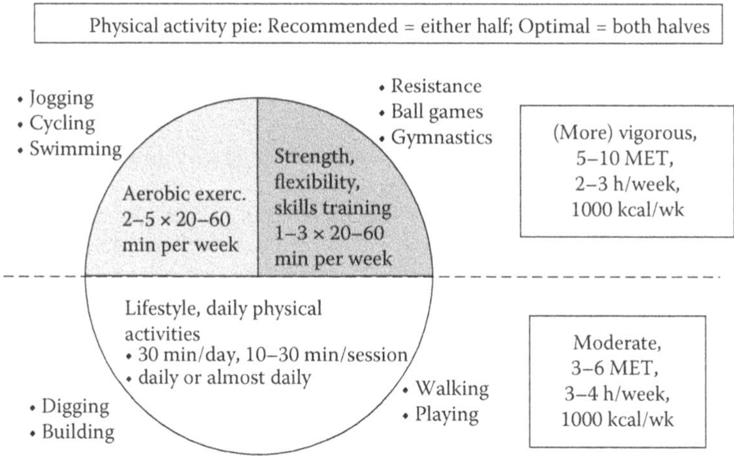

FIGURE 29.9 Physical activity pie: a graphical presentation of recommendations for health-enhancing physical activity.

REFERENCES

1. Klausen B, Toubro S, Astrup A. Age and sex effects on energy expenditure. *Am J Clin Nutr* 1997; 65(4):895–907.
2. Astrup A, Buemann B, Christensen NJ, Madsen J, Gluud C, Bennett P, et al. The contribution of body composition, substrates, and hormones to the variability in energy expenditure and substrate utilization in premenopausal women. *J Clin Endocrinol Metab* 1992; 74:279–286.
3. Toubro S, Sorensen TI, Ronn B, Christensen NJ, Astrup A. Twenty-four-hour energy expenditure: the role of body composition, thyroid status, sympathetic activity, and family membership. *J Clin Endocrinol Metab* 1996 Jul; 81:2670–2674.
4. Svendsen OL, Hassager C, Christiansen C. Impact of regional and total body composition and hormones on resting energy expenditure in overweight postmenopausal women. *Metabolism* 1993; 42(12):1588–1591.
5. Gilliat–Wimberly M, Manore MM, Woolf K, Swan PD, Carroll SS. Effects of habitual physical activity on the resting metabolic rates and body compositions of women aged 35 to 50 years. *J Am Diet Assoc* 2001; 101(10):1181–1188.
6. Foster GD, McGuckin BG. Estimating resting energy expenditure in obesity. *Obesity Res* 2001; 9 Suppl 5:367S–372S
7. Ferrannini E. The theoretical bases of indirect calorimetry: a review. *Metabolism* 1988; 37(3):287–301.
8. WHO. Energy and protein requirements. Report of a joint FAO/WHO/UNU expert consultation. WHO Technical Report Series; 724. Geneva: WHO, 1985.
9. Ainsworth BE, Haskell WL, Whitt MC, Irwin ML, Swartz AM, Strath SJ, O'Brien WL, Bassett DR Jr, Schmitz KH, Emplaincourt PO, Jacobs DR Jr, Leon AS. Compendium of physical activities: an update of activity codes and MET intensities. *Med Sci Sports Exercise* 2000; 32(9 Suppl):S498–504.
10. Tataranni PA, Larson DE, Snitker S, Ravussin E. Thermic effect of food in humans: methods and results from use of a respiratory chamber. *Am J Clin Nutr* 1995; 61(5):1013–1019.
11. Hellerstein MK. No common energy currency: *de novo* lipogenesis as the road less traveled. *Am J Clin Nutr* 2001; 74:707–708.
12. Caspersen CJ, Powell K, Christenson G. Physical activity, exercise and physical fitness: Definitions and distinctions for health-related research. *Pub Health Rep* 1985; 100:126–131.
13. Fogelholm M, Männistö S, Vartiainen E, Pietinen P. Determinants of energy balance and overweight in Finland 1982 and 1992. *Int J Obesity* 1996; 20:1097–1104.
14. Kraemer WJ, Ratamess NA. Fundamentals of resistance training: progression and exercise prescription. *Med Sci Sports Exercise* 2004; 36:674–688.

15. Jakicic JM. Exercise in the treatment of obesity. *Endocrinol Metab Clin North Am* 2003; 32(4):967–980.
16. Dunn AL, Marcus BH, Kampert JB, Garcia ME, Kohl HW 3rd, Blair SN. Comparison of lifestyle and structured interventions to increase physical activity and cardiorespiratory fitness: a randomized trial. *JAMA* 1999; 281(4):327–334.
17. Levine JA. Nonexercise activity thermogenesis (NEAT): environment and biology. *Am J Physiol Endocrinol Metab* 2004; 286(5):E675–E685.
18. Pate RR, Pratt M, Blair SN, Haskell WL, Macera AA, Bouchard C, Buchner D, Ettinger W, Health GW, King A, Kriska A, Leon AS, Marcus BH, Morris J, Pafenbarger RS, Patrick K, Pollock ML, Rippe JM, Sallis J, Wilmore JH. Physical activity and public health: a recommendation from the Centers for Disease Control and Prevention and the American College of Sports Medicine. *JAMA* 1995; 273:402–407.
19. Fogelholm M, Himberg J-J, Alopaeus K, Gref C-G, Laakso J, Lehto J, Mussalo–Rauhamaa H. Dietary and biochemical indices of nutritional status in male athletes and controls. *J Am Coll Nutr* 1992; 11:181–191.
20. Westerterp KR, Saris WH, van Es M, ten Hoor F. Use of the doubly labeled water technique in humans during heavy sustained exercise. *J Appl Physiol* 1986; 61 (6):2162–2167.
21. Sjödin AM, Andersson AB, Hogberg JM, Westerterp KR. Energy balance in cross-country skiers: a study using doubly labeled water. *Med Sci Sports Exercise* 1994; 26:720–724.
22. Romijn JA, Coyle EF, Sidossis LS, Gastaldelli A, Horowitz JF, Endert E, Wolfe RR. Regulation of endogenous fat and carbohydrate metabolism in relation to exercise intensity and duration. *Am J Physiol* 1993; 265:E380–E391.
23. Wiborg Lange KH. Fat metabolism in exercise — with special reference to training and growth hormone administration. *Scand J Med Sci Sports* 2004; 14:74–99.
24. Lemon PWR. Is increased dietary protein necessary or beneficial for individuals with a physically active lifestyle? *Nutr Rev* 1996; 54:S169–S175.
25. Wagenmakers AJM, Beckers EJ, Brouns F, Kuipers H, Soeters PB, van der Vusse GJ, Saris WHM. Carbohydrate supplementation, glycogen depletion, and amino acid metabolism during exercise. *Am J Physiol* 1991; 260:E883–E890.
26. Tikkanen HO, Näveri H, Härkönen M. Skeletal muscle fiber distribution influences serum high-density lipoprotein cholesterol level. *Atherosclerosis* 1996; 120:1–5.
27. Van Loon LJC, Jeukendrup AE, Saris WHM, Wagenmakers AJM. Effect of training status on fuel selection during submaximal exercise with glucose ingestion. *J Appl Physiol* 1999; 87:1413–1420.
28. Coyle EF, Jeukendrup AE, Wagenmakers AJ, Saris WHM. Fatty acid oxidation is directly regulated by carbohydrate metabolism during exercise. *Am J Physiol* 1997; 273:E268–E275.
29. Melby CL, Scholl G, Edwards G, Bullough R. Effect of acute resistance exercise on postexercise energy expenditure and resting metabolic rate. *J Appl Physiol* 1993; 75:1847–1853.
30. Burleson MA, O'Bryant H, Stone MH, Collins MA, Triplett–McBride T. Effect of weight training exercise and treadmill exercise on post-exercise oxygen consumption. *Med Sci Sports Exercise* 1998; 30:518–522.
31. Gore CJ, Whither RT. The effect of exercise intensity and duration on the oxygen deficit and excess post-exercise oxygen consumption. *Eur J Appl Physiol* 1990; 60:169–174.
32. Saris WHM, Schrauwen P. Substrate oxidation differences between high- and low-intensity exercise are compensated over 24 hours in obese men. *Int J Obesity* 2004; 28:759–765.
33. Schrauwen P, van Marken Lichtenbelt WD, Saris WHM, Westerterp KR. Role of glycogen-lowering exercise in the change of fat oxidation in response to a high-fat diet. *Am J Physiol* 1997; 273:E623–E629.
34. Martinez–Gonzalez MA, Martinez JA, Hu FB, Hu FB, Gibney MJ, Kearney J. Physical inactivity, sedentary lifestyle and obesity in the European Union. *Int J Obesity* 1999; 23:1192–1201.
35. Fogelholm M, Kukkonen–Harjula K. Does physical activity prevent weight gain — a systematic review. *Obesity Rev* 2000; 1:95–111.
36. Klesges RC, Klesges LM, Haddock CK, Eck LH. A longitudinal analysis of the impact of dietary intake and physical activity on weight change in adults. *Am J Clin Nutr* 1992; 55:818–822.
37. Owens JF, Matthews KA, Wing RR, Kuller LH. Can physical activity mitigate the effects of aging in middle-aged women? *Circulation* 1992; 85:1265–1270.

38. Haapanen N, Miilunpalo S, Pasanen M, Vuori I. Association between leisure time physical activity and 10-year body mass change among working-aged men and women. *Int J Obesity* 1997; 21:288–296.
39. Bild DE, Sholinsky P, Smith DE, Lewis CE, Hardin JM, Burke GL. Correlates and predictors of weight loss in young adults: the CARDIA study. *Int J Obesity* 1996; 20:47–55.
40. Williamson DF, Madans J, Anda RF, Kleinman JC, Kahn HS, Byers T. Recreational physical activity and 10-year weight change in a US national cohort. *Int J Obesity* 1993; 17:279–286.
41. Parker DR, Gonzalez S, Derby CA, Gans KM, Lasater TM, Carleton RA. Dietary factors in relation to weight change among men and women from two southeastern New England communities. *Int J Obesity* 1997; 21:103–109.
42. Crawford DA, Jeffery RW, French SA. Television viewing, physical inactivity and obesity. *Int J Obesity* 1999; 23:437–440.
43. Rissanen AM, Heliovaara M, Knekt P, Reunanen A, Aromaa A. Determinants of weight gain and overweight in adult Finns. *Eur J Clin Nutr* 1991; 45:419–430.
44. Barefoot JC, Heitmann BL, Helms MJ, Williams RB, Surwit RS, Siegler IC. Symptoms of depression and changes in body weight from adolescent to mid-life. *Int J Obesity* 1998; 22:688–694.
45. Heitmann BL, Kaprio J, Harris JR, Rissanen A, Korkeila M, Koskenvuo M. Are genetic determinants of weight gain modified by leisure-time physical activity? A prospective study of Finnish twins. *Am J Clin Nutr* 1997; 66:672–678.
46. Taylor CB, Jatulis DE, Winkleby MA, Rockhill BJ, Kraemer HC. Effects of lifestyle on body mass index change. *Epidemiology* 1994; 5:599–603.
47. Coakley EH, Rimm EB, Colditz G, Kawachi I, Willett W. Predictors of weight change in men: results from the health professionals follow-up study. *Int J Obesity* 1998; 22:89–96.
48. Guo SS, Zeller C, Chumlea WC, Siervogel RM. Aging, body composition, and lifestyle: the Fels Longitudinal Study. *Am J Clin Nutr* 1999; 70:405–411.
49. Fogelholm M, Kujala U, Kaprio J, Sarna S. Predictors of weight change in middle-aged and old men. *Obesity Res* 2000; 8:367–373.
50. Garrow JS, Summerbell CD. Meta-analysis: effect of exercise, with or without dieting, on the body composition of overweight subjects. *Eur J Clin Nutr* 1995; 49:1–10.
51. Ballor DL, Keesey RE. A meta-analysis of the factors affecting exercise-induced changes in body mass, fat mass and fat-free mass in males and females. *Int J Obesity* 1991; 15:717–726.
52. Wing RR. Physical activity in the treatment of the adulthood overweight and obesity; current evidence and research issues. *Med Sci Sports Exercise* 1999; 31(11 suppl):S547–S552.
53. Ross R, Janssen I. Physical activity, total and regional obesity; dose–response considerations. *Med Sci Sports Exercise* 2001; 33(6 suppl):S521–S527.
54. Jeffery RW, Wing RR, Sherwood NE, Tate DF. Physical activity and weight loss: does prescribing higher physical activity goals improve outcome? *Am J Clin Nutr* 2003; 78:684–9.
55. Leon AS, Casal D, Jacobs D. Effects of 2000 kcal per week of walking and stair climbing on physical fitness and risk factors for coronary heart disease. *J Cardiopulm Rehabil* 1996; 16:183–92.
56. Borg P, Kukkonen-Harjula K, Fogelholm M, Pasanen M. Effects of walking or resistance training on weight loss maintenance in obese, middle-aged men: a randomized trial. *Int J Obesity* 2002; 26:676–83.
57. Ross R, Dagnone D, Jones PJ, Smith H, Paddags A, Hudson R, Janssen I. Reduction in obesity and related comorbid conditions after diet-induced weight loss or exercise-induced weight loss in men. A randomized, controlled trial. *Ann Intern Med* 2000; 133(2):92–103.
58. Hardman A. Issues of fractionization of exercise (short vs. long bouts). *Med Sci Sports Exercise* 2001; 33:S421–S427.
59. Fogelholm M. Walking for the management of obesity. *Dis Manage Health Outcomes* 2005; 13:9–18.
60. Jeffery RW, Epstein LH, Wilson GT, Drewnowski A, Stunkard AJ, Wing RR. Long-term maintenance of weight loss: current status. *Health Psychol* 2000; 19(suppl.):5–16.
61. Pavlou KN, Krey SK, Steffee WP. Exercise as an adjunct to weight loss and maintenance in moderately obese subjects. *Am J Clin Nutr* 1989; 49:1115–1123.
62. King AC, Frey-Hewitt B, Dreon DM, Wood PD. Diet vs. exercise in weight maintenance. *Arch Intern Med* 1989; 149:2741–2746.
63. Van Dale D, Saris WHM, ten Hoor F. Weight maintenance and resting metabolic rate 18 to 40 months after a diet/exercise treatment. *Int J Obesity* 1990; 14:347–359.

64. Perri MG, McAdoo WG, McAllister DA, Lauer JB, Yancey DZ. Enhancing the efficacy of behavior therapy for obesity: effects of aerobic exercise and a multicomponent maintenance program. *J Consult Clin Psychol* 1986; 54:670–675.
65. Skender ML, Goodrick K, Del Junco DJ, Reeves RS, Darnell L, Gotto AM, Foreyt JP. Comparison of 2-year weight loss trends in behavioral treatments of obesity: diet, exercise, and combination interventions. *J Am Diet Assoc* 1996; 96:342–346.
66. Wadden TA, Vogt RA, Foster GD, Anderson DA. Exercise and the maintenance of weight loss: 1-year follow-up of a controlled trial. *J Consult Clin Psychol* 1998; 66:429–433.
67. Wing RR, Venditti E, Jakicic JM, Polley BA, Lang W. Lifestyle intervention in overweight individuals with a family history of diabetes. *Diabetes Care* 1998; 21:350–359.
68. Perri MG, McAllister D, Gange JJ, Jordan RC, McAdoo WG, Nezu AM. Effects of four maintenance programs on the long-term management of obesity. *J Consult Clin Psychol* 1988; 56:529–534.
69. Leermakers EA, Perri MG, Shigaki CL, Fuller PR, Effects of exercise-focused versus weight-focused maintenance programs on the management of obesity. *Addict Behav* 1999; 24:219–227.
70. Fogelholm M, Kukkonen-Harjula K, Nenonen A, Pasanen M. Effects of walking training on weight maintenance after a very-low-energy diet in premenopausal obese women. A randomized controlled trial. *Arch Int Med* 2000; 160:2177–2184.
71. Andersen RE, Wadden TA, Bartlett SJ, Zemel B, Verde TJ, Franckowiak SC. Effects of lifestyle activity vs structured aerobic exercise in obese women. A randomized trial. *JAMA* 1999 Jan 27; 281(4):335–340.
72. McGuire MT, Wing RR, Klem ML, et al. What predicts weight regain in a group of successful weight losers? *J Consult Clin Psychol* 1999; 67(2):177–185.
73. Schoeller DA, Shay K, Kushner RF. How much physical activity is needed to minimize weight gain in previously obese women? *Am J Clin Nutr* 1997; 66:551–556.
74. Saris WH, Blair SN, Van Baak MA, Eaton SB, Davies PS, Di Pietro L, Fogelholm M, Rissanen A, Schoeller D, Swinburn B, Tremblay A, Westerterp KR, Wyatt H. How much physical activity is enough to prevent unhealthy weight gain? Outcome of the IASO 1st Stock Conference and consensus statement. *Obesity Rev* 2003; 4:101–114.
75. U.S. Department of Health and Human Services. Physical activity and health: a report from the Surgeon General. Atlanta: U.S. Department of Health and Human Services, Centers for Disease Control and Prevention, National Center for Chronic Disease Prevention and Health Promotion, 1996.
76. Kesaniemi YK, Danforth E Jr, Jensen MD, Kopelman PG, Lefebvre P, Reeder BA. Dose–response issues concerning physical activity and health: an evidence-based symposium. *Med Sci Sports Exercise* 2001; 33(Suppl 6):S351–S358.
77. Leon AS, Sanchez OA. Response of blood lipids and lipoproteins to exercise training alone or combined with dietary intervention. *Med Sci Sports Exercise* 2001; 33 (Suppl. 6):S502–S515.
78. Durstine JL, Grandjean PW, Davis PG, Ferguson MA, Alderson NL, DuBose KD. Blood lipid and lipoprotein adaptations to exercise. *Sports Med* 2001; 31(5):1033–1062.
79. Halbert JA, Silagy CA, Finucane P, Withers RT, Hamdorf PA. Exercise training and blood lipids in hyperlipidemic and normolipidemic adults: A meta-analysis of randomized, controlled trials. *Eur J Clin Nutr* 1999; 53:514–522.
80. Kraus WE, Houmard JA, Duscha BD, Knetzger KJ, Wharton MB, McCartney JS, Bales CW, Henes S, Samsa GP, Otvos JD, Kulkarni KR, Slentz CA. Effects of the amount and intensity of exercise on plasma lipoproteins. *N Engl J Med* 2002; 347:1483–1492.
81. Katsanos CS, Grandjean PW, Moffatt RJ. Effects of low and moderate exercise intensity on postprandial lipemia and postheparin plasma lipoprotein lipase activity in physically active men. *J Appl Physiol* 2004; 96:181–188.
82. Kelley DE, Goodpaster DH. Effects of exercise on glucose homeostasis in type-2 diabetes mellitus. *Med Sci Sports Exercise* 2001; 33 (Suppl. 6):S495–S501.
83. Boule NG, Haddad E, Kenny GP, Wells GA, Sigal RJ. Effects of exercise on glycemic control and body mass in type-2 diabetes mellitus: a meta-analysis of controlled clinical trials. *JAMA* 2001; 286(10):1218–1227.
84. Houmard JA, Tanner CJ, Slentz CA, Duscha BD, McCartney JS, Kraus WE. Effect of the volume and intensity of exercise training on insulin sensitivity. *J Appl Physiol* 2004; 96:101–106.

85. Thompson, PD, Crouse SF, Goodpaster B, Kelley D, N Moyna N, Pescatello I. The acute vs. the chronic response to exercise. *Med Sci Sports Exercise* 2001; 33(Suppl. 6):S438–S445.
86. Fagard RH. Exercise characteristics and the blood pressure response to dynamic physical training. *Med Sci Sports Exercise* 2001; 33(Suppl. 6):S484–S492.
87. Hagberg JM, Park J-J, Brown MD. The role of exercise training in the treatment of hypertension. *Sports Med* 2000; 30:193–206.
88. Visser M, Langlois J, Guralnik JM, Cauley JA, Kronmal RA, Robbins J, Williamson JD, Harris TB. High body fatness, but not low fat-free mass, predicts disability in older men and women: the Cardiovascular Health Study. *Am J Clin Nutr* 1998; 68:584–590.
89. Kelley GA, Kelley KS. Progressive resistance exercise and resting blood pressure. A meta-analysis of randomized controlled trials. *Hypertension* 2000; 35:838–843.
90. Poehlman ET, Dvorak RV, DeNino WF, Brochu M, Ades PA. Effects of resistance training and endurance training on insulin sensitivity in nonobese, young women: a controlled randomized trial. *J Clin Endocrinol Metab* 2000; 85:2463–2468.
91. Goodyear LJ, Kahn BB. Exercise, glucose transport, and insulin sensitivity. *Annu Rev Med* 1998; 49:235–261.
92. Mujika I, Padilla S. Muscular characteristics of detraining in humans. *Med Sci Sports Exercise* 2001; 33(8):1297–1303.
93. Mujika I, Padilla S. Cardiorespiratory and metabolic characteristics of detraining in humans. *Med Sci Sports Exercise* 2001; 33(3):413–421.
94. Croteau KA. A preliminary study on the impact of a pedometer-based intervention on daily steps. *Am J Health Promot* 2004; 18(3):217–220.
95. Tudor–Locke C, Bassett Jr DR. How many steps/day are enough? *Sports Med* 2004; 34(1):1–8.
96. Manson JE, Greenland P, LaCroix AZ, Stefanick ML, Mouton CP, Oberman A, Perri MG, Sheps DS, Pettinger MB, Siscovick DS. Walking compared with vigorous exercise for the prevention of cardiovascular events in women. *N Engl J Med* 2002; 347(10):716–725.
97. Klem ML, Wing RR, McGuire MT, et al. A descriptive study of individuals successful at long-term maintenance of substantial weight loss. *Am J Clin Nutr* 1997; 66:239–246.
98. Schneider PL, Crouter SE, Bassett DR. Pedometer measures of free-living physical activity: comparison of 13 models. *Med Sci Sports Exercise* 2004; 36(2):331–335.
99. Westerterp KR. Assessment of physical activity in relation to obesity: current evidence and research issues. *Med Sci Sports Exercise* 1999; 31(suppl. 11):S522–S525.
100. Jakicic JM, Marcus BH, Gallagher KI, et al. Effect of exercise duration and intensity on weight loss in overweight, sedentary women. A randomized trial. *JAMA* 2003; 290(10):1323–1330.
101. Perri MG, Martin AD, Leermakers EA, et al. Effects of group- vs. home-based exercise in the treatment of obesity. *J Consult Clin Psychol* 1997; 65:278–285.
102. American College of Sports Medicine. Position statement on the recommended quantity and quality of exercise for developing and maintaining fitness in healthy adults. *Med Sci Sports Exercise* 1978; 10:viii–x.
103. The 10,000 Steps Rockhampton Project [online]. Available from URL: http://www.10000steps.cqu.edu.au. Accessed June 20, 2005.
104. America on the move [online]. Available from URL: http://www.americaonthemove.org. Accessed June 20, 2005.

30 Diet and Other Means of Energy Balance Control

David Heber and Susan Bowerman

CONTENTS

INTRODUCTION

Obesity results from an imbalance of energy intake and expenditure. Currently, the obesity research community has placed a great deal of emphasis on energy balance as the key to achieving and maintaining optimum weight. However, energy balance depends on a number of physiological and behavioral factors other than total calories ingested or expended through exercise. Understanding these factors will provide new directions for nutritional intervention strategies that can be tested for their efficacy in cancer prevention. These factors include:

- Protein intake
- Fiber intake
- Total fruit and vegetable intake
- Glycemic load of the diet
- Dietary fat intake
- Special foods such as meal replacements and portion-controlled meals
- Dietary supplements that have an impact on energy expenditure, such as green tea, caffeine, and capsaicin

In turn, energy excess can stimulate numerous hormonal and inflammatory pathways that can promote the multistep process of carcinogenesis. The quality of the diet has some effects on these processes as well. For example, omega-6 fatty acids are proinflammatory by comparison to omega-3 fatty acids. The nature of the proteins, fats, and carbohydrates found in different foods and supplements has physiological effects, including the anti-inflammatory effects of phytochemicals and the effects of indigestible carbohydrates on hormonal balance. For example, soluble and insoluble fibers can affect the enterohepatic recirculation of estrogens and the size of the body estrogen pool.

Insights on how to control energy balance through diet and other means may be of interest to those studying nutritional strategies for cancer prevention in populations and in individuals who have already survived the primary treatment of a common form of cancer.

UNDERSTANDING EPIDEMIOLOGICAL EVIDENCE

Epidemiological studies suggest that populations eating so-called traditional low-fat diets have a far lower incidence of many common forms of cancer than populations eating typical modern diets in industrialized nations. However, traditional diets have many other characteristics outside of their overall lower percent of energy from fat than diets eaten in industrialized nations to which they are compared. Among the differences are greater ingestion of fruits, vegetables, and whole grains. This difference in dietary pattern leads to a greater ingestion of soluble and insoluble dietary fiber and thousands of phytochemicals with cellular effects beyond antioxidation. In addition, the fibers from whole grains and lower intakes of red meat, sugar, added fat, and starch lead to reduced energy density of the diet, which has been shown to lead to satiety at a lower level of total calorie intake.

In the U.S., the intake of hidden fats in processed foods has increased over the past 20 years. At the same time, the intake of high fructose corn syrup has increased from processed foods. The result of these trends has been an increase in overall energy intake, which, in the absence of increases in physical activity, predictably leads to an increase in body fat.

DIETARY FACTORS AFFECTING ENERGY BALANCE

Protein Intake Effects on Body Composition and Satiety

Protein provides a stronger signal to the brain to satisfy hunger than carbohydrate or fat does and is needed for muscle deposition, which can increase the lean body mass that, in turn, raises resting metabolic rate. A number of amino acids, including tryptophan, phenylalanine, and tyrosine, have been theorized to affect the hunger control mechanisms once they cross the blood–brain barrier. Although the mechanism of action is unknown, it has been suggested that single amino acids or small peptides enter the brain to elicit their effects. Also, the small differences in the rates at which proteins release their amino acids into the blood stream can affect satiety. Voluntary reduction in energy consumption has been noted in subjects consuming high-protein meals compared with high-carbohydrate meals when fed *ad libitum*.

Researchers in the Netherlands [1] have studied the effects of protein on hunger perceptions by studying subjects in a whole-body energy chamber under controlled conditions for over 24 hours. Subjects were divided into two groups and were fed isocaloric diets that were high-protein/high-carbohydrate (protein/carbohydrate/fat, percentage of calories 30/60/10) or high-fat (protein/carbohydrate/fat, percentage of calories 10/30/60). Subjects reported significantly more satiety on the high-protein/high-carbohydrate diet, and hunger, appetite, desire to eat, and estimated quantity of food eaten were significantly lower. Less hunger was experienced during and after the high-protein meals. A higher diet-induced thermogenesis was also observed with the high-protein diet.

Westerterp–Plantenga further investigated the effects of dietary protein on body weight maintenance after weight loss. After following a very low energy diet for 4 weeks, 148 male and female subjects were randomly assigned to receive diets with either 18 or 15% of total energy from protein, representing a 20% higher intake of protein in the additional protein group. During this 3-month maintenance period, those receiving additional protein showed a 50% lower body weight regain, only consisting of fat-free mass, with increased satiety and decreased energy efficiency [2].

Another research team [3] compared a high-protein diet (25% calories from protein, 45% from carbohydrate, and 30% from fat) to a control diet (12% protein, 58% carbohydrate, and 30% fat) to evaluate weight loss over 27 weeks. Two groups of 25 moderately obese subjects were allowed to eat as much of either of two diets as they wanted. Weight loss (8.9 vs. 5.1 kg) and fat loss (7.6 vs. 4.3 kg) were significantly higher in the higher protein group, due to a reduction in daily calorie intake of approximately 16%.

Another study comparing the effects of a high-protein, low-fat diet (32% of energy from protein, <30% from fat) with a high-carbohydrate, low-fat diet (66% of calories from carbohydrate, 15% of calories from protein, 30% of energy from fat) reported that the higher protein diet improved utilization of body fat while maintaining lean body mass. This study concluded that the increased proportion of protein to carbohydrate had positive effects on body composition as well as on blood lipids, glucose homeostasis, and satiety during weight loss [4]. A similar study comparing diets with 15 vs. 30% of calories from protein found that weight loss in the two groups was similar over the 6-week trial, but diet satisfaction was significantly greater in those consuming the higher protein diet [5].

Brehm [6] studied the effects of a very low carbohydrate diet and a calorie-restricted low-fat diet on body weight and heart disease risk factors in healthy women over a 6-month period. The very low carbohydrate diet group lost more weight (8.5 vs. 3.9 kg; $p < 0.001$) and more body fat (4.8 vs. 2.0 kg; $p < 0.01$) than the low-fat group. This study emphasized that the group with more weight loss was eating a low-carbohydrate diet; however, the protein content as a percentage of calories of the low carbohydrate diet was also much higher than that of the low-fat diet (28 vs. 16% of calories), which could also account for more weight loss due to increased satiety. In addition, the group eating more protein maintained a higher lean body mass while losing weight and a greater percentage of the weight that they lost came from excess body fat.

A meta-analysis by Eisenstein et al. [7] concluded that, on average, high-protein diets were associated with a 9% decrease in total calorie intake. The role of protein in affecting overall calorie intake and in body weight regulation in comparison to fat and carbohydrate needs further investigation. However, the evidence is strong that protein affects hunger-signaling mechanisms in the brain, induces thermogenesis, and contributes to the building and maintenance of lean body mass.

Fiber Intake Effects on Satiety

It has been suggested that the increase in obesity in Western countries since 1900 may be related to changes in dietary fiber. Recommended fiber intakes of 20 to 35 g per day for healthy adults, and age plus 5 g per day for children, are not being met because intakes of fruits, vegetables, whole grains and legumes are below recommended amounts [8]. Fiber-rich meals promote early satiety, are usually less calorie dense, lower in fat and added sugars than meals typical of a Western dietary pattern, and characteristic of a pattern to prevent and treat obesity.

In clinical trials and observational studies, the intake of whole-grain foods, rich in fiber, is inversely associated with plasma biomarkers of obesity, including insulin, C-peptide, and leptin concentrations. Fiber-rich foods have a low glycemic index and glycemic load, resulting in lower postprandial glucose and insulin levels. In addition to promoting satiety due to their bulk, high-fiber foods containing soluble fiber found in some fruits, oats, and barley may delay gastric emptying and intestinal absorption of macronutrients and may affect secretion of gut hormones to act as satiety factors.

Few direct studies on the relationship between whole-grain intake and obesity have been undertaken, although several studies report an association between whole-grain intake and insulin sensitivity, which provides indirect support for the role of whole grains in body weight regulation. The relationship between obesity and fiber has been evaluated epidemiologically. Using food frequency questionnaires, obese men and women have been shown to have significantly more fat and less fiber in their diets than lean men and women [9]. In a study of normal weight, moderately obese, and severely obese subjects, total fiber intake was higher in the lean than in the obese groups and the grams of fiber/1000 kcal were inversely related to body mass index [10].

The association between dietary fiber intake and weight gain over time was examined in a prospective cohort study of over 74,000 female nurses. Their dietary habits were followed for 12 years and assessed and validated with food-frequency questionnaires. Women who consumed more whole grains consistently weighed less than those who consumed fewer whole grains; over the 12-year period, those with the greatest intake of dietary fiber gained an average of 1.52 kg less body weight than those with the smallest increase in dietary fiber [11]. Similar findings were reported in the Iowa Women's Health Study [12] and the CARDIA study in which whole grain intake was inversely related to BMI after following subjects for 7 years [13]. Epidemiological studies also report that whole-grain intake is protective against cardiovascular disease, cancer, and diabetes and has diverse potential mechanisms, including antioxidation and mediation of insulin and glucose responses.

The bulk of evidence suggests that dietary fiber decreases food intake and decreases hunger and that water-soluble fiber may be more efficient in this regard than water-insoluble fiber. Dietary fiber supplements (5 to 40 g/day) lead to small (1 to 3 kg) weight losses greater than placebo. Although the weight loss obtained with dietary fiber is less than the 5% of initial body weight felt to confer clinically significant health benefits, the safety of dietary fiber and its other potential benefits on cardiovascular risk factors recommend it for inclusion in weight reduction diets.

Total Fruit and Vegetable Intake

Because fruits and vegetables are high in water and fiber, incorporating them in the diet can reduce energy density, promote satiety, and decrease energy intake while at the same time providing phytonutrients. Few interventions have specifically addressed fruit and vegetable consumption and weight loss, but evidence suggests that the recommendation to increase these foods while decreasing total energy intake is an effective strategy for weight management. Although obesity is often considered synonymous with overnutrition, it is more accurately depicted as overnutrition of calories but undernutrition of many essential vitamins, minerals, and phytonutrients.

The increased incidence of obesity has been associated with an increased incidence of heart disease, breast cancer, prostate cancer, and colon cancer by comparison with populations eating a dietary pattern consisting of less meat and more fruits, vegetables, cereals, and whole grains. The intake of 400 to 600 g/day of fruits and vegetables is associated with a reduced incidence of many common forms of cancer and heart disease and many chronic diseases of aging [14–16].

The common forms of cancer, including breast, colon, and prostate cancers, are the result of genetic-environmental interactions. Most cancers have genetic changes at the somatic cell level, which lead to unregulated growth through activation of oncogenes or inactivation of tumor suppressor genes. Reactive oxygen radicals are thought to damage biological structures and molecules including lipids, protein, and DNA, and some evidence indicates that antioxidants can prevent this damage.

Fruits and vegetables provide thousands of phytochemicals to the human diet and many of these are absorbed into the body. Although these are commonly antioxidants, based on their ability to trap singlet oxygen, they have been demonstrated scientifically to have many functions beyond antioxidation. These phytochemicals can interact with the host to confer a preventive benefit by regulating enzymes important in metabolizing xenobiotics and carcinogens, by modulating nuclear receptors and cellular signaling of proliferation and apoptosis, and by acting indirectly through antioxidant actions that reduce proliferation and protect DNA from damage [17].

Phytochemicals found in fruits and vegetables demonstrate synergistic and additive interactions through their effects on gene expression, antioxidation, and cytokine action. Fruits and vegetables are 10- to 20-fold less calorie dense than grains. They provide increased amounts of dietary fiber compared to refined grains as well as a balance of omega-3 and omega-6 fatty acids and a rich supply of micronutrients.

Several studies have sought to characterize dietary patterns and relate these patterns to body weight and other nutritional parameters. A prospective study of 737 nonoverweight women in the Framingham Offspring/Spouse cohort explored the relationship between dietary patterns and the development of overweight over a 12-year period. Participants were grouped into one of five dietary patterns at baseline:

- A heart-healthy pattern (low fat, nutritionally varied)
- Light eating (lower calories, but proportionately more fat and fewer micronutrients)
- A wine and moderate eating pattern
- A high-fat pattern
- An empty calorie pattern (rich in sweets and fat, low in fruits and vegetables)

Women in the heart-healthy cluster consumed more servings of vegetables and fruits than women in each of the other four clusters. Over the 12-year period, 214 cases of overweight developed in this cohort. Compared with women in the heart-healthy group, women in the empty calorie group were at a significantly higher risk for developing overweight (relative risk 1.4) [18].

In another analysis of dietary patterns among 179 older rural adults, those in the high-nutrient-dense cluster (higher intake of dark green/yellow vegetables, citrus/melons/berries, and other fruits and vegetables) had lower energy intakes and lower waist circumferences than those in the low-nutrient-dense cluster (higher intake of breads, sweets, desserts, processed meats, eggs, fats, and oil). Those with a low-nutrient-dense pattern were twice as likely to be obese [19]. Similar observations were reported utilizing data from the Canadian Community Health Survey from 2000 to 2001. The frequency of eating fruits and vegetables was positively related to being physically active and not being overweight [20].

In a controlled clinical trial, families with obese parents and nonobese children were randomized into a comprehensive behavioral weight management program featuring encouragement to increase fruit and vegetable consumption or to decrease intake of high-fat, high-sugar foods. Over a 1-year period, parents in the increased fruit and vegetable group showed significantly greater decreases in percentage of overweight than in the group attempting to reduce fat and sugar [21].

Current NCI dietary recommendations emphasize increasing the daily consumption of fruits and vegetables from diverse sources such as citrus fruits, cruciferous vegetables, and green and yellow vegetables [22]. The concept of selecting foods by color was extended in a book for the public to seven different groups, based on their content of a primary phytochemical family for which there is evidence of cancer prevention potential (see Table 30.1) [23].

Glycemic Index and Glycemic Load of the Diet

Due to its high-calorie density, a decrease in dietary fat has been a target in conventional approaches to weight loss. However, the relationship between dietary fat and obesity has been brought into question for several reasons. Weight loss on low-fat diets has been shown to be modest, and prospective epidemiological studies have not been able consistently to correlate dietary fat intake with weight. In addition, obesity prevalence in the U.S. has risen dramatically since the 1970s, despite a decrease in fat consumption as a percent of total energy and the increase in availability of reduced-fat or fat-free foods [24]. Although dietary fat has decreased as a percentage of calories, carbohydrate consumption has increased; most of this increase has been in the form of refined

TABLE 30.1
Color Codes for Groups of Fruits and Vegetables

Color	Fruits and vegetables	Phytochemical
Red	Tomatoes, tomato soups, juices, or sauces, pink grapefruit, watermelon	Lycopene
Red/purple	Red grapes, blueberries, blackberries, cherries, plums, prunes, raspberries, strawberries, red apples	Anthocyanins and polyphenols
Orange	Apricots, acorn and winter squash, butternut and yellow squash, carrots, mangoes, cantaloupes, pumpkin, sweet potatoes	Alpha- and beta-carotene
Orange/yellow	Clementines, Mandarin oranges, oranges and orange juice, peaches, pineapple and pineapple juice, nectarines, papayas, tangerines, tangelos	Beta-cryptoxanthin and flavonoids
Yellow/green	Collard greens, green and yellow peppers, green beans, kale, beets and mustard greens, green peas, avocado, honeydew melon, yellow corn	Lutein and zeaxanthin
Green	Broccoli and broccoli sprouts, bok choy, Brussels sprouts, cabbage, Chinese cabbage, kale	Glucosinolates and indoles
White/green	Asparagus, celery, chives, endive, garlic, leeks, mushrooms, pearl onions, pears, shallots	Allyl sulfides and flavonoids

starches and concentrated sweets with a high glycemic index and/or glycemic load. This has led to increased interest in the role of refined carbohydrates in the current obesity epidemic.

In 1981, Jenkins et al. introduced the glycemic index as a system for classifying carbohydrate-containing foods based upon their effect on postprandial glycemia [25]. In this system, the glycemic response to the ingestion of 50 g of available carbohydrate from the test food is compared to the response from the ingestion of 50 g of the reference food (glucose or white bread). This is expressed as the area under the glucose response curve for the test food, divided by the area under the curve for the standard, and then multiplied by 100.

However, because the amount of carbohydrate in a typical serving of a given food will vary depending upon the food, the concept of glycemic load was introduced. This is an expression of the glycemic index of the food multiplied by the carbohydrate content of the food and takes into account the differences in carbohydrate content among foods [26]. For example, a carrot has a relatively high glycemic index but, due to its low total carbohydrate content, has a low glycemic load. In general, fruits, nonstarchy vegetables, nuts, and legumes have a low glycemic load.

The intake of high glycemic index/glycemic load meals induces a sequence of hormonal changes, including an increased ratio of insulin to glucagon, that limit the availability of metabolic fuels in the postprandial period and promote nutrient storage [27]. This in turn would be expected to stimulate hunger and promote food intake. Short-term feeding studies have demonstrated less satiety and greater voluntary food intake after consumption of high glycemic index meals as compared to low glycemic index meals.

In one study of obese teenage boys, *ad libitum* food intake was measured for 5 hours following a low, medium, or high glycemic index lunch. Voluntary energy intake after the high glycemic index meal was 53% greater than after the medium glycemic index meal and 81% greater than after the low glycemic index meal [28]. Similar outcomes have been seen in other single-meal studies — for example, demonstrating prolonged satiety after consumption of a low glycemic index bean puree vs. a high glycemic index potato puree [29].

Weight loss on a low-calorie, reduced-fat diet may be enhanced if the diet also has a low glycemic index [30]; even when energy intake is not restricted, low glycemic index and/or low glycemic load diets have been shown to produce greater weight loss than conventional low-fat diets. Ebbeling et al. [31] compared the effects of an *ad libitum*, reduced glycemic load diet with an energy-restricted, reduced-fat diet in obese adolescents and found significantly greater loss of weight and fat mass among subjects consuming the reduced glycemic load diet. At 12 months, mean BMI and fat mass had decreased significantly more in the low glycemic load experimental group compared with the conventional low-fat group.

In another short-term (6 days) study, 12 men with abdominal obesity were treated with an *ad libitum* low glycemic index, low-fat, high-protein diet or with a low-fat American Heart Association Step 1 diet consumed *ad libitum* to observe the nutritional and metabolic effects. Men on the low glycemic index diet, but not the low-fat diet, had a spontaneous 25% reduction in energy intake, with significant reductions in body weight and waist and hip circumference [32].

Other data suggest that low glycemic index/glycemic load diets may confer protection against certain forms of cancer, cardiovascular disease and the metabolic syndrome, and type-2 diabetes. In the Women's Health Study, a high glycemic load dietary pattern was associated with an increased risk for colon cancer [33], and data from the Iowa Women's study indicated that a higher glycemic load pattern may be a risk factor for endometrial cancer incidence in nondiabetic women [34]. In a study of 244 healthy women, a strong and statistically significant positive association was found between dietary glycemic load and plasma C-reactive protein, a plasma marker for chronic inflammation associated with an increased risk for heart disease [35]. In large prospective epidemiological studies, the glycemic index and the glycemic load of the overall diet have been associated with a greater risk of type-2 diabetes in men and in women [36,37].

Effects of Dietary Fat on Calorie Balance and Inflammation

Given that fat has more than twice the calorie density of carbohydrate or protein on a per-gram basis, the relationship between dietary fat and body weight has been of research interest for decades. Several reports have demonstrated a positive relationship between dietary fat intake and body weight [38–40]; however, others have noted a decrease in dietary fat as a percentage of calories with a higher overall calorie intake in the U.S. with increasing obesity in the population [41–43]. Reports regarding the efficacy of low-fat diets to reduce body weight are inconsistent and, as yet, the role of dietary fat in the regulation of food intake is not fully understood. In short-term trials, a modest reduction in body weight is seen in individuals randomized to diets with a lower percentage of calories from fat.

Randomized, controlled, *ad libitum* low-fat, high-carbohydrate studies have demonstrated a range of weight loss in the range of 0 to 10 kg in the intervention groups, as compared to controls consuming their usual diet or a medium- to high-fat diet. Because of the large variability in outcome, the role of dietary fat in weight reduction has come into question. However, Bray and Popkin [44] found that a reduction of 10% in the proportion of calories from fat was associated with weight loss of 16 g/day, or 2.9 kg over 6 months, based on 28 intervention trials.

In a meta-analysis of *ad libitum* low-fat dietary intervention studies, Astrup et al. analyzed the relationship between initial body weight and weight loss. The analysis included data from 16 trials lasting 2 to 12 months and included 1728 individuals. Weight loss was positively and independently related to reduction in the percentage of calories from fat, although weight loss was not the primary aim of 12 of the 16 studies. It was concluded that *ad libitum* low-fat diets prevent weight gain in normal-weight subjects and consistently cause weight loss in overweight subjects [45]. A longitudinal study in 54 postmenopausal women demonstrated that a very low fat diet (<15% of energy intake) consumed *ad libitum* over an 8-month period produced a mean weight loss of 8% and a 2.7% reduction in body fat [46].

Obese individuals are at an increased risk for a number of diseases related to inflammation, and adipose tissue is an important endocrine organ that secretes a range in inflammatory mediators. Circulating concentrations of these cytokines are increased in obesity, and it has been shown that plasma levels of tumor necrosis factor-α (TNF-α) are associated with obesity [47] and decrease with weight loss [48,49]. Abdominal obesity is specifically associated with increases in cytokine concentrations in addition to the effects of body weight [47] and is one of the defining features of the metabolic syndrome.

Human beings evolved on a diet with a favorable balance of ω-6:ω-3 of approximately 4:1, but the current Western diet has a ratio estimated at 16.74 [50]. The ω-3 polyunsaturated fatty acids possess the most potent immunomodulatory activities; among the ω-3 polyunsaturated fatty acids (PUFA), those from fish oil (eicosapentaenoic acid [EPA] and docosahexaenoic acid [DHA]) are more biologically potent than α-linolenic acid (ALA). Animal experiments and clinical intervention studies have indicated that ω-3 fatty acids have anti-inflammatory properties and, therefore, might be useful in the management of inflammatory and autoimmune diseases.

There are various sources of ω-3 and ω-6 PUFA in the diet. Green leafy vegetables and nuts are rich in α-linolenic acid (a precursor of ω-3 PUFA), and the long-chain ω-3 PUFAs (EPA and DHA) are found in fish oils such as salmon, mackerel, and herring. The ω-6 PUFAs occur mostly in the diet as linoleic acid and can be found in vegetable oils, with corn oil contributing the majority of lineoleic acid in the American diet.

In animal studies, the anti-inflammatory effects of ω-3 PUFA have been demonstrated by the measurement of the cytokines TNF-α and IL-6 [51,52]. Human ω-3 PUFA intervention studies have shown anti-inflammatory effects in patients with chronic inflammatory conditions, including rheumatoid arthritis [53] and Crohn's disease [54], and ω-3 PUFA has been shown to alleviate symptoms of these diseases.

Inflammation may be an important modulator of the relationship between obesity and the metabolic syndrome. The mechanisms through which obesity is associated with insulin resistance and cardiovascular disease may in part be mediated through inflammation. Some preliminary evidence now suggests that dietary ω-3 PUFA can modulate at least some aspects of disease risk.

Meal Replacements and Portion-Controlled Meals

Portion control is one of the primary strategies in calorie control. Many people do not take the time to weigh and measure foods or they may abandon this practice after a period of time, thinking that they can estimate portions fairly well. Typical diet plans specify what foods are to be consumed for meals and snacks, and portion sizes are usually specified in standard weights and measures. Practical problems may arise with patients, such as whether to weigh foods before or after cooking or failure to account for condiments or ingredients used in cooking.

A few small mistakes over the course of a day or week can have a significant impact on weight loss progress. For example, an extra few ounces of meat could add an extra 200 cal to a day's intake, and calories in cereals range widely — from 50 to over 400 cal per cup. In restaurants, portions are almost always much larger than those specified on a meal plan, and fats and oils, sauces, dressings, gravies, and other high-fat ingredients are not always evident.

Meal replacements are foods designed to take the place of a meal while at the same time providing nutrients within a known calorie limit. These can take the form of shakes, bars, soups, or frozen portion-controlled meals; they provide security to the patient due to a defined calorie and nutrient content. Meal replacements have been shown to produce weight loss results superior to calorie counting. In a study by Ditschuneit et al. [55], patients were divided into two groups: one consumed an all-food diet of between 1200 and 1500 cal per day and the other consumed two meal replacements as part of an overall diet plan of 1200 to 1500 cal.

The all-food group lost approximately 3 lb over the first 12 weeks, and the meal replacement group lost approximately 17 lb. The markedly increased weight loss in the meal replacement group over the first 12 weeks was attributed to the enhanced dietary compliance mediated by the use of meal replacements. Both groups were then given one meal replacement per day over the course of 2 years and both groups lost additional weight. Ditschuneit and colleagues have shown that this approach can be maintained for up to 4 years [56].

In a 1994 study, 300 men and women at six sites throughout the U.S. took two meal replacement shakes per day as part of a 1200-cal/day diet plan for 12 weeks. For the next 24 months, they consumed one shake per day as part of a 1200-cal diet plan. Weight loss was about 7% of the starting weight, and subjects who continued to the end of the study (approximately 56% of the initial group) maintained much of their weight loss [57].

Heymsfield et al. [58] used primary data for meta- and pooling analyses from studies that compared partial meal replacement plans (in which one or two meal replacements were used daily) to reduced-calorie diet plans. Subjects prescribed the partial meal replacement or reduced-calorie diet treatment plans lost significant amounts of weight at the 3-month and 1-year evaluation time points; however, all methods of analysis indicated a significantly greater weight loss in subjects receiving the partial meal replacement plan compared to that in the reduced-calorie diet group. Additionally, the dropout rate for partial meal replacement and reduced-calorie diet groups was equivalent at 3 months and significantly less in the partial meal replacement group at 1 year.

Recent research has demonstrated that, with the exception of fruits and vegetables, increased variety of intake in all categories of foods promotes obesity [59]. By reducing variety, meal replacements help patients maintain a structured diet and portion control. Some meal replacements are excellent sources of protein, fiber, vitamins, and minerals and may be superior to simply restricting conventional food intake if careful food choices, which would ensure nutritional adequacy, are not made.

Dietary Supplements that Affect Energy Expenditure

Caffeine

Obesity has been associated with low sympathetic activity [60] and caffeine has been studied in animals and humans because it can increase sympathetic nervous system activity. In genetically obese mice without endogenous leptin production (ob/ob mice), caffeine has been shown to decrease body fat and improve sympathetic activity, suggesting a possible role in the treatment of human obesity [61]. In a study of obese and lean humans acting as their own controls, caffeine in an oral dose of 250 mg increased free fatty acids and glucose, but not cortisol levels, compared to a water placebo [62]. Increases in oxygen consumption and fat oxidation have been demonstrated in normal subjects given caffeine 8 mg/kg orally compared to 0.5 gm glucose, as well as in seven normal and six obese subjects after 4 mg/kg of caffeinated coffee compared to a decaffeinated control after fasting and after a mixed meal [63].

In small studies, administration of caffeine has been shown to increase lipolysis, circulating fatty acid levels and oxygen consumption [64–67]. In one study, caffeine administration significantly elevated systolic blood pressure 4.5 to 6.6 mm Hg, but diastolic blood pressure or pulse rate did not change [66]; subjects reported no symptoms or side effects. The increase in resting metabolic rate induced by 4 mg/kg of caffeine predicts the amount of weight lost in response to a diet and exercise program, and the dose–response characteristics have been carefully documented [68–71]. Therefore, the scientific evidence in animals and humans supports a potential role for caffeine in weight reduction through increases in oxygen consumption and fat oxidation.

Several epidemiological studies have addressed the safety of caffeine. The positive correlation found between heavy coffee drinking and elevated cholesterol is felt to be due to factors other than caffeine in coffee because caffeine consumption in the form of tea or cola has no effect on cholesterol [72,73]. A clinical trial with 288 healthy subjects evaluated the effects of a single 200-mg/day dose of caffeine compared to placebo. Caffeine gave a 2.2 mm Hg rise in diastolic blood pressure, which was felt to be clinically insignificant. Pulse rate or systolic blood pressure [74] did not change. Similarly, in women, the negative effects on osteoporosis of drinking more than two cups of coffee per day are associated with factors other than caffeine in coffee [75]. The FDA approves caffeine for sale without a prescription for use as a stimulant [76] by persons 12 years of age or older at a dose up to 200 mg every 3 hours (1600 mg/day) and as an ingredient in pain medications, which gives further support to its safety.

Green Tea Catechins

Green tea prepared by heating or steaming the leaves of *Camelia sinensis* is widely consumed on a regular basis throughout Asia. However, the most widely consumed tea is the black tea consumed by more than 80% of the world's population [77]. Black tea is made by allowing the green tea leaves to auto-oxidize enzymatically, leading to the conversion of a large percentage of green tea catechins to theaflavins. The catechins are a family of compounds including epigallocatechin gallate (EGCG), considered to be the most potent antioxidant in the family of compounds. Drinking one cup of tea per day has been reported to decrease the odds ratio of suffering a myocardial infarction to 0.56 compared to that for those who do not drink tea [78].

These compounds are flavonoids in the class of polyphenols and have many activities, including inhibition of the catechol-O-methyl transferase (COMT) enzyme, which degrades norepinephrine [79]. The catechins appear to be able to enhance sympathetic nervous system activity at the level of the fat cell adrenoreceptor. *In vitro*, a green tea extract containing catechins and caffeine was more potent in stimulating brown adipose tissue thermogenesis than equimolar concentrations of caffeine alone [80]. The use of ephedrine to release norepinephrine increased the thermogenic effect noted with green tea catechins. Oolong tea or placebo was orally administered to mice over a 10-week period during high-fat feeding. Mean food consumption was not different between the groups, but oolong tea prevented the obesity and fatty liver induced by the high-fat diet. Noradrenaline-induced lipolysis was shown to increase and pancreatic lipase activity to be inhibited by the oolong tea [81].

Because caffeine occurs naturally in green tea extract, it has been difficult to separate the effects of green tea from caffeine in humans. However, a study by Dulloo et al. [65] gave subjects green tea extract capsules, three times per day, providing a total of 150 mg caffeine and 375 mg total catechins, of which 270 mg was epigallocatechin gallate. Subjects spent three 24-hour periods in an energy chamber during which they received the green tea extract, 150 mg of caffeine, or placebo. In the 24 hours when green tea was administered, 24-hour urinary excretion of norepinephrine but not epinephrine was noted compared to the caffeine or placebo-treatment periods. Energy expenditure was higher by 4.5% in the green tea period compared to placebo and 3.2% higher than when the same dose of caffeine was given alone. In addition, fat oxidation was increased. The net effect attributable to green tea could be estimated at 328 kJ/day or approximately 80 cal/day. Clearly, it is difficult to demonstrate the effects of green tea catechins alone, but a synergistic interaction with ephedrine independent of the caffeine content of green tea is possible and should be evaluated.

Capsaicin

Capsaicin from chili peppers and red peppers has been shown to stimulate fat oxidation and thermogenesis [82,83]. The exact mechanism for this effect is not known, but the constituents appear to activate neural signals that result in vasodilation and endorphin release. Ohnuki et al.

[84] have investigated the effects of capsiate, a nonpungent capsaicin analog found in the fruits of a nonpungent cultivar of pepper, CH-19 Sweet, on oxygen consumption and fat accumulation in mice. Capsaicin as well as capsiate increased oxygen consumption and serum adrenalin levels vs. controls. Additionally, after the administration of capsaicin and capsiate for 2 weeks, capsiate suppressed body-fat accumulation as well as capsaicin vs. control.

The effects of the same cultivar were tested in humans in whom core body temperature, body surface temperature, and oxygen consumption were measured after ingestion of CH-19 or a control pepper that contained neither capsaicin nor capsiate. The core body temperature and forehead temperature were higher in the CH-19 group vs. control, and body surface temperature increased for approximately 20 minutes after consumption of the CH-19. Oxygen consumption was significantly higher in the CH-19 group, suggesting that the nonpungent cultivar increased thermogenesis and energy consumption [85].

Tsi et al. studied the combined effect of capsaicin, green tea extract, and essence of chicken vs. placebo on body-fat content in healthy overweight subjects. The supplement contained 0.4 mg capsaicin, 625 mg green tea extract, and 800 mg essence of chicken. Subjects were instructed to maintain their usual dietary and exercise habits and, after 2 weeks, showed a decrease in mean body fat percentage and an increase in resting energy expenditure in the treatment group compared to controls [86].

CONCLUSION

In clinical intervention trials of low-fat diets designed to test the ability of nutrition to affect cancer incidence, the total caloric intake has not changed significantly due to the continued and increased intake of refined carbohydrates in compensation of lower fat intake. Typically, in studies such as the Women's Health Initiative, overall mean changes in body weight have been small, reflecting little change in overall energy intake or balance. Similarly, high-protein diets based on increased animal protein intake with controlled intakes of refined carbohydrates have not led to sustained reductions in body weight.

There are a number of strategies for affecting the overall dietary pattern while restricting energy intake through calorie restriction. The control of energy balance will continue to be of interest to those studying the relationship between obesity and cancer. Overweight increases the risk for several cancers, including esophageal, colorectal, breast, endometrial, and kidney cancers, and maintenance of healthy body weight and avoidance of weight gain in adulthood are advised. Further research into strategies for cancer prevention and the role of energy balance control is critical, given the current national epidemic of obesity.

REFERENCES

1. Westerterp-Plantenga MS, Rolland V, Wilson SAJ, Westerterp KR. Satiety related to 24-h diet-induced thermogenesis during high protein/carbohydrate vs. high-fat diets measured in a respiration chamber. *Eur J Clin Nutr* 1999; 53:495–502.
2. Westerterp-Plantenga MS, Lejeune MP, Nihs I, van Ooijen M, Kovacs EM. High-protein intake sustains weight maintenance after body weight loss in humans. *Int J Obesity Relat Metab Disord* 2004; 28:57–64.
3. Skov AR, Toubro S, Ronn B, Holm L, Astrup A. Randomized trial on protein vs. carbohydrate in *ad libitum* fat reduced diet for the treatment of obesity. *Int J Obesity Related Metab Disord* 1999; 23:528–536.
4. Layman DK, Boileau RA, Erickson DJ, Painter JE, Shiue H, Sather C, Christou DD. A reduced ratio of dietary carbohydrate to protein improves body composition and blood lipid profiles during weight loss in adult women. *J Nutr* 2003; 133:411–417.

5. Johnston CS, Tjonn SL, Swan PD. High-protein, low-fat diets are effective for weight loss and favorably alter biomarkers in healthy adults. *J Nutr* 2004; 134:586–591
6. Brehm BJ, Seeley RJ, Daniels SR, D'Alessio DA. A randomized trial comparing a very low carbohydrate diet and a calorie-restricted low fat diet on body weight and cardiovascular risk factors in healthy women. *J Clin Endocrinol Metab* 2003; 88:1617–1623.
7. Eisenstein J, Roberts SB, Dallal G, Saltzman E. High protein weight loss diets: are they safe and do they work? A review of experimental and epidemiologic data. *Nutr Rev* 2002; 60:189–200.
8. Marlett JA, McBurney MI, Slavin JL. Position of the American Dietetic Association: health implications of dietary fiber. *J Am Diet Assoc* 2002; 102:993–1000.
9. Miller WC, Niederpruem MG, Wallace JP, Lindeman AK. Dietary fat, sugar, and fiber predict body fat content. *J Am Diet Assoc* 1994; 94:612–615.
10. Alfieri MA, Pomerleau J, Grace DM, Anderson L. Fiber intake of normal weight, moderately obese and severely obese subjects. *Obesity Res* 1995; 3:541–547.
11. Liu S, Willett WC, Manson JE, Hu FB, Rosner B, Colditz G. Relation between changes in intakes of dietary fiber and grain products and changes in weight and development of obesity among middle-aged women. *Am J Clin Nutr* 2003; 78:920–927.
12. Jacobs DR Jr, Meyer KA, Kushi LH, Folsom AR. Whole-grain intake may reduce the risk of ischemic heart disease death in postmenopausal women: the Iowa Women's Health Study. *Am J Clin Nutr* 1998; 68:248–257.
13. Pereira A, Jacobs D, Slattery M, Ruth K, Van Horn L, Hilner J, Kushi L. The association of whole grain intake and fasting insulin in a biracial cohort of young adults: the CARDIA study. *CVD Prev* 1998; 1:231–242.
14. Temple NJ. Antioxidants and disease: more questions than answers. *Nutr Res* 2000; 20:449–559.
15. Willett WC. Diet and health: what should we eat? *Science* 1994; 254:532–537.
16. Willett WC. Diet, nutrition and avoidable cancer. *Environ Health Perspect* 1995; 103:165–170.
17. Blot WJ, Li J-Y, Taylor PR, Guo W, Dawsey S, Wang G-Q, Yang CS, Zheng S-F, Gail M, Li G-Y, Yu Y, Liu B-Q, Tangrea J, Sun Y-H, Liu F, Fraumeni JF, Zhang Y-H, Li B. Nutrition intervention trials in Linxiang, China: supplementation with specific vitamin/mineral combinations, cancer incidence, and disease-specific mortality in the general population. *J Nat Cancer Inst* 1993; 85:1483–1492.
18. Quatromoni PA, Copenhafer DL, D'Agostino RB, Millen BE. Dietary patterns predict the development of overweight in women: the Framingham Nutrition Studies. *J Am Diet Assoc* 2002; 102:1240–1246.
19. Ledikewe JH, Smiciklas-Wright H, Mitchell DC, Miller CK, Jensen GL. Dietary patterns of rural older adults are associated with weight and nutritional status. *J Am Geriatr Soc* 2004; 52:589–595.
20. Perez CE. Fruit and vegetable consumption. *Health Rep* 2002; 13:23–31.
21. Epstein LH, Gordy CC, Raynor HA, Beddome M, Kilanowski CK, Paluch R. Increasing fruit and vegetable intake and decreasing fat and sugar intake in families at risk for childhood obesity. *Obesity Res* 2001; 9:171–178.
22. Steinmetz KA, Potter JD. Vegetables, fruits, and cancer. I. Epidemiology. *Cancer Causes Control* 1991; 2:325–337.
23. Heber D, Bowerman S. *What Color is Your Diet*? New York: Harper Collins, 2001.
24. Putnam JJ, Allshouse JA. Food consumption, prices, and expenditures, 1970–1997. U.S. Department of Agriculture: Washington, D.C., 1999.
25. Jenkins DJ, Wolever TM, Taylor RH, Barker H, Fielden H, Baldwin JM, Bowling AC, Newman HC, Jenkins AL, Goff DV. Glycemic index of foods: a physiological basis for carbohydrate exchange. *Am J Clin Nutr* 1981; 34:362–366.
26. Salmeron J, Manson JE, Stampfer MJ, Colditz GA, Wing AL, Willett WC. Dietary fiber, glycemic load, and risk of non-insulin-dependent diabetes mellitus in women. *JAMA* 1997; 254:472–477.
27. Ludwig DS. The glycemic index: physiological mechanisms relating to obesity, diabetes, and cardiovascular disease. *JAMA* 2002; 287:2414–2423.
28. Ludwig DS, Majzoub JA, Al-Zahrani A, Dallal GE, Blanco I, Roberts SB. High glycemic index foods, overeating, and obesity. *Pediatrics* 1999; 103:E26.
29. Leathwood P, Pollett P. Effects of slow release carbohydrates in the form of bean flakes on the evolution of hunger and satiety in man. *Appetite* 1988; 10:1–11.

30. Slabber M, Barnard HC, Kuyl JM, Dannhauser A, Schall R. Effects of a low-insulin-response, energy-restricted diet on weight loss and plasma insulin concentrations in hyperinsulinemic obese females. *Am J Clin Nutr* 1994; 60:48–53.
31. Ebbeling CB, Leidig MM, Sinclair KB, Hangen JP, Ludwig DS. A reduced-glycemic load diet in the treatment of adolescent obesity. *Arch Pediatr Adolesc Med* 2003; 157:773–779.
32. Dumesnil JG, Turgeon J, Tremblay A, Poirier P, Gilbert M, Gagnon L, St-Pierre S, Garneau C, Lemieux I, Pascot A, Bergeron J, Despres JP. Effect of a low-glycemic index–low-fat–high-protein diet on the atherogenic metabolic risk profile of abdominally obese men. *Br J Nutr* 2001; 86:557–568.
33. Higginbotham S, Zhang ZF, Lee IM, Cook NR, Giovannucci E, Buring JE, Liu S. Dietary glycemic load and risk of colorectal cancer in the Women's Health Study. *J Natl Cancer Inst* 2004; 96:229–233.
34. Folsom AR, Demissie Z, Harnack L. Glycemic index, glycemic load and incidence of endometrial cancer: The Iowa Women's Health Study. *Nutr Cancer* 2003; 46:119–124.
35. Liu S, Manson JE, Buring JE, Stampfer MJ, Willett WC, Ridker PM. Relation between a diet with a high glycemic load and plasma concentrations of high-sensitivity C-reactive protein in middle-aged women. *Am J Clin Nutr* 2002; 75:492–498.
36. Salmeron J, Ascherio A, Rimm EB, et al. Dietary fiber, glycemic load, and risk of NIDDM in men. *Diabetes Care* 1997; 20:545–550.
37. Salmeron J, Manson JE, Stampfer MJ, Colditz GA, Wing AL, Willett WC. Dietary fiber, glycemic load, and risk of non-insulin-dependent diabetes mellitus in women. *JAMA* 1997; 277:472–477.
38. Harnack LJ, Jeffery RW, Boutelle KN. Temporal trends in energy intake in the United States: an ecologic perspective. *Am J Clin Nutr* 2000; 71:478–484.
39. Lissner L, Heitmann Bl. Dietary fat and obesity: evidence from epidemiology. *Eur J Clin Nutr* 1995; 49:79–90.
40. Lichtenstein AH, Kennedy E, Barrier P, Danford D, Ernst ND, Grundy SM, Leveille GA, Van Horn L, Williams CL, Booth SL. Dietary fat consumption and health. *Nutr Rev* 1998; 56:S3–19.
41. Heini AF, Weinsier RL. Divergent trends in obesity and fat intake patterns: the American paradox. *Am J Med* 1997; 102:259–264.
42. Willett WC, Leibel RL. Dietary fat is not a major determinant of body fat. *Am J Med* 2002; 113 Suppl 9B:47S–59S.
43. Arnett DK, McGovern PG, Jacobs DR Jr, Shahar E, Duval S, Blackburn H, Luepker RV. Fifteen-year trends in cardiovascular risk factors (1980–1982 through 1995–1997): the Minnesota Heart Survey. *Am J Epidemiol* 2002; 156:929–935.
44. Bray GA and Popkin BM. Dietary fat intake does affect obesity. *Am J Clin Nutr* 1998; 68:1157–1173.
45. Astrup A, Ryan L, Grunwald G, Storgaard M, Saris W, Melanson E, Hill JO. The role of dietary fat and body fatness: evidence from a preliminary meta-analysis of *ad libitum* low-fat dietary intervention studies. *Br J Nutr* 2000; 83:S25–S32.
46. Mueller-Cunningham WM, Quintanta R, Kasim-Karakas, SE. An *ad libitum*, very low-fat diet results in weight loss and changes in nutrient intakes in postmenopausal women. *J Am Diet Assoc* 2003; 103:1600–1606.
47. Tsigos C, Kyrou I, Chala E, Tsapogas P, Stavridis JC, Raptis SA & Katsilambros N. Circulating tumor necrosis factor alpha concentrations are higher in abdominal vs. peripheral obesity. *Metabolism* 1999; 48:1332–1335.
48. Kern PA, Saghizadeh M, Ong JM, Bosch RJ, Deem R, Simsolo RB. The expression of tumor necrosis factor in human adipose tissue. Regulation by obesity, weight loss, and relationship to lipoprotein lipase. *J Clin Invest* 1995; 95:2111–2119.
49. Dandona P, Weinstock R, Thusu K, Abdel-Rahman E, Aljada A, Wadden T. Tumor necrosis factor-alpha in sera of obese patients: fall with weight loss. *J Clin Endo Metab* 1998; 83:2907–2910.
50. Simopoulos AP. N-3 fatty acids and human health: defining strategies for public policy. *Lipids* 2001; 36:S83–89.
51. Mulrooney HM, Grimble RF. The influence of butter, and corn, coconut and fish oils on the effects of recombinant human tumour necrosis factor alpha in rats. *Clin Sci* 1993; 84:105–112.
52. Sadeghi S, Wallace FA, Calder PC. Dietary lipids modify the cytokine response to bacterial lipopolysaccharide in mice. *Immunology* 1999; 96:404–410.

53. Geusens P, Wouters C, Nijs J, Jiang Y, Dequeker J. Long-term effect of omega-3 fatty acid supplementation in active rheumatoid arthritis. A 12-month, double blind, controlled study. *Arthritis Rheum* 1994; 37:824–829.
54. Belluzzi A, Brignola C, Campieri M, Pera A, Boschi S, Miglioli M. Effect of an enteric-coated fish-oil preparation on relapses in Crohn's disease. *N Eng J Med* 1996; 334:1557–1560.
55. Ditschuneit HH, Flechtner-Mors M, Johnson TD, Adler G. Metabolic and weight-loss effects of a long-term dietary intervention in obese patients. *Am J Clin Nutr* 1999 Feb; 69(2):198–204.
56. Flechtner-Mors M, Ditschuneit HH, Johnson TD, Suchard MA, Adler G. Metabolic and weight loss effects of long-term dietary intervention in obese patients: 4-year results. *Obesity Res* 2000; 8:399–402.
57. Heber D, Ashley, JM, Wang, H-J, Elashoff, RM. Clinical evaluation of a minimal intervention meal replacement regimen for weight reduction. *J Am Coll Nutr* 1994; 13:608–614.
58. Heymsfield SB, van Mierlo CA, van der Knaap HC, Heo M, Frier HI. Weight management using a meal replacement strategy: meta- and pooling analysis from six studies. *Int J Obesity Relat Metab Disord* 2003; 27:537–549.
59. Roberts S. Multiple components contribute to dietary risk for obesity (abstract). *Obesity Res* 1999; 7(Suppl 1):13S.
60. Macdonald IA. Advances in our understanding of the role of the sympathetic nervous system in obesity. *Int J Obesity Relat Metab Disord* 1995; 19 Suppl 7:S2–S7.
61. Chen MD, Lin WH, Song YM, Lin PY, Ho LT. Effect of caffeine on the levels of brain serotonin and catecholamine in the genetically obese mice. *Chung Hua I Hsueh Tsa Chih* (Taipei) 1994; 53:257–261.
62. Oberman Z, Herzberg M, Jaskolka H, Harell A, Hoerer E, Laurian L. Changes in plasma cortisol, glucose and free fatty acids after caffeine ingestion in obese women. *Isr J Med Sci* 1975; 11:33–36.
63. Acheson KJ, Zahorska-Markiewicz B, Pittet P, Anantharaman K, Jequier E. Caffeine and coffee: their influence on metabolic rate and substrate utilization in normal weight and obese individuals. *Am J Clin Nutr* 1980; 33:989–997.
64. Jung RT, Shetty PS, James WP, Barrand MA, Callingham BA. Caffeine: its effect on catecholamines and metabolism in lean and obese humans. *Clin Sci* 1981; 60:527–535.
65. Dulloo AG, Geissler CA, Horton T, Collins A, Miller DS. Normal caffeine consumption: influence on thermogenesis and daily energy expenditure in lean and postobese human volunteers. *Am J Clin Nutr* 1989; 49:44–50.
66. Bracco D, Ferrarra JM, Arnaud MJ, Jequier E, Schutz Y. Effects of caffeine on energy metabolism, heart rate, and methylxanthine metabolism in lean and obese women. *Am J Physiol* 1995; 269:E671–678.
67. Bondi M, Grugni G, Velardo A, et al. Adrenomedullary response to caffeine in prepubertal and pubertal obese subjects. *Int J Obesity Relat Metab Disord* 1999; 23:992–996.
68. Yoshida T, Sakane N, Umekawa T, Kondo M. Relationship between basal metabolic rate, thermogenic response to caffeine, and body weight loss following combined low-calorie and exercise treatment in obese women. *Int J Obesity Relat Metab Disord* 1994; 18:345–350.
69. Abernethy DR, Todd EL, Schwartz JB. Caffeine disposition in obesity. *Br J Clin Pharmacol* 1985; 20:61–66.
70. Cheymol G. Clinical pharmacokinetics of drugs in obesity. An update. *Clin Pharmacokinet* 1993; 25:103–114.
71. Caraco Y, Zylber-Katz E, Berry EM, Levy M. Caffeine pharmacokinetics in obesity and following significant weight reduction. *Int J Obesity Relat Metab Disord* 1995; 19:234–239.
72. Haffner SM, Knapp JA, Stern MP, Hazuda HP, Rosenthal M, Franco LJ. Coffee consumption, diet, and lipids. *Am J Epidemiol* 1985; 122:1–12.
73. La Vecchia C, Franceschi S, Decarli A, Pampallona S, Tognoni G. Risk factors for myocardial infarction in young women. *Am J Epidemiol* 1987; 125:832–843.
74. Noble R. A controlled clinical trial of the cardiovascular and psychological effects of phenylpropanolamine and caffeine. *Drug Intell Clin Pharm* 1988; 22:296–299.
75. Barrett-Connor E, Chang JC, Edelstein SL. Coffee-associated osteoporosis offset by daily milk consumption. The Rancho Bernardo Study. *JAMA* 1994; 271:280–283.
76. Sawynok J. Pharmacological rationale for the clinical use of caffeine. *Drugs* 1995; 49:37–50.

77. Steele VE, Kelloff GJ, Balentine D, Boone CW, Mehta R, Bagheri D, Sigman CC, Zhu S, Sharma S. Comparative chemopreventive mechanisms of green tea, black tea and selected polyphenol extracts measured by *in vitro* bioassays. *Carcinogenesis*. 2000; 21:63–67.
78. Sesso HD, Gaziano JM, Buring JE, Hennekens CH. Coffee and tea intake and the risk of myocardial infarction. *Am J Epidemiol* 1999; 149:162–167.
79. Borchardt RT, Huber JA. Catechol O-methyltransferase. 5. Structure–activity relationships for inhibition by flavonoids. *J Med Chem* 1975; 18:120–122.
80. Dulloo AG, Seydoux J, Giradier L. Tealine and thermogenesis: interactions between polyphenols, caffeine and sympathetic activity. *Int J Obesity Relat Metab Disord* 1996; 20 (Suppl 4):71.
81. Han LK, Takaku T, Li J, Kimura Y, Okuda H. Antiobesity action of oolong tea. *Int J Obesity Relat Metab Disord* 1999; 23:98–105.
82. Henry CJ, Emery B. Effect of spiced food on metabolic rate. *Hum Nutr Clin Nutr* 1986; 40:165–168.
83. Yoshioka M, St-Pierre S, Suzuki M, Tremblay A. Effects of red pepper added to high-fat and high-carbohydrate meals on energy metabolism and substrate utilization in Japanese women. *Br J Nutr* 1998; 80:503–510.
84. Ohnuki K, Haramizu S, Oki K, Watanabe T, Yazawa S, Fushiki T. Administration of capsiate, a nonpungent capsaicin analog, promotes energy metabolism and suppresses body fat accumulation in mice. *Biosci Biotechnol Biochem* 2001; 65:2735–2740.
85. Ohynuki K, Niwa S, Maeda S, Inoue N, Yazawa S, Fushiki T. H-19 sweet, a nonpungent cultivar of red pepper, increased body temperature and oxygen consumption in humans. *Biosci Biotechnol Biochem* 2001; 65:2033–2036.
86. Tsi D, Nah AK, Kiso Y, Moritani T, Ono H. Clinical study on the combined effect of capsaicin, green tea extract and essence of chicken on body-fat content in human subjects. *J Nutr Sci Vitaminol* (Tokyo) 2003; 49:437–441.

31 Population-Based Approaches to Increasing Physical Activity

Fiona Bull

CONTENTS

INTRODUCTION

The case for physical inactivity as an important lifestyle risk factor for several site-specific cancers as well as other chronic diseases is now well established. Although research into the preventive health benefits of physical activity commenced as early as the 1950s [1], it has been only in recent years that the body of evidence has positioned inactivity as a major public health issue. In 2002, the World Health Organization estimated that 1.9 million deaths and 19 million disability adjusted life years (DAYLs) were attributable to inactivity [2]. Conservative calculations estimate that 10% of breast cancer and 16% of colon cancer worldwide could be attributed to physical inactivity alone [3]. These are similar to other estimates; Mezzetti et al. [4] estimated that 11% of breast cancer risk and Slattery et al. [5] estimated that 13% of colon cancer risk could be attributable to physical inactivity. It is, however, likely that all these estimates grossly underestimate the true magnitude of burden due to physical inactivity because of the wide variation in measurement used and the unaccounted-for contribution of physical inactivity to increased body mass [6].

The economic cost of low levels of activity is also being recognized despite the measurement difficulties. Recent estimates suggest that, in the U.S., physical inactivity alone contributes as much as $75 billion to U.S. medical costs (year 2000) [7,8], and costs associated with inactivity and obesity accounted for 9.4% of the national health expenditure (in 1995). In Canada, physical inactivity is estimated to cost about 2.5% ($2.1 billion) of the direct total health care expenditures; a 10% reduction in inactivity has the potential to reduce these costs by $150 million [9]. In England, total costs of inactivity due to the direct costs of treatment for major lifestyle diseases and the indirect costs through sickness absence has been estimated to be £8.2 billion a year [10].

The public health response to physical inactivity has varied widely around the world. Several countries, notably Canada and Finland, have implemented major national initiatives for well over two decades [11,12]; however, for others, public health involvement and action at national and state/regional levels is much more recent. In 2002, the World Health Organization commenced the development of a global strategy on physical activity, diet, and health and this was endorsed by the member states in 2004 [13]. This reflects the growing recognition by government and nongovernment organizations of the role of physical activity in reducing noncommunicable disease and their need to help address levels of inactivity in the whole population. Evidence-based reviews of effectiveness of interventions have proliferated in response [14–16] and these summaries of what is known to work can assist governments in prioritizing their actions. Growing awareness of the trends in overweight and obesity, evidence of chronic disease in young children and adolescents, rates of urbanization, and changing patterns of transportation have helped accelerate the agenda for population-based programs aimed at physical activity. Media interest also has focused attention on these issues so that, now, countries around the world are beginning to take the importance of active lifestyles across the life course much more seriously.

This chapter provides a summary of the evidence base for public health action, an overview of the principles and content of a population-based approach, and a review of selected initiatives. This includes examples of communication campaigns, efforts aimed at creating supportive environments, programs in different settings, and a summary of recent developments in the policy arena. It is not possible to provide a comprehensive review of all intervention research on physical activity, nor is it needed. Interested readers are referred to other recent reviews mentioned earlier for critiques of interventions aimed at specific settings and populations.

WHAT IS A POPULATION HEALTH APPROACH?

Population (or public) health is the organized, collective, or social efforts of society to protect, promote, and restore the health of the population [17]. It represents not a single action, but rather a combination of sciences, skills, and activities directed to the maintenance and improvement of the health of all people. The actions can and do change with changing technology and shifting threats to health, but the primary goal of improving the health status of the entire population remains the same [17]. In contrast, health care has as its aim the treatment or rehabilitation of illness.

The discipline and practice of public health has a long history, evolving over time to meet the health needs brought about by industrialization, urbanization, and, most recently, globalization [18]. Many countries with rapidly developing economies face the challenges of treatment and prevention of communicable and noncommunicable diseases. Although the priorities and foci of public health action vary around the world, the core functions of population health can be broadly summarized as (adapted from National Public Health Partnership [19]):

- Measurement, analysis and communication of the health status and health needs of a population
- Prevention and control of communicable and noncommunicable disease and injury through risk factor reduction, education, screening, immunization, and other interventions
- Development, promotion, and support of: healthy lifestyles and behaviors; healthy public policy (which includes legislation, regulation, and fiscal measures); safe and healthy environments; and healthy growth and development throughout all life stages
- Strengthen skills, competencies, systems, and infrastructure to achieve measurable improvements in health status
- Strengthen communities through consultation, participation, and empowerment

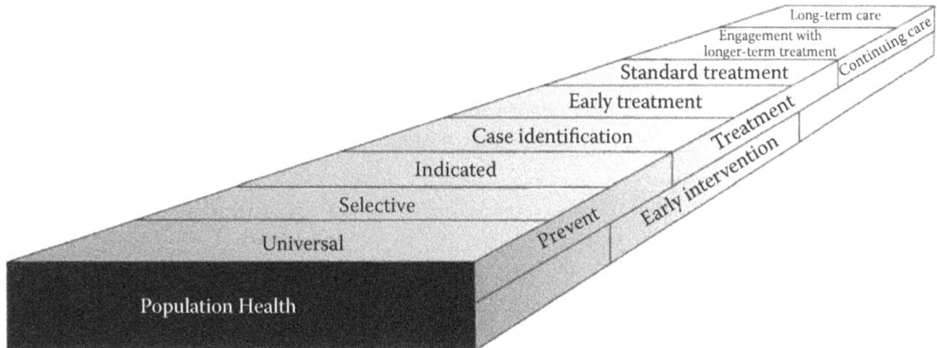

FIGURE 31.1 A schema of the continuum of population health through to clinical care. (Adapted from South Eastern Sydney Area Health Service, Population Health Directions for South East Health, http://www.sesahs.nsw.gov.au/index.htm. Accessed February 2005.)

Translation of information on the patterns of ill health and its causes into practical interventions delivered in the community, including the development of supportive public policy, is central to disease prevention and health promotion. Figure 31.1 shows the relationship between and reach of prevention and treatment aspects of the health care continuum [20].

PRINCIPLES OF A POPULATION-BASED APPROACH

A population-based approach involves thinking in aggregate terms rather than as individuals, which is more familiar to physicians and clinicians. The approach recognizes the multiple determinants of health and their complex interactions that affect health status and involves implementing strategies that address the entire range of factors that determine health. A population approach also includes identifying vulnerable populations and directing efforts to address the differences in health status between groups within populations. More recently, the pressing need to accelerate understanding of and intervention on the social, behavioral, economic, and political inequalities that generate health inequalities is being recognized [18].

The underlying principles of a population health-based approach in practice include a strong commitment to working in partnership with communities and other organizations, the use of the best available evidence for action, and a focus on achieving sustained action and investment in long-term health outcomes [21]. In practice, a population-based approach comprises universal strategies aimed at all people and targeted programs for those who are most vulnerable [19]. The latter aims at addressing the identified gaps in health status between subgroups in the population.

CASE FOR A POPULATION-BASED APPROACH TO PHYSICAL ACTIVITY FOR PREVENTION OF SITE-SPECIFIC CANCERS

The role of physical activity in the prevention of specific cancers has received considerable attention in recent years [6,22–25]. Overall, the findings are consistent. Colon cancer risk decreases with increased levels of physical activity. The risk reduction for physically active men and women is around 30 to 40%, compared with that for inactive people [6]. Although the evidence base on the exact amount of activity required is modest, it appears that 30 to 60 minutes per day of moderate to vigorous exercise is required to decrease risk [25]. Furthermore, a dose–response relationship is apparent, with risk declining with higher levels of activity. Available evidence indicates that physical activity is not associated with a reduced risk of developing rectal cancer [6].

There is clear evidence on the preventive effect of physical activity on breast cancer risk. Physically active women have about a 20 to 30% reduction in risk compared with inactive women [6]. It appears that 30 to 60 minutes per day of moderate to vigorous exercise is required to decrease the risk of breast cancer and that a dose–response relation probably occurs [25]. These associations have been reported for pre- and postmenopausal women and in studies measuring total activity, fitness, and levels of walking.

No consistent evidence on an association between physical activity and endometrial, prostate, testicular, ovarian, or lung cancers has been found [6,24]. Further research is required to understand the possible associations with these cancers as well as to clarify the dose–response relationship between specific cancers and different types (frequency, intensity, and duration) of activity. The most recent evidence suggests that more intense activity, and increased frequency and duration of activity, may provide more protection. Although physical activity is associated with reduced risk of cancer, the mechanisms are still being investigated.

This brief summary of research indicates a substantial evidence base underpinning the need for a coordinated agenda of action at the population level to increase levels of physical activity for the prevention and treatment of cancer. For more comprehensive coverage of the evidence, readers are directed to other chapters in this volume and recent reviews [6,24].

POPULATION LEVELS OF PHYSICAL ACTIVITY

Nationally representative data on levels of participation in physical activity are available from less than one third of the countries [3]. Although most countries in Western Europe, along with North America, Australia, and New Zealand, have such data, in many other countries data are available only from selected regions or cities or not at all. Significant efforts to improve the assessment of key risk factors of cancer and chronic disease, including physical inactivity, are under way internationally and regionally [26]. The development of measurement instruments and methods (e.g., the STEPwise approach to risk factor monitoring) as well as the central collation of risk factor data worldwide [27] are supported by the World Health Organization. At a regional level, the first data on inactivity from several countries in South and Central America are now available [28,29].

The ability to track trends in risk factors over time has been hampered by the use of different measures and this is particularly true for levels of inactivity. However, again only in recent years, a concerted effort has been made to increase consistency between surveys and, when possible, comparability between countries. The international physical activity questionnaire [30] and the global physical activity questionnaire [31] are two different instruments developed for use as a brief assessment tool in population health monitoring systems. They provide overall and domain-specific estimates of activity, respectively [32].

In countries with data, notably the more advanced economies, the current pattern of participation is of great concern. In the U.S., the U.K. and elsewhere, less than half of the adult population achieve the current recommended levels of at least 150 minutes of activity per week. The proportion of adults reporting no physical activity can range from 15% in Australia [33] to 80% in Brazil [29]. Few countries have good trend data; however, where they are available, the results show mostly declining levels of activity (Australia) or at best no change (U.S.) [32].

Low levels of activity in many countries are of concern, as are notable differences between subgroups within the population. In general, findings from the national surveys show that levels of activity are highest for younger adults (e.g., the 18 to 29 years), but this declines sharply with age. Men are more likely than women to meet current recommended levels of activity, although it is known that these differences can disappear when different domains and types of activity are assessed. Adults with higher educational attainment are more likely to be more active compared with those with lower levels of education. However, this is seen most often with measures of leisure-time activity and may also diminish if other types of activity, such as transport-related activity (e.g., walking and cycling) and home-based activities, are included.

POPULATION-BASED INTERVENTIONS — WHAT WORKS FOR PHYSICAL INACTIVITY?

Increased levels of participation in physical activity through a population-based approach comprising initiatives aimed at reaching everyone in the community, combined with targeted programs in selected settings to reach specific subpopulations based on need and inequalities, has considerable potential. Recent reviews have examined the effectiveness of various intervention approaches [14,15,35,36]. Furthermore, at least two ongoing systematic review processes are under way, one in the U.S. under the guidance of the Task Force on Community Preventive Services [37] and the other in the U.K. as part of the Health Development Agency's Evidence and Guidance Collaborating Centre work program [38]. The most recent recommendations from the work completed in the U.S. are shown in Table 31.1. Six of the eleven interventions reviewed to date are recommended for widespread implementation.

It is widely recognized that no single strategy or intervention will produce large changes in population levels of an activity. Instead, it is necessary to implement a coordinated, comprehensive set of strategies for investment over the medium to long term. Like other lifestyle risk factors, patterns of individual and population levels of activity are difficult to change, and isolated, short-term quick fixes will not be sufficient.

A successful comprehensive approach to increasing physical activity requires action at the policy level combined with program interventions and a supportive environment. Gaining political and professional support as well as necessary community awareness and engagement is needed and can be achieved through the use of mass media (television, radio, and print) combined with strategic lobbying and public relations activities. The need to create healthy public policy and the need for increased provision of programs require action in areas outside the health sector (notably in transport and urban planning); therefore, it is particularly important that a comprehensive approach be undertaken in partnership with relevant government and nongovernment agencies and community groups. For instance, after-school activity programs may require the combined efforts of public and private education authorities, schools, teachers, parents, sport and recreation services, and local or municipal government.

TABLE 31.1
Summary of Recommendations from the U.S. Guide to Preventive Services

Type of intervention	Recommendation
Informational approaches	
Point of decision prompts to promote stair use	Recommended
Community wide campaigns	Strongly recommended
Mass media campaigns	Insufficient evidence
Classroom-based health education focused on information provision and skills related to decision-making	Insufficient evidence
Behavioral and social approaches	
School-based PE	Strongly recommended
College-based health education and PE	Insufficient evidence
Classroom-based health education focused on reducing TV watching and video playing	Insufficient evidence
Family-based social support	Insufficient evidence
Social support interventions in community settings	Recommended
Individually adapted health behavior change programs	Recommended
Environmental and policy approaches	
Creation of or enhanced access to places for activity combined with information outreach activities	Strongly recommended

Source: Produced from results presented in Kahn, E.B. et al., *Am J Prev Med* 22, 73, 2002.

Developing a population-based approach to increasing physical activity can appear daunting. The demands of a comprehensive approach with multiple strategies and need to work in collaboration with nontraditional partners (i.e., those outside the health sector) are new and complex. Nonetheless, excellent examples of this approach are being put into practice in Europe, Australia, New Zealand, the U.S., Brazil, and elsewhere in South and Central America. Figure 31.2 shows one example of a planning and organizational framework for a statewide initiative to increase levels of physical activity.

The work in Western Australia (population 2 million) follows similar work in New South Wales, where a task force commenced in 1997 [39] soon after the release of the U.S Surgeon General's Report on Physical Activity and Health [40]. In Western Australia, a multisector task force was created representing a collaboration across state-level government [41]; it was positioned within central government (the premier's office) rather than within a single participating government department (e.g., Sport and Recreation, Education, Health, Transport and Planning). Such a move was strategically very important for several reasons:

- It positioned the initiative in close proximity of the highest decision-maker (the premier).
- It avoided the perception of the "problem" and/or the "solutions" being viewed as the responsibility of a single government department — in other words, it made the high levels of physical inactivity "everybody's business."
- The relevance of the issue to many government departments' agendas provided a real opportunity for action at a cross-government level or, in current terminology, "joined-up government."

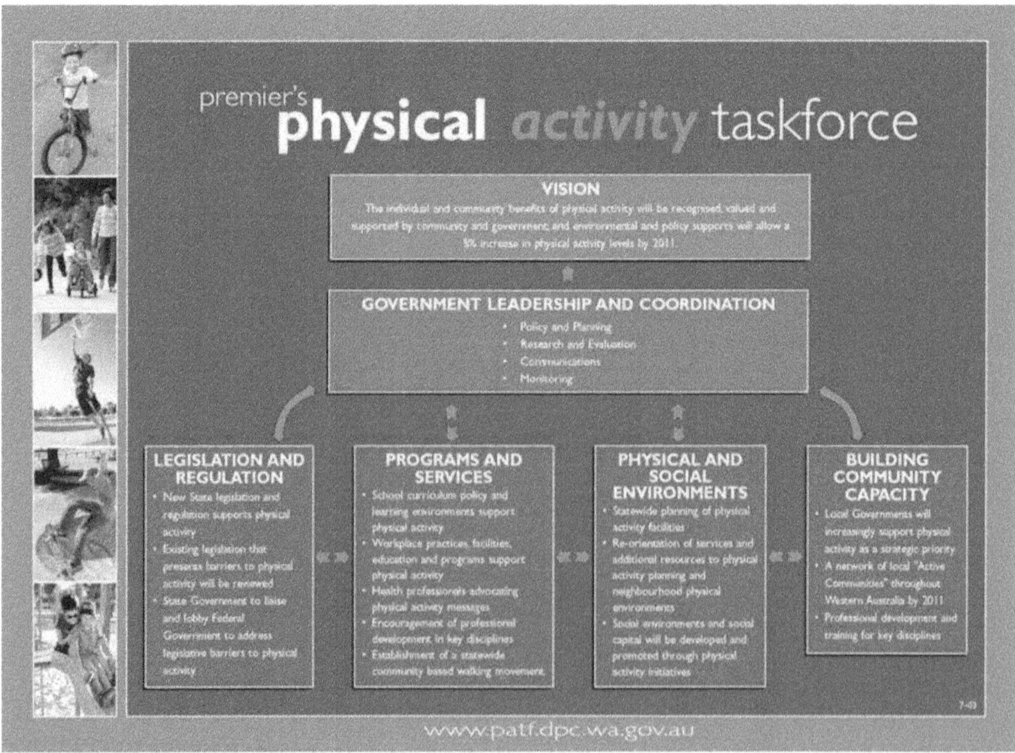

FIGURE 31.2 The strategic plan of the Western Australian Premier's task force on physical activity. (From http://www.asnsw.health.nsw.gov.au/public-health/health-promotion/activity/taskforce/index.html.)

In addition to senior government support, a strategic plan is an essential component to guide the direction and work of a multisector task force, along with a clear program of work with set timeframes, lead agencies, and identified partners. In Western Australia, day-to-day implementation of the work is undertaken by the Taskforce secretariat and three working groups (I Local Government, II Communication, and III Monitoring and Evaluation) comprising representatives from government departments, relevant nongovernment agencies, and academic institutions. More details on the work and progress in Western Australia are available [41]. Other examples of similar regional or state coalitions exist in Australia and elsewhere [42,43].

NATIONAL PHYSICAL ACTIVITY POLICY

Although the development of national policy on physical activity is a relatively new endeavor, several countries have a policy in place or under development. This has been strongly encouraged by the World Health Organization in its Global Strategy on Diet, Physical Activity, and Health [13]. A national policy on physical activity has been defined as [44]

> ... a formal statement that defines physical activity as a priority area, states specific goals and provides a specific plan or framework for action. It describes the procedures of institutions in the government, nongovernment and private sectors to promote physical activity in the population and should define the accountability of the involved partners.

A recent comparative study of several emerging national policies in 13 countries revealed a number of similarities in their approaches. For example, intersectoral consultation and partnership were considered an integral part of policy development process; multiple individual-oriented behavior change interventions and, to a lesser extent, environmentally focused interventions were proposed in various combinations. Leadership for policy development and coordination was usually within health or/and sport departments. Although links to other policies such as healthy nutrition and obesity were evident, connections to transport and environmental policies were less developed [44]. Notable gaps were present in policies in terms of specifying timeframes and accountabilities for implementation and no evidence of long-term funding to support implementation. To date, national policy on physical activity is rare and the most recent developments have yet to be evaluated.

CREATING SUPPORTIVE ENVIRONMENTS

The role of the environment on individual behavior has long been recognized in theories of health behavior (e.g., social cognitive theory), but it is only in the past 5 years that it has become a major focus for those working on increasing levels of physical activity. In contrast, the development of behavioral interventions aimed at individuals in different settings (e.g., worksite, health care, schools) has received considerable attention from researchers and practitioners. However, a prominent paradigm shift has occurred [45] and now researchers and practitioners are keenly interested in defining, understanding, and ultimately influencing the design of buildings, neighborhoods, and whole communities to create places that support engaging in physical activity [46]. This shift toward influencing the places in which people live and work has the potential to reach all members of the population and represents a real shift from the clinical (individual)-based model of health promotion and disease prevention to a truly population health-based approach.

The scale of interest in the role of the physical environment varies. Patterns of use of stairs in buildings have received attention along with simple interventions aimed at increasing use (such as point-of decision posters); these have proved to be quite successful in the short term [47]. The design of parks and public open space is also being explored — in particular, to understand and increase the provision of safe places for children to play [48] —because of their potential to provide opportunities for active recreation and leisure for adults [49,50] and improve public health [51,52]. On an even larger scale, the relationship between transportation systems and concomitant infrastructure (roads, highways/freeways, bike paths, rail and bus links, and public footpaths/ sidewalks) has attracted interest at the city or metropolitan regional level [53,54].

Despite the explosion of interest in the environment, understanding and empirical evidence are still at the formative stage of development. This is frustrating for practitioners who want to know today where to invest effort and resources and what urban design interventions represent the best buy. Significant progress has been made on the measurement challenges of this new field and some of the early findings across a variety of studies are consistently showing that density of population, level of traffic, proximity to destinations and the aesthetic nature of the local environment are associated with higher levels of physical activity.

It is also apparent that the physical attributes of an environment that influence participation may differ for different subgroups and for different behaviors. In other words, what influences a young mother and child to walk to school will differ from what influences an older person to walk for recreation and a young man to cycle for fitness. These differences require future research to target specific behaviors in specific environmental contexts [49,55]. Meanwhile it remains too early for definitive advice on what interventions are more or less effective.

Although this is a new field, there are examples of initiatives aimed at improving the physical and social environment in different countries and at least one review [55]. Interventions aimed at increasing the use of stairs and walking trails have been tested. In the U.S., trails have been built in local communities in southern Missouri, a deprived rural region. These have been built in partnership with the local communities and, in some cases, with private sector sponsorship; the results have shown increased levels of walking [56].

Large-scale changes to the urban environment are neither easy to gain support for nor quick to do. Moreover, they are usually costly. Therefore, it is recommended that these be undertaken opportunitistically and that they capitalize on the shared concerns within governments and in communities around issues with potential synergy with physical activity (and particularly walking), such as: improving air quality, reducing traffic and noise pollution, attracting business and building the economy, and enhancing the sense of community [57]. All these agendas share a common goal — namely, contributing to the improvement of quality of life and quality of a community. Increasing physical activity (as part of travel or for recreation) can be used to bring seemingly disparate groups and agendas together.

CASE STUDIES OF POPULATION-BASED APPROACH TO PHYSICAL ACTIVITY

Figure 31.3 and Figure 31.4 showcase two recent examples of how combining components to form a comprehensive population-based approach to raise levels of physical activity can work [58,59]. Both examples use media strategies (television, print, and radio) as an overarching strategy aimed at communicating a clear, simple, and consistent message. Coincidentally, Rockhampton (Queensland, Australia) and Wheeling (West Virginia, U.S.) focus on the specific activity of walking. Along with the mass media communication strategy, other program activities included:

- Environmental improvements (in Rockhampton)
- Signage strategies
- Involvement of health care professionals, notable doctors and nurses providing advice
- Use of walking challenges and other programs in the worksite and other community settings to raise motivation and incentives
- Links with faith-based organizations

Ten Thousand Steps Rockhampton

10,000 steps Rockhampton is a multi-strategy health promotion program which aims to increase levels of health-related physical activity in this Central Queensland community (60,000 pop). The central coordinating theme of the project is the promotion of pedometer use to raise awareness and provide motivation for physical activity, through *accumulation* of steps throughout the day.

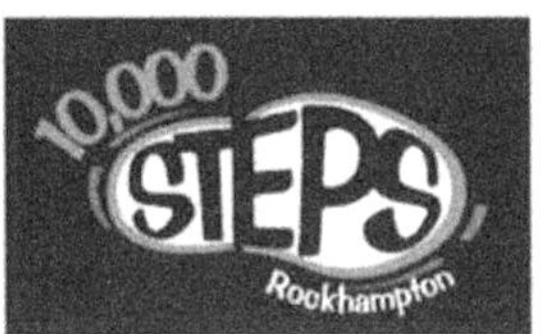

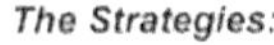

The Strategies:

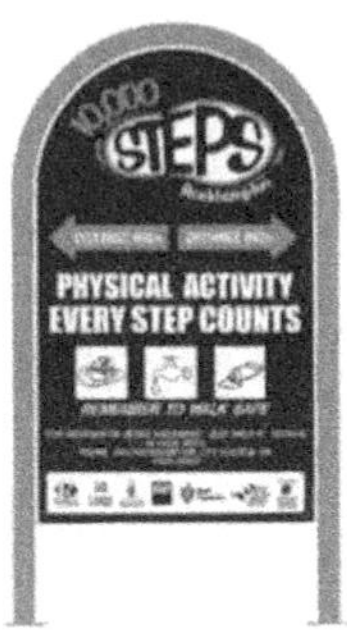

- Media campaign: TV adverts for 2 months and continuous print media aimed at raising awareness
- Promotion of physical activity by GPs (n=63) and other health professionals using prescription pads
- Liaison with Local Government to create more 'walkable' environments (included signage and distance markers in 'steps') and to promote dog walking (with leaflets – see left);
- Improving social support for activity (with walking groups)
- Community micro-grant scheme to develop innovative ways of increasing daily steps.

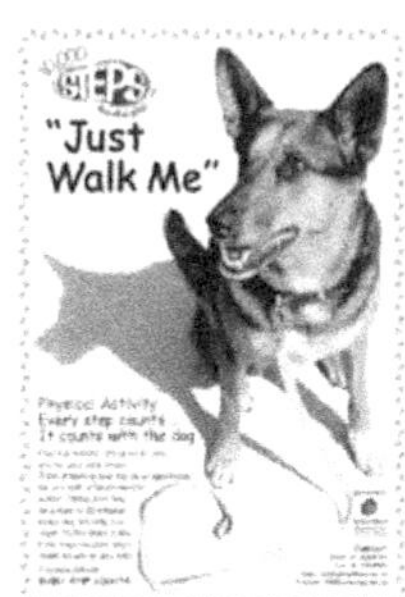

Results:

At 24 months:

- Project awareness has reached 97% in the Rockhampton community
- 5% increase (from 35% to 40%) in the proportion of adult women achieving activity levels sufficient for health benefit.

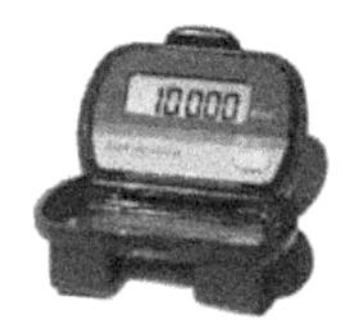

For more information see http://www.10000steps.cqu.edu.au/index.php

FIGURE 31.3 Case study, 10,000 STEPS Rockhampton, Queensland, Australia. (From Brown WJ et al. 10,000 steps Rockhampton: establishing a multistrategy physical activity promotion project in a Queensland community. *Health Promot J Austr* 14, 95, 2003. With permission.)

Both programs combined top-down and bottom-up approaches. That is, a set of planned strategies were implemented in partnership with community agencies but there was scope to respond and integrate community ideas and assistance during the programs. Both initiatives showed promising increases in physical activity levels after 12- or 24-month evaluation. However, there were limitations in the duration and magnitude of change in behavior and more whole-of-community demonstration projects testing the implementation of comprehensive population health-based approaches are urgently needed.

One example of such a program with a particularly strong community development component is in Sao Paulo, Brazil [60]. *Agita* is a multilevel, community-wide intervention aimed at increasing knowledge of benefits and levels of participation in physical activity. Mass media and program activities are coordinated across three target settings (home, transport, and leisure). Working with a large partnership of government and nongovernment organizations provides strong support, leverages resources, and builds co-ownership of the initiative. Agita has been ongoing for over 6 years and its success has influenced developments nationally in Brazil and in neighboring countries in the region [61].

CONCLUSION

The contribution of physical inactivity to noncommunicable disease is now well established. The need to take action at a population level is recognized within the international and national health

Wheeling Walks – A community campaign to encourage walking among sedentary adults

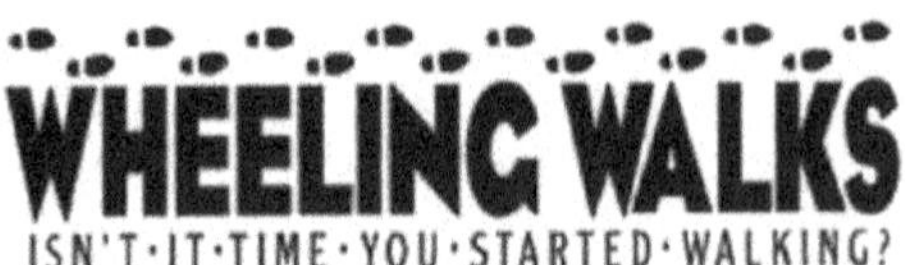

What did they do?

An 8-week intensive, paid media-based community physical activity campaign using paid advertising, public relations and public health education activities to deliver a targeted public health message on physical activity (namely 30 minutes or more of moderate-intensity walking almost every day)

Goals

- 10% increase in proportion of adults meeting recommendations
- 15% improvement in intention or stage of behaviour change

Target Population

City of Wheeling, West Virginia (pop 31,400); sedentary and irregularly active adults aged 50-65 years

Program Components

Paid Media: 2 newspaper adverts (printed 14 x _ page adverts); 2 30-second TV adverts (aired 683 times), 2 60 second radio adverts (aired 1988 times on 12 stations) developed to address a pre-identified key conceptual barrier 'I don't have time'

Public Relations: weekly press conferences and campaign events added news coverage

Worksite: worksite wellness walking challenge with walking packs

Website: community volunteer designed and maintained providing information on events and activities (www.wheelingwalks.org)

Primary Health Care: doctor prescriptions for walking with prescription pads (involved 270 of 400 local doctors)

Other: local health professionals trained to give presentations at worksites, civic organizations; 6 ministers including walking message in church bulletins /worship services

Evaluation

Random sample population telephone survey assessed total physical activity and walking at baseline in Wheeling (n=719) and Control city (Parkersburg; n=753). Using panel design at follow up 517 (Wheeling) and 571 (Parkersburg) were re- interviewed (74% response)

Outcomes

14% net increase in the number of sedentary adults reporting achieving 30 minutes of moderate walking on at least 5 days; progression in stages of change; positive (predicted) changes in perceived control and intention; earned extensive media coverage (>170 radio, TV and newspaper stories); reached 90% of target population.

Conclusions

This pilot demonstration was successful in showing how community wide promotion using paid advertising combined with community support and theory-based media messages can generate significant un-paid media coverage, impact on mediators of behaviour change and produce increases in physical activity among sedentary older adults.

FIGURE 31.4 Case study, Wheeling Walks West Virginia, U.S. (From Reger B et al. Wheeling walks: a community campaign using paid media to encourage walking among sedentary older adults. *Prev Med* 35, 285, 2002. With permission.)

agenda of developed and developing countries. Concerns of rising levels of obesity and diabetes and aging populations and greater recognition of the impact of the rapid changes taking place in the social and urban environment have focused attention on what action can be taken to halt and reverse the decline in activity levels.

Recent evidence-based reviews provide sign posts for the types of programs likely to be effective and, although not tested in every region of the world, they represent some of the current "best buys." It is very clear from the evidence collated over the past decade that isolated, short-term ad hoc efforts are not effective. In contrast, comprehensive community-wide programs adopting the principles and practice of a population health approach offer the most promise. When such approaches are implemented at a national level for a sustained period of time, positive trends are possible (for example, in Finland, Canada, Brazil). Although most reviews of interventions on physical activity usually identify at least some successful elements, there is a call consistently for implementation of them within a comprehensive framework with sustained commitment.

In conclusion, strong evidence supports the importance of inactivity as a major risk factor for some cancers and other chronic diseases. However, more work is needed to improve the science and art of population-based approaches to promoting physical activity and calls for more research abound. Research into the biological mechanisms and the dose–response relationship should continue to inform public health recommendations. Measurement and comparability of data will hopefully improve. However, the greatest challenge remains in translating what is learned into effective population health approaches. Applied researchers, clinicians, and health practitioners, along with partners in nonhealth sectors, are encouraged to pursue the evaluation and, when successful, dissemination of innovative approaches, applying the growing evidence base to reducing the rising levels of inactivity.

REFERENCES

1. Morris JN et al. Coronary Heart-Disease and physical activity of work. *Lancet* 21, 1054–1057; 1111–1120, 1953.
2. World Health Organization. World Health Report 2002: Reducing risks promoting healthy life. Geneva: World Health Organization, 2002.
3. Bull FC et al. Physical inactivity. In Ezzati M, Lopez A, Rodgers A, Murray C., Eds. *Comparative Quantification of Health Risks: Global and Regional Burden of Disease due to Selected Major Risk Factors*. Geneva: World Health Organization, 2005.
4. Mezzetti M et al. Population attributable risk for breast cancer: diet, nutrition, and physical exercise. *J Natl Cancer Inst* 90, 389, 1998.
5. Slattery ML et al. Energy balance and colon cancer — beyond physical activity. *Cancer Res* 57, 75, 1997.
6. International Agency for Research on Cancer [IARC]. *Weight Control and Physical Activity. IARC Handbook of Cancer Prevention* (Vol. 6). Lyon: IARC Press, 2002.
7. Wang G, Pratt M, Macera CA, et al. Physical activity, cardiovascular disease, and medical expenditures in U.S. Adults. *Ann Behav Med* 28, 88, 2004.
8. http://www.who.int/hpr/physactiv/economic.benefits.shtml (accessed January 2005).
9. Katzmarzyk PT; Gledhill N, and Janssen I. The economic costs associated with physical inactivity and obesity in Canada: an update. *Can J Appl Physiol* 29, 90, 2004.
10. Department of Culture, Media and Sport/Strategy Unit (DCMS). Game plan: a strategy for delivering governments' sport and physical activity objectives. London: Strategy Unit 2002.
11. Rootman I and Edwards P. The best laid schemes of mice and men. ParticipACTION's legacy and the future of physical activity promotion in Canada. *Can J Public Health* 95, S37, 2004.
12. Vuori I, Lankenau B, and Pratt M. Physical activity policy and program development: the experience in Finland. *Public Health Rep* 119, 331, 2004.
13. World Health Organization. A global strategy for diet, physical activity and health, Geneva: World Health Organization, 2004.

14. Kahn EB et al. The effectiveness of interventions to increase physical activity: a systematic review. *Am J Prev Med* 22, 73, 2002.
15. Hillsdon M et al. The effectiveness of public health interventions for increasing physical activity among adults: a review of reviews. London: National Health Service and Health Development Agency, 2004. Available at www.hda.nhs.uk/evidence.
16. Brown W. Physical activity and health: updating the evidence 2000–2003. *J Sci Med Sport* 7(Suppl), 1, 2004.
17. Last JM. *A Dictionary of Epidemiology.* 3rd ed. Oxford, Oxford University Press, 1995.
18. McMichael A and Beaglehole R. *The Global Context for Public Health.* Oxford University Press, Oxford, 2003.
19. National Public Health Partnership (NPHP) Secretariat. Public health practice today: a statement of core functions. Melbourne, Victoria, Australia. September 2000.
20. South Eastern Sydney Area Health Service. Population Health Directions for South East Health. http://www.sesahs.nsw.gov.au/index.htm Accessed February 2005.
21. Health Canada. Taking action on population health. Population Health Directorate, Health Promotion and Programs Branch. Ottawa, Canada. 1998. http://www.phac-aspc.gc.ca/ph-sp/phdd/pdf/tad_e.pdf.
22. McTiernan A et al. Recreational physical activity and the risk of breast cancer in postmenopausal women: the Women's Health Initiative Cohort Study. *JAMA* 290, 1331, 2003.
23. McTiernan A et al. Physical activity and cancer etiology: associations and mechanisms. *Cancer Causes Control* 9, 487, 1998.
24. Thune I and Furberg AS. Physical activity and cancer risk: dose–response and cancer, all sites and site specific. *Med Sci Sports Exercise* 33, S530, 2001.
25. Lee IM Physical activity and cancer prevention — data from epidemiologic studies. *Med Sci Sports Exercise* 35, 1823, 2003.
26. Armstrong T, Bonita R. Capacity building for an integrated noncommunicable disease risk factor surveillance system in developing countries. *Ethnic Dis* 13, S13, 2003.
27. Strong KL and Bonita R. Investing in surveillance: a fundamental tool of public health. *Soz Praventivmed* 49, 269, 2004.
28. Jacoby E, Bull FC, and Neiman A. Rapid change in lifestyle make "Move for Health" a priority for the Americas. *Rev Panam Salud Publica/Pan Am J Public Health* 14, 226, 2003.
29. Monteiro CA et al. A descriptive epidemiology of leisure-time physical activity in Brazil, 1996–1997. *Rev Panam Salud Publica /Pan Am J Public Health* 14, 246, 2003.
30. www.ipaq.ki.se.
31. http://www.who.int/ncd_surveillance/en/steps_framework_dec03.pdf.
32. Craig C L et al. International Physical Activity Questionnaire: 12-country reliability and validity. *Med Sci Sports Exercise* 35, 1381, 2003.
33. Armstrong T, Bauman A, and Davies J. Physical activity patterns of Australian adults. Results of the 1999 National Physical Activity Survey. Canberra: Australian Institute of Health and Welfare, 2000.
34. Craig CL et al. Twenty-year trends in physical activity among Canadian adults. *Can J Public Health* 95, 59, 2004.
35. Bull FC, Bauman AE, Bellew B, Brown W. (Eds.) Getting Australia Active II: An update of evidence on physical activity. Melbourne, Australia, National Public Health Partnership, 2004.
36. Dishman RK, and Buckworth J. Increasing physical activity: a quantitative synthesis meta-analysis. *Med Sci Sports Exercise* 28:706–719, 1996.
37. Briss PA, Brownson RC, Fielding JE. Developing and using the Guide to Community Preventive Services: lessons learned about evidence-based public health. *Annu Rev Public Health*; 25, 281, 2004.
38. http://www.hda.nhs.uk/html/about/collaboratingcentres.html#pa.
39. http://www.asnsw.health.nsw.gov.au/public-health/health-promotion/activity/taskforce/index.html.
40. U.S. Department of Health and Human Services. *Physical Activity and Health: A Report of the Surgeon General.* Atlanta: Department of Health and Human Services, Centers for Disease Control and Prevention, National Center for Chronic Disease Prevention and Health Promotion, 1996.
41. http://www.patf.dpc.wa.gov.au/.
42. http://www.physicalactivity.tas.gov.au.
43. http://www.show.scot.nhs.uk/sehd/patf/index.htm.

44. Bull FC, Bellew B, Schöppe S, Bauman AE. Developments in national physical activity policy: an international review and recommendations towards better practice. *J Sci Med Sport* 7(Suppl), 93, 2004.
45. O'Donnell M. Health promoting community design. *Am J Health Promot* 18, 1, 2003.
46. Stokols D, Grzywacz JG, McMahan S. Increasing the health promotive capacity of human environments. *Am J Health Promot* 18, 4, 2003.
47. Kerr NA, Yore MM, Ham SA. Increasing stair use in a worksite through environmental changes. *Am J Health Promot* 18, 312, 2004.
48. Molnar B, Gortmaker SL, Buka SL, and Bull FC. Unsafe to play? Neighborhood disorder predicts reduced physical activity among urban children and adolescents. *Am J Prev Med* 18, 378, 2004.
49. Giles-Corti B, Broomhall MH, Knuiman M, Collins C, Douglas K, Ng K, Lange A, Donovan RJ. Increasing walking: how important is distance to, attractiveness and size of public open space? *Am J Prev Med* 28, 199, 2005.
50. Giles-Corti B, Donovan RJ. SES differences in recreational PA levels and real and perceived access to a supportive physical environment. *Prev Med* 35, 601, 2002.
51. Department for Transport Local Government and the Regions (DTLGR). Improving urban parks, play areas and open spaces. London: Department for Transport Local Government and the Regions, 2002.
52. Maller C, Townsend M, Brown P, St Leger L. Healthy parks healthy people. The benefits of contact with nature in the park context. Deakin University and Parks Victoria, Melbourne, Australia, November 2002.
53. Frank LD, Andresen MA, Schmid TL. Obesity relationships with community design, physical activity, and time spent in cars. *Am J Prev Med* 27, 87, 2004.
54. Dannenberg AL, Jackson RJ, Frumkin H. The impact of community design and land-use choices on public health: a scientific research agenda. *Am J Public Health* 93, 1500, 2003.
55. Foster C, Hillsdon M. Changing the environment to promote health-enhancing physical activity. *J Sports Sci* 22, 755, 2004.
56. Brownson RC, Baker EA, Boyd RL. A community-based approach to promoting walking in rural areas. *Am J Prev Med* 27, 28, 2004.
57. Frank LD, Engelke PO, Schmid TL. *Health and Community Design: The Impact of the Built Environment on Physical Activity*. Washington D.C.: Island Press, 2003.
58. Brown WJ et al. 10,000 steps Rockhampton: establishing a multistrategy physical activity promotion project in a Queensland community. *Health Promot J Austr* 14, 95, 2003.
59. Reger B et al. Wheeling walks: a community campaign using paid media to encourage walking among sedentary older adults. *Prev Med* 35, 285, 2002.
60. Matsudo V et al. Promotion of physical activity in a developing country: the Agita São Paulo experience. *Pub Health Nurtr* 51, 253, 2002.
61. Matsudo S et al. Physical activity promotion: experiences and evaluation of the Agita São Paulo program using the ecological mobile model. *J Phys Activity Health* 1, 81, 2004.

32 Incorporating Exercise and Diet Recommendations into Primary Care Practice

Nicolaas P. Pronk

CONTENTS

INTRODUCTION

Many powerful and interacting forces in the current social and cultural environment have an impact on the physiological traits of individuals. The ability to maintain sufficient levels of physical activity (i.e., energy expenditure) successfully in order to counterbalance the excess of energy intake in modern society is a challenging proposition for many, if not most, of us. As a result, excess body weight is no longer the exception; rather, because more than 65% of the population is currently defined as overweight, it has become the norm [1–3]. Due to their increasing prevalence, overweight and obesity may be the most common conditions encountered in the primary care setting. However, patients are not visiting the clinic for their obesity per se. Because excess weight is so strongly associated with a host of medical conditions, many patients are seen in the primary care setting for treatment of obesity-related sequelae [4].

Primary care practitioners can support their patients in a variety of ways to address the challenges of dealing with overweight and obesity. Control of body weight depends upon a balance between food consumed and energy expended in the context of the natural tendency of the body to accumulate body fat. Thus, clinicians can help raise awareness of the importance of healthy nutrition and physical activity, motivating their patients to take action and facilitating access to appropriate programs.

It is the purpose of this chapter to consider the opportunity that resides within primary care to address overweight and obesity through physical activity and diet. It will discuss the clinical burden associated with obesity in the context of administrative and operational challenges and financial realities of clinical practice that call for extended care teams, identification of patients, counseling and referral tools, and efficient and effective operational clinic systems. A discussion of specific content related to diet and physical activity recommendations appropriate for weight loss and weight maintenance is beyond the scope of this chapter because they have been addressed in other chapters.

THE MAGNITUDE OF OBESITY

Overweight and obesity are recognized as major public health concerns in the U.S. and many other countries. Since the mid-1980s, overweight and obesity rates have steadily increased among children, adolescents, and adults of all ages. Based on measured height and weight among a representative sample of noninstitutionalized U.S. civilians, the National Health and Nutrition Examination Survey (NHANES) studies have monitored the prevalence of overweight and obesity since 1960 [1]. Current estimates of the prevalence of overweight and obesity among children and adults using NHANES 1999–2002 data are outlined in Table 32.1.

Among adults (age 20 years and over) and children (age 2 through 19 years), the prevalence of overweight in 2002 was 65.7 and 16.5%, respectively [2]. In addition, obesity rates among low-income adults are estimated to be almost twice as high compared to those of adults with higher incomes; rates are disproportionately high among African American and Latino women. Whereas the increase in prevalence of obesity has been rapid over the past two decades, the increase in prevalence of severe obesity (defined as body mass index (BMI) ≥ 40 kg/m^2) has outpaced all other classes of obesity. Between 1986 and 2000, the prevalence of severe obesity quadrupled from a rate of about 1 in 200 to 1 in 50, compared to a doubling in the prevalence of obesity rates of a BMI of 30 kg/m^2 or greater (from 1 in 10 to 1 in 5) [3].

THE CLINICAL BURDEN OF OBESITY

The clinical burden associated with overweight and obesity has been well documented by numerous studies. One of the most compelling examples is the rising prevalence of type 2 diabetes mellitus, which appears to be on a parallel track with the rising rates of overweight and obesity [5,6]. Indeed,

TABLE 32.1
Prevalence of Overweight and Obesity in the U.S. among Children and Adults, 2002

Children		**At risk for overweight (BMI for age ≥ 85th percentile)**	**Overweight (BMI for age ≥ 95th percentile)**
2–5 years		22.6 ± 1.5	10.3 ± 1.2
6–19 years		31.0 ± 1.1	16.0 ± 0.8
Adults	**Overweight (BMI ≥ 25 kg/m^2)**	**Obesity (BMI ≥ 30 kg/m^2)**	**Extreme obesity (BMI ≥ 40 kg/m^2)**
20 years and over	65.1 ± 0.8	30.4 ± 0.9	4.9 ± 0.4

Notes: BMI = body mass index; data presented as percent ± standard error.

Source: Data adapted from Hedley, A.A. et al., *JAMA* 2004; 291(23):2847–2850.

its prevalence in obese adults is three to seven times that in normal-weight adults. Those with a BMI > 35 kg/m^2 are 20 times more likely to develop diabetes compared to those with a BMI in a healthy range [7]. However, overweight and obesity are associated with several other medical concerns as well.

Obesity and Medical Conditions

In addition to type 2 diabetes mellitus, excess weight has been associated with increased risks of metabolic disorders such as hypertension, dyslipidemia, insulin resistance, and glucose tolerance [8]. Increased risk for cardiovascular disease is related to the association between excess weight and increases in inflammatory markers such as C-reactive protein and fibrinogen in adults and children [9–11]. In addition, overweight and obesity have been linked to increased risks of coronary heart disease, ischemic stroke, osteoarthritis, gallbladder disease, and several types of cancer including cancer of the breast, endometrium, colon, kidney, esophagus, stomach, and gallbladder [12]. Some studies have also reported links between obesity and cancers of the prostate, ovaries, and pancreas [13–15], although these relationships remain unclear.

Obesity, Physical Activity, Utilization, and Costs

The relationship between obesity and medical conditions has a significant impact on primary care as evidenced by data from Quesenberry and colleagues [4], who reported on health care utilization rates according to BMI categories among members of a large health plan. Significant utilization rates were related to inpatient and outpatient services for BMI categories ≥ 30 kg/m^2. In addition, this study showed a direct effect of obesity on inpatient, pharmacy, laboratory, and outpatient costs. The burden of obesity is economic as well as clinical.

The overall economic impact of obesity on health care expenditures is clearly substantial. Colditz [16] presented data based on prevalence statistics of obesity derived from NHANES III that estimated the direct costs of obesity to be around $70 billion, or approximately 7% of the total health care costs for the U.S. Quesenberry and associates [4] had also estimated the total health care expense related to obesity for the health plan and reported it to be approximately 6% of total health plan costs.

Although total costs associated with obesity are high, excess charges appear to be incurred in a short timeframe as well. In a series of studies, Pronk and colleagues reported on the excess health care costs associated with obesity among older health plan members aged 40 years and over and active employees aged 18 to 65 years, and finally the indirect costs related to decrements in productivity that are associated with obesity. First, they studied the relationship between modifiable health risks and short-term health care charges in a random sample of older adult health plan members [17]. Results indicated that, after adjustment for age, sex, race, and chronic disease status, each BMI unit was prospectively related to 1.9% higher charges. In other words, for each incremental unit of BMI, excess health care charges increased by 1.9% during the course of the year.

Next, among active employees, the annualized health care costs associated with excess weight were studied based on BMIs calculated from self-report health assessment surveys [18]. In a sample of 8822 employees, after statistically controlling for age, sex, asthma, breast cancer, other cancers, diabetes, heart disease, hypercholesterolemia, hypertension, back pain, lung disease, and emotional and physical function, average health care costs for overweight and obese employees were 8% higher per year.

Finally, a study was conducted to examine the association between obesity and work performance, or productivity [19]. Work performance was considered in the absenteeism and "presenteeism" domains — that is, work loss days as well as decrements in performance among employees while at work. Obesity was significantly related to work loss days as well as an interpersonal relationship variable expressed as "getting along with coworkers." Due to these studies, it is concluded that obesity increases not only direct medical care expenses, but also the indirect costs associated with reduced productivity due to decrements in work performance.

Reduction of the Clinical Burden by Weight Loss and Physical Activity

It is important to determine whether advice to lose weight through diet and physical activity results in an improvement of health status and management of associated medical conditions. Based on a variety of studies [20–24], it appears that modest weight loss and increases in physical activity are associated with a significant reduction in disease-related risks. Table 32.2 presents a summary of the positive impact that weight loss and physical activity increases have on a variety of diseases and chronic conditions. Detailed information on the recommendations to follow regarding physical activity and weight management is beyond the scope of this chapter; however, the following statement, as put forth by Blair et al. [25], represents advice supported by current knowledge that fits with clinical approaches to implement preventive counseling guidelines based on systematic reviews of scientific literature:

> Current public health recommendations for physical activity are for 30 min of moderate-intensity activity/d, which provides substantial benefits across a broad range of health outcomes for sedentary adults. This dose of exercise may be insufficient to prevent unhealthful weight gain for some, perhaps many, but probably not all, persons. For persons who are exercising 30 min/d and consuming what appears to be an appropriate number of calories, but are still having trouble controlling their weight, additional exercise or caloric restriction is recommended to reach energy balance and minimize the likelihood of further weight gain. For persons exercising 30 min/d who are weight stable, we recommend that they try to build up to 60 min activity/d, which will provide additional benefit. In addition to aerobic

TABLE 32.2
Summary of Weight Loss and Physical Activity Studies on Beneficial Changes in Risks Associated with Medical Conditions

Disease or health risk factor	Benefit of weight loss	Benefit of increased physical activity
Breast cancer	Mild	Mild
Coronary artery disease	Moderate	Strong
Colorectal cancer	Mild	Moderate
Dyslipidemia	Moderate	Moderate
Gallbladder disease	Mild	Mild
Hypertension	Strong	Strong
Mental health/depression	Unknown	Strong
Osteoarthritis	Moderate	Mild
Osteoporosis	No benefit	Strong
Sleep apnea	Moderate	Unknown
Stroke	Mild	Moderate
Type-2 diabetes mellitus	Strong	Strong

Source: Data summarized from National Cancer Institute. http://cancerweb.ncl.ac.uk/cancernet/400387.html.; National Institutes of Health, National Heart, Lung, and Blood Institute, Obesity Education Initiative. Clinical guidelines on the identification, evaluation, and treatment of overweight and obesity in adults. Available at: http://www.nhlbi.nih.gov/guidelines/obesity/ob_gdlns.htm (accessed March, 2004); Halbert, J.A. et al., *J Hum Hypertension* 1997; 11(10):641–649; Stefanick, M.L. In: Hennekens, C.H., Ed. *Clinical Trials in Cardiovascular Disease: a Companion Guide to Braunwald's Heart Disease*. Philadelphia, PA: WB Sanders Co; 1999:375–391; and U.S. Dept. of Health and Human Services Centers for Disease Control and Prevention. *Physical Activity and Health: A Report of the Surgeon General*. Washington, DC; 1996.

exercise, it is desirable that people engage in activities that build musculoskeletal fitness, such as resistance training and flexibility exercises, at least twice a week. These additional exercises will promote maintenance of lean body mass, improvements in muscular strength and endurance, and preservation of function, all of which enable long-term participation in regular physical activity and promote quality of life.

The basic elements of effective weight reduction and weight management include dietary changes that produce a reduction in energy intake, increased physical activity, and behavior modification [20,24]. Long-term maintenance of weight loss is strongly associated with sustained increased physical activity, normalized eating patterns, a healthful diet low in fat content, and the adoption of specific behavioral strategies strongly related to problem-solving mastery [26–29]. For example, in a cross-sectional study of individuals who had maintained a 30-lb (14-kg) weight loss for at least 5 years, over 80% had adopted behavior changes in the areas of nutrition, physical activity, and the use of specific behavioral strategies [26].

ROLE OF CLINICIANS IN ADDRESSING OBESITY, DIET, AND PHYSICAL ACTIVITY

Based on the knowledge that weight loss and increased physical activity confer benefit on the patient, clinicians should consider addressing these adverse health risk factors in the clinical setting. However, to do so, physicians and other clinical personnel would need to overcome significant barriers related to addressing weight and physical activity issues [30]. These barriers, among others, include:

- Limited training in counseling techniques
- Lack of training and background in nutrition, exercise science, and obesity management
- Lack of confidence in ability to change patient behavior
- Lack of time to provide counseling
- Financial reimbursement
- An overwhelmingly large number of obese patients
- Lack of supporting evidence that weight management is efficacious
- The view that obesity is simply willful misconduct by obese individuals
- Questions about safety and efficacy of pharmacological and surgical treatment options

The primary care physician is in an excellent position to help patients address their overweight- or obesity-related concerns. Routine contact provides ongoing, longer term opportunities for intervention and repeated advice and motivation. Patients who are advised by their physician to lose weight, increase their physical activity, or adjust their diet tend to be more willing to attempt weight loss compared to those who do not receive such advice [31,32].

PHYSICIAN COUNSELING FOR OBESITY AND PHYSICAL ACTIVITY

Brief interventions in diet and exercise in primary care settings have proven to be effective for weight loss. Among U.S. adults, 28 to 48% reported receiving physician advice on physical activity [33–36], although physicians from several specialties did not feel qualified or successful in treating obese patients. In general, counseling tends to be done more often and for a longer duration by physicians who feel comfortable and successful at counseling as compared to those who do not [37]. It is therefore not surprising that physicians who receive training in counseling their patients for weight loss have a higher rate of success in obesity management than those who do not receive training [38]. When the physician provides advice regarding weight loss, the odds of the patient acting upon such advice were nearly three times greater than those for patients who did not receive this advice [39].

As it turns out, some factors or patient characteristics appear to be related to a higher likelihood of receiving counseling or advice about weight. These factors include [40]:

- Being a woman
- Living in the Northeastern U.S.
- Being below 60 years of age
- Having a higher level of education
- Having a higher socioeconomic status
- Being married
- Having a chronic disease (e.g., diabetes, cardiovascular disease, hypertension, etc.)
- Being severely obese

Figure 32.1 presents an overview of the results of two studies that support the notion that higher risk patients or those with diagnosed conditions are more likely to receive counseling advice about their weight and the importance of physical activity [34,39].

Another aspect of the counseling practices among physicians in the U.S. is the noted positive association between a physician's personal habits and the likelihood to counsel patients about weight-related lifestyle behaviors, such as physical activity or diet. Lewis and Wells [41] showed that physicians attempting to lose weight were significantly more likely to provide advice to their patients about weight loss and those who perceived themselves as overweight were less likely to counsel their patients. The majority (~90%) of family physicians in the U.S. believe that they should be role models to their patients when it comes to healthy weight. Unfortunately, overweight physicians were also much less likely to refer obese patients to dietitians and nutritionists [42].

Multiple Risk Factors in Primary Care

In addressing obesity through diet and physical activity, it is recognized that the approach is no longer a single- but rather a multiple-risk factor approach. This creates some additional issues and considerations: the clinician needs a better understanding of each of the risks prior to counseling;

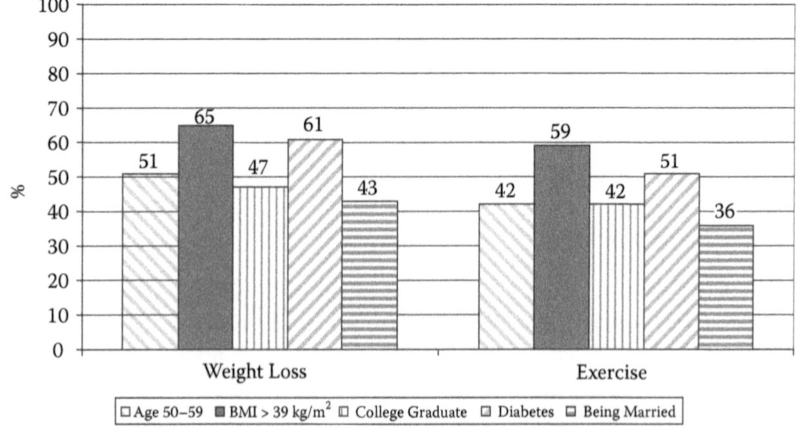

FIGURE 32.1 Likelihood of adults receiving physician counseling for weight loss and exercise. (Data from Wee CC. Physical activity counseling in primary care: the challenge of effecting behavioral change. *JAMA* 2001; 286(6):717–719; Galuska DA, Will JC, Serdula MK, Ford ES. Are health care professionals advising obese patients to lose weight? *JAMA* 1999; 282(16):1576–1578.)

however, this approach also needs to be tailored to the willingness or readiness of the patient to take action on any or all of the risk factors that may be modified. Thus, the physician needs to be able to:

- Measure each of the risk factors and document whether advice is needed
- Understand whether changes can be made in the risk factor that will improve the patient's health status
- Provide counsel and advice to the patient about the options available or the action that may be taken
- With the patient, work toward a collaboratively agreed-upon plan to take next steps
- Support the patient in implementing the action plan
- Provide an avenue for periodic follow-up

These steps can be summarized in the context of the "5As" approach that has been extensively used in addressing tobacco use and smoking in the primary care practice setting [43,44]. The 5As stand for assess, advise, agree, assist, and arrange for follow-up. Table 32.3 outlines the steps involved in this approach and a brief discussion of their content.

When integrated into an office system, elements of the 5As (i.e., assess, advise, agree, assist, and arrange follow-up) can be delivered at various points in the process of care (i.e., previsit, during the visit, after the visit, or between visits) by various members of the clinical care team (e.g., medical assistant, physician, nurse, health educator) across multiple visits or contacts. Thus, the role of the primary care clinician might be to use data obtained from a previsit risk assessment (assess) to provide a brief personalized motivational message tied to the patient's health concerns (advise). The primary care clinician might also encourage the patient to choose a behavioral goal and, if the patient agrees, address a specific risk behavior (agree); he or she can refer the patient to a system-based counseling service staffed by a health educator or other member of the health care team (assist and arrange follow-up) [45].

This type of integrated approach to addressing multiple risk factors in a clinical setting, in which multiple clinic team members have responsibility for different aspects of the 5As, eases the burden on the primary care physician within the context of time-pressured primary care practice. Limiting primary care clinicians' roles and responsibility to the advise and agree components of the 5As may be the most efficient way to utilize their influence while also enhancing their confidence regarding intervening successfully.

The assessment of a patient's readiness to change is another opportunity to optimize success. Because multiple risk factors are addressed, it is unlikely that the patient is ready to take action on all of them. For some, the patient may be contemplating making changes in his or her diet but not be ready to sign up for several sessions with the dietitian. However, the patient is ready to enroll and participate actively in a program specific to a single behavior (say, physical activity) by joining a walking club. In order to ensure that this opportunity is not lost, the physician should make sure not to overemphasize one solution over another and thereby lose the interest of the patient.

The stages of readiness-to-change model, which is the central construct in the transtheoretical model as outlined by Prochaska and Velicher [46], can be used to identify the stage that a patient is in. Table 32.4 outlines this staging process in a way that clinicians can use very efficiently during the course of the conversation as opposed to a more time-consuming method [47].

THE PATIENT-CENTERED VIEW

As outlined by the Institute of Medicine (IOM), a chasm exists between the care patients deserve and the care patients receive in the U.S. today [48]. In order to transform the care provided to patients, the Institute of Medicine has proposed several recommendations, including one in which all health care organizations, professional groups, and private and public purchasers should pursue

TABLE 32.3
The "5As" for Addressing Obesity-Related Risk Factors in Primary Care

5As	Tasks	Tools	Talking points
Assess	Measure height, weight, physical activity, dietary practices	Health risk appraisal, balance beam scale, stadiometer, paper and pencil tests	"Based on your body mass index and a consideration of your activity level, it may be a good idea for us to talk about your weight. Are you okay with that?"
Advice	Review BMI recommendations, consider baseline weight of the patient, and recommend lifestyle changes	Give respectful, clear advice and connect the health risk factor with health outcomes. Explain why certain actions are needed and what to expect in terms of results. Be empathetic. Consider the patient's readiness to change the behaviors under discussion.[a]	"I know you have been trying to lose weight in the past, but there may be some approaches you have not tried before, such as the combination of physical activity and cutting back on food portion seizes. Are you ready to try such an approach if there is a program that fits your learning style and interests?"
Agree	Gain explicit agreement with the patient on taking action. This important step of collaboratively identifying behavioral and self-management goals is critical in the process. Active participation of patients in the goal-setting process is associated with improved outcomes.	Present options for the patient to take action on. Use handouts and educational materials to have the patient understand the options. Emphasize achievable goals and ongoing maintenance of the changes. Focus in on a collaborative agreement to take action.	"As you see, there are various options available that seem to fit your style. Tell me if you agree and what your thoughts are about participating in one of these."
Assist	Discuss the program, the resources that the patient will have access to, and the skills that will help achieve success. Focus on continued motivation.	Provide skills training; use a variety of counseling techniques such as motivational interviewing cognitive reframing, and verbal encouragement. Use clear and concise handouts.	"Most people who successfully lose weight and keep it off use a combination of changes in their eating and physical activity habits. Keeping track of those changes by using a log is very helpful. The handouts you received have activities in them that you work through yourself and we'll review those the next time we meet. Do you think this approach will work for you? Do you have any other questions?"
Arrange	Schedule the next visit. Provide contact information. Make referrals as needed.	Agree on a specific time and date for the follow-up time. Decide how to follow up by phone, in person, or via the Internet.	"I'd like to make sure you have enough time to work through the material and try out the new behaviors as you work with the dietitian and the exercise physiologist. How about we visit again in 6 months? Does that work for you?"

[a]For additional information on readiness to change, see Table 32.4.

Note: For the purpose of this chart, the tasks are limited to addressing weight, height, body mass index, physical activity and dietary practices. Other obesity-related risk factors do exist and may need to be addressed, given the complexity and uniqueness of each individual patient.

Source: Adapted from HealthPartners, Center for Health Promotion, 2002 [66].

TABLE 32.4
Summary of Stages of Readiness-to-Change Construct for Clinician Use with Physical Activity as the Example Behavior

Precontemplation: "I won't"	Contemplation: "I might"	Preparation: "I will"	Action: "I am"	Maintenance: "I have"	Termination: "I did"
How to recognize the stage of readiness to change in a patient[a]					
Patient is in denial, cannot see the problem, does not want to become physically active. He or she will say no when asked, "Are you seriously intending to increase your level of physical activity in the next six months?"	Patient acknowledges the problem and is thinking about solving it and has an indefinite plan to take action in the next 6 months. He or she is not quite ready to increase level of physical activity yet and may stall.	Patient plans to make a change within the next month and is making final adjustments.	Patient has been following a plan for making the change. He or she may be terrified or exhilarated and may change his or her level of awareness, emotions, self-image, or thinking	Patient may be struggling to prevent relapse into sedentary behavior. He or she is reaping rewards of the change, but may also complain of the "cost."	Maintaining change is effortless; no temptations; total confidence.
How to help a patient move to the next stage[b]					
Give information. Ask patient to list as many benefits as possible related to changing his or her level of physical activity. Write them down. Ask patient to take a list and add to it before next appointment. Be patient. Follow up at next appointment.	Help patient begin to develop an attitude of "want" rather than "have" to become physically active. Focus on a solution, rather than the problem. Have him or her compare pros and cons of staying sedentary vs. initiating regular physical activity.	Help patient select the best course of action — one that is acceptable, accessible, appropriate, and effective. Help patient focus on plan of increasing physical activity and to anticipate pitfalls and ways to overcome them. Help him or her to choose incentive rewards.	Provide positive support. Encourage relaxation and positive self-statements. Reaffirm patient's decision and focus on activity. Ask whether he or she has announced the change to others, to show commitment. Discuss relapse triggers.	Let patient know the time it takes to accomplish sustained change in physical activity behavior. Remind him or her to review benefits. Focus on successes! Provide positive support. Encourage relaxation and positive self-statements.	Provide positive support.

[a]With a relapse, patient returns to a less active stage.

[b]When relapse occurs, help patient to start over with slight adaptations in the strategy used. Avoid discouragement and continue to think about change.

Note: The "action" stage is defined as: "accumulation of 30 minutes of mild to moderate physical activity on most days of the week."

Source: Adapted from Behavior Change Counseling Guide. Center for Health Promotion, HealthPartners, 1998 [67].

six major aims: specifically health care should be safe, effective, timely, efficient, equitable, and patient centered. The patient-centeredness aim is particularly salient to the issue of obesity because it has been observed that gaps remain in the way in which physicians and other clinicians provide medical care services to obese patients. As defined by the Institute of Medicine [48], patient centeredness relates to providing care that is respectful of and responsive to individual patient preferences, needs, and values and ensuring that patient values guide all clinical decisions.

According to the Centers for Disease Control and Prevention [49], approximately 29% of men and 44% of women are trying to lose weight. Furthermore, among men who consider themselves to be overweight or obese, 36 and 60% are trying to lose weight, respectively. Among women who consider themselves to be overweight or obese, 60 and 70% are trying to lose weight. Even among those who consider themselves to be at a weight that is about right for them, 7% of men and 27% of women are trying to lose weight. Although the combination of diet and physical activity is the preferred method for weight loss, most attempt to lose weight by diet alone, fewer by physical activity alone, and even fewer use the combination.

Patients tend to value the interaction with their physician highly; often they view their primary care physician as a "trusted guide." However, in the context of addressing obesity, the studies appear to be equivocal. Overweight patients were significantly less satisfied with the care that they received for obesity and with the physician's expertise in this area compared to the care that they received in the areas of their general health or medical needs, as well as their physician's expertise in these other areas of medicine and health [50]. Among the reasons cited, 50% of patients reported that their physician had not mentioned any of ten common weight loss methods; 65% of patients reported a lack of understanding on the physician's part about the difficulty of being overweight; and about 35% indicated that the doctor did not believe them when they talked about their food consumption. More worrisome findings included the reporting of overweight and obese patients' feelings that they were treated with disrespect by their health care providers based on their weight status [51].

On the other hand, patients also report the importance of feeling that their physician helps them in achieving their weight-related goals. Dietary advice, help in setting realistic goals, and exercise recommendations are among the most appreciated reasons for advice [52]. Yet, the denial of a patient's weight problem or the avoidance of addressing the issue of obesity by the physician is not appreciated by the patient at all. Patients want to discuss their obesity-related issues with their physician and would like more rather than less physician involvement; however, almost two-thirds of patients report that their physician did not bring up the subject at their last visit [52].

It is clear that the patient wants to be supported by the primary care physician in attempts to address concerns about excess weight. However, it appears that, in general, advice is often lacking and the approach taken to address weight-related issues may not be the most empathetic or respectful in some cases. A more thoughtful and systematic method of including this topic in the arsenal of clinical tools and strategies for dealing with patient care may be needed.

TRANSLATING WHAT WE KNOW INTO WHAT WE DO

Despite best intentions, the integration of counseling for diet, physical activity, and excess weight into clinical care is below par. The reality of busy clinic schedules, limited time for a physician to spend time with the patient, the issue of financial reimbursement, and other reasons result in missed opportunities to talk to patients about taking action on these modifiable adverse health risks [53,54]. It is also unlikely that physicians will ever have more time to devote to counseling for health behaviors due to the high cost of physician time and the time pressures under which they do their work [53].

Therefore, a promising approach is to consider how best to extend the reach of the primary care physician into an extended care team that is inclusive of nurses, but also dietitians, exercise physiologists, health educators, and behavior change counselors. This approach would require an office-based system that may be viewed as a recognizable organized process supporting the systematic delivery of counseling and interventions that address obesity, nutrition, and physical activity [54]. Such systems should not be limited to the clinics, but extend beyond the clinic walls and employ multiple technologies, including mail, telephone, and Web-based solutions [55].

Extending the Clinical Care Team

Creating a system, or organized process, around the provision of effective obesity care that operates efficiently on a day-to-day basis is extremely important. Such a system should be integrated and be designed around a patient care team that places the patient's needs at the core of its work. Because teamwork needs coordination, delegation of tasks, and ongoing feedback, key steps and referrals and hand-offs need to be delineated and systematized so that they may be documented, tracked, and monitored to allow for continuous improvement. Starfield [56] defines a patient care team as "a group of diverse clinicians who communicate with each other regularly about the care of a defined group of patients and participate in that care." Such teams ensure that all elements of care are performed competently [57].

The optimal team composition is also important to consider and will certainly vary among practices. The physician should be positioned as the team leader and source of the common philosophy of care [58] based on the notion that critical success factors include physician commitment and leadership and a supportive organizational structure [59]. Prior to patient–physician clinical interaction, however, support staff plays a role in meeting and greeting the patient and setting the tone for the visit. Registered nurses review the patient chart and obtain vital signs that should include height and weight measurement. In a paper-based practice, height and weight can be converted easily into BMI with the use of BMI charts; in practices that employ electronic medical records, the BMI can be calculated immediately as preprogrammed into the computer applications. Alternatively, BMI information may be already available if the patient had a chance to complete a more in-depth assessment of health risks behaviors such as a health risk appraisal. The nurse may also include additional measurements, such as the waist circumference.

Armed with this information, which completes the first of the 5As, the physician has a chance to initiate a dialogue with the patient, provide advice, and gain agreement for action. In a typical, busy clinic schedule, the physician has approximately 1 minute available to address prevention-related topics [60]; thus, a referral to another member of the extended care team should be made to do the "assist" and "arrange" for follow-up. This referral may be made to a clinical registered dietitian or to a centralized service that provides the counseling needed to support behavior changes. The health professionals in such a centralized program include registered dietitians, health educators, counseling psychologists, pharmacists, and exercise physiologists. Few examples of such systems are available in the literature, although some are emerging [61].

Connecting the Dots

As discussed earlier, the integration of such organized preventive systems is important. Integration of documentation of the patient data, referrals, action steps taken, program participation, results and outcomes, and evaluation data, and the tracking of such data in robust databases can create efficient office-based systems. To do this effectively, systems designs should optimize the use of interactive technologies. Interactive technology approaches have great potential to enhance primary care behavior change counseling and support [62–64]. Computer-based strategies can help clinicians to "systematize" repetitive aspects of practice, such as repeated assessments and identification of individual goals. In addition, they can help avoid systematic errors in the process by consistently following a predetermined pathway of actions. Such approaches can be integrated into the visit process and result in more consistent implementation of the 5As.

A Protocol to Integrate "in-Clinic" and "between-Clinic" Visits

A combination of clinic-based resources and the use of an extended care team that includes resources available for "between visit care" may well be an optimal form of treatment design because most of the behavior changes will happen outside the clinic walls. Figure 32.2 depicts a protocol that combines the in-clinic "assess," "advise", and "agree" steps of the 5As with the "assist" and "arrange" steps that may be provided by an extended care team. This team includes allied health professionals associated with the clinic and the physician but located in a centralized department, such as a health plan health education department or a contracted vendor arrangement. The clinic personnel, including the nursing staff and the physicians, stay connected with the behavior change staff using interactive technology such as a secure Website, telephone, and fax. The use of a Website is of interest because physicians and their nursing team can be provided access to a portion of the site specific to their patient only. At the time of the next visit, the patient's records can be reviewed and advice can be tailored to progress in the treatment program.

This type of approach is used by the National Center for Lifestyle Management (NCLM) project as implemented by the Health Partners Health Behavior Group [45]. This project utilizes a secure Website (www.nclm.us) that houses a physician-training program and referral and documentation information for patients referred to a telephone-based intervention for weight management that has a walking program integrated in its curriculum. The training module presents an overview of the problem of obesity in the U.S. that also provides Continuing Medical Education (CME) credit when completed. In addition, clinical staff can use the Website to refer patients into the phone course.

The physician or nurse enters key information into the Website that allows the centralized NCLM staff to contact the patient proactively. Once the staff member connects by phone with the patient, a choice is available to enroll in the program or — based upon more detailed information regarding learning style and other interests — a match can be made to an available community-based resource that has previously been identified by clinic staff. Because the referrals are made following the "agree" step in the 5As process, the enrollment rate into the phone-based program is relatively high based upon early results of the project — i.e., over 70% of referred patients enroll in the program. In addition, the average weight of the referred patients is relatively high, i.e., a BMI over 35 kg/m^2.

Once the patient enrolls in the program, periodic calls averaging ~15 minutes in length connect him or her to the behavior change counselors. The course consists of ten lessons that are typically completed in approximately 6 months. Average weight loss associated with this program is ~6 kg at 6 months [65].

On an ongoing basis, counselors document patient progress into the Website in a format that allows the physician to review this information by patient or by his or her panel of referred patients. Thus, following a referral into this program, when a patient is scheduled for a follow-up clinic visit, the updated information on progress can be reviewed prior to the visit and included in the chart so that reinforcement can be provided based on current and accurate data.

SUMMARY

Addressing obesity in the primary care practice setting represents an important opportunity for health improvement. Despite recognition that obesity is an important health concern, efforts to provide advice, counseling, and referrals into credible programs are currently underutilized. Using an approach that integrates the "5As" as an organizing principle for interventions design, a patient-centered method of implementing an office-based protocol for weight management has been outlined.

In this protocol, a clinical care delivery team (physician, nurse, clinical dietitian, and receptionist) extend their reach by collaborating with more centralized functions provided by allied health personnel (health educator, exercise physiologist, pharmacist, and dietitian). Together, this extended care team can support the patient during the clinic visit and during the time between two visits.

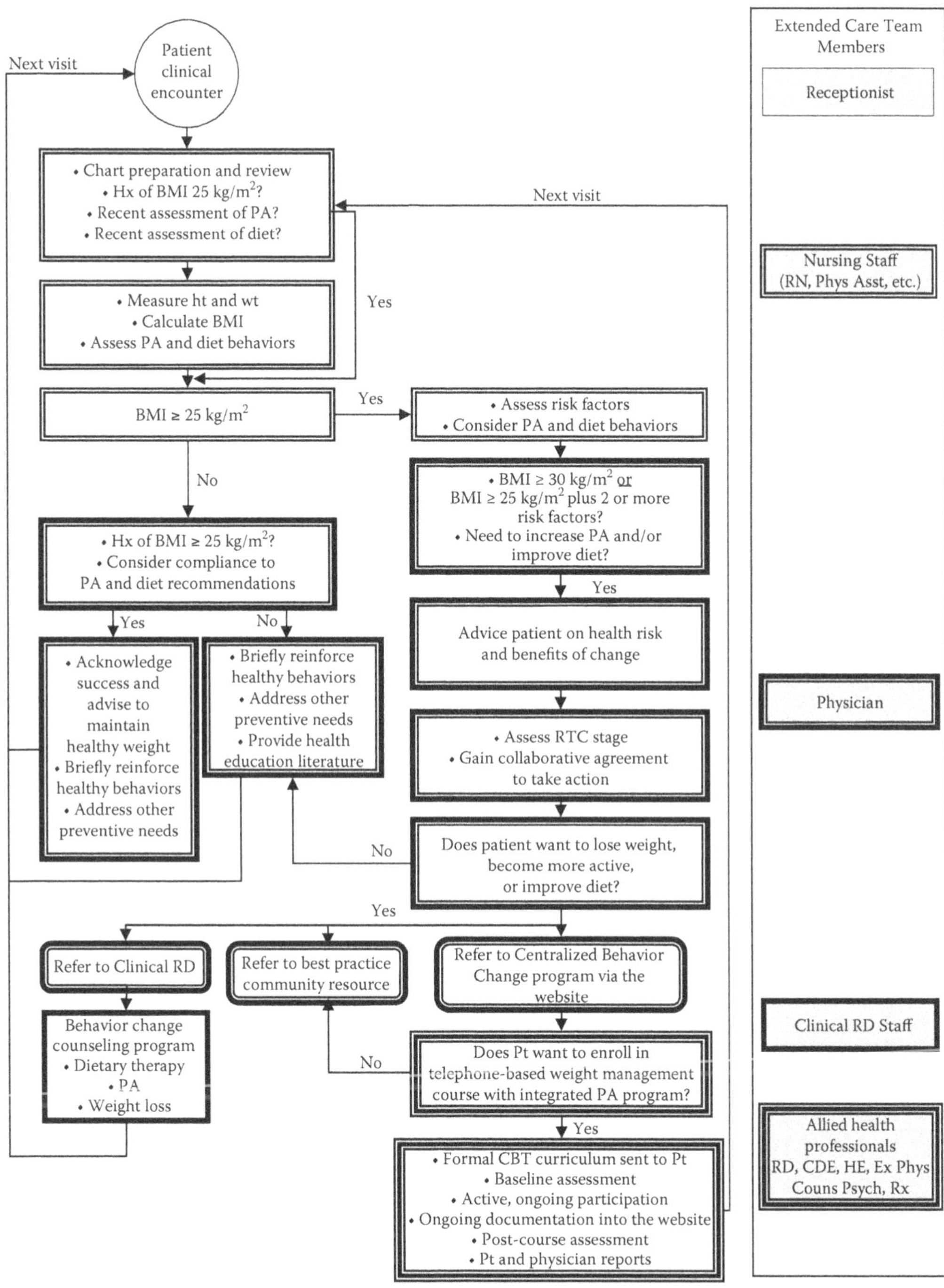

Note: Protocol based on NHLBI Clinical Guidelines (20) and the National Center for Lifestyle Management Project (45); Hx = history; BMI = body mass index; Ht = height; wt = weight; RD = registered dietitian; CDE = certified diabetes educator; HE = health educator; Ex Phys = exercise physiologist; Couns Psych = counseling psychologist; Rx = pharmacist; PA = physical activity; RTC = readiness to change; Pt = patient

FIGURE 32.2 A protocol to integrate "in-clinic" and "between-clinic" visits. (Adapted from HealthPartners, Center for Health Promotion, 2004 [68].)

Ongoing motivation and monitoring of clinical outcomes can be provided during the clinic visits. On the other hand, behavior change and ongoing health education can be provided during the time between the visits. This approach efficiently and effectively integrates exercise and diet recommendations into busy primary care practice settings without overburdening the primary care providers.

ACKNOWLEDGMENTS

This work was supported in part by the Robert Wood Johnson Foundation, Princeton, NJ (Grant # 046929).

REFERENCES

1. Flegal KM, Carroll MD, Ogden CL, Johnson CL. Prevalence and trends in obesity among U.S. adults, 1999–2000. *JAMA* 2002; 288(14):1723–1727.
2. Hedley AA, Ogden CL, Johnson CL, Carroll MD, Curtin LR, Flegal KM. Prevalence of overweight and obesity among U.S. children, adolescents, and adults, 1999–2002. *JAMA* 2004; 291(23):2847–2850.
3. Sturm R. Increases in clinically severe obesity in the United States, 1986–2000. *Arch Intern Med* 2003; 163(18):2146–2148.
4. Quesenberry CP Jr, Caan B, Jacobson A. Obesity, health services use, and health care costs among members of a health maintenance organization. *Arch Intern Med* 1998; 158(5):466–472.
5. Harris MI, Flegal KM, Cowie CC, Eberhardt MS, Goldstein DE, Little RR, Wiedmeyer HM, Byrd-Holt DD. Prevalence of diabetes, impaired fasting glucose, and impaired glucose tolerance in U.S. adults. The Third National Health and Nutrition Examination Survey, 1988–1994. *Diabetes Care* 1998; 21(4):518–524.
6. Mokdad AH, Bowman BA, Ford ES, Vinicor F, Marks JS, Koplan JP. The continuing epidemics of obesity and diabetes in the United States. *JAMA* 2001; 286(10):1195–1200.
7. Field AE, Coakley EH, Must A, Spadano JL, Laird N, Dietz WH, Rimm E, Colditz GA. Impact of overweight on the risk of developing common chronic diseases during a 10-year period. *Arch Intern Med* 2001; 161(13):1581–1586.
8. Willett WC, Dietz WH, Colditz GA. Guidelines for healthy weight. *N Engl J Med* 1999; 341(6):427–434.
9. Ford ES, Galuska DA, Gillespie C, Will JC, Giles WH, Dietz WH. C-reactive protein and body mass index in children: findings from the Third National Health and Nutrition Examination Survey, 1988–1994. *J Pediatr* 2001; 138(4):486–492.
10. Visser M, Bouter LM, McQuillan GM, Wener MH, Harris TB. Elevated C-reactive protein levels in overweight and obese adults. *JAMA* 1999; 282(22):2131–2135.
11. Duncan BB, Schmidt MI, Chambless LE, Folsom AR, Carpenter M, Heiss G. Fibrinogen, other putative markers of inflammation, and weight gain in middle-aged adults — the ARIC study. Atherosclerosis Risk in Communities. *Obesity Res* 2000; 8(4):279–286.
12. National Cancer Institute. http://cancerweb.ncl.ac.uk/cancernet/400387.html.
13. Cerhan JR, Torner JC, Lynch CF, Rubenstein LM, Lemke JH, Cohen MB, Lubaroff DM, Wallace RB. Association of smoking, body mass, and physical activity with risk of prostate cancer in the Iowa 65+ Rural Health Study (United States). *Cancer Causes Control* 1997; 8(2):229–238.
14. Farrow DC, Weiss NS, Lyon JL, Daling JR. Association of obesity and ovarian cancer in a case-control study. *Am J Epidemiol* 1989; 129(6):1300–1304.
15. Michaud DS, Giovannucci E, Willett WC, Colditz GA, Stampfer MJ, Fuchs CS. Physical activity, obesity, height, and the risk of pancreatic cancer. *JAMA* 2001; 286(8):921–929.
16. Colditz GA. Economic costs of obesity and inactivity. *Med Sci Sports Exercise* 1999; 31(11 Suppl):S663–667.
17. Pronk NP, Goodman MJ, O'Connor PJ, Martinson BC. Relationship between modifiable health risks and short-term health care charges. *JAMA* 1999; 282(23):2235–2239.

18. Pronk NP, Tan AW, O'Connor P. Obesity, fitness, willingness to communicate and health care costs. *Med Sci Sports Exercise* 1999; 31(11):1535–1543.
19. Pronk NP, Martinson B, Kessler RC, Beck AL, Simon GE, Wang P. The association between work performance and physical activity, cardiorespiratory fitness, and obesity. *J Occup Environ Med* 2004; 46(1):19–25.
20. National Institutes of Health, National Heart, Lung, and Blood Institute, Obesity Education Initiative. Clinical guidelines on the identification, evaluation, and treatment of overweight and obesity in adults. Available at: http://www.nhlbi.nih.gov/guidelines/obesity/ob_gdlns.htm (accessed March, 2004).
21. Halbert JA, Silagy CA, Finucane P, Withers RT, Hamdorf PA, Andrews GR. The effectiveness of exercise training in lowering blood pressure: a meta-analysis of randomized controlled trials of 4 weeks or longer. *J Hum Hypertension* 1997; 11(10):641–649.
22. Stefanick ML. Exercise and weight loss. In: Hennekens CH, Ed. *Clinical Trials in Cardiovascular Disease: a Companion Guide to Braunwald's Heart Disease*. Philadelphia, PA: WB Saunders Co; 1999: 375–391.
23. Manson JE, Skerrett PJ, Greenland P, VanItallie TB. The escalating pandemics of obesity and sedentary lifestyle. A call to action for clinicians. *Arch Intern Med* 2004; 164(3):249–258.
24. U.S. Dept of Health and Human Services Centers for Disease Control and Prevention. Physical activity and health: a report of the Surgeon General. Washington, D.C.; 1996.
25. Blair SN, LaMonte MJ, Nichaman MZ. The evolution of physical activity recommendations: how much is enough? *Am J Clin Nutr* 2004; 79(5):913S–920S.
26. Klem ML, Wing RR, McGuire MT, Seagle HM, Hill JO. A descriptive study of individuals successful at long-term maintenance of substantial weight loss. *Am J Clin Nutr* 1997; 66(2):239–246.
27. McGuire MT, Wing RR, Klem ML, Hill JO. Behavioral strategies of individuals who have maintained long-term weight losses. *Obesity Res* 1999; 7(4):334–341.
28. Shick SM, Wing RR, Klem ML, McGuire MT, Hill JO, Seagle H. Persons successful at long-term weight loss and maintenance continue to consume a low-energy, low-fat diet. *J Am Diet Assoc* 1998; 98(4):408–413.
29. Perri MG, Sears SF, Jr., Clark JE. Strategies for improving maintenance of weight loss. Toward a continuous care model of obesity management. *Diabetes Care* 1993; 16(1):200–209.
30. Rippe JM, McInnis KJ, Melanson KJ. Physician involvement in the management of obesity as a primary medical condition. *Obesity Res* 2001; 9 Suppl 4:302S–311S.
31. Sciamanna CN, Tate DF, Lang W, Wing RR. Who reports receiving advice to lose weight? Results from a multistate survey. *Arch Intern Med* 2000; 160(15):2334–2339.
32. O'Connor PJ, Rush WA, Prochaska JO, Pronk NP, Boyle RG. Professional advice and readiness to change behavioral risk factors among members of a managed care organization. *Am J Managed Care* 2001; 7(2):125–130.
33. Glasgow RE, Eakin EG, Fisher EB, Bacak SJ, Brownson RC. Physician advice and support for physical activity: results from a national survey. *Am J Prev Med* 2001; 21(3):189–196.
34. Wee CC. Physical activity counseling in primary care: the challenge of effecting behavioral change. *JAMA* 2001; 286(6):717–719.
35. Eakin EG, Glasgow RE, Riley KM. Review of primary care-based physical activity intervention studies: effectiveness and implications for practice and future research. *J Fam Pract* 2000; 49(2):158–168.
36. Damush TM, Stewart AL, Mills KM, King AC, Ritter PL. Prevalence and correlates of physician recommendations to exercise among older adults. *J Gerontol A Biol Sci Med Sci* 1999; 54(8):M423–427.
37. Lewis CE, Clancy C, Leake B, Schwartz JS. The counseling practices of internists. *Ann Intern Med* 1991; 114(1):54–58.
38. Simkin–Silverman LR, Wing RR. Management of obesity in primary care. *Obesity Res* 1997; 5(6):603–612.
39. Galuska DA, Will JC, Serdula MK, Ford ES. Are health care professionals advising obese patients to lose weight? *JAMA* 1999; 282(16):1576–1578.
40. Taira DA, Safran DG, Seto TB, Rogers WH, Tarlov AR. The relationship between patient income and physician discussion of health risk behaviors. *JAMA* 1997; 278(17):1412–1417.
41. Lewis CE, Wells KB, Ware J. A model for predicting the counseling practices of physicians. *J Gen Intern Med* 1986; 1(1):14–19.

42. Price JH, Desmond SM, Krol RA, Snyder FF, O'Connell JK. Family practice physicians' beliefs, attitudes, and practices regarding obesity. *Am J Prev Med* 1987; 3(6):339–345.
43. Whitlock EP, Orleans CT, Pender N, Allan J. Evaluating primary care behavioral counseling interventions: an evidence-based approach. *Am J Prev Med* 2002; 22(4):267–284.
44. Glynn TJ, Manley MW. *How to Help Your Patients Stop Smoking. A National Cancer Institute Manual for Physicians*. Bethesda, MD: Smoking, Tobacco and Cancer Program, Division of Cancer Prevention and Control, National Cancer Institute; 1989.
45. National Center for Lifestyle Management. http://www.nclm.us (accessed June, 2004).
46. Prochaska JO, Velicer WF. The transtheoretical model of health behavior change. *Am J Health Promot* 1997; 12(1):38–48.
47. Pronk NP, O'Connor PJ, Martinson BC. Population health and active living: economic potential of physical activity promotion. *Am J Sports Med* 2002; 4:51–57.
48. Committee on Quality Health Care in America, Institute of Medicine. *Crossing the Quality Chasm: a New Health System for the 21st Century.* Washington, D.C.; National Academy Press; 2001.
49. Serdula MK, Mokdad AH, Williamson DF, Galuska DA, Mendlein JM, Heath GW. Prevalence of attempting weight loss and strategies for controlling weight. *JAMA* 1999; 282(14):1353–1358.
50. Wadden TA, Anderson DA, Foster GD, Bennett A, Steinberg C, Sarwer DB. Obese women's perceptions of their physicians' weight management attitudes and practices. *Arch Fam Med* 2000; 9(9):854–860.
51. Rand CS, Macgregor AM. Morbidly obese patients' perceptions of social discrimination before and after surgery for obesity. *South Med J* 1990; 83(12):1390–1395.
52. Potter MB, Vu JD, Croughan–Minihane M. Weight management: what patients want from their primary care physicians. *J Fam Pract* 2001; 50(6):513–518.
53. Kottke TE, Edwards BS, Hagen PT. Counseling: implementing our knowledge in a hurried and complex world. *Am J Prev Med* 1999; 17(4):295–298.
54. Solberg LI, Kottke TE, Brekke ML, Conn SA, Magnan S, Amundson G. The case of the missing clinical preventive services systems. *Eff Clin Pract* 1998; 1(1):33–38.
55. O'Connor PJ, Pronk NP. Integrating population health concepts, clinical guidelines, and ambulatory medical systems to improve diabetes care. *J Ambul Care Manage* 1998; 21(1):67–73.
56. Starfield B. *Primary Care Concepts, Evaluation, and Policy.* New York: Oxford University Press; 1992.
57. Wagner EH. The role of patient care teams in chronic disease management. *Br Med J* 2000; 320(7234):569–572.
58. Dickey L, Frame P, Rafferty M, Wender RC. Providing more — and better — preventive care. *Patient Care* 1999; November:198–210.
59. Crabtree BF, Miller WL, Aita VA, Flocke SA, Stange KC. Primary care practice organization and preventive services delivery: a qualitative analysis. *J Fam Pract* 1998; 46(5):403–409.
60. Stange KC, Woolf SH, Gjeltema K. One minute for prevention: the power of leveraging to fulfill the promise of health behavior counseling. *Am J Prev Med* 2002; 22(4):320–323.
61. Pronk NP, Boucher JL, Gehling E, Boyle RG, Jeffery RW. A platform for population-based weight management: description of a health plan-based integrated systems approach. *Am J Managed Care* 2002; 8(10):847–857.
62. Bodenheimer T, Grumbach K. Electronic technology: a spark to revitalize primary care? *JAMA* 2003; 290(2):259–264.
63. Rice RE, Katz JE. *The Internet and Health Communication.* Sage Publications, Inc.; 2001.
64. Street JL, Gold WR, Manning TE. *Health Promotion and Interactive Technology: Theoretical Applications and Future Directions*. London: Lawrence Erlbaum Associates; 1997.
65. Boucher JL, Schaumann JD, Pronk NP, Priest B, Ett T, Gray CM. The effectiveness of telephone-based counseling for weight management. *Diabetes Spectrum* 1999; 12:121–123.
66. HealthPartners Center for Health Promotion. *Addressing Obesity in Primary Care*. Health Partners Minneapolis, MN, 2002.
67. HealthPartners Center for Health Promotion. *Behavior Change Counseling Guide*. HealthPartners, Minneapolis, MN, 1998.
68. HealthPartners Center for Health Promotion. *National Center for Lifestyle Management Project.* HealthPartners, Minneapolis, MN, 2004.

33 Promoting Physical Activity in Cancer Survivors

Anna L. Schwartz and Kerri Winters-Stone

CONTENTS

Motivating people to exercise is one of the greatest challenges in helping people adopt physical activity. The threat of cancer is life-shaking enough that most patients are willing to try anything to recover more quickly or improve their odds of survival, even if that includes beginning an exercise program. Exercise is reported as the most frequently used (21%) alternative therapy for management of diseases.[1] Although a diagnosis of cancer may be a trigger to increase physical activity, numerous barriers can lead to noncompliance.

PHYSICAL ACTIVITY, MOTIVATION, AND NONCOMPLIANCE

Because exercise is a voluntary activity, people often lose their motivation when faced with the challenges of lack of time, demands by family and work, and even the discomfort of exercise when a program progresses too quickly or a participant is pushed, or pushes himself or herself, beyond capacity. People begin and maintain an exercise program if the outcomes of their physical activity efforts are valued, and to many cancer patients, the outcomes of improved quality of life, and physical and emotional well-being are sufficient to persist in an exercise program.

Three key concepts are related to adherence: (1) the activity must be meaningful; (2) the benefits need to be connected to the survivor's personal goals (e.g., maintain mobility); and (3) the goals need to be realistic so that results can be seen in a step-by-step fashion.[2] Outcome expectancies for each survivor need to be consistent, reasonable, and systematically set up to guide the individual toward his or her desired goals. A survivor may not have been physically active in many years or may actually be averse to physical activity. Self-confidence and belief in their ability to complete the exercise and achieve their goals successfully must be considered when developing physical activity programs for cancer survivors. Breast cancer survivors who were successful in adhering to a 6-month strength and weight training program used self-efficacy to stay motivated and comply with the program.[3]

Part of promoting an individual's confidence and self-efficacy to exercise is to help in understanding what must be done to attain desired goals. If beliefs and behaviors are consistent with the exercise program, the individual will be moving in the direction of goal attainment. Cancer patients and survivors appear to have different beliefs about the benefits of exercise and may be motivated to exercise for difference reasons.[4] Exercise programs that build confidence and slowly increase the level of intensity appear to be most appealing to survivors.[5]

Social influences can impede or enhance a patient's decision to participate in an exercise program and continue with it in the long run.[6] The beliefs and attitudes of family and friends, work colleagues and health care professionals, as well as the subtle persuasion of the media, all influence a person's interest and willingness to exercise. Social influence is powerful and can have negative outcomes. Cancer survivors have reported that well-meaning family and friends discouraged them from exercise and that health care professionals did not support their decisions to exercise.[7–9] These negative factors affect how well a patient will adhere to physical activity. Conversely, survivors who report positive interactions with family, friends, colleagues, and health care providers are more likely to begin an exercise program and adhere to it in the long term.[8]

An awareness of the value of physical activity for cancer survivors is growing rapidly in the lay community and numbers of exercise groups and hospital-based programs for survivors are growing. Team Survivor is a national program to promote physical activity among women with a diagnosis of cancer. This program helps women, many of whom have never been physically active, to begin to exercise. The supportive environment of exercising with other cancer survivors provides a positive social influence and reinforcement to exercise.

Patients who are having a difficult time adhering to an exercise program need special attention. A discussion with the patient about conflicts and barriers can be enormously helpful in developing an appropriate exercise prescription and assisting the individual in building strategies to overcome barriers. A study testing the theory of planned behavior observed that intention to exercise among breast and prostate cancer survivors was influenced by attitude, subjective norms, and perceived behavioral control.[10] Another study of breast cancer survivors training for dragon boat racing also supported the theory of planned behavior, demonstrating that intention determined adherence to the program.

Although most cancer survivors use exercise as a way to feel in control, feel better, look better and improve their health, the age of a patient may have some bearing on choice of exercise.[11] Patients in their 20s or younger may be more motivated to improve their looks and physique, and want to feel strong and healthy again, whereas patients in their 30s, 40s, and 50s may choose to exercise so that they can maintain their ability to work, raise their family, and ward off some of the effects of aging. Patients over 60 years old often elect to exercise to maintain their physical strength and independence and slow the aging process. Older patients who are retired tend to have more time to devote to exercise, and this population is often willing and excited about joining an exercise program or adding specific exercises tailored to their daily regimen and particular needs.[8] Conversely, older patients may have significant comorbidities that limit their exercise capacity.

PATIENT INTERACTIONS

One's approach to the cancer patient is important.[12,13] The majority of survivors (85%) report that they would prefer to meet in person to receive exercise counseling, and 77% preferred that information about exercise be provided by an exercise specialist associated with a cancer center, indicating a strong desire for trustworthy and professional information.[5] Maintaining a patient's privacy and confidentiality is imperative to developing a trusting relationship in which the patient feels comfortable asking potentially sensitive questions.

Information to review with patients includes their health history, exercise history, and results from fitness evaluations. Regular meetings to review individual progress can increase a survivor's motivation and interest and provide time for the individual to discuss any challenges experienced with the exercise prescription, social pressures, or personal concerns. The exercise leader who can project sensitivity, concern, and trust while imparting information about an exercise prescription developed in collaboration with the survivor will help him or her feel comfortable and informed and may even increase satisfaction and encourage greater compliance with the program.

APPROACH TO EXERCISE PRESCRIPTION

A challenge confronting the professional developing an exercise prescription is individualizing it to the patient.[14] In the cancer setting, this concept is further complicated by the myriad side effects that patients may experience during cancer treatments and the long-term side effects that may influence mobility, strength, balance, cardiac and pulmonary function, and tactile sensations. Considering the acute and chronic side effects of therapy when organizing a group exercise program presents additional challenges. A collaborative relationship with the patient's health care team can mitigate the risks of prescribing exercise to individuals with complex medical backgrounds and possibly other comorbid conditions, which may further affect their ability to exercise.

Inherent in developing an exercise prescription for patients is determining the appropriate activities. Survivors are more likely to comply with an exercise program over time if they participate in activities that they enjoy. At this point in time, it is not known whether aerobic is superior to resistance exercise, or vice versa; therefore, it is unwise to guide a patient in one direction or another. The ideal exercise program may prove to be a combination of aerobic and resistance exercise to help patients maintain and improve their cardiopulmonary function while strengthening muscles that may have been disrupted from surgery or need strengthening to improve balance and ambulation.

Providing specific individualized guidelines for target heart rate ranges during aerobic exercise helps patients stay within a reasonable exercise intensity so that physical activity is fun and challenging, rather than aversive. However, when patients are receiving chemotherapy or other treatments, it is more difficult to prescribe exercise using heart rate because anemia and fluid shifts can dramatically influence heart rates. Starting patients very slowly and even breaking exercise sessions into different times of the day may be important to help them succeed without getting overly tired. Patients who keep records or logs of their exercise can see their progress, which is motivating. Logs help patients see gradual increments of improvement. They can chart the increase in duration and intensity of exercise.

One of the hardest concepts for patients, whether previous exercisers or not, is that they must start slowly and build an aerobic base. As people age, it takes longer to build this base and the process of physiological adaptation needs to be given about 40% more time.[15] The slow rate of progress is difficult for people who want to see instant results or who think that they should be able to exercise the way that they did when they were 20 years old. Jones' 2002 survey of cancer survivors' preferences observed that survivors prefer to exercise at a moderate intensity; this must be taken into consideration when developing exercise programs. Most survivors prefer to walk and engage in other moderate-intensity exercises.[5,16]

Another approach to monitoring exercise intensity is using subjective measures of effort. Scales, such as Borg's Perceived Exertion Scale, can help patients to monitor their efforts. However, using subjective measures has its limits, especially among patients new to exercise. Individuals who are just beginning to exercise may find themselves focusing more on the scale and how they feel then on the exercise. Focusing on physical sensations and symptoms leads to increased perceived work intensity relative to actual workload and may result in individuals working at too low an intensity.[17]

PROMOTING SURVIVOR'S COMMITMENT TO EXERCISE

Making exercise meaningful is key to promoting a patient's commitment to and enthusiasm for exercise. It is critical to establish, with the patient, positive outcomes that are individualized, specific, realistic, and objective. When working with survivors, it is important to catch their attention and make them aware of the significance of the changes that will occur with exercise. Work to help the individual fit exercise into his or her life and select activities that are appropriate and ideally linked to other interests.

Teach survivors to counter negative beliefs and self-talk about exercise by helping them to redirect their thinking in a more positive and constructive direction. That is, instead of thinking that exercise takes too much time, think that exercise provides more energy and strength to do important activities. Pinto et al. observed that overweight and obese breast cancer survivors were more likely to have low self-efficacy than their nonoverweight peers regarding their ability to succeed with exercise.[18] These patients may need individualized interventions to increase their self-efficacy and refocus their negative self-talk. Finally, educate patients about the negative consequences of not exercising — focusing on what an important role exercise has in combating the debilitating effects of inactivity and how exercise will keep them strong enough to play with their grandchildren or continue working or pursuing goals.

A common precursor to noncompliance is lack of social support. Help survivors identify positive and negative sources of support and plan ways to build support from people who are positive and encouraging. Assist the individual in developing strategies to manage negative support and prevent problems before they occur. Organize exercise sessions so that family and friends can join in. Suggest that individuals use exercise time to walk the dog or spend quality time with children or friends. Help the survivor identify where he or she would prefer to exercise and with whom. Survivors have diverse and different needs and preferences, with 44% choosing to exercise alone and 40% favoring exercise programs performed at home.[5]

Breast cancer survivors participating in dragon boat racing reported that support from their physician, spouse, and friends was key to their success, as was the belief and confidence that they could attend the program given the time constrains of daily life, fatigue, and other health problems.[19] Determinants of exercise for survivors of colon cancer were also intention and perceived control.[20] This study observed that colon cancer survivors' beliefs about the benefits of exercise are substantially different from those of their healthy counterparts. Survivors reported exercising to improve well-being, gain control over cancer and life, improve recovery, help cope with stress of treatment and disease, and get their mind off their disease.

Establishing a step-by-step approach that leads the individual toward a regular exercise program can help those who are hesitant and unsure about starting an exercise program. This three-phase approach, called shaping,[21] (1) helps the patient build confidence; (2) ensures that the patient paces activities to stay within the comfort zone; and (3) avoids overexertion and getting sore or injured and provides a personalized exercise program. Behavioral contracting is another approach to motivating exercise adherence. The contract to exercise must clearly spell out the objectives, the timeframe, and any consequences of failing to uphold the agreement.[22] Contracting works best when it is made between two people because then it becomes a formal commitment and there is an obligation to fulfill the agreement in the contract.

GOAL SETTING AND FEEDBACK

Goal setting is an effective motivator if it is individualized, manageable, and directed toward the ultimate goals of the survivor. Well-developed goals point the survivor in a positive direction and minimize disappointment and discouragement. Short-term goals that move the individual toward the long-term goal are optimal in promoting success because the survivor can see that goals are being achieved, step by step. Although long-term adherence to exercise programs appears to be more strongly influenced by survivor's perceived success rather than actual objective success, the exercise professional's responsibility is to guide the patient in selecting reasonable, realistic, and attainable goals.

Success with goal setting is connected to providing positive and constructive feedback. For feedback to be useful, it must be specific to the individual's goals, objective, and provided on a regular basis or formal schedule. Providing feedback based on objective measures is most helpful and can help survivors to identify even modest gains. Feedback on a 6- or 12-week basis is most helpful. The individual knows when to expect it and can use the information for motivation and reinforcement of the new lifestyle. Reiterate to the individual that the goals may need to be modified and revised at various times depending on progress, toleration of the exercise regimen, unanticipated changes in the treatment plan, and unexpected life events. Goal setting needs to be viewed as a fluid means to an end. For inactive survivors, providing reassurance that exercise is safe and educating them to understand the many benefits of exercise may help with exercise initiation and long-term adherence.

ADHERENCE RATES IN RESEARCH STUDIES

It is a challenge to determine adherence rates in research on exercise in cancer patients and survivors because these studies vary in duration of the intervention, measures of adherence, and type of exercise program. Adherence rates were included in 12 studies; however, the methods of reporting the data varied. Adherence rates were reported by percentage of total subjects (ranging from 61 to 100% adhering) to percentage of attendance per subject (ranging from 72 to 98% adherence) to percentage of total training in exercise group (66 to 89% adherence).[16,19,23–32] Although the research on adherence rate is limited, it is clear that cancer survivors exercise at a higher adherence rate than their healthy counterparts.

SUMMARY

Until relatively recently, exercise programs for cancer patients were not sought by patients or recommended by physicians. A growing body of research has established that, in fact, exercise may be an important component of an overall treatment plan for survivors. Promoting physical activity in the cancer setting is based on meeting the survivor's immediate and long-term goals. Developing a reasonable, realistic, and individualized program that is of a moderate intensity and not unduly physically challenging is important. It may be beneficial to help survivors identify ways to make exercise more pleasurable — whether that is to have music in the background, participate in an activity that they like, or exercise with friends and family. Although the body of research in cancer and exercise is growing, more work is needed to determine factors related to promoting exercise for survivors during and following cancer treatment.

REFERENCES

1. Huber, R., Koch, D., Beiser, I., Zschocke, I., & Luedtke, R. (2004). Experience and attitudes towards CAM — a survey of internal and psychosomatic patients in a German university hospital. *Alternative Ther Health Med*, 10(1), 32–36.
2. Bandura, A. (1977). Self-efficacy: toward a unifying theory of behavioral change. *Psychological Rev*, 84, 191–215.
3. Ott, C.D., Lindsey, A.M., Waltman, N.L., Gross, G.J., Twiss, J.J., Berg, K., Brisco, P.L., & Hendrickson, S. (2004). Facilitative strategies, psychological factors, and strength/weight training behaviors in breast cancer survivors who are at risk for osteoporosis. *Orthoped Nursing* 23(1), 45–52.
4. Courneya, K.S. & Freidenreich, C.M. (1999). Utility of the theory of planned behavior for understanding exercise during breast cancer treatment. *Psychooncology*, 8(2), 112–122.
5. Jones, L.W. & Courneya, K.S. (2002). Exercise counseling and programming preferences of cancer survivors. *Cancer Pract*, 10(4), 208-215.
6. Rotter, J.B. (1954). *Social Learning and Clinical Psychology*. Englewood Cliffs, NJ: Prentice Hall.
7. Cooper, H. (1995). The role of physical activity in the recovery from breast cancer. *Melpomene J*, 14, 18–20.

8. Schwartz, A.L. (1998). Patterns of exercise and fatigue in physically active cancer survivors. *Oncology Nursing Forum*, 25(3), 485–491.
9. Young-McCoughan, S. & Sexton, D.L. (1991). A retrospective investigation of the relationship between aerobic exercise and quality of life in women with breast cacner. *Oncology Nursing Forum*, 18, 751–757.
10. Blanchard, C.M., Courneya, K.S., Rodgers, W.M., & Murnaghan D.M. (2002). Determinants of exercise intention and behavior in survivors of breast and prostate cancer: an application of the theory of planned behavior. *Cancer Nursing*, 25(2), 88–95.
11. Ajzen, I. & Fishbein, M. (1980). *Understanding Attitudes and Predicting Social Behavior*. Englewood Cliffs, NJ: Prentice Hall.
12. Dishman, R.K. (1982). Compliance/adherence in health-related exercise. *Health Psychol*, 1(3), 237–267.
13. Zimbardo, P.G., Ebbesen, E.B., & Maslach, C. (1977). *Influencing Attitudes and Changing Behavior* (2nd ed.). Reading, MA: Addison–Wesley.
14. Skinner, J.S. (Ed.). (1987). *Exercise Testing and Exercise Prescription for Special Cases*. Philadelphia: Lea & Febiger.
15. Pollock, M.L., Wilmore, J.H., & Fox, S.M. (1984). *Exercise in Health and Disease*. Philadelphia: W.B. Saunders.
16. Schwartz, A.L., Thompson, J.A., & Masood, N. (2002). Interferon-induced fatigue in patients with melanoma: a pilot study of exercise and methylphenidate. *Oncology Nursing Forum*, 29(7), E85–90.
17. Pennebaker, J.W. (1982). *The Psychology of Physical Symptoms*. New York: Springer–Verlag.
18. Pinto, B.M., Maruyama, N.C., Clark, M.M., Cruess, D.G., Park, E., & Roberts, M. (2002). Motivation to modify lifestyle risk behaviors in women treated for breast cancer. *Mayo Clin Proc*, 77(2), 122–129.
19. Courneya, K.S., Blanchard, C.M., & Laing, D.M. (2001). Exercise adherence in breast cancer survivors training for a dragon boat race competition: a preliminary investigation. *Psychooncology*, 10(5), 444–452.
20. Courneya, K.S. & Freidenreich, C.M. (1997). Determinants of exercise during colorectal cancer treatment: an application of the theory of planned behavior. *Oncology Nursing Forum*, 24(10), 1715–1723.
21. Martin, J.E. & Dubbert, P.M. (1984). Behavioral management strategies for improving health and fitness. *J Cardiopulm Rehabil*, 4, 200–208.
22. Epstein, L.H., Wing, R.R., Thompson, J.K., & Griffin, W. (1980). Attendance and fitness in aerobic exercise: the effect of contract and lottery procedures. *Behav Modification*, 4, 464–479.
23. Coleman, E.A., Hall-Barrow, J., Coon, S., & Stewart, C.B. (2003). Facilitating exercise adherence for patients with multiple myeloma. *Clin J Oncol Nursing*, 7(5), 529–534, 540.
24. Courneya, K.S., Friedenreich, C.M., Quinney, H.A., Fields, A.L., Jones, L.W., & Fairey, A.S. (2003). A randomized trial of exercise and quality of life in colorectal cancer survivors. *Eur J Cancer Care* (Engl), 12(4), 347–357.
25. Courneya, K.S., Mackey, J.R., Bell, G.J., Jones, L.W., Field, C.J., & Fairey, A.S. (2003). Randomized controlled trial of exercise training in postmenopausal breast cancer survivors: cardiopulmonary and quality of life outcomes. *J Clin Oncol*, 21(9), 1660–1668.
26. Courneya, K.S., Friedenreich, C.M., Sela, R.A., Quinney, H.A., Rhodes, R.E., & Handman, M. (2003). The group psychotherapy and home-based physical exercise (GROUP-HOPE) trial in cancer survivors: physical fitness and quality of life outcomes. *Psychooncology*, 12(4), 357–374
27. Pickett, M., Mock, V., Ropka, M.E., Cameron, L., Coleman, M., & Podewils, L. (2002). Adherence to moderate-intensity exercise during breast cancer therapy. *Cancer Pract*, 10(6), 284–292.
28. Schwartz, A.L., Mori, M., Gao, R., Nail, L.M., & King, M.E. (2001). Exercise reduces daily fatigue in women with breast cancer receiving chemotherapy. *Med Sci Sports Exercise*, 33(5), 718–723.
29. Schwartz, A.L. (1999). Fatigue mediates the effects of exercise on quality of life. *Qual Life Res*, 8(6), 529–538.
30. Segal, R., Evans, W., Johnson, D., Smith, J., Colletta, S., Gayton, J., Woodard, S., Wells, G., & Reid, R. (2001). Structured exercise improves physical functioning in women with stages I and II breast cancer: results of a randomized controlled trial. *J Clin Oncol*, 19(3), 657–665.

31. Segal, R.J., Reid, R.D., Courneya, K.S., Malone, S.C., Parliament, M.B., Scott, C.G., Venner, P.M., Quinney, H.A., Jones, L.W., D'Angelo, M.E., & Wells, G.A. (2003). Resistance exercise in men receiving androgen deprivation therapy for prostate cancer. *J Clin Oncol*, 21(9), 1653–1659.
32. Waltman, N.L., Twiss, J.J., Ott, C.D., Gross, G.J., Lindsey, A.M., Moore, T.E. & Berg, K. (2003). Testing an intervention for preventing osteoporosis in postmenopausal breast cancer survivors. *J Nursing Scholarship*, 35(4), 333–338.

34 Obesity and Early Stage Breast Cancer Outcome

Rowan T. Chlebowski and Michelle L. Geller

CONTENTS

The preponderance of reports indicates that obese women have a worse prognosis following a breast cancer diagnosis compared to nonobese women.[1] However, the area has remained controversial because of contradictory results from studies relying on relatively small patient samples.[2,3] Most recently, a number of recent reports involving larger patient populations, which control for more potential confounding factors, have provided additional information regarding this question.[4]

BODY WEIGHT AND BREAST CANCER OUTCOME (COHORTS)

In a study of 5204 Nurses Health Study (NHS) participants diagnosed with invasive localized breast cancer in which 860 total deaths and 681 recurrences were seen, clinical outcomes were related to body mass index (BMI) at diagnosis.[5] In a multivariate-adjusted analysis, weight at baseline was associated with increased risk for breast cancer recurrence and death, but these associations were seen only in participants who had never smoked. In addition, among those who had never smoked, breast cancer patients who gained weight after diagnosis had a significantly elevated risk of breast cancer death ($p = 0.03$). In this report, detailed information regarding systemic therapy received was not available. This report identified a negative prognostic role for obesity in women with resected breast cancer and suggested an interaction with smoking as well. In this regard, smoking has been previously associated with breast cancer incidence[6] and lung metastases from breast cancer.[7,8]

In a report from Fox Chase Cancer Center, clinical outcome from 2010 patients diagnosed with stages I to II breast cancer were determined and related to BMI categories.[9] At diagnosis, 22% of the patients were normal weight, 43% were overweight, and 35% were obese. The three weight groups showed no differences in terms of tumor size or lymph-node involvement, providing control for an important prognostic variable. The 5-year rates of distant metastases were 7% for patients with normal weight, 6% for overweight women, and 10% for obese individuals. Similarly, 5-year survival rates were lower in obese women compared to other groups (88 vs. 92%, respectively).

Enger and colleagues reported on body weight correlates with risk of breast cancer death in a population of 1376 breast cancer patients with stages I to II disease seen at one medical center.[10] After 6.8 years of follow-up, 240 patients had died from breast cancer. A dose–response was seen; increasing weight also increased the likelihood of dying of breast cancer with a twofold increased risk when the lowest category of weight was compared to the highest category (hazard ratio [HR] 2.54, 95% confidence interval [CI], 1.08 to 6.00; $P = 0.02$). In subgroup analyses, women in the upper 50th percentile of weight with estrogen receptor (ER) negative cancers were at nearly a fivefold increase mortality risk (HR 4.99, 95% CI, 2.17 to 11.48; P for interaction = 0.10) compared with women in the lower 50th percentile for weight with receptor-positive tumors. In this report influence on breast cancer recurrence was not provided.

In a cohort of 512 women reported by Goodwin and Colleagues,[11] a J-shaped relationship between body weight and breast cancer prognosis was described. In this group of early stage breast cancer patients, women with low or high BMI (<20 (low) or >25 (high) kg/m^2) had the worst outcome. These more recent reports in larger populations suggest a role of higher body weight in adversely influencing prognosis. Questions raised by the exploratory analyses performed regarding a role for smoking and receptor status, as well as lower weight extremes in this process, remain unanswered. Also, methodology differences preclude direct comparison of these reports.

BODY WEIGHT AND BREAST CANCER OUTCOME (IN COOPERATIVE GROUP TRIALS)

Most recently, the relationship between obesity and early stage breast cancer outcome has been addressed in analyses from randomized adjuvant breast cancer therapy trials performed by multicenter, cooperative clinical trial groups. The associations among obesity, tamoxifen use, and clinical outcomes in estrogen receptor positive early stage breast cancer have been examined in a cohort of 3385 women in the National Surgical Adjuvant Breast Project (NSABP) BP-14 — a randomized trial comparing tamoxifen to placebo. With long-term follow-up exceeding 166 months, breast cancer recurrence, contralateral breast cancers, and overall survival were compared in women who were obese (BMI > 30) at diagnosis compared to normal weight women at diagnosis (BMI < 25).[12]

The presence or absence of obesity had no effect on tamoxifen efficacy because reduced recurrence risk and increased survival were seen with tamoxifen regardless of BMI. In this population of receptor-positive patients, breast cancer recurrence was not influenced by obesity (HR 95% CI, 0.98, 0.80 to 1.18 for obese vs. not obese). However, contralateral breast cancer risk and all-cause mortality were significantly greater in women diagnosed when they were obese (for contralateral breast cancer, HR 1.59, 95% CI, 1.10 to 2.25 and for all-cause mortality, HR 1.31, 95% CI, 1.12 to 1.54). Thus, although obesity had no effect on recurrence risk in this population, overall mortality was significantly greater for obese breast cancer patients compared with those with normal weight.

Quite similar results have been reported from an analysis conducted by the International Breast Cancer Study Group of their trials.[13] This group evaluated outcome of 6792 pre- and postmenopausal patients randomized to International Breast Cancer Study Group Trials and related outcome to BMI, which was categorized as normal (<25), intermediate (25 to 29.9), or obese (≥30). In these analyses, eight other conventional prognostic factors incorporating tumor stage and characteristics were also considered. In studies involving chemotherapy and hormonal therapy, patients with normal BMI had significantly longer overall survival and disease-free survival than patients with intermediate or obese BMI. However, when adjusted for other prognostic factors, higher BMI was associated with decreased overall survival ($p = 0.03$), but not decreased disease-free survival ($p = 0.12$).

These two retrospective analyses of outcome in randomized cooperative group clinical trials have considerable strengths — namely, carefully defined information on tumor stage, systemic therapy delivered, and cancer outcomes. However, it is not clear how protocol eligibility requirements may have excluded individuals with extremes of weight indirectly through comorbidity exclusions. In any event, taken together (see Table 34.1), these data suggest that body weight represents an independent prognostic factor for breast cancer patient survival. These cooperative reports do not exclude a potential influence of obesity or related factors on breast cancer recurrence outcome, given the limitation of their retrospective design and protocol entry requirements.

CLINICAL SIGNIFICANCE: OBESITY IN BREAST CANCER PATIENTS

Delay in breast cancer recurrence is important; however, improved survival and quality of life are among the major objectives of therapies provided for early stage breast cancer patients. The observed statistically significant adverse influence of obesity on overall survival and non–breast cancer-related survival in these clinical trials — initiated decades ago in some cases — will be of increasing importance in determining outcome of currently diagnosed breast cancer patients.[14] Currently, the more widespread use of mammography is diagnosing patients at an earlier stage and therapeutic improvements related to chemotherapy and hormonal therapy are substantially reducing a woman's risk of death related to breast cancer recurrence. Therefore, appropriate management of obesity in breast cancer patients will become a major factor in determining clinical outcome of women with resected early stage breast cancer.[15,16]

OBESITY AND BREAST CANCER PATIENT OUTCOMES: POTENTIAL MEDIATING MECHANISM

When one compares obese to nonobese individuals, many differences can be seen. Correlates of obesity with potential factors that could influence breast cancer growth are outlined in Table 34.2. Among these factors, fasting insulin has received the most attention with respect to prognostic significance. Goodwin and colleagues[11] reported that, in a cohort of 512 women without known diabetes, clinical outcome was related to fasting insulin levels. In this population of early stage breast cancer patients, higher fasting insulin was significantly associated with an increased risk for distant disease recurrence and death (HR, 95% CI, for those in the highest [>51.9 pmol/L] vs. the

TABLE 34.1
Breast Cancer Clinical Outcomes (Obese vs. not Obese) in Analyses from Multicenter Clinical Trial Groups

Endpoint	NSABP (HR, 95% CI) obese vs. not	IBCSG (HR, 95% CI, obese vs. not obese)	
		Pre/peri menopausal	Post menopausal
Breast cancer recurrence	0.98 (0.80, 1.18)	Not reported	Not reported
Contralateral breast cancer	1.58 (1.10, 2.25)	Not reported	Not reported
Disease-free survival	Not reported	1.16 (1.02, 1.33)	1.06 (0.96–1.17)
Overall survival	1.31 (1.12, 1.54)	1.22 (1.05, 1.42)	1.11 (0.97–1.24)

Note: Disease-free survival time from randomization to relapse, second cancer, or death from any cause.

Source: IBCSG: International Breast Cancer Study Group[13]; NSABP: National Surgical Adjuvant Breast Cancer Project[12].

TABLE 34.2
Associations with Obesity with Factors Having Potential Influence on Breast Cancer Patient Outcome

Lifestyle association
Higher caloric intake
Higher fat intake
Lower physical activity
Hormone association
Higher estrogens (estradiol, estrone)
Higher testosterone
Higher insulin
Higher IGF-1

Source: Chlebowski, R. et al. *J Clin Oncol* 2002; 20:1128.

lowest [<27.0 pmol/L] insulin quartile was 2.0, 1.2 to 3.3, and 3.1, 1.7 to 5.7, respectively). Although insulin was significantly correlated with BMI, insulin remained an independent predictor for adverse clinical outcome.[11] Estrogen levels were not correlated with recurrence risk or mortality risk in these pre- and postmenopausal breast cancer patients.

Recently, Borugian and colleagues have reported similar findings from a British Columbia Tumor Registry cohort of 603 early stage breast cancer patients in which 112 deaths have occurred.[17] Using a Cox Proportional Hazard Regression Model, they reported a statistically significant correlation with high insulin tertile and increased mortality risk in postmenopausal breast cancer patients (relative risk [RR] 1.9, 95% CI, 0.7 to 6.6). In this regard, the previously mentioned report by Enger and colleagues, which found that obesity was most strongly related to mortality in women with estrogen-receptor negative breast cancers, suggests that factors other than estrogen may mediate the effect.[10] In addition, cross-sectional analyses in postmenopausal women without cancer suggest that low physical activity and high caloric intake are related to higher fasting insulin levels, suggesting a role for insulin in obesity-mediated change in breast cancer outcome.[18] Although obesity has been linked to higher estrogen levels as potential mediator of its adverse influence on breast cancer incidence in postmenopausal women,[19] a role for obesity-induced estrogen increase has not been linked to breast cancer recurrence risk.

Women who are obese are more likely to have higher caloric and dietary fat intakes and be less physically active compared to leaner women. These factors of increased energy intake, increased dietary fat intake, and reduced physical activity have been correlated with risk of at least breast cancer incidence in some reports.[20–22] More recently, several of these lifestyle factors have been related to recurrence risk as well. In a cohort of a 122,000 women for the Nurses' Health Study with 2100 breast cancers and 209 deaths from cancer, the risk of breast cancer death was significantly less in women with more physical activity.[28] Walking 1 hour at 3 miles per hour expends 3 MET-hours. Women with 3 to 9 MET-hours per week of physical activity had a relative risk for breast cancer death of 0.80% compared to those with >9 to 14 MET-hours/week, who had a risk of breast cancer death of 0.50%.

RACE/ETHNICITY OBESITY AND BREAST CANCER OUTCOME

Consideration of breast cancer outcomes in African American women has raised issues regarding the potential role of obesity — particularly in this population. Although age-adjusted incidence of breast cancer is lower in African American compared that of white women, African American women have higher breast cancer mortality,[24] a phenomenon that has been largely unexplained.[25,26]

We have recently explored this issue in the 156,570 postmenopausal women participating in the Women's Health Initiative.[27]

Following collection of breast cancer risk factors, women were prospectively followed for breast cancer incidence, breast cancer characteristics, and breast cancer mortality. Adjustment for multiple breast cancer risk factors accounted for differences in breast cancer incidence in all minorities except for African Americans, in whom the HR 0.75, 95% CI, 0.61 to 0.92 continued to indicate a lower breast cancer incidence risk. African American women were nearly twice as likely to be obese (BMI ≥ 30; seen in 51% of African Americans compared to 28% of whites, $p = 0.001$) and breast cancers in African Americans had unfavorable characteristics; 32% of those in African Americans but only 10% in white women were high-grade and estrogen receptor-negative (adjusted odds ratio 4.70; 95% CI, 3.12 to 7.09).

To examine the relative contribution of ethnicity/race and obesity to these results, multinomial logistic regression models of the influence on breast cancer histology of age, BMI, menopausal hormone therapy use, socioeconomic factors, and ethnicity/race were performed. In these models, BMI was only a modest nonstatistically significant ($p = 0.10$) predictor of the unfavorable high-grade, ER-negative cancers; ethnicity/race was highly correlated ($p < 0.001$) with this histology. In addition, after adjustment for prognostic factors, a higher mortality after breast cancer diagnosis was identified in African American compared to white women (HR 1.79, 95% CI, 1.05 to 3.05). Thus, comprehensive analyses suggest that factors other than obesity may contribute to the adverse outcome of African American women with breast cancer. Such findings suggest that detailed biologically based subgroup analyses may be needed to dissect relationships between obesity and breast cancer outcome correctly.

OBESITY AND BREAST CANCER OUTCOME: POTENTIAL INTERVENTION STRATEGIES

Obesity[2] and associated factors of increased dietary fat intake[22,23] and decreased physical activity[28] have been related to adverse clinical outcome, at least in some reports, for women with breast cancer.

Given the already identified factors that vary together with obesity,[29] it is unlikely that retrospective analyses of existing patient populations will provide definitive information regarding a role for weight loss or weight maintenance as a breast cancer management strategy. Currently, no ongoing full-scale trials of weight loss or weight management in women with diagnosed breast cancer are being conducted. Because randomized trials and other patient populations have identified a strategy to achieve and maintain moderate weight loss that incorporates dietary counseling, increased physical activity, behavioral therapy, and ongoing medical suppression,[30] weight loss programs incorporating these elements could be recommended for evaluation in obese breast cancer patients. The status of lifestyle intervention strategies currently under evaluation in clinical trials involving breast cancer patients is outlined next.

Although full-scale outcome studies of weight loss in women with breast cancer have not been conducted, several small randomized trials support the feasibility of weight loss intervention in this population.[31–34] With respect to exercise, moderately sized randomized trials suggest that increased physical activity can be achieved with favorable influence — at least on physical functioning parameters including fatigue symptoms.[35,36]

Dietary fat intake has received the most concerted attention. Two full-scale outcome studies have been funded by the National Cancer Institute and accruals to these efforts have been completed. The Women's Intervention Nutrition Study (WINS) has randomized 2437 breast cancer patients ≥ 48 years of age receiving standard breast cancer management to a control condition or a program consisting of dietary fat intake reduction. The feasibility of this intervention as been established[37,38] and results suggest that the dietary fat intake reduction may improve relapse free survival of post menopausal breast cancer patients, particularly in patients who were ER receptor negative ($p < 0.018$).[39]

The Women's Healthy Eating Lifestyle (WHEL) study has randomized over 3000 pre- and postmenopausal women with early stage resected breast cancer to a control condition vs. a program of dietary fat intake reduction plus fruits and vegetable increase.[40,41] The feasibility of this intervention has also been reported; however, substantial weight loss (not an intervention target) has not been seen.[42] Clinical outcome results of this ongoing study are anticipated in the near future.

INCORPORATING EXERCISE AND DIET RECOMMENDATIONS INTO CLINICAL ONCOLOGY PRACTICE

While awaiting definite results from clinical trials, current clinical management can perhaps be best guided[43] by the recently updated American Cancer Society guide for informed choice, nutrition, and physical activity during and after cancer treatment.[44] These guidelines provide specific recommendations for exercise and nutrition for patients with breast cancer and can be used to make recommendations to patients in clinical practice. Women should attempt, at least, to maintain weight after breast cancer diagnosis. Weight gain after diagnosis is a common occurrence[45] and clinicians should recommend that patients avoid or reverse this type of weight gain. If a patient is unable to achieve ideal body weight, it is postulated that 5 to 10% weight loss over 6 to 12 months may also have benefits, as seen in reduction of biomarkers associated with risk.[44] Weight loss of 1 to 2 lb per week is considered safe for overweight women[46,47] as long as it does not interfere with treatment.

DIET

In general, the American Cancer Society recommends that individuals eat a variety of healthy foods with an emphasis on plant sources for cancer prevention — specifically,[44]

- Eating five or more servings of a variety of vegetables and fruits daily
- Choosing whole grains over processed (refined) grains and sugars
- Limiting consumption of red meats (especially high-fat or processed meat)
- Choosing foods to help maintain a healthy weight

The Department of Health and Human Services (HHS) and the U.S. Department of Agriculture (USDA) have put forth the 2005 Dietary Guidelines for Americans.[48] For healthy adults, the recommendation is to consume less than 10%t of calories from saturated fatty acids and less than 300 mg/day of cholesterol, and to keep *trans* fatty acid consumption as low as possible. It is also recommended that individuals keep total fat intake between 20 to 35% of calories, with most fats coming from sources of polyunsaturated and monounsaturated fatty acids. Recent results from ongoing randomized trials suggest that more specific recommendations regarding further reduction of dietary fat intake to reduce recurrence risk and increase survival of patients with early stage breast cancer may be present.[39]

Alcohol Intake

Alcohol intake has been associated with an increased risk for breast cancer[49]; however, the effect is unclear for risk of recurrence and survival for patients with breast cancer. Modest alcohol intake (one to two drinks per day) may lower the risk for cardiovascular disease,[50] which would be beneficial in these patients. Because increased risk of breast cancer with alcohol is associated with lower folate intake,[51–53] adequate folic acid intake might decrease this risk. This association is not known for women diagnosed with breast cancer.

Soy Products

Little evidence has been found that soy intake in regular amounts has beneficial or harmful effects in women with breast cancer.[54] Higher amounts of soy may have estrogenic effects, which could increase risk and should be avoided in women with diagnosed breast cancer. This is also true of soy and isoflavone supplements.

Exercise

The USDA/HHS Dietary Guidelines for Americans[48] suggest that healthy adults engage in regular physical activity to promote well-being and healthy body weight. To reduce the risk of chronic disease in adulthood, these guidelines recommend that adults engage in at least 30 minutes of moderate-intensity physical activity on most days of the week. To help prevent unhealthy weight gain in adulthood, it is suggested to engage in approximately 60 minutes of moderate- to vigorous-intensity activity on most days of the week without exceeding caloric intake. To sustain weight loss in adulthood, one should participate in at least 60 to 90 minutes of daily moderate-intensity activity without exceeding caloric intake. Activities recommended include cardiovascular conditioning, flexibility exercises, and resistance training.

Although few randomized clinical trials have been conducted, most studies suggest that exercise improves quality of life in patients with breast cancer during as well as after treatment. As mentioned, increased physical activity is associated with a decreased risk of primary breast cancer and new evidence suggests a reduction in recurrence risk in women with breast cancer.[44] The American Cancer Society recommends that individuals adopt an active lifestyle and engage in physical activity at least 5 or more days per week possibly to reduce risk of primary breast cancer.[44] This same principle may apply to women with diagnosed breast cancer, given the new evidence. Aerobic training may help with reducing or maintaining weight after diagnosis.[31,55,56]

REFERENCES

1. Chlebowski RT. Obesity and early stage breast cancer. *J Clin Oncol* 2005; 23(7):481–482.
2. Chlebowski RT, Aiello E, McTiernan A. Weight loss in breast cancer patient management. *J Clin Oncol* 2002; 20:1128–1143.
3. Goodwin PJ, Boyd NF. Body size and breast cancer prognosis: a critical review of the evidence. *Breast Cancer Res Treat* 1990; 16:205–214.
4. Dignam JJ, Mamounas EP. Obesity and breast cancer prognosis: an expanding body of evidence. *Ann Oncol* 2004; 15:850–851.
5. Kroenke CH, Chen WY, Rosner B, Holmes MD. Weight, weight gain and survival after breast cancer diagnosis. *J Clin Oncol* 2005; 23(7):683–694.
6. Reynolds P, Hurley S, Goldberg DE, et al. Active smoking, household passive smoking, and breast cancer: evidence from the California Teachers Study. *J Natl Cancer Inst* 2004; 96(1):29–37.
7. Scanlon FA. Suh O, Murthy SM, et al. Influence of smoking on the development of lung metastases from breast cancer. *Cancer* 1995; 75:2693–2699.
8. Murin S, Inciardi J. Cigarette smoking and the risk of pulmonary metastasis from breast cancer. *Chest* 2001; 119(6):1635–1640.
9. Anderson PR, Freedman G, Hanlon A, et al. Obesity at diagnosis confers worse outcome in patients with early stage breast cancer treated with breast conservation therapy. *Proc Am Soc Thera Rad Oncol* 2004; abstract 132.
10. Enger SM, Greif JM, Polikoff J, Press M. Body weight correlates with mortality in early stage breast cancer. *Arch Surg* 2004; 139:954–960.
11. Goodwin PJ, Ennis M, Pritchard KI, et al. Fasting insulin and outcome in early-stage breast cancer: results of a prospective cohort study. *J Clin Oncol* 2001; 20:42–51.
12. Dignam JJ, Wieand K, Johnson K, et al. Obesity, tamoxifen use, and outcomes in women with estrogen receptor-positive early stage breast cancer. *J Natl Cancer Inst* 2003; 95: 1467–1476.

13. Berclaz G, Li S, Price KN, et al. Body mass index as a prognostic feature in operable breast cancer: the International Breast Cancer Study Group experience. *Ann Oncol* 2004; 15:875–884.
14. Joensuu H, Lehtimaki T, Holli K, et al. Risk for distant recurrence of breast cancer detected by mammography screening or other methods. *JAMA* 2004; 292(9):1064–1073.
15. Manson JE, Willet WC, Stampfer MJ, et al. Body weight and mortality among women. *N Engl J Med* 1995; 333:677–685.
16. Yancik R, Wesley MN, Ries LA, et al. Effect of age and morbidity and cancer in older patients: approaches to expand the knowledge base. *JAMA* 2001; 285:885–892.
17. Borugian MJ, Shep SB, Kim-Sing C, et al. Insulin, macronutrient intake, and physical activity: potential indicators of insulin resistance associated with mortality from breast cancer? *Cancer Epidemiol Biomarkers Prev* 2004; 13(7):1163–1172.
18. Chlebowski RT, Pettinger M, Stefanick M, Howard BV, Mossavar–Rahmani Y, McTiernan A. Insulin levels, physical activity and energy intake in postmenopausal women: implications for breast cancer. *J Clin Oncol* 2004; 22(22):4518–4521.
19. Key TJ, Applyby PN, Reeves GK, Roddam A, et al. Body mass index, serum sex hormones, and breast cancer risk in postmenopausal women. *J Natl Cancer Inst* 2003; 95(16):1218–1226.
20. Michels KB, Ekbom A. Caloric restriction and incidence of breast cancer. *JAMA* 2004; 291(10):1226–1230.
21. Jain M, Miller AB, To T. Premorbid diet and the prognosis of women with breast cancer. *J Natl Cancer Inst* 1994; 86:1390–1397.
22. Zhang S, Folsom AR, Sellers TA, Kushi LH, Potter JD. Better breast cancer survival for postmenopausal women who are less overweight and eat less fat. The Iowa Women's Health Study. *Cancer* 1995; 76:275–283.
23. Holmes MD, Stampfer MJ, Colditz GA, et al. Dietary factors and the survival of women with breast carcinoma. *Cancer* 1999; 86:826–835.
24. Ghafoor A, Jemal A, Ward E, Cokkinides V, Smith P, Thun M. Trends in breast cancer by race and ethnicity. *Calif Cancer J Clin* 2003; 53:342–355.
25. Weir HK, Thun MJ, Hankey BF, Ries LA, Howe HL, Wingo, et al. Annual report to the nation on the status of cancer, 1975–2000, featuring the uses of surveillance data for cancer prevention and control. *J Natl Cancer Inst* 2003; 95:1276–1299.
26. Vastag B. Breast cancer racial gap examined: no easy answers to explain disparities in survival. *JAMA* 2003; 290:1838–1842.
27. Chlebowski RT, Chen Z, Anderson GL, Rohan T, Aragaki A, Lane D, Dolan NC, Paskett ED, McTiernan A, Hubbell FA, Adams–Campbell LL, Prentice R. Ethnicity and breast cancer: factors influencing differences in incidence and outcome. *J Natl Cancer Inst* 2005; 97:439–448.
28. Holmes MD, Chen WY, Feskanich D, Colditz GA. Physical activity and survival after breast cancer diagnosis. *JAMA* 2005; 293(20):2479–2486.
29. McTiernan A, Kooperberg C, White E, et al. Recreational physical activity and the risk of breast cancer in postmenopausal women: the Women's Health Initiative Cohort Study. *JAMA* 2003; 290(10):1331–1336.
30. McTigue KM, Harris R, Hemphill B, et al. Screening and interventions for obesity in adults: summary of the evidence for the U.S. Preventive Services Task Force. *Ann Intern Med* 2003; 139(11):933–949.
31. Goodwin PJ, Esplen MJ, Butler K, et al. Multidisciplinary weight management in locoregional breast cancer: results of a phase II study. *Breast Cancer Res Treat* 1998; 48:53–64.
32. Dujuric Z, Dilaura NM, Jenkins I, et al. Weight loss in obese breast cancer survivors: novel strategies. *Breast Cancer Res Treat* 2000; 64:49 (abstr).
33. Dujuric Z, Dilaura NM, Jenkins I, et al. Combining weight-loss counseling with the Weight Watchers plan for obese breast cancer survivors. *Obesity Res* 2002; 10:657–665.
34. DeWaard F, Ramlan R, Mulders Y, et al. A feasibility study on weight reduction in obese postmenopausal breast cancer patients. *Eur J Cancer Prev* 1993; 2:233–238.
35. Segal R, Evans W, Johnson D, Smith J, Colletta S, Gayton J, Woodard S, Wells G, Reid R. Structured exercise improves physical functioning in women with stages I and II breast cancer: results of a randomized controlled trial. *J Clin Oncol* 2001; 19(3):657–665.
36. Mock V, Frangakis C, Davidson NE, et al. Exercise manages fatigue during breast cancer treatment: a randomized controlled trial. *Psychooncology* 2005; 14:464–477.

37. Chlebowski RT, Blackburn GL, Buzzard IM, et al. Adherence to a dietary fat intake reduction program in postmenopausal women receiving therapy for early breast cancer. *J Clin Oncol* 1993; 11:2072–2080.
38. Chlebowski RT, Blackburn G, Winters B, et al. Long term adherence to dietary fat reduction in the Women's Intervention Nutrition Study (WINS). *Proc Am Soc Clin Oncol* 2000; 15:302.
39. Chlebowski RT, Blackburn GL, & Lashoff RE, Dietary fat reduction in postmenopausal women with primary breast cancer: Phase III Women's Intervention Nutrition Study (WINS) *Proc Amer Soc Clin Oncol* 2005; 24:10 (abstract).
40. Pierce JP, Faeber S, Wright FA, et al. Feasibility of a randomized trial of a high-vegetable diet to prevent breast cancer recurrence. *Nutr Cancer* 1997; 28:282–288.
41. Pierce JP. Faerber S, Wright FA, et al. for the Women's Healthy Eating and Living (WHEL) study group. A randomized trial of the effect of a plant-based dietary pattern on additional breast cancer events and survival: the Women's Healthy Eating and Living (WHEL) Study. *Control Clin Trials* 2002; 23:728–756.
42. Rock CL, Thomson C, Caan BJ, et al. Reduction in fat intake is not associated with weight loss inmost women after breast cancer diagnosis. *Cancer* 2001; 91:25–34.
43. Chlebowski RT. The ACS guide for nutrition and physical activity for cancer survivors: a call to action for clinical investigators. *Calif Cancer J Clin* 2003; 53(5):253–254 (editorial).
44. Brown JK, Byers T, Doyle C, Courneya KS, Demark–Wahnefried W, Kushi LH, McTiernan A, et al. Nutrition and physical activity during and after cancer treatment: an American Cancer Society Guide for informed choices. *Calif Cancer J Clin* 2003; 53(5):268–291.
45. Rock CL, Demark–Wahnerfried W. Nutrition and survival after the diagnosis of breast cancer: a review of the evidence. *J Clin Oncol* 2002; 20:3302–3316.
46. McTiernan A, Ulrich C, Slate S, Potter J. Physical activity and cancer etiology. Associations and mechanisms. *Cancer Causes Control* 1998; 9:487–509.
47. Irwin M, Yasui Y, Ulrich CM, et al. Effect of moderate and vigorous intensity exercise on total and intra abdominal body fat in postmenopausal women: a one year randomized controlled trial. *JAMA* 2003; 289:323–333.
48. Dietary Guidelines for Americans 2005. U.S. Department of Health and Human Services. U.S. Department of Agriculture. http://www.health.gov/dietaryguidelines/dga2005/document/pdf/DGA2005.pdf
49. Smith-Warner SA, Spiegelman D, Yuan SS, et al. Alcohol and breast cancer on women: a pooled analysis of cohort studies. *JAMA* 1998; 279:535–540.
50. Rimm R. Alcohol and cardiovascular disease. *Curr Atherosler Rep* 2000; 2:529–535.
51. Sellers TA, Kushi LH, Cerhan RD, et al. Dietary folate intake, alcohol, and risk of breast cancer in a prospective study of postmenopausal women. *Epidemiology* 2001; 12:420–428.
52. Feigelson HS, Jonas CR, Roberson AS, et al. Alcohol, folate, methionine, and risk of incident breast cancer in the American Cancer Society Cancer Prevention Study II nutrition cohort. *Cancer Epidemiol Biomarkers Prev* 2003; 12:161–164.
53. Zhang S, Willett W, Selhub J, et al. Plasma folate, vitamin B6, vitamin B12, homocysterine, and risk of breast cancer. *J Natl Cancer Inst* 2003; 95:373–380.
54. Messma M, Loprinzi C. Soy for breast cancer survivors: a critical review of the literature. *J Nutr* 2001; 131:3905s–3908s.
55. Demark-Wahnerfried W, Kenyon AJ, Eberle P, et al. Preventing sarcopenic obesity among breast cancer patients who receive adjuvant chemotherapy: results of a feasibility study. *Clin Exercise Physiol* 2002; 4:44–49.
56. McTiernan A, Ulrich C, Kumai C, et al. Anthrometric and hormone effects of an 8-week exercise–diet intervention in breast cancer patients: results of a pilot study. *Cancer Epidemiol Biomarkers Prev* 1998; 7:477–481.

35 Incorporating Weight Control into Management of Patients with Early Breast Cancer in the U.K.

Michelle Harvie and Anthony Howell

CONTENTS

Weight problems are common among breast cancer patients in the U.K. An estimated 64% of patients commencing endocrine therapy and 51% commencing adjuvant chemotherapy are overweight or obese. One third of patients experience significant weight gain (>5 kg) over the course of adjuvant chemotherapy, and those receiving endocrine therapy also appear to experience gains in fat, particularly central fat. Weight gain is a major concern to patients. They often seek further information, advice, and support in their endeavors to control their weight. The ideal way of delivering weight management advice in this group is not resolved. It is likely that, for some patients, successful weight management would require a multidisciplinary team, including a dietitian and a specialist breast care nurse, with further psychological support available wherever appropriate. Low staffing levels within U.K. cancer centers mean that these services are not widely available. The use of slimming on referral, exercise on prescription, and pharmacotherapy in nonspecialist weight management services has increased. The relevance of these approaches to the management of patients with cancer needs to be investigated.

TRENDS IN INCIDENCE OF AND MORTALITY FROM BREAST CANCER IN THE U.K.

Breast cancer is the most common malignancy among women in the U.K. affecting an estimated 41,000 women and accounts for 25 to 30% of female cancers. The incidence of breast cancer has increased by 11% over the past decade. Age-standardized mortality rates from breast cancer over this time have been reduced dramatically. The annual breast cancer death rate per 100,000 women at ages 20 to 49, 50 to 69, and 70 to 79 decreased by 22, 22, and 12% respectively [1]. The increasing incidence and greater proportion of patients surviving breast cancer means that the population of cancer survivors in the U.K. is growing (Figure 35.1). The long-term health and well-being of cancer patients are thus an increasingly important consideration for health care professionals.

PREVALENCE OF OVERWEIGHT AND OBESITY IN CANCER PATIENTS IN THE U.K.

Over the past 20 years in the U.K., the prevalence of overweight (body mass index, BMI, of 25 to 29.9) and obesity (BMI ≥ 30) for males and females has increased dramatically. The proportion of women estimated to be overweight or obese has increased from 32% in 1984 to 56% in 2002 (Figure 35.2). It is not therefore surprising that prevalence of overweight and obesity of breast

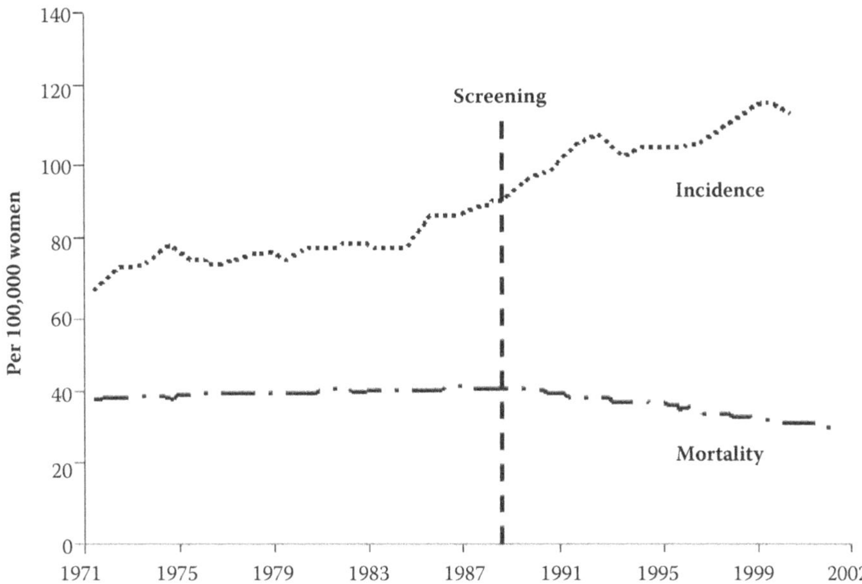

FIGURE 35.1 Trends in incidence and 5-year age standardized survival for breast cancer in the U.K. (From http://www.statistics.gov.uk, accessed July 2004 [62].)

cancer patients has also increased over the last 20 years. Data from our institution shows that only 25% of women receiving adjuvant therapy were overweight or obese in 1975 through 1979, compared to 51% of women treated in 2003. The age profiles of women receiving treatment at these two time points were not different. The dramatic increase in the prevalence of overweight and obesity appears to reflect the secular trend of greater weight in the population. The prevalence of overweight and obesity among patients receiving adjuvant chemotherapy and endocrine therapy in the U.K. are reported in Table 35.1. Of women going on to adjuvant endocrine therapy, 64% were overweight or obese at the time of commencing treatment; 51% of those receiving adjuvant endocrine therapy were.

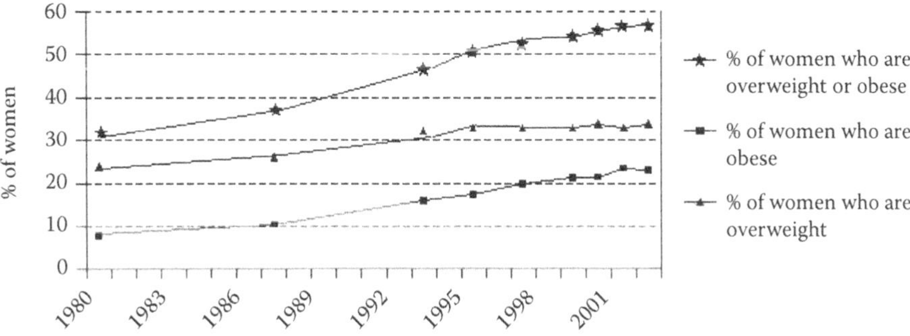

FIGURE 35.2 Prevalence of overweight and obesity in women in the U.K. between 1980 and 2002. (From http://www.publications.doh.gov.uk, accessed July 2004 [63].)

TABLE 35.1
Prevalence of Overweight and Obesity in Early Breast Cancer Patients and Age-Matched Population Controls from Health Survey England

		Percentage of population		
	Age (years)	Normal weight (BMI < 25 kg/m^2)	Overweight (BMI 25–29.9 kg/m^2)	Obese (BMI ≥ 30 kg/m^2)
Endocrine therapy (n = 3228)[b]	64.1 (9)[a]	36.5	39.1	24.4
Age matched population (n = 1896)	55-74	31	40.2	28.8
Adjuvant chemotherapy (n = 128)[c]	52(10)[a]	39	36	25
Age-matched population (n = 1109)	44–64	35.5	37.2	27.3

[a]Mean (SD).

[c]H Flint and C Price, Christie Hospital NHS Trust, personal communication.

[b]ATAC Trialists' Group personal communication.

Source: http://www.publications.doh.gov.uk (accessed July 2004 [63].)

SIGNIFICANCE OF EXCESS WEIGHT AND WEIGHT IN BREAST CANCER PATIENTS

Excess weight at diagnosis has been linked to a poorer prognosis in patients with breast cancer. Much of this increased risk is thought to be linked to later detection and increased nodal involvement among heavier women. Based on 6792 women, the largest analysis to date found BMI to be an independent, albeit weak, prognostic factor predicting disease free and overall survival irrespective of tumor characteristics in the overall group [2]. The adverse effects of excess weight in this study, however, were mainly seen among pre- and perimenopausal women treated with chemotherapy without endocrine therapy. Relative risk (RR) of relapse in this group was 1.23 (95% confidence interval (CI) 1.08 to 1.39) for obese women and 1.07 (0.97 to 1.18) for overweight women compared to normal weight women. Likewise RR of overall mortality over 10 years in this group was 1.24 (95% CI 1.08 to 1.43) for obesity and 1.10 (95% CI 0.98 to 1.23) for overweight compared to normal weight women [2].

Similarly a recent analysis among 3144 patients from the French Adjuvant Study Group (FASG) trial, found BMI to be an independent prognostic factor for relapse in patients receiving chemotherapy only or combined with tamoxifen [3]. Newman et al. found higher BMI to have a negative impact on survival among women who were estrogen receptor-positive and negative, suggesting weight may have an impact on survival via nonestrogen receptor-mediated mechanisms [4].

The effects of excess weight among postmenopausal women receiving endocrine therapy are not resolved. In the French Adjuvant Study Group analysis BMI did not have an impact on prognosis among women receiving tamoxifen alone [3]. In contrast, although the National Surgical Adjuvant Breast and Bowel Project did not associate excess weight at diagnosis with increased rate of breast cancer recurrence among women receiving tamoxifen, risk of contralateral breast cancer was greater in obese (RR 1.58; 95% CI 1.1 to 1.25) and in overweight (RR 1.22 (0.87 to 1.71) compared to normal weight women. Noncancer deaths were also more likely among obese (RR 1.49; 95% CI 1.15 to 1.92) and overweight (RR 1.19; 95% CI 0.94 to 1.92) compared to normal weight women [5].

PREVALENCE OF OBESITY-RELATED COMORBIDITIES IN BREAST CANCER PATIENTS

Few data on the prevalence of comorbidities among breast cancer patients are available. Recent data from the British Women's Heart Study, a community-based cohort study, reported that 10% of women diagnosed with postmenopausal breast cancer had non-insulin-dependent diabetes [6]. Data from the Malmo study, a community-based cohort study in Sweden, found hypertension (systolic blood pressure > 135 mm Hg) in a significant proportion of the women diagnosed with pre- (18%) and post- (26%) menopausal breast cancer. Similarly, hypercholesterolaemia (cholesterol > 6.9 mmol/l) occurred in 25% of the premenopausal and in 74% of the postmenopausal breast cancer cases. Notably, 23% of the postmenopausal cancer cases had an impaired glucose tolerance test [7].

WEIGHT GAIN AFTER DIAGNOSIS FOR EARLY BREAST CANCER

Patients Receiving Adjuvant Chemotherapy

Weight gain is a well documented unwanted side effect of adjuvant chemotherapy for early breast cancer. The prognostic effect of weight gain during chemotherapy remains uncertain. The largest study to date, based predominately on premenopausal women in the U.S., linked weight gains in excess of 5.9 kg to relative risks of relapse of 1.5 and mortality of 1.6 over 6.6 years of follow-up [8]. A recent U.K. series found approximately one third of patients gained more than 5 kg over the course of commencing chemotherapy [9]. Aside from the potential effects on prognosis of breast cancer and other comorbidities, weight gain will most likely be a major concern to these patients that will have an adverse effect on their quality of life and self esteem.

We have previously reported a prospective study of weight change and energy balance among patients receiving adjuvant fluorouracil (or 5FU), epirubicin, and cyclophosphamide (FEC) cyclophosphamide, methotrexate, and fluorouracil (5-FU) (CMF) chemotherapy. The principal findings were the significant weight gain occurred during chemotherapy and in the 6 months after treatment. After 1 year, mean (±SE) weight gain in patients during adjuvant chemotherapy was 5.0 (1.0) kg. Body fat increased significantly (mean (±SE) 7.1 (1.0) kg) — particularly central fat — with a mean gain in waist circumference of 5.0 (1.0) cm (Table 35.2). Gains in fat were partly accounted

TABLE 35.2
Change in Body Mass and Composition over 1 Year[a]

	Pre	Mid	Post	1 year
Weight (kilograms)	70.3 (2.2)	1.0 (0.6)	3.3 (1.0)[b]	5.0 (1.0)[c]
Body fat (kilograms)	25.8 (1.5)	0.2 (0.6)	4.0 (0.8)[c]	7.1 (1.0)[c]
FFM (kilograms)	44.5 (2.0)	0.79 (0.4)	–0.5 (0.6)	–1.7(0.6)[b]
Waist (centimeters)	84.8 (1.0)	0.8 (1.0)	3.5 (1.0)[b]	5.1 (1.0)[b]

[a] $N = 17$.
[b] $p < 0.05$.
[c] Mean (SE) $p < 0.01$.

Source: Adapted from Harvie, M.N. et al., *Breast Cancer Res Treat*, 2004; 83, 201–210.

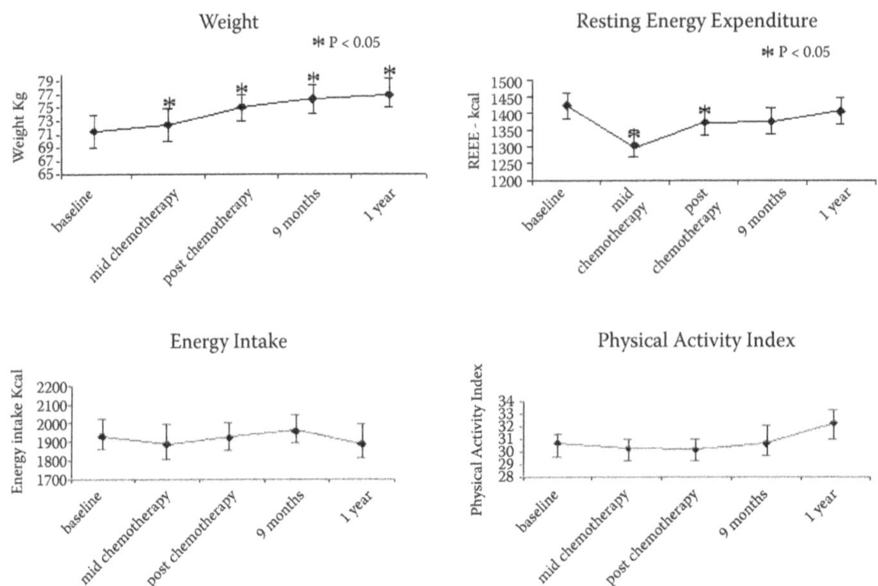

FIGURE 35.3 Energy balance over 1 year in patients receiving adjuvant chemotherapy, n = 17. (Adapted from Harvie, M.N. et al., *Breast Cancer Res Treat* 2004; 83, 201–210.)

for by a decline in resting energy expenditure during and in the 3 months after chemotherapy and a failure to reduce energy intake (Figure 35.3). Patients also reported low activity levels in the year after diagnosis of breast cancer [10].

Women Receiving Neoadjuvant Chemotherapy

Few data on weight change during neoadjuvant chemotherapy have been reported. Data from our small series (n = 6) showed weight loss occurred during neoadjuvant chemotherapy, mean (±SE) to 2.3 (2.3) kg, but weight gain rebounded in the postchemotherapy period. At 1 year, patients had gained 2.3 (2.6) kg. They had experienced significant gains in total fat 4.7 (2.5) kg- and a 4.7 (2.5) cm increase in waist circumference.

Women Receiving Adjuvant Endocrine Therapy

Endocrine therapies such as tamoxifen and anastrazole are widely used as adjuvant treatment for prevention of breast cancer in the U.K. Among patients, the perception is that these therapies lead to weight gain, yet randomized studies have shown modest weight gains of 1 to 2 kg in study and control patients [11]. Weight change is a poor predictor of the amounts of fat and lean body mass and the distribution of fat, particularly among postmenopausal women [12].

We determined changes in body composition, body fat, and fat-free mass from skinfolds, waist and hip circumference, and abdominal skinfold over the first year of treatment among 23 postmenopausal women receiving adjuvant anastrozole or tamoxifen [13]. Mean (±SE) age of the group was 54.7 (0.8) years; mean (±SE) BMI after surgery was 27.8 (1.2) kg/m^2; percentage body fat was 39.0 (1.3)%. The modest weight gain in the endocrine group 2.6 (0.8) kg was comparable to published figures among healthy women: 2.1 (0.4) kg. Women receiving endocrine therapy appeared to have comparatively greater gains in total fat, particularly central fat, i.e., waist circumference and abdominal skinfold and a greater loss of fat-free mass compared to published data among healthy women (Table 35.3) [14,15]. Changes in body composition in women receiving adjuvant

TABLE 35.3
Changes in Weight and Body Composition among Women Receiving Adjuvant Endocrine with Tamoxifen (n = 7) or Anastrozole (n = 8) or Combined Anastrazole and Arimidex Therapy (n = 8) and in Healthy Menopausal Women over 1 Year

	Baseline in the endocrine group	Change over 12 months in endocrine group	Change over 12 months in healthy women
Weight (kilograms)	71.7 (4.3)[a]	2.6 (0.8)	2.1 (0.4)[b]
Body fat (kilograms)	28.7 (2.6)	4.2 (0.8)	0.3 (0.2)[c]
Fat free mass (kilograms)	42.9 (1.7)	−1.6 (0.5)	−0.14 (0.1)[c]
Waist (centimeters)	89.3 (3.5)	4.4 (1.3)	2.8 (0.4)[b]
Hip (centimeters)	103.6 (3.1)	2.4 (1.1)	1.1 (0.5)[b]
Abdominal skinfold (millimeters)	45.6 (2.4)	11 (1.4)	No data

[a]Mean (standard error).
[b]Published data from Espeland, M.A. et al., *J Clin Endocrinol Metab* 1997; 82:1549–1556.
[c]Published data from Dawson–Hughes, B. and Harris, S. *Am J Clin Nutr* 1992; 56: 307–313.

endocrine therapy were largely independent of weight change and highlight the importance of assessing body composition in addition to weight postoperatively.

The absence of a control group means that conclusions cannot be drawn as to whether the changes relate to the therapies or simply reflect the normal effects of inactivity among women recently diagnosed with breast cancer, recovering from breast surgery, and undergoing radiotherapy. It is possible that changes may specifically relate to the effects of the associated lower estrogen levels (anastrozole) or the estrogen agonist/antagonist action (tamoxifen) on body composition. However, an earlier prospective randomized prevention study among healthy women reported minimal weight change, but significant increases in central fat among study patients on tamoxifen and control patients [16].

The propensity to increase fat, particularly central fat, and lose lean body mass among women receiving endocrine therapy may have adverse metabolic and prognostic effects. Gains in body fat and waist circumference will be perceived by women and may explain the large numbers of women (40%) who complain of "weight gain" during adjuvant endocrine therapy [17] when seemingly only modest changes in body mass occur. The concern of weight gain among women may decrease compliance with these adjuvant agents.

SUBGROUPS OF EARLY BREAST CANCER PATIENTS IN WHICH WEIGHT MANAGEMENT MAY BE IMPORTANT

British South Asian women

Although rates of breast cancer in British South Asian women are lower than in their British native counterparts, they are increasing rapidly. A recent survey estimated a 37% increase in the incidence of breast cancer over the past decade among South Asians from the city of Leicester [18]. A further report suggested that Pakistani or Indian Muslims have a significantly higher risk of breast cancer compared to Gujarati Hindi women (RR 2.32 [95% confidence intervals 1.38–3.88]; Figure 35.4), which was attributed to higher levels of central obesity, higher intakes of dietary fat, and lower intakes of dietary fiber [19]. Pakistani or Indian Muslim breast cancer patients are groups who may well benefit from weight control advice.

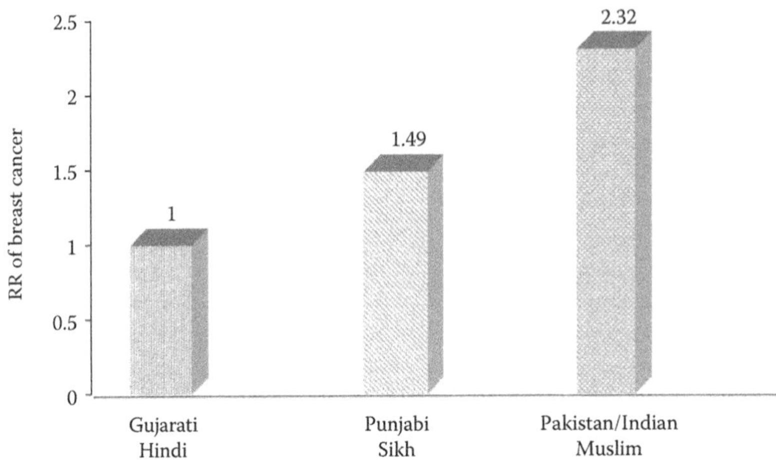

FIGURE 35.4 Breast cancer risk among different ethnic groups in the U.K. (Adapted from McCormack, V.A. et al., *Br J Cancer* 2004; 90(1):160–166.)

Women from Lower Social Classes

Breast cancer occurs most frequently among women in the higher social classes. Typically, only 15% of the breast cancer patients diagnosed are from lower social classes, although lower social class is well known to be linked to a poorer survival (relative risk of death from breast cancer of 1.32 [CI 1.12 to 1.55]) [20].

Strategies to improve survival among socially deprived women are an identified priority for cancer services in the U.K. Part but by no means all of the adverse prognosis is attributed to later stage of presentation and more advanced disease in these socially disadvantaged women. Some believe that the greater prevalence of obesity among women from lower social classes may also be a contributory factor to their poorer survival (Figure 35.5) [21]. Weight management may be particularly applicable to women from the lower social classes.

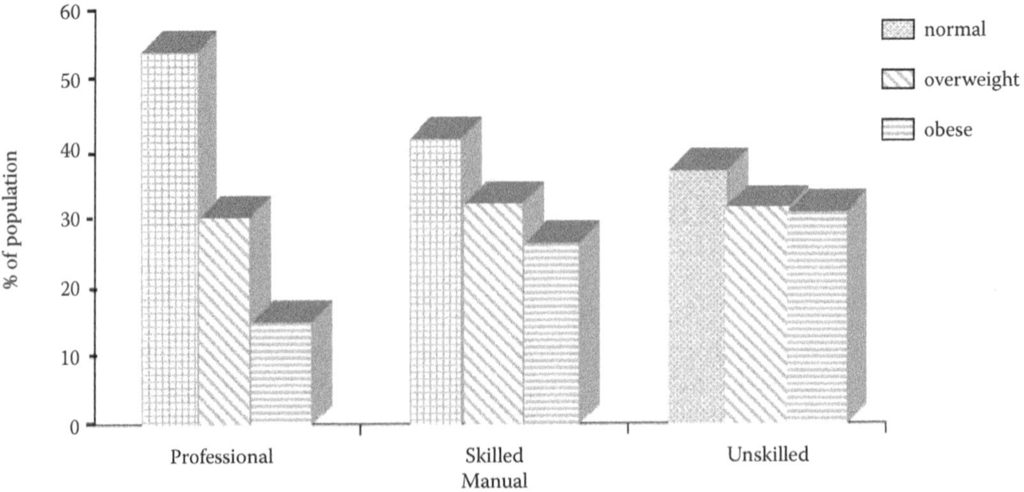

FIGURE 35.5 Prevalence of overweight and obesity by social class in England. (Adapted from http://www.publications.doh.gov.uk/public/hse98.htm, accessed July 2004 [64].)

Patients Who Stop Smoking

The widely perceived links between smoking and cancer and the motivation to change health behaviors at the time of diagnosis mean a number of patients cease smoking around the time of cancer diagnosis. Smoking cessation will undoubtedly improve their overall health, but will most likely also lead to weight gain. Typically, weight gains of between 3.5 to 6 kg are reported after smoking cessation [22]. Diet and exercise weight management advice are often used as an adjunct to smoking cessation advice to limit weight gain and increase adherence with smoking cessation. Weight gain after quitting smoking is frequently cited as a reason for relapsing after smoking cessation, particularly among women [23].

Overweight Patients with Lymphedema

Lymphedema is an undesirable complication following axillary clearance or radiotherapy to the axilla that has negative physical and psychological impacts on women [24]. Obesity has been cited as an additional risk factor for the development of lymphedema [25], possibly due to increased risk of postoperative infections, coupled with the increased likelihood of technical problems during axillary surgery among heavier women. Higher failure rates of the less invasive sentinel node biopsy among heavier women mean heavier women are more likely to undergo complete axillary dissection for staging.

Little work has been done on the effects of weight loss on existing lymphedema. A recent randomized, controlled study undertaken at The Royal Marsden Hospital, London, examined the effects of a weight reduction diet compared to no dietary intervention in overweight women with lymphedema following treatment for breast cancer. The dietary intervention was delivered by a state-registered dietician. Women wore compression hosiery as part of their usual lymphedema management. Arm volume, as measured by circumference measurements, was significantly reduced in the weight reduction group when compared with the control group. Further research is planned by this group to examine the mechanism whereby weight reduction helps to reduce arm volume (C. Shaw, personal communication, 2004).

CURRENT PRACTICE AND ATTITUDES TO WEIGHT MANAGEMENT OF BREAST CANCER PATIENTS AMONG HEALTH CARE PROFESSIONALS IN U.K. CANCER CENTERS

Nutritional management of the cancer patient has traditionally focused on malnutrition and nutrition support rather than weight management. An increasing body of evidence indicates that disease progression and quality of life of breast cancer patients may be modified through weight control and exercise [26]. We conducted a structured interview questionnaire by telephone with oncology dieticians ($n = 20$) in randomly selected cancer hospitals within the U.K.; current practice and their views on the potential benefits and appropriateness, as well as potential problems of implementing diet and exercise weight management interventions for breast cancer patients, were assessed. We also interviewed specialist breast care nurses ($n = 8$), medical oncologists ($n = 3$), and breast surgeons ($n = 2$) in these hospitals to provide a multidisciplinary perspective on weight management for breast cancer patients.

Current weight management practice by dieticians in the U.K. is shown in Table 35.4. There was little current dietetic input to breast cancer patients. Dieticians were not routinely involved in advising patients with breast cancer. The majority of dieticians interviewed advised the occasional patient (75%) and dieticians in other centers had no involvement with breast cancer patients (25%). Patients seen were mainly seen at the request of the patients (92%) rather than of the medical oncologist or surgeon (8%). The majority of patients had received adjuvant chemotherapy (66%), although those receiving endocrine therapy (34%) were also seen. The majority of patients were

TABLE 35.4
Current Weight Management Practice for Breast Cancer Patients in 20 Cancer Centers in the U.K.

		Percentage of centers
Level of weight management service provided by dietetic department	Small numbers of breast cancer patients seen	75
	Do not give weight management advice	25
Source of referral	Self-referral by patients	92
	Referred by medical oncologist	8
Patient groups referred for weight management advice	Chemotherapy	66
	Endocrine therapy	34
Timing and type of advice given	Weight maintenance during treatment	26
	Weight loss during treatment	13
	Weight loss after treatment	61
	General healthy eating leaflets provided in treatment areas	50
	Healthy eating talks to breast cancer support groups	25
Routine monitoring of weight	Patients receiving chemotherapy	90
	Patients receiving endocrine therapy	10
	Monitoring of body fat or waist circumferences	0
Treatment program	Dietetic advice — one-off consultation	55
	Dietetic advice — repeated visits	15
	Multidisciplinary weight loss program within oncology center (dietitian, psychologist, breast cancer nurses, physiotherapist)	15
	Specialist multidisciplinary general weight loss program	15
	Use of exercise on prescription	15

given weight management advice after treatment had finished (61%), although some centers did provide weight maintenance (26%) and weight loss advice (13%) during treatment. The majority of patients received weight loss advice as a single dietetic consultation (55%). Others offered a multidisciplinary weight loss program for these breast cancer patients within the oncology center (15%) or in a general weight management clinic (15%).

Although current dietetic input was quite low, the majority of dieticians felt that further weight management service should ideally be provided within the specialist oncology center (76%). Some of the reasons to support weight management and caveats to providing weight management are cited in Table 35.5. The limited funding for oncology dietetic services is one of the major barriers to the development of weight management services within oncology centers. The remaining

TABLE 35.5
Health Care Professionals' Views on Weight Control in the Management of Breast Cancer Patients

Dieticians' reasons to incorporate weight control management	Percentage of dieticians
Breast cancer patients are interested in diet and health and particularly receptive to health promotion advice.	40
Weight gain is a major source of distress for cancer patients.	30
Provision of weight loss services within the specialist center means the unique expertise of cancer. patients and their treatments allow advice to be tailor made to cancer patients' needs.	30
Weight control should improve body image, which is important for breast cancer patients. Patients want advice and thus may well seek less considered advice elsewhere.	30
Need to provide sensible nutrition advice to offset less balanced advice that may be received from the media, Internet, friends, and family.	20
Absence of sensible weight loss advice may lead to erratic eating patterns, omission of important food groups, and inadequate diets.	20
Important to educate families of patients to help prevent weight gain; families may be overprotective and may feed the patient up and discourage exercise.	6
Dieticians' reasons not to incorporate weight control management	
Weight management is labor intensive. Dietetic departments are already under-resourced and cannot currently provide such a service. Large increases in staffing levels would be required.	94
Discourage attempts to lose weight until patients had finished their treatment because they felt it could jeopardize the cancer patients.	30
Weight management is not a priority in the management of cancer patients.	20
Alerting patients to their weight and diet may be an additional and unwelcome burden for patients as they go through cancer treatment.	20
Dieticians who perceived a poor success rate with weight reduction advice viewed weight management as a poor use of limited dietetic resources.	20
Concern about recommending weight loss because they felt this might jeopardize future health of the cancer patients.	20
The evidence base for the beneficial effects of weight reduction advice is not strong enough to make recommendations.	20
Weight loss is not part of the recommended National Institute Clinical Excellence (NICE) care pathways and not likely to become common practice.	20
They do not see relevance of weight management in the care pathway of cancer patients.	15
Oncology dieticians aim to get patients through treatment and are not involved in the future health of the patients.	15
Eating is a coping strategy for some women with breast cancer. Restricting food intake during chemotherapy may remove this coping strategy.	7
Breast care nurses' views of weight management for breast cancer patients	
Weight control is an important issue with regard to breast reconstruction and matching of prosthesis.	
Weight is likely to be a sensitive subject particularly in the overweight/obese woman. Women recently diagnosed with breast cancer may not be able to deal with the weight issue as well.	
Encouraging women to try to lose weight and exercise is reassuring women that they can return to normal life and function.	
It may be difficult for women to limit their food intake during chemotherapy. Overeating is a function of comfort eating; alterations in taste are often driven by fatigue and boredom.	
Promoting exercise is good for women who exercised prior to diagnosis.	
It is likely to be difficult to motivate previous nonexercisers to take up exercise.	

(continued)

TABLE 35.5 (CONTINUED)
Health Care Professionals' Views on Weight Control in the Management of Breast Cancer Patients

Patients and health care professionals may consider weight issues as trivial compared to the diagnosis of cancer.
Diet and exercise interventions will only be effective in motivated individuals and should be provided for those who express an interest but not imposed on all breast cancer patients.
Burdening patients with additional worry of weight is a concern. The role of the breast cancer nurse is to promote the psychological well-being of the patient and he or she does not want to add to their anxiety and stress.

Medical oncologists' and breast surgeons' views of weight management for breast cancer patients
Patients believe that all weight gain is due to the drug treatments and not in their control. It may be difficult to convince them otherwise.
Patients are fixated with dietary components — i.e., milk-free, vitamin supplements rather than weight.
There are inadequate staffing resources to address these issues in cancer centers.
Weight management services are unlikely to attract funding within the National Health Service. It is necessary to demonstrate tangible benefits and cost effectiveness of such a service to attract adequate resources.
Weight management is not a clinical priority within cancer centers.

dieticians (24%) felt that weight management was not the domain of the specialist oncology centers, stating that primary care teams should address weight management once the patient had been discharged from the specialist oncology center.

The majority of breast cancer nurses routinely counseled all women receiving adjuvant breast cancer to adhere to a healthy diet and try to exercise to limit weight gain during treatment (63%). Others only raised the issue of weight management if asked by the patients (25%) or not all (12%). Among breast care nurses, concerns were that raising the issue of weight was adding an additional burden to breast cancer patients when they were already dealing with the stress of a recent diagnosis. Medical oncologists were aware that weight management was an issue among women with early breast cancer. This was not considered a clinical priority within the cancer service compared to more pressing issues of securing funding for appropriate chemotherapy treatments.

EXERCISE INTERVENTIONS IN THE U.K.

A growing body of evidence indicates the potential benefits of exercise among breast cancer patients. The effects of exercise on survival and prognosis are not well established. Recent data from the Nurse's Health Study, however, suggest that moderate activity in excess of 3 hours per week may promote survival among women with stages I through III breast cancer [27]. Exercise has been consistently shown to have beneficial effects on body composition [28], physical function [29], well-being, and fatigue in cancer patients [30].

A recent postal survey of oncology nurses in U.K. hospitals was conducted to ascertain the extent to which exercise has a role in cancer care [31]. This survey was not specifically examining the provision for breast cancer patients; nevertheless, it showed that, in general, use of exercise within cancer care in the U.K. is currently rare. The sample of 221 hospitals had a 62% response rate. Some kind of exercise program or class for patients was offered by 19 hospitals (9%). In a further 17 (8%), other opportunities for exercise were available (e.g., an exercise bicycle for inpatients). Among nurses, 65% were in favor of the idea of providing a specific exercise rehabilitation service for patients. Scarce resources and lack of awareness and expertise were identified as common barriers to establishing such a service. More than half (58%) of nurses were unaware of or unfamiliar with the published research on exercise for cancer rehabilitation and 33% reported receiving no training relating to exercise and health. The survey results indicate that some hospitals include exercise in the services offered to patients and that the majority of nurses favor adopting exercise as a rehabilitation intervention.

CLINICAL PRACTICE IN THE U.K. — AUDIT OF A WEIGHT LOSS SERVICE FOR BREAST CANCER PATIENTS

Few oncology dieticians are involved in weight management of breast cancer patients. An audit of a weight loss service for breast cancer patients managed by a dedicated oncology dietician in Ormskirk, N West England, suggests that this can be a successful approach (Table 35.6). Weight was lost by 80% of patients and a further 12.5% maintained current weight; only 6% of patients continued to gain weight. Average weight loss was 3.6 (1 to 11) kg. The dietician saw patients fortnightly or monthly; 27% of the patients were also referred to the psychologist for counseling (H. Lugton, Southport and Ormsmirk Primary Care Trust, personal communication).

INFORMATION NEEDS OF CANCER PATIENTS

Patients cope better with cancer when they are provided with clear, adequate information tailored to their needs. Awareness of the importance of meeting the information needs of cancer patients is increasing within the U.K. The need for better information was a patient-identified priority in the recent national cancer patient survey [32].

Breast cancer patients are well known to seek information regarding their disease, particularly in relation to the potential benefits of diet. Salminen et al. [33] recently reported on the dietary information currently available and the need for dietary counseling among breast cancer patients from Australia (n = 215) and Finland (n = 139). Approximately 30% of these women expressed the need for more information on dietary factors relating to disease. The health care professionals did not currently meet their needs for nutritional advice. Only 24% of patients had received dietary advice from health care professionals; the majority had instead received their dietary advice from the media (44%).

TABLE 35.6
Audit of a Weight Management Service among Women with Breast Cancer[a]

Organization of clinic	New patients scheduled for 30- to 60-minute consultation Review patients scheduled for 15- to 30-minute consultation Patients are seen fortnightly or monthly
Weight at time of referral	Average weight gain since diagnosis: 9.7 (4.5–27.5) kg Average BMI: 27.9 (21–36) kg/ m^2
Aims of dietetic management	To achieve weight loss: 86% To achieve weight maintenance: 14%
Weight loss achieved	Mean (range) 3.6 (1–11) kg
Patients requiring additional counseling with psychologist	27%

[a] N = 30.

Source: H. Lugton, personal communication.

The limited access to dietetic advice for breast cancer patients within the U.K. most likely means that the number of patients with unmet dietary information needs is even higher. We examined changes made to diet since diagnosis of breast cancer and the sources of information that prompted these changes among 37 consecutive patients with metastatic breast cancer attending clinic in our institution. Women had a median (range) age of 53 (36 to 76) years and had been diagnosed a median (range) of 3 (0.5 to 20) years previously. Thirteen of the women (35%) had changed their diet since diagnosis of breast cancer, and 12 (36%) had commenced vitamin or other nutritional supplements. Only one of the women had changed her diet on the basis of advice from a health care professional. The most common sources of advice were the mass media (55%) and family and friends (22%). Dietary changes, use of vitamin supplements, and sources of dietary information are reported in Figure 35.6A through Figure 35.6D.

There is a move toward developing information leaflets in collaboration with patient support groups to increase their relevance to the patient experience. However, there is also awareness that simply providing information leaflets may not meet patients' needs. A recent focus group of cancer patients examining the information provided on cancer fatigue revealed that many patients found it difficult to access written resources. More importantly, they preferred to receive advice directly from a health care professional. Written information was no substitute for this personal advice [34].

Women from lower social classes and women from ethnic minorities are poorly served with appropriate information. These groups are traditionally a minority of the patients diagnosed with breast cancer; however, they are increasing in number and are likely to be overweight [18]. These patients are far more likely to depend on high-quality information from within the cancer service because they are less able to access information from external sources such as charities or the Internet. A recent survey showed that information needs of British Asian cancer patients were

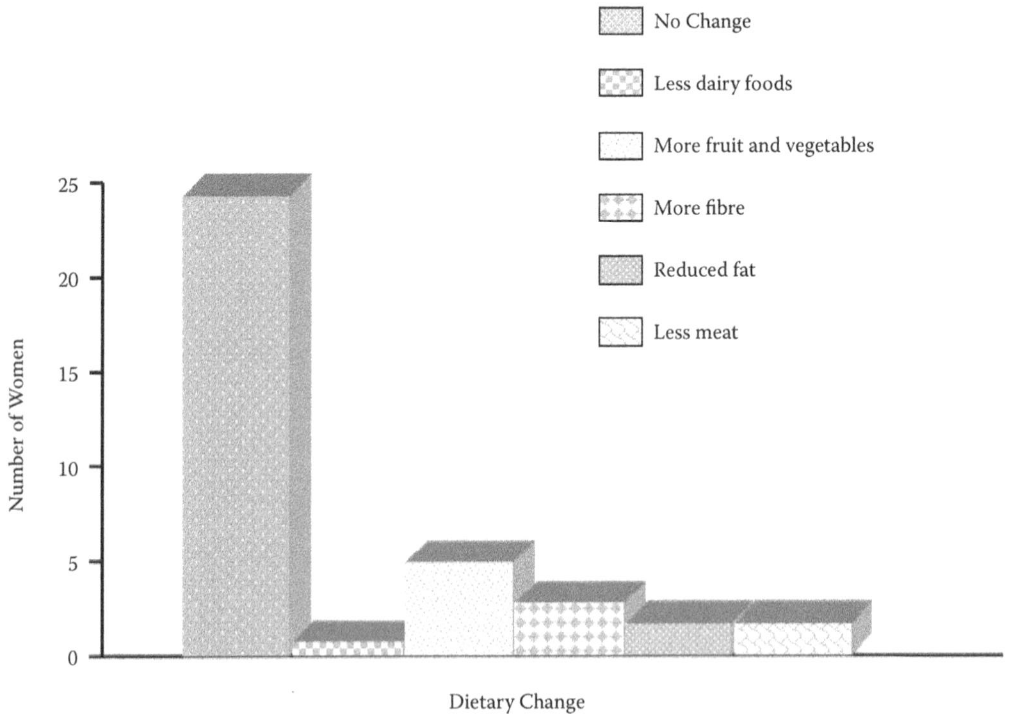

FIGURE 35.6A Dietary change since diagnosis among patients with metastic breast cancer.

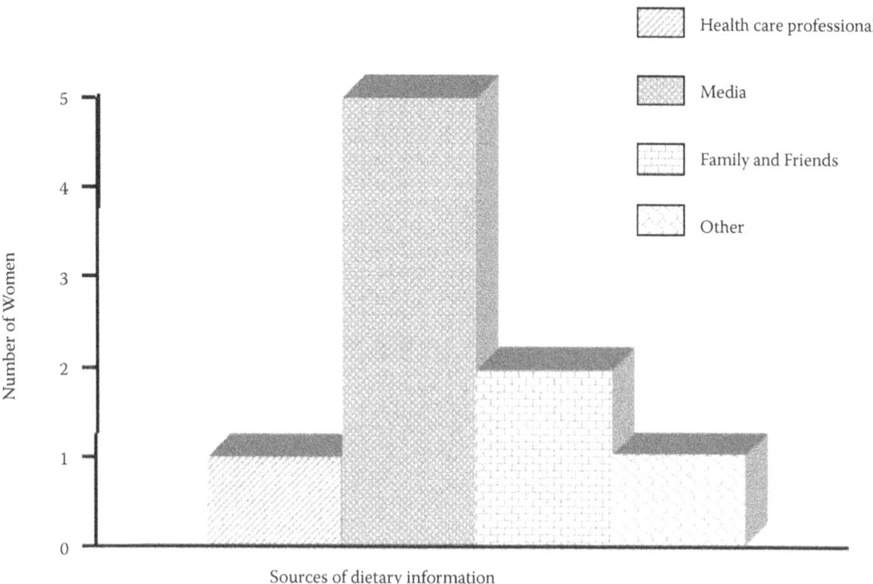

FIGURE 35.6B Sources of dietary advice since diagnosis among patients with metastasic breast cancer.

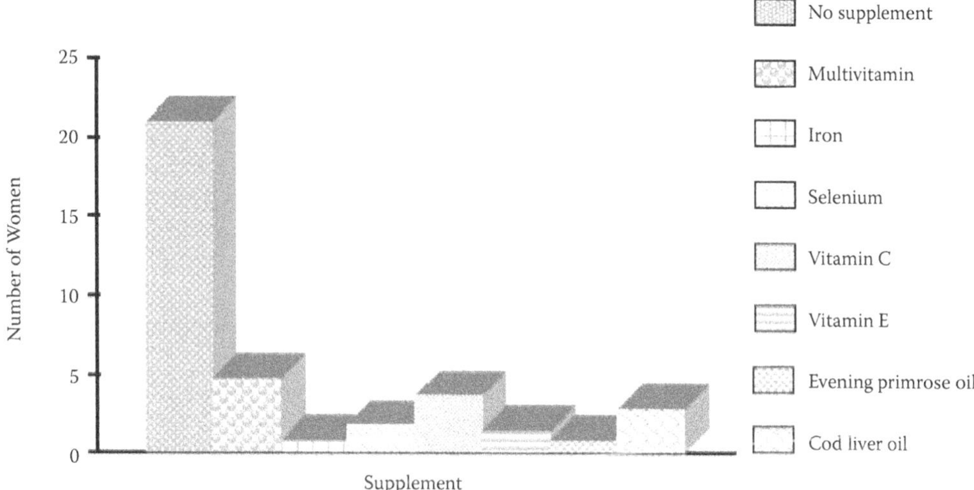

FIGURE 35.6C Use of nutritional supplements since diagnosis among patients with metastatic breast cancer.

poorly served. Patients in this survey expressed a need for verbal and written information conveyed in their own language. This information should be provided within the oncology service or via their general practitioner [35].

CURRENT RESEARCH PROGRAMS WITHIN THE U.K.

- Supervised exercise program as a rehabilitation treatment for women receiving early stage breast cancer treatment — Anna Campbell, Nanette Mutrie, Fiona White, Fiona McGuire and Nora Kearney, MRC Social and Public Health Sciences Unit, Institute of

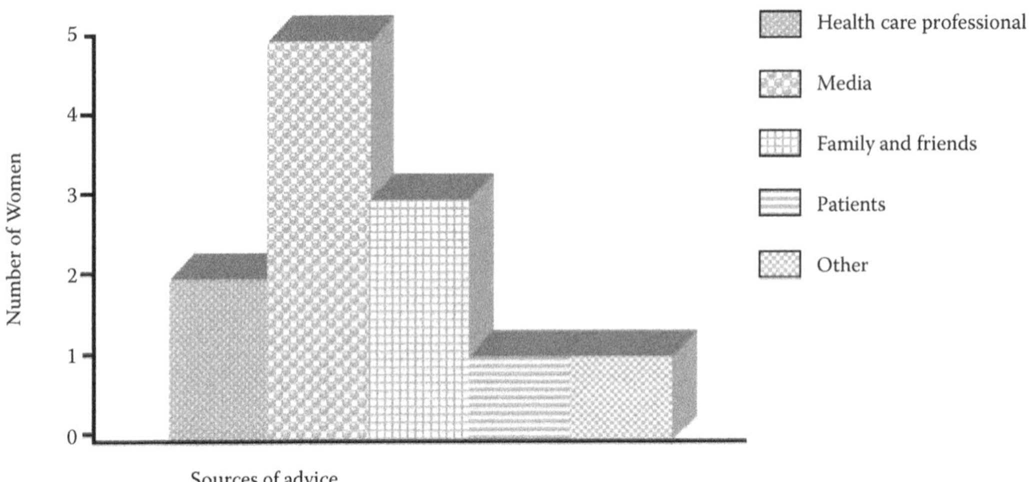

FIGURE 35.6D Source of advice on nutritional supplements among patients with metastic breast cancer.

Biomedical and Life Sciences Glasgow, University of Glasgow, and University of Stirling.

This group recently undertook a randomized controlled pilot study to examine whether exercise as an adjunctive rehabilitation therapy could benefit women who have early stage breast cancer and are currently receiving chemotherapy/radiotherapy. Physical functioning, fatigue, and quality of life (QoL) outcomes were evaluated before and after a 12-week intervention. The results showed that after 12 weeks the women who participated in the exercise program (n = 12) displayed higher levels of physical functioning and reported higher quality of life scores than the controls did (n = 10). Changes favored the intervention group but did not reach statistical significance. This pilot study did not allow appropriately powered analyses of fatigue and satisfaction with life and favored relatively young and socioeconomically advantaged women [36].

- Randomized controlled trial of a supervised exercise program as rehabilitation treatment for women receiving early stage breast cancer treatment

  This follow up study by the Glasgow group is examining the effects of a supervised exercise program (twice weekly exercise classes for 12 weeks) on a number of psychological/quality of life (FACT B FACT F — fatigue) and physical (fitness — 12-minute walk test, 7-day recall of activity, BMI) outcome measures. The study will be conducted in 182 women currently undergoing treatment for early breast cancer. Eligible women will have received breast surgery and will currently be receiving adjuvant radiotherapy, chemotherapy, or tamoxifen treatment. Women will be recruited around the time of the second or third chemotherapy cycle or during the second or third week of radiotherapy. Focus groups among women attending a high and low number of classes are planned to examine the issues of adherence to exercise interventions. The results of this study are expected in August, 2005.

- Exercise therapy in women who have had breast cancer — Sheffield Women's Exercise and Well-Being Project — A.J. Daly, N. Mutrie, H. Crank, R. Coleman, and J. Saxton, Department of Primary Care and General Practice, University of Birmingham.

  This is a randomized controlled trial to evaluate the effects of exercise therapy on quality of life in 120 women who have completed chemotherapy or radiotherapy within the past 12 to 36 months. Participants will be randomized to one of three groups: exercise therapy (one-to-one counseling, 30 minutes of aerobic exercise and 20 minutes of exercise counseling three times a week); body conditioning (50 minutes of low-intensity body conditioning); or a control group (usual patient care) over 8 weeks. Outcome measures are quality of life, physical self-perceptions, depression, satisfaction with life, aerobic capacity, and percent of body fat (bioelectrical impedance). Follow-up assessments at 3 and 6 months postintervention are planned to assess the long-term impact of these interventions. This study seeks to examine the use of the theory of planned behavior to predict exercise behavior over the study period [37].

- Women's Intervention Nutrition Study (U.K.): stage 1 — B. Parry, R. Rainsbury, and J. Cade, Royal Hampshire County Hospital, Winchester.

  This multicenter randomized controlled trial is examining whether it is possible for women in the U.K. who have been treated for early breast cancer diagnosed after menopause to reduce their current fat intake by at least half and continue to follow this very low fat diet over 2 years, given advice and support. The study has currently recruited 150 of the 240 women required. Women are aged 48 to 78 years, 1 year after breast surgery with invasive and noninvasive ductal carcinoma *in situ*. Women are divided into two groups: one is given advice and support to maintain a healthy way of eating and the other is given advice and support to follow a very low fat diet. Women meet regularly in small groups for advice about their eating. These small groups support the women following the very low fat diet separately from those following the general healthy eating advice. The amount of fat eaten is measured using 4-day food diaries, completed on seven occasions during the study period. All women will have their weight, waist and hip circumferences, quality of life (FACT – B), and lipid profile measured regularly throughout the study.

GUIDELINES FOR WEIGHT MANAGEMENT IN EARLY BREAST CANCER PATIENTS

NICE Guidelines for Best Clinical Practice

Clinical practice in the U.K. is mainly led by evidence-based guidelines from the National Institute of Clinical Excellence (NICE). No NICE guidelines currently address the provision of diet and exercise advice among breast cancer patients. Recent guidelines on improving outcomes in breast cancer [38] recommended that a multidisciplinary team, which must include a specialist breast care nurse, should treat breast cancer patients. This document acknowledged that some patients may also require access to a physiotherapist, but does not mention the need for dietetic support. Further NICE guidelines for improving supportive care for adults with cancer recognized the important role of the professions allied to medicine — i.e., physiotherapists, dietitians, and occupational therapists — in the rehabilitation of cancer patients and highlighted the need for more therapists [39].

Recommended Guidelines for Weight Management in Early Breast Cancer

A recommended treatment pathway for the weight management of early breast cancer patients is shown in Figure 35.7. Weight management advice can be delivered during active chemotherapy or radiotherapy treatment, in the immediate post-treatment recovery phase, at any time after treatment, or at any point after commencing adjuvant endocrine therapy.

During Chemotherapy or Radiotherapy and Endocrine Therapy

All patients should receive counseling regarding healthy eating and weight maintenance and be encouraged to be physically active during treatment. High-quality nutritional information should be available to answer nutritional queries that the patient may have. Patients with existing weight problems may be a group at particularly high risk of weight gain as they undergo treatment, but this is not resolved [40,41]. Patients wishing to lose weight at this stage with a BMI ≥ 25 kg/m^2 or a waist circumference ≥ 88 cm should be referred to the dietitian for assessment and entered into a weight loss program wherever appropriate.

Recovery Phase

Weight loss should be advised when relevant in individuals who are seeking this advice. Exercise should be promoted to foster rehabilitation.

Health Maintenance

To avoid recurrence of breast cancer, the occurrence of other preventable diseases (i.e., osteoporosis, cardiovascular disease, diabetes), and to promote good psychological health and well-being, healthy eating, exercise, and weight control should be promoted at follow-up appointments after treatment to encourage lifelong habits. Patients who report significant gains in weight since diagnosis (>5 kg) or who have larger waist or BMI should be referred for dietetic assessment and entered into a weight loss program wherever appropriate.

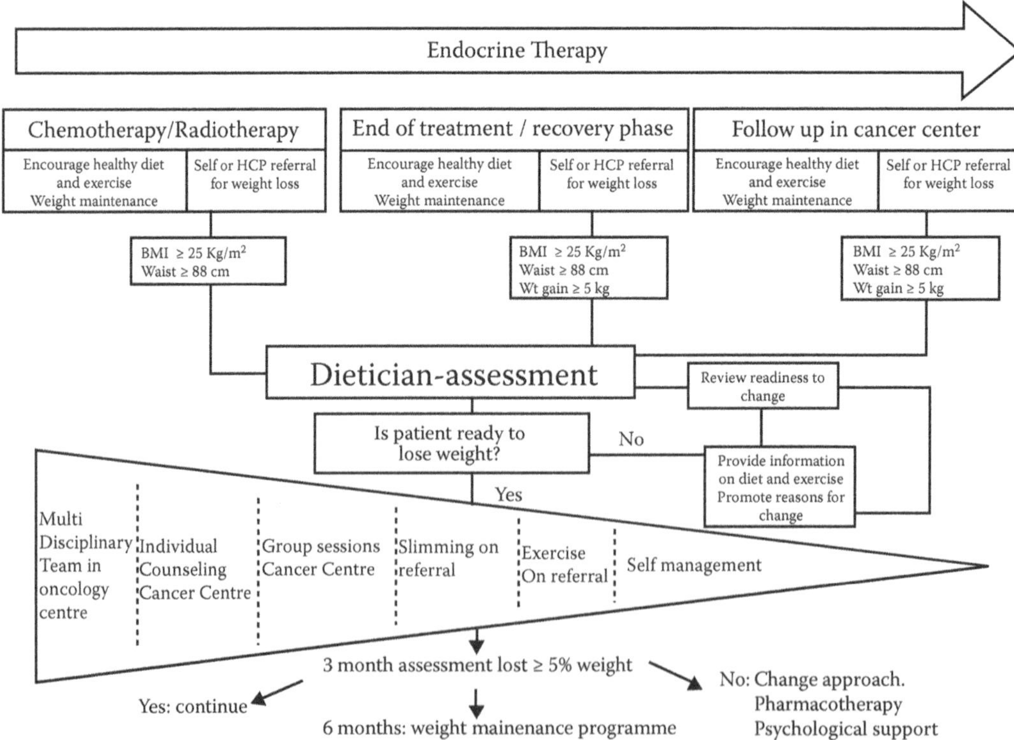

FIGURE 35.7 Suggested treatment pathway for weight management of breast cancer patients.

Assessment of Body Weight and Body Composition in Breast Cancer Patients

The amount of fat and lean tissue should ideally be assessed in breast cancer patients. Weight is a poor predictor of changes in body fat, particularly among patients receiving chemotherapy or endocrine therapy for breast cancer. Bioelectrical impedance is increasingly used to assess body composition in weight management settings. Impedance is the resistance of the body to the flow of an alternating current. This technique is based on the fact that lean tissues have a high water and electrolyte content and are good conductors, whereas fat is a poor conductor. Impedance measurements are thus related to the volume of the conductor, which relates to total body water, fat-free mass, and fat mass. However, impedance does not appear to be a good predictor of changes in body fat among women receiving adjuvant chemotherapy [10] because they may have unpredictable changes in fluid and electrolyte distribution and the ratio of extracellular to intracellular fluid. A further limitation of impedance among women receiving adjuvant or endocrine therapy is that impedance is insensitive to measure changes in central fat stores [42].

In noncancer settings, focus has increasingly been on the importance of waist measurements rather than BMI as a marker of risk for weight-related comorbidity. Specifically, waist measurements predict aspects of the metabolic syndrome, i.e., insulin resistance, hypertension, and dyslipidemia [43]. The avoidance of metabolic syndrome is relevant among breast cancer patients. This will reduce the likelihood of comorbidities such as heart diseases and diabetes. Aspects of the metabolic syndrome — i.e., insulin resistance [44] and a greater waist to hip ratio [45] — have been linked to a poorer prognosis.

Waist and hip circumferences should be measured alongside weight measurements among breast cancer patients. For non-Asian women, a waist circumference > 32 in. (80 cm) is considered to place women at an increased risk of metabolic syndrome, and a waist circumference > 35 in. (88 cm) places women at high risk of metabolic syndrome. For Asian women, a waist greater than 32 in. (80 cm) places women at high risk of metabolic syndrome. In our studies among early breast cancer patients, the proportion of women who had a "high-risk" waist measurement at 1 year from commencing adjuvant chemotherapy (70% of patients at 1 year compared to 40% at baseline) or adjuvant endocrine therapy (53% of patients at 1 year compared to 40% at baseline) increased significantly.

Identifying Patients Suitable for Weight Loss Interventions

Patients

Women may self-refer or be referred by a health care professional to lose weight. Weight management should be prioritized for women who have a BMI ≥ 25 kg/m^2, gained ≥5 kg of body weight over the course of treatment, or have a waist measurement ≥ 88 cm.

Motivation for and Barriers to Success for Successful Weight Loss

Motivation is pivotal to the success of any diet and exercise weight loss interventions. Motivation to make necessary changes to diet and exercise behaviors should be explored from discussion with the dietitian — i.e., how willing, able, and ready the patient is to make these changes. The relative benefits and problems of making changes to these behaviors should also be explored. Patients who are not able to make changes at present should be counseled to promote reasons to change and reviewed at a later stage.

Patients should also be screened for depression and other psychiatric disorders (General Health Questionnaire, GHQ) and referred for psychiatric input wherever appropriate. The prevalence of depression among breast cancer patients is estimated to be between 25 to 35% using screening tools like the GHQ [46]. The number of depressed overweight women breast cancer survivors is likely to be even greater because obesity increases the risk of depression. This is particularly relevant for women entering a weight loss program; the presence of depression or other psychiatric disorders is known to limit the success of weight loss interventions in breast cancer survivors [47].

Weight Management Advice

Need for an Individualized Approach

Loss of body fat is an inevitable consequence of a reduction in intake of energy and/or an increase in energy expenditure — i.e., an increase in the level of physical activity. The relative benefits of the different weight loss approaches and the level of support required for successful weight loss have been the subject of much debate. The success of any dietary and exercise intervention in an individual mainly depends on the level of adherence to the regimen, which in turn reflects individual preferences and lifestyles and the level of support required. Not surprisingly, it is becoming increasingly evident that the best way to achieve and maintain weight loss is to choose an approach suited to individual lifestyle and preferences, with the appropriate level of support [48].

Goal Setting

Treatment goals may focus on attaining a specific weight loss (typically, ≥5%), maintaining current weight, or changing specific diet and exercise behaviors. Weight loss of 5% is linked to significant reductions in risk of diabetes [49] and cardiovascular disease [50]. The effects of weight loss on risk of breast cancer recurrence are not known. Modest weight loss of 5% has reduced serum levels of estradiol (17%) among healthy postmenopausal women [51] and serum levels of testosterone (23%) alongside increases in sex hormone binding globulin (22%) among healthy premenopausal women [52].

Weight Loss Advice

A combined diet and exercise approach should be used to achieve weight loss or maintenance among breast cancer patients. The benefits of exercise among breast cancer survivors — aside from the effect of exercise on weight control — mean that exercise is a pivotal component in any weight loss intervention. Diet and exercise advice should be personalized and tailored to a woman's individual needs.

Patients should be counseled on ways to achieve a nutritionally balanced, calorie-restricted diet based on a range of foods that include high intakes of cereal fiber, fruit, and vegetables and low intake of saturated fat and refined sugar. The benefits of a high-fiber intake for breast cancer patients were recently supported by observations that an increase in fiber intake led to declines in estradiol among breast cancer patients in the Women's Healthy Eating and Living Study [WHEL] [53]. Patients should be counseled to avoid nutritionally inadequate fad diets, particularly calorie-controlled diets that are high in saturated fat, and low in fiber, fruit, and vegetables.

Factors to Promote Adherence to Weight Loss Program

Self-Monitoring

The use of food and exercise diaries to self-monitor diet and exercise patterns is well known to help promote and sustain beneficial changes in diet and exercise behaviors [42].

Self-Management

The level of support required to achieve and maintain weight loss varies widely between patients. Although supported programs tend to give better results overall, some sufficiently motivated individuals may opt to lose weight on their own after discussing the options with the health care practitioner. A recent audit among 1256 obese patients in primary care (74% female, 26% male) found that 8.8% of patients opted for self-management rather than the group or individualized services available [54]. Additional telephone support from a health care professional may be beneficial for these patients.

One-to-One vs. Group Counseling — Hospital Based

In the noncancer setting, the tendency has been to promote the use of group therapy above individualized counseling for weight loss. Groups were believed to provide better weight loss outcomes and a cost-effective way of addressing patient numbers. It is clear that patients will prefer a group or an individual approach. Matching treatment to their preferences will therefore provide better results [55].

Slimming on Prescription

In the noncancer setting, referring patients to commercial slimming groups can be an effective and sustainable way to successful weight loss and maintenance. A 12-week pilot scheme among 107 obese subjects (88% women, mean BMI 36 kg/m^2, range 30 to 47) reported that 36% of participants achieved a weight loss of 5% or greater. A number of schemes have been established between primary care trusts and the three main commercial slimming organizations within the U.K.: Slimming World, Weight Watchers, and Rosemary Conley Diet and Fitness Clubs.

The efficacy of slimming on prescription for cancer patients has not yet been demonstrated. Data from a pilot study in the U.S. suggested that slimming groups alone were by no means as effective in achieving weight loss as individual counseling from a specialist dietitian. In a group of obese cancer survivors, 48 were randomized to a control group, a Weight Watchers' group, one-to-one counseling with a specialist dietitian, and combined Weight Watchers and individualized counseling. Subjects in the three intervention groups lost weight over 12 months:

- Control: 1.1 ± 1.7 kg
- Weight Watchers group: –2.7 ± 2.1 kg
- Individually counseled group: –8.0 ± 1.9 kg
- Combined group: –9.5 ± 2.7 kg

Interestingly, the combined approach of the individual counseling and the commercial group was the most effective method of achieving weight loss in this study. Such an approach would allow individual problems of the cancer patients to be addressed and also provide the motivational benefits of commercial weight loss groups [56]. The potential role of slimming groups for the management of weight among breast cancer patients requires further investigation, but may be applicable for some patients.

Specialist Multidisciplinary Oncology Teams

It is likely that, for many patients with breast cancer, successful weight loss will require good diet and exercise advice to be underpinned with psychological support. This advice should be delivered from a multidisciplinary team that works in oncology and has a unique insight into the complexities of weight management and the treatments and psychological effects of the diagnosis of cancer and its treatment.

Pharmacotherapy for Weight Management

Two agents are currently available as part of a weight management program for overweight and obese patients in the U.K. Neither agent has been linked to the development of breast cancer; however, their different pharmacological properties, contraindications, and side effects require consideration for patients with breast cancer (Table 35.7).

Orlistat

Orlistat is a specific inhibitor of gastric and pancreatic lipases. The inactivated enzymes are thus unavailable to hydrolyse dietary fat, allowing 30% of dietary fat to pass through the gut unabsorbed. Patients are counseled to follow a hypocaloric diet containing less than 30% of energy from fat because high-fat diets lead to steatorrhea, flatus, and fecal urgency. Treatment with orlistat may potentially impair the absorption of fat-soluble vitamins (A, D, E, and K), although the vast majority of patients receiving up to 4 full years of treatment with orlistat in clinical studies had vitamin A, D, E, and K and beta-carotene levels that stayed within normal range. Diets rich in fruit and vegetables should be encouraged. Recent proteomic work suggested that orlistat might halt the proliferation of pancreatic tumor cells via an inhibitory effect on fatty acid synthetase [57]. This finding is not directly clinically relevant because orlistat exerts its therapeutic activity in the lumen of the stomach and has no defined systemic pharmacokinetic effects.

Sibutramine

Sibutramine inhibits the uptake of serotonin and noradrenalin in the brain. Weight loss is achieved through early satiety, with a reported 20% reduction in food intake; sympathetically mediated thermogenesis maintains original basal metabolic rate, which normally falls as weight is lost.

TABLE 35.7
Eligibility for Initiation and Continuation of Orlistat and Sibutramine for Weight Management

	Orlistat	Sibutramine
	Criteria for eligibility	
Age (years)	18–75	18–6 5
BMI (kg/m^2)	BMI > 30 BMI > 28 + comorbidity[a]	BMI > 30 BMI > 27 + comorbidity[b]
Weight loss required prior to first prescription	2.5 kg with diet and exercise	5% in the past 3 months
Contraindications	Malabsorptive conditions Cholestasis	BP > 145/90 mm Hg History of psychiatric illness, depression, eating disorder Patients taking antipsychotics/antidepressants History of stroke or heart failure
	Criteria for continuation of therapy	
1-Month criteria		Check blood pressure fortnightly; 2-kg weight loss
3-Month criteria	5% weight loss	5% weight loss
6-Month criteria	10% weight loss	10% weight loss
Maximum length of treatment	24 months	12 months

[a]Diabetes, hyperlipidaemia, hypertension, coronary heart disease, stroke.
[b]Diabetes, hyperlipidaemia. Sibutramine is contraindicated if BP > 145/90 mm Hg.

Source: Adapted from National Obesity Forum, www.nationalobesityforum.org.uk (accessed July 2004 [65].)

Sibutramine is contraindicated among patients with a history of psychiatric illness, depression, and eating disorder and in those with hypertension [43]. The prevalence of these psychiatric disorders [46] and hypertension [47] among obese breast cancer survivors may preclude use of sibutramine for a significant number of them.

Exercise on Prescription

Exercise on prescription schemes have existed in the U.K. since the early 1990s. These schemes refer patients to a 10- to 12-week cost-free or cost-reduced center (private or public gym and/or swimming facilities) based exercise program with an aim of promoting lifelong physical activity. Currently, 816 schemes are estimated to be operating in the U.K. [58]. Schemes are based in primary care settings, with general practitioners referring sedentary patients with a range of conditions, including obesity and cardiovascular disease.

The benefits of these schemes among breast cancer survivors have not been evaluated. Moreover, the effectiveness of these schemes in the noncancer setting is not resolved. In common with many interventions aimed at promoting physical activity, low uptake (41%) and adherence (28%) to the schemes have been reported [59]. Further uncertainty surrounds any long-term improvements in level of exercise achieved with these schemes [60]. The acceptability and efficacy of such schemes among the overweight and obese and in different cultural groups are not resolved [61]. Schemes, which make provision for the perceived barriers to exercise among these groups, are identified as research priorities.

FUTURE RESEARCH PRIORITIES

Currently, little data have been collected on the prevalence of weight problems and obesity-related comorbidities within breast cancer patients within the U.K. Breast cancer treatment units should maintain comprehensive databases recording weight, body composition (waist and hip measurements), and the prevalence of comorbidities at the time of diagnosis and throughout treatment.

The success of any weight management approach varies between individuals; thus, randomized studies comparing different approaches will not reveal the best way to manage the weight of an individual. The efficacy of a pragmatic weight management program using a range of approaches, as outlined earlier, on weight loss and maintenance among early breast cancer patients should be evaluated in a number of cancer centers. This weight management program should also be evaluated from a patient perspective, using qualitative data obtained from structured interviews and measures of health-related quality of life.

REFERENCES

1. Peto R, Boreham J, Clarke M, Davies C, Beral V. U.K. and USA breast cancer deaths down 25% in year 2000 at ages 20–69 years. *Lancet*. 2000; 355:1822.
2. Berclaz G et al. Body mass as a prognostic factor in operable breast cancer. The International Breast Cancer Study Group experience. *Ann Oncol* 2004; 15:875–884.
3. Gladieff L, Fumoleau P, Kerbrat P, Bonneterre J, Mayer F, Namer M, Monnier A, M-J Goudier, Luporsi E, Roche H. Which are the interactions between baseline body mass index, toxicity of chemotherapy and efficacy of adjuvant treatment? 9-year follow-up results of French Adjuvant Study Group (FASG) trials. ASCO 40th Annual Meeting 2004; A550.
4. Newman SC, Lees AW, Jenkins HJ. The effects of body mass index and oestrogen receptor level on survival of breast cancer patients International *J Epidemiol* 1997; 26:484–490.
5. Dignam JJ, Wieand K, Johnson KA, Fisher B, Xu L, Mamoumas EP. Obesity, tamoxifen use, and outcomes in women with oestrogen receptor-positive early stage breast cancer. *J Natl Cancer Inst* 2003; 95:1467–1476.

6. Lawlor DA, Smith GD, Ebrahim S. Hyperinsulinaemia and increased risk of breast cancer: findings from the British Women's Heart and Health Study. *Cancer Causes Control* 2004; 15:267–275.
7. Manjer J, Kaaks R, Riboli E, Berglund G. Risk of breast cancer in relation to anthropometry, blood pressure, blood lipids and glucose metabolism: a prospective study within the Malmo Preventive Project. *Eur J Cancer Prev* 2001; 10:33–42.
8. Camoriano JK, Loprinzi CL, Ingle JN, Therneau TM, Krook JE, Veeder MH. Weight change in women treated with adjuvant therapy or observed following mastectomy for node-positive breast cancer. *J Clin Oncol* 1990; 8:1327–1334.
9. Lankester KJ, Philips JE, Lawton PA. Weight gain during adjuvant and neoadjuvant chemotherapy for breast cancer: an audit of 100 women receiving FEC or CMF chemotherapy. *Clin Oncol* 2002; 14: 64–67.
10. Harvie MN, Campbell IT, Baildam A, Howell A. Energy balance in early breast cancer patients receiving adjuvant chemotherapy. *Breast Cancer Res Treat* 2004; 83, 201–10.
11. Baum M, Buzdar AU, Cuzick J, Forbes J, Houghton JH, Klijn JG, Sahmoud T, ATAC Trialists' Group. Anastrozole alone or in combination with tamoxifen versus tamoxifen alone for adjuvant treatment of postmenopausal women with early breast cancer: first results of the ATAC randomized trial. *Lancet* 2002; 359: 2131–2139.
12. Gallagher D, Visser M, Sepulveda D, Pierson RN, Harris T, Heymsfield SB. How useful is body mass index for comparison of body fatness across age, sex, and ethnic groups? *Am J Epidemiol* 1996; 143: 228–239.
13. Harvie MN, Campbell IT, Howell A, Thatcher N, and Baildam A. Changes in body composition in postmenopausal women receiving endocrine therapy. *Proc Nutr Soc* 2001; 60:90A.
14. Espeland MA, Stefanick ML, Kritz–Silverstein D, Feinberg E, Waclawiw MA, James MK, Greendale GA. Effect of postmenopausal hormone therapy on body weight and waist and hip girths. *J Clin Endocrinol Metab* 1997; 82:1549–1556.
15. Dawson–Hughes B, Harris S. Regional changes in body composition by time of year in healthy post menopausal women. *Am J Clin Nutr* 1992; 56: 307–313.
16. Grey AB, Stapleton JP, Evans MC, Reid IR. The effect of the antiestrogen tamoxifen on cardiovascular risk factors in normal postmenopausal women. *J Clin Endocrinol Metab* 1995; 80:3191–3195.
17. Fallowfield L, Fleissig A, Edwards R, et al. Tamoxifen for the prevention of breast cancer: psychosocial impact on women participating in two randomized controlled trials. *J Clin Oncol* 2001; 19:1885–1892.
18. Smith LK, Botha JL, Benghiat A, Steward WP. Latest trends in cancer incidence among U.K. South Asians in Leicester. *Br J Cancer* 2003; 89(1):70–733.
19. McCormack VA, Mangtani P, Bhakta D, McMichael AJ, dos Santos Silva I. Heterogeneity of breast cancer risk within the South Asian female population in England: a population-based case-control study of first-generation migrants. *Br J Cancer* 2004;90(1):160–166.
20. Kaffashian F, Godward S, Davies T, Solomon L, McCann J, Duffy SW. Socioeconomic effects on breast cancer survival: proportion attributable to stage and morphology. *Br J Cancer* 2003; 89(9):1693–1696.
21. Carmichael AR, Bates T. Obesity and breast cancer: a review of the literature. *Breast* 2004; 13(2):85–92.
22. Filozof C, Fernandez Pinilla MC, Fernandez–Cruz A. Smoking cessation and weight gain. *Obesity Rev* 2004; 5(2):95–103.
23. Klesges RC, Brown K, Pascale RW, Murphy M, Williams E, Cigrang JA. Factors associated with participation, attrition, and outcome in a smoking cessation program at the workplace. *Health Psychol* 1988; 7(6):575–589.
24. Tobin MB, Lacey HJ, Meyer L, Mortimer PS. The psychological morbidity ofbreast cancer-related arm swelling. Psychological morbidity of lymphoedema. *Cancer* 1993; 72(11):3248–3252.
25. Werner RS, McCormick B, Petrek J, Cox L, Cirrincione C, Gray JR, Yahalom J. Arm edema in conservatively managed breast cancer: obesity is a major predictive factor. *Radiology* 1991; 180(1):177–184.

26. Brown JK, Byers T, Doyle C, Coumeya KS, Demark-Wahnefried W, Kushi LH, McTierman A, Rock CL, Aziz N, Bloch AS, Eldridge B, Hamilton K, Katzin C, Loonce A, Main J, Mobley C, Morra ME, Pierce MS, Sawyer KA. American Cancer Society. Nutrition and physical activity during and after treatment: an American Cancer Society guide for informed choices. *Calif Cancer J Clin* 2003; 53(5):268–291.
27. Holmes MD, Chen WY, Feskanich D, Colditz GA. Physical activity and survival after breast cancer diagnosis. *Proc AACR*. 2004; 45:A1462.
28. Schmitz KH, Ahmed RL, Yee D. Effects of a 9-month strength training intervention on insulin, insulin-like growth factor (IGF)-1, IGF-binding protein (IGFBP)-1, and IGFBP-3 in 30- to 50-year-old women. *Cancer Epidemiol Boimarkers Prev* 2002; 11(12):1597–1604.
29. Segal R, Evans W, Johnson D, Smith J, Collettas, GJ, Woodard S, Wells S, Wells G, Reid R. Structured exercise improves physical functioning in women with stages I and II breast cancer: results of a randomized controlled trial. *J Clin Oncol* 2002; 19(3): 657–665.
30. Courneya KS, Mackey JR, Bell GJ, Jones LW, Field CJ, Fairey AS. Randomized controlled trial of exercise training in postmenopausal breast cancer survivors: cardiopulmonary and quality of life outcomes. *J Clin Oncol* 2003; 21(9):1660–1668.
31. Stevenson C, Fox KR. Role of exercise for cancer rehabilitation in hospitals: a survey of oncology nurses. *Eur J Cancer Care* 2005; 14(1): 63–69.
32. http://www.modern.nhs.uk/cancer/5628/6022/9203/CSC%20%Section% pdf (accessed July 2004).
33. Salminen E, Bishop M, Poussa T, Drummond R, Salminen S. Breast cancer patients have unmet needs for dietary advice. *Breast* 2002; 11(6):516–521.
34. Ream E, Browne N, Glaus A, Knipping C, Frei IA. Quality and efficacy of educational materials on cancer-related fatigue: views of patients from two European countries. *Eur J Oncol Nursing* 2003; 7(2):99–109.
35. Muthu Kumar D, Symonds RP, Sundar S, Ibrahim K, Savelyich BS, Miller E. Information needs of Asian and White British cancer patients and their families in Leicestershire: a cross-sectional survey. *Br J Cancer* 2004; 90(8):1474–1478.
36. Campbell A, Mutrie N, White F, McGuire F, Kearney N. Supervised exercise program as a rehabilitation treatment for women receiving early stage breast cancer treatment. *Eur J Oncol Nursing* 2005; 9(1): 55–63.
37. Daley AJ, Mutrie N, Crank H, Coleman R, Saxton J. Exercise therapy in women who have had breast cancer: design of the Sheffield Women's Exercise and Well-Being Project. *Health Educ Res* 2004; 19(6): 636–697.
38. Improving outcomes breast cancer, http://www.nice.org.uk/pdf/ (accessed July 2004).
39. http://www.nice.org.uk/pdf/csgspmanual.pdf (accessed July 2004).
40. Rock CL, Mc Eligot AJ, Flatt SW, Sobo EJ, Wilfley DE, Jones VE, Hollenbach KA, Marx RD. Eating pathology and obesity in women at risk for breast cancer recurrence. *Int J Eat Disord* 2000; 27(2):172–179.
41. Rock CL, Flatt SW, Newman V, CaanBJ, Haan MN, Stefanick ML, Faerber S, Pierce JP. Factors associated with weight gain in women after diagnosis of breast cancer. Women's Healthy Eating and Living Study Group. *J Am Diet Assoc* 1999; 99(10):1212–1221.
42. Baumgartner RN. Electrical impedence and total body conductivity. In *Human Body Composition*. Roche AF, Heymsfield SB, Lohman TH (Eds.). Human Kinetic Books, Champaign, (IL) 79–107, 1996.
43. www.nationalobesityforum.org.uk (accessed July 2004).
44. Goodwin PJ, Ennis M, Pritchard KI, Trudeau ME, Koo J, Madarnas Y, Hartwick W, Hoffman B, Hood N. Fasting insulin and outcome in early stage breast cancer: results of a prospective cohort study. *J Clin Oncol* 2002; 20(1):42–51.
45. Borugian MJ, Sheps SB, Kim-Sing C, Olivotto IA, Van Patten C, Dunn BP, Coldman AJ, Potter JD, Gallagher RP, Hislop TG. Waist-to-hip ratio and breast cancer mortality. *Am J Epidemiol* 2003; 158(10):963–968.
46. Fallowfield L, Ratcliffe D, Jenkins V, Saul J. Psychiatric morbidity and its recognition by doctors in patients with cancer. *Br J Cancer* 2001; 84(8):1011–1015.
47. Jenkins I, Djuric Z, Darga L, DiLaura NM, Magnam M, Hryniuk WM. Relationship of psychiatric diagnosis and weight loss maintenance in obese breast cancer survivors. *Obesity Res* 2003; 11(11):1369–1375.

48. Millward DJ, Tothill P, deLooy A, Fox K, Logan C, Macdonald L, Morgan L, Truby H. Diet trials, weight and fat loss in a randomized controlled trial of commercially available slimming diets. *Proc Nutr Soc* Summer Meeting 2004. Abstract.
49. Tuomilehto J, Lindstrom J, Eriksson JG, Valle TT, Hamalainen H, Ilanne–Parikka P, Keinanen–Kiukaanniemi S, Laasko M, Louheranta A, Rastas M, Salimen V, Uusitupa M: Finnish Diabetes Prevention Study Group. Prevention of type 2 diabetes mellitus by changes in lifestyle among subjects with impaired glucose intolerance. *N Eng J Med* 2001; 344(18):1343–1350.
50. National Heart Lung Blood Institute. Clinical guidelines on the identification, evaluation, and treatment of overweight and obesity in adults. Executive summary. USA 1998.
51. Prentice R, Thompson D, Clifford C, Gorbach S, Goldin B, Byar D. Dietary fat reduction and plasma estradiol concentration in healthy postmenopausal women. The Woman's Health Trial Study Group. *J Natl Cancer Inst* 1990; 82(2):129–134.
52. Harvie MH, Mercer T, Alford D, Malik R, Adams J, Howell A. The effects of weight loss and weight gain on biomarkers of breast cancer risk. Proceedings of American Association of Cancer research 2nd frontiers in *Cancer Epidemiol Biomarkers Prev* November 2003 Abstract 196.
53. Rock CL, Flatt SW, Thompson CA, Stefanick ML, Newman VA, Jones LA, Natarajan L, Ritenbaugh C, Hollenbach KA, Pierce JP, Chang RJ. Effects of a high-fiber, low-fat diet intervention on serum concentrations of reproductive steroid hormones in women with a history of breast cancer. *J Clin Oncol* 2004; 22(12):2379–2387.
54. Laws R. Counterweight Project Team. Current approaches to obesity management in U.K. primary care: the Counterweight Program. *J Hum Nutr Diet* 2004; 17(3):183–190.
55. Renjilian DA, Perri MG, Nezu A M, McElvey WF, Shermer RL, Anton SD, Individual versus group therapy for obesity: effects of matching participants to their treatment preferences. *J Consult Clin Psychol* 2001; 69(4):717–721.
56. Jen KL, Djuric Z, DiLaura NM, Buison A, Redd JN, Maranci V, Hryniuk WM. Improvement of metabolism among obese breast cancer survivors in differing weight loss regimens. *Obesity Res* 2004; 12(2):306–312.
57. Kridel SJ, Axelrod F, Rozenkrantz N, Smith JW. Orlistat is a novel inhibitor of fatty acid synthase with antitumor activity. *Cancer Res* 2004; 64(6):2070–2075.
58. http://www.wrightfoundation.com (accessed July 2004).
59. Taylor AH, Doust J, Webborn N. Randomized controlled trial to examine the effects of a GP exercise referral program in Hailsham, East Sussex, on modifiable coronary heart disease risk factors. *J Epidemiol Community Health* 1998; 52(9):595–601.
60. http://www.dh.gov.uk/assetRoot/04/07/90/09/04079009.pdf (accessed July 2004).
61. Carroll R, Ali N, Azam N. Promoting physical activity in South Asian Muslim women through "exercise on prescription." *Health Technol Assess* 2002; 6(8):1–101.
62. http://www.statistics.gov.uk (accessed July 2004).
63. http://www.publications.doh.gov.uk (accessed July 2004).
64. http://www.publications.doh.gov.uk/public/hse98.htm (accessed July 2004).
65. Health Survey England, htttp://www.publications.doh.gov.uk/stats/tables/adults2002tab6.xls.

Index

B

C

H

I

J

K

L

M

Q

R

S

T

Y

Z

Milton Keynes UK
Ingram Content Group UK Ltd.
UKHW050308111024
449327UK00044B/2481